Breast and Gynecological Cancers

Mahesh K. Shetty
Editor

Breast and Gynecological Cancers

An Integrated Approach for Screening and Early Diagnosis in Developing Countries

Foreword by Edward L. Trimble, MD, MPH

Springer

Editor
Mahesh K. Shetty, MD, FRCR, FACR, FAIUM
Chief Physician, Woman's Center and MRI
Woman's Hospital of Texas
Clinical Professor of Radiology,
Baylor College of Medicine
Houston, TX, USA

ISBN 978-1-4614-1875-7 ISBN 978-1-4614-1876-4 (eBook)
DOI 10.1007/978-1-4614-1876-4
Springer New York Heidelberg Dordrecht London

Library of Congress Control Number: 2013932875

Printed on acid-free paper

Springer is part of Springer Science+Business Media (www.springer.com)

To women who have suffered the devastation of breast and gynecological cancers and to their families who have had to endure the agony of the suffering or loss of a beloved.

To my father, mother, brothers, and sisters

To Ambika, Sarika, and Veena

Foreword

Breast and gynecologic cancers comprise the leading causes of cancer deaths among women worldwide. According to IARC estimations, breast cancer is both the most frequent cancer diagnosed among women as well as the leading cause of cancer deaths among women in both the developed and the developing world. In 2008, the International Agency for Research on Cancer (IARC) estimated that there were 1.38 million new cases of breast cancer. Cervical cancer is the third most common cancer among women. The burden of cervical cancer lays heavier upon women in the developing world, in which 85% of cervical cancer cases and 88% of cervical cancer deaths occur. In 2008, IARC estimated that there were 50,000 new cases of cervical cancer and 275,000 deaths from cervical cancer. When diagnosed early, both breast and cervical cancers are generally curable by inexpensive, standard interventions. Treatment for women diagnosed with either breast or cervical cancers at advanced stages is much more complex and expensive, with far lower rates of cure and control. Other gynecologic cancers, such as endometrial cancer, ovarian cancer, and gestational trophoblastic neoplasia, also convey major cancer burdens on women around the world.

This volume provides state-of-the-art overviews, encompassing cancer burden, risk factors, prevention, screening, diagnosis, and treatment for breast and gynecologic cancers in low- and middle-income countries. The critical topics of integrating cancer screening and prevention within well-women care, training in detection of women's cancers across different levels of health workers, improving the quality of and access to health care through telemedicine, and coordinating research and care across national health programs, NGOs, philanthropy, and international agencies are all addressed. The readers of this book will gain insight into which interventions are "ready for prime time," which interventions need validation in different populations, and what is in need of additional research.

As Dr. Shetty and his contributors make clear, through ongoing collaboration we have the opportunity to make major reductions in the burden of cancer among women around the globe.

Rockville, MD, USA — Edward L. Trimble, MD, MPH

Preface

The rising incidence and disproportionately higher mortality resulting from breast and gynecological cancers in developing countries call for urgent healthcare intervention strategies aimed at dealing with and rectifying the existing disparity. Remarkably, there has been minimum allocation of funds in the national healthcare budgets of developing countries for programs for cancer control as well as such allocation in the aid from affluent nations to developing countries. Recently, however, there has been much needed recognition of the need to increase funding for noncommunicable diseases such as cancer, diabetes, and heart disease to reflect the changing patterns of disease incidence.

Cancer control programs in developing countries must be matched to resources available and the existing disease burden. Organized screening of the eligible population using mammography, for instance, as is practiced in developing countries for breast cancer screening is neither a feasible nor a desired option. There is no one-size-fits-all solution. It also must be noted that even within a low- or mid-resource country, the urban-based population may have access to higher quality cancer care than the majority of the population that is rural-based, so that even within a country, strategies adopted may vary depending upon the particular needs. This is particularly true in large densely populated countries such as India, China, and Brazil. In low resource settings, the challenges of competing healthcare priorities have to be overcome in order to focus on reducing cancer mortality in women. Methodologies that are proven to have passed the risk benefit analysis test must be adopted.

The vision of this text book is to promote integration of screening and early detection of breast and gynecological cancers utilizing cost-effective modalities that are more appropriate for implementation in developing countries. A single-visit approach for breast and cervical cancer screening and diagnosis is presented to improve compliance and as a cost-effective intervention to reduce mortality. The concept and project design of such an integrated strategy, delivered through a well-woman clinic setting, are discussed in detail. The effectiveness of such an approach must be validated by conducting large-scale observational studies so that national policies can be influenced to adopt such a program. It is important to have a robust system of treating screen positive cases that are diagnosed in such cancer screening programs, without which there will not be any impact on outcomes and mortality rates. Resources must be allocated for screening/early diagnosis programs as well as for effective treatment strategies and palliative care.

An international group of experts in the field of breast and gynecological cancer screening and early detection has contributed to a comprehensive review of the pathology, of tested and proven methods for screening and early diagnosis, and of training of healthcare professionals involved in screening and early diagnosis of these cancers. The cancer prevention group of the International Agency for Research on Cancer has contributed two excellent chapters on the disease burden and challenges faced in cancer control intervention programs in developing countries. Funding is a key challenge for implementation of programs aimed at cancer control; the roles of NGOs and philanthropy in this area are addressed, and an excellent review of cost effectiveness of screening strategies is presented. Cancer prevention is an important aspect in this strategy, and its role is discussed by the cancer prevention group of NCI. Also included is a chapter outlining future strategies for screening of breast cancer and prevention of cervical cancer.

I would like to thank the contributors for sharing their expertise, knowledge, and vast experience in the field of breast and gynecological cancer control and providing readers with a much needed resource with an array of topics that deals with cancers affecting women worldwide.

Houston, TX, USA Mahesh K. Shetty, MD, FRCR, FACR, FAIUM

Contents

Contributors

Benjamin O. Anderson, MD, FACS Fred Hutchinson Cancer Research Center, Department of Surgery, University of Washington, Seattle, WA, USA

Gustavo S. Azenha, PhD Department of Global Health, American Cancer Society, New York, NY, USA

William Kofi Bosu, MB, ChB, MPH, MSc, DTMH, FWACP, FGCP Disease Control and Prevention Department, Ghana Health Service, Accra, Ghana

Kelli A. Cohen, MD Diagnostic Radiologist, Locum Tenens, McGovern Center for Humanities and Ethics University of Texas, Houston, TX, USA

Terri L. Cornelison, MD, PhD Division of Cancer Prevention, National Cancer Institute, Rockville, MD, USA

Alessandra Durstine, MBA Department of Global Health, American Cancer Society, New York, NY, USA

Laurie Elit, MD, MSc, FRCS(C) Department of Obstetrics and Gynecology, Hamilton Health Sciences Centre, Hamilton, ON, Canada

J. Ferlay, ME Section of Cancer Information (CIN), International Agency for Research on Cancer (IARC), Lyon, France

Adhemar Longatto Filho, PhD Department of Pathology, São Paulo State University, São Paulo, Brazil

José Humberto Tavares Guerreiro Fregnani, MD, PhD Center for Research Support, Teaching and Research Institute, Barretos Cancer Hospital, Barretos, Brazil

K. Grosse Frie, PhD Early Detection and Prevention Section (EDP), Screening Group (SCR), International Agency of Research on Cancer (IARC), Lyon, France

Jennifer C. Garza, MS Edinburg Regional Medical Center, Edinburg Children's Hospital, Edinburg, TX, USA

Yun Gong, MD Department of Pathology, University of Texas MD Anderson Cancer Center, Houston, TX, USA

Nalini Gupta, MD, DNB Department of Cytology and Gynaecological Pathology, Postgraduate Institute of Medical Education and Research, Chandigarh, India

Raphael Luiz Haikel Jr., MD, PhD Department of Cancer Prevention, Barretos Cancer Hospital, Barretos, Brazil

Brandy M. Heckman-Stoddard, PhD, MPH Division of Cancer Prevention, National Cancer Institute, Rockville, MD, USA

Jose Jeronimo, MD Instituto Nacional de Enfermedades Neoplasicas—INEN, Direccion de Control de Cancer, Lima, Peru

John Kavanagh, BSc Economy, MD Department of Obstetrics and Gynecology, University, Bangkok, Thailand

Kevin M. Kelly, MD Pasadena Breast Ultrasound Center, Pasadena, CA, USA

Carrie L. Kovarik, MD Hospital of the University of Pennsylvania, Perelman School of Medicine at the University of Pennsylvania, Philadelphia, PA, USA

Y.L. Qiao, MD Department of Cancer Epidemiology, Cancer Institute/Hospital, Chinese Academy of Medical Sciences, Peking Union Medical College, Beijing, China

Kelly E. Quinley, BA Hospital of the University of Pennsylvania, Perelman School of Medicine at the University of Pennsylvania, Philadelphia, PA, USA

Arvind Rajwanshi, MD, FRCPATH Department of Cytology and Gynaecological Pathology, Postgraduate Institute of Medical Education and Research, Chandigarh, India

K. Ramadas, MD, FAMS Regional Cancer Centre, Trivandrum, India

Silvana Rodrigues, BSc Department of Cancer Prevention, Barretos Cancer Hospital, Barretos, Brazil

R. Sankaranarayanan, MD Early Detection and Prevention Section (EDP), Screening Group (SCG), International Agency for Research on Cancer (IARC), Lyon, France

Gustavo Javier Sarria Bardales, MC Instituto Nacional de Enfermedades Neoplasicas—INEN, Director de la Direccion de Control de Cancer, Lima, Peru

Rola M.S.K. Shaheen, MD, MBBS Department of Radiology, Harrington Memorial Hospital—BIDMC, Harvard Medical School, Boston, MA, USA

Mahesh K. Shetty, MD, FRCR, FACR, FAIUM Woman's Center for Breast Care and MRI, Woman's Hospital of Texas, Houston, TX, USA

Laura Sichero, PhD Molecular Biology Laboratory, Center for Translational Oncology, Cancer Institute of São Paulo Av Dr Arnaldo, São Paulo, Brazil

Thiago Buosi Silva, MSc Department of Cancer Prevention, Barretos Cancer Hospital, Barretos, Brazil

Sujha Subramanian, PhD RTI International, Waltham, MA, USA

Siriwan Tangjitgamol, BSc Pharm, MD Department of Obstetrics and Gynecology, Vajira Hospital, Bangkok, Thailand

Trevor Tejada-Bergés, MD Department of Obstetrics and Gynecology, Women and Infants' Hospital, Providence, RI, USA

Edward L. Trimble, MD, MPH Department of Health and Human Services, Center for Global Health, National Cancer Institute, National Institutes of Health, Rockville, MD, USA

Vivien D. Tsu, PhD, MPH Reproductive Health, PATH, Seattle, WA, USA

Luisa Lina Villa, PhD Molecular Biology Laboratory, Center for Translational Oncology, Cancer Institute of Säo Paulo Av Dr Arnaldo, Säo Paulo, Brazil

Karolyn A. Wanat, MD Hospital of the University of Pennsylvania, Perelman School of Medicine at the University of Pennsylvania, Philadelphia, PA, USA

Jennifer L. Winkler, MPH PATH, Seattle, WA, USA

Burden of Breast and Gynecological Cancers in Low-Resource Countries

1

R. Sankaranarayanan and J. Ferlay

Abstract

Information on cancer patterns and burden is valuable for formulating policies and planning health services for efficient cancer control. Of the 12.7 million new cancer cases and 7.6 million cancer deaths estimated globally around 2008, about 6.0 million cases and 3.4 million deaths occurred in women. The IARC *Cancer Incidence in Five Continents* series, GLOBOCAN 2008, and the WHO mortality database are the major sources of cancer patterns and burden worldwide. Almost half of 1.4 million new breast cancer cases, two-thirds of 458,000 breast cancer deaths, and 2.4 million of the 5.2 million prevalent cases occurred in less-developed countries where breast cancer incidence is rising steadily, with an annual percentage increase ranging between 1 and 2 %. Five-year survival from breast cancer in less-developed countries ranges between 12 and 60 %. Given the challenges in organizing screening programs, improving breast awareness and ensuring access to basic care seem to be the only feasible control strategies in less-developed countries. Four-fifths of the global burden of cervical cancer (530,000 new cases and 275,000 deaths) is experienced in less-developed countries. The discovery of persistent oncogenic HPV infection as the cause of cervical cancer has led to HPV vaccination and HPV testing as promising prevention measures. An integrated approach combining vaccination of young girls and screening middle-aged women at least once can lead to substantial reduction in cervical cancer burden in less-developed countries. Cancer of uterine corpus accounted for 144,800

R. Sankaranarayanan (✉)
Early Detection and Prevention Section (EDP), Screening Group (SCR), International Agency for Research on Cancer (IARC), Lyon 69008, France
e-mail: sankarR@iarc.fr

J. Ferlay
Section of Cancer Information (CIN), International Agency for Research on Cancer (IARC), Lyon 69008, France
e-mail: ferlayJ@iarc.fr

M.K. Shetty (ed.), *Breast and Gynecological Cancers: An Integrated Approach for Screening and Early Diagnosis in Developing Countries*, DOI 10.1007/978-1-4614-1876-4_1,

cases and 41,000 deaths, whereas ovarian cancer accounted for 125,200 cases and 75,700 deaths in less-developed countries. Current ovarian cancer screening tests suffer from high false-positive rates, and it is not yet clear if screening can reduce ovarian cancer mortality. Advocacy and political will to invest in creating awareness and accessible as well as efficient health services hold the key for effectively reducing the burden and suffering from these major cancers in women.

Abbreviations

CBE	Clinical breast examination
CERs	Cost-effectiveness ratios
DALY	Disability-adjusted life-years lost
HPV	Human papillomavirus
IARC	International Agency for Research on Cancer
ICD-10	International classification of disease
NCCP	National Cancer Control Program
UN	United Nations
VIA	Visual inspection with acetic acid
WHO	World Health Organization
WHO-AFRO	WHO-Regional Office for Africa
WHO-SEARO	WHO-Regional Office for South-East Asia
YLDs	Years of life lived with a disability
YLLs	Years of life lost

Introduction

Information on the burden of cancer in terms of incidence, mortality, and prevalence is valuable for formulating policies and planning health services for efficient cancer control. It is a valuable resource to define priorities for preventive, diagnostic, therapeutic, and palliative care services, to assess demands of care, to evaluate the outcomes of targeted interventions, and for comparing disease burden between different populations. International comparisons of disease burden by area and time period can provide important clues to the underlying causes and to the effects of natural or planned interventions, and serve as indicators of the scope for preventive strategies.

Cancer is one of the major causes of morbidity and mortality globally, with 12.7 million new cancer cases and 7.6 million cancer deaths estimated worldwide in 2008 [1, 2]. There were an estimated 6.0 million new cases and 3.4 million cancer deaths among women. Cancer has become one of the major causes of ill health and death globally, and the number of new cases and cancer deaths is increasing due to population growth and aging as well as to varying distribution of cancer risk determinants and vast disparities in prevention, early detection and treatment, and health services organization and efficiency.

In this chapter, we will describe the incidence, mortality, and prevalence of cancers of the breast (International classification of disease (ICD-10) code C50), uterine cervix (ICD-10 C53), uterine corpus (corpus uteri, ICD-10 C54), and ovary (ICD-10 C56) in order to quantify the global and regional breast and major gynecological cancer burden around the year 2008, and we discuss briefly data sources, data validity, and methods of estimation and the implications for cancer control and health services investments in low-resource countries.

Indicators of Cancer Burden

Incidence, mortality, and prevalence are considered the standard set of indicators to describe cancer burden. Cancer incidence refers to the number of newly diagnosed cases in a specified period in a given population; it is expressed as the total number of cases per year or as number of cases per 100,000 persons per year. Incidence refers to the average risk of developing a cancer in a population and reflects the load of new cancer patients diagnosed in a given region [2–4]. The impact of prevention strategies based on modulating exposure of populations to risk factors (e.g., reducing tobacco/alcohol use or preventing human papillomavirus (HPV) infection or hepatitis B infection by vaccination) or early detection and treatment of precancerous lesions (e.g., cervical cancer screening and colorectal cancer screening) can be evaluated using trends in cancer incidence and mortality rates.

Cancer mortality indicates the number of deaths occurring in a specified time period in a given population and is expressed as the total number of deaths per year or as number of cancer deaths per 100,000 persons per year. Mortality is the product of case fatality (the proportion of incident cancer patients that die) and incidence, and reflects the outcome of disease [2, 3]. Cancer mortality rates measure the average risk of dying from cancer in a population, while fatality reflects the probability of an individual with cancer dying from it. Mortality rates are influenced by the trends in incidence rates as well as by screening, early diagnosis, and treatment practices. Mortality rate should not be used as a proxy measure of cancer incidence when comparing different populations, assuming equal survival/fatality in the populations is compared. Survival duration of a cancer patient refers to the time interval between the diagnosis and death.

Prevalence refers to the total number of persons in a population affected by the disease in a defined time period (e.g., 2 or 5 years). Prevalence pertains to the number of persons in a defined population who have had cancer diagnosed at some time in the past, during a given period of time [3, 4]. Prevalence of cancer cases diagnosed within 1, 3, and 5 years provides useful supplementary information for different phases of cancer management, such as initial treatment (1-year prevalence) and treatment of residual/recurrent disease and clinical follow-up (3- or 5-year prevalence, respectively).

Other indicators of disease burden include "disability-adjusted life-years lost" (DALY) which incorporates both the years of life lost (YLL) as well as the years lived with poor quality of life between diagnosis and death [5–7]. DALYs measure the loss of health as a result of illness in the population relative to the ideal scenario where everyone in the population lives to an old age in full health. It combines the time lost due to premature mortality (YLLs) and the duration of disability (years of life lived with a disability or YLDs) in survivors. One lost DALY equates to one lost year of "healthy" life, either as a result of premature death from the disease or because of disease-related illness or disability. Although DALYs link data on disease occurrence to health outcomes and they are a useful aid in establishing country-specific agendas regarding cancer control, their compilation at the global level is challenging. They are not available for many low-resource countries due to paucity of information on multiple variables required for their computation [6, 7]. Thus, we discuss the burden of disease predominantly in terms of incidence, mortality, and prevalence in this chapter.

Sources and Methods of Estimation of Data

The information given in this chapter is based on the data from the ninth volume of the *Cancer Incidence in Five Continents,* published by the International Agency for Research on Cancer (IARC) of the World Health Organization (WHO) [8], which contains comprehensive and comparable incidence data for the period 1998–2002 from 225 population-based cancer registries and 300 populations in 60 countries and on the country-specific cancer incidence, mortality, and prevalence estimates for 2008 extracted from the GLOBOCAN database [1, 2, 4]. The methods of estimation used in GLOBOCAN 2008 have been described elsewhere [1–4], and the estimates for different countries and regions vary in accuracy, depending upon the extent and validity of the data available; for several developing countries from which no data are available (e.g., Laos, Cameroon, and Mozambique), the estimates are derived from neighboring countries. While the currently available incidence, survival, and mortality data from low-resource countries might be of varying quality, this information is still of considerable importance as it remains the only relatively unbiased and accessible information on the patterns of burden of cancer. Mortality statistics in GLOBOCAN 2008 are, wherever possible, based on WHO data [9], although not all national datasets in the WHO mortality database are of the same quality and completeness. While almost all the high- and middle-income countries in Europe and the Americas have comprehensive death registration systems, most African and Asian countries (including the large populous countries of Nigeria, India, and Indonesia) do not. Survival probabilities have been used to estimate mortality from incidence in the absence of mortality data. Recently, survival data have been available from selected low- and middle-income countries in Asia, Africa, and Central America [10, 11]. Prevalence was estimated from incidence estimates and observed survival by cancer and age group. National population estimates for 2008 were extracted from the United Nations (UN) population division, the 2008 revision [12].

The 2008 Estimates of Breast and Gynecological Cancer Burden

The estimated total number of annual incident cases, age-standardized incidence rates, annual number of deaths, age-standardized mortality rates, and 5-year prevalence of breast, uterine cervix, uterine corpus, and ovarian cancers for the world, more-developed regions, less-developed regions, the WHO regions, Africa, and sub-Saharan Africa around 2008 are given in Table 1.1. More-developed regions include North America, Europe (including all of Russia), Australia, New Zealand, and Japan, and those in the remaining regions are grouped under "less-developed regions."

Burden and Control of Breast Cancer

Worldwide, around 1.4 million new cases of female breast cancers are diagnosed each year (Table 1.1). It is the most common cancer in women, accounting for 23 % of the estimated annual six million cancers diagnosed in them, and the second most common cancer, after lung cancer, in both sexes [1, 2]. It is also the most common cancer in women in both developing and developed countries, with similar numbers of cancer cases (692,600 in more-developed regions; 690,900 in less-developed regions), where age-standardized rates are 2.5 times higher in developed areas as compared to developing areas (96.3/100,000 women-years in more-developed regions; 39.2 in less-developed regions) [1, 2]. The highest and lowest age-standardized incidence and the range in selected population of countries in the different continents during 1998–2002, as measured by population-based cancer registries, are given in Fig. 1.1 [8]. There is at least a tenfold variation in breast cancer incidence rates worldwide [8], largely as a consequence of a range of socioeconomically correlated differences in the population prevalence of several reproductive, hormonal, and nutritional factors. In general, high incidence rates are observed in high-income countries, intermediate rates in middle-income, and low rates in low-income countries. Differences in various socioeconomic, reproductive and hormonal factors, as well as in early detection services, contribute to the international variation in incidence. In high-resource countries, mammographic screening and efficient treatment have considerably affected breast cancer diagnosis and mortality. In absolute terms, about half of the breast cancer cases and 60 % of the breast cancer deaths occur in developing countries.

As a consequence of changing exposures to reproductive- and nutrition-related determinants over time, women are at increasingly high risk of breast cancer, with incidence rates rising in most low- and middle-income countries in the past few decades. Although there is a paucity of sufficiently

Table 1.1 Estimated incidence, mortality, and 5-year prevalence from four gynecological cancers in 2008

	Breast					Cervix uteri					Corpus uteri					Ovary				
	Incidence		Mortality		5-Year	Incidence		Mortality		5-Year	Incidence		Mortality		5-Year	Incidence		Mortality		5-Year
Population	Number	(ASR)	Number	(ASR)	prevalence	Number	(ASR)	Number	(ASR)	prevalence	Number	(ASR)	Number	(ASR)	prevalence	Number	(ASR)	Number	(ASR)	prevalence
World	1,384,155	38.9	458,503	12.4	5,189,028	530,232	15.2	275,008	7.8	1,555,341	288,387	8.2	73,854	1.9	1,097,620	224,747	6.3	140,163	3.8	549,850
More-developed regions	692,634	66.4	189,455	15.3	2,808,718	76,701	9.1	32,931	3.1	266,655	143,518	13.0	32,689	2.3	555,307	99,521	9.3	64,439	5.1	244,387
Less-developed regions	691,521	27.1	269,048	10.7	2,380,310	453,531	17.7	242,077	9.7	1,288,686	144,869	5.9	41,165	1.7	542,313	125,226	4.9	75,724	3.1	305,463
WHO Africa region (AFRO)	68,012	26.5	37,182	15.4	216,830	75,827	30.7	50,571	21.7	194,039	5,866	2.6	1,899	0.9	21,451	10,400	4.0	7,815	3.2	23,730
WHO Americas region (PAHO)	320,413	57.2	82,515	13.7	1,272,545	80,711	15.3	36,125	6.5	270,426	59,281	10.5	14,123	2.2	232,617	40,876	7.2	26,909	4.4	105,616
WHO East Mediterranean region (EMRO)	61,525	29.3	31,632	16.0	215,532	18,291	9.0	11,123	5.7	52,652	4,722	2.5	1,463	0.8	17,436	9,846	4.7	7,214	3.7	24,016
WHO Europe region (EURO)	450,322	62.8	139,829	16.7	1,770,814	61,397	10.1	28,181	3.9	206,110	93,562	12.3	23,528	2.5	353,442	69,565	9.5	44,280	5.3	166,781
WHO South-East Asia region (SEARO)	203,929	26.1	93,979	12.5	630,253	188,242	24.4	102,693	13.7	498,867	19,223	2.6	8,093	1.1	71,664	47,689	6.2	32,960	4.4	107,348
WHO Western Pacific region (WPRO)	279,499	26.3	73,194	6.7	1,081,664	105,577	9.9	46,217	4.1	332,870	105,668	10.0	24,728	2.2	400,770	46,309	4.4	20,962	1.9	122,212
Africa	92,613	28.0	49,991	16.0	302,310	80,419	25.2	53,334	17.6	206,411	7,379	2.5	2,371	0.9	26,908	13,976	4.2	10,443	3.4	32,186
Sub-Saharan Africa	64,620	26.3	35,427	15.3	204,371	75,141	31.7	50,233	22.5	191,809	5,733	2.6	1,856	0.9	20,985	9,961	4.0	7,484	3.2	22,575

Created using data from Ferlay J, Shin HR, Bray F, Forman D, Mathers C, Parkin DM. GLOBOCAN 2008 v2.0, Cancer Incidence and Mortality Worldwide: IARC CancerBase No. 10 [Internet]. Lyon, France: International Agency for Research on Cancer; 2010. Available from: http://globocan.iarc.fr, accessed on 9 Sept 2012

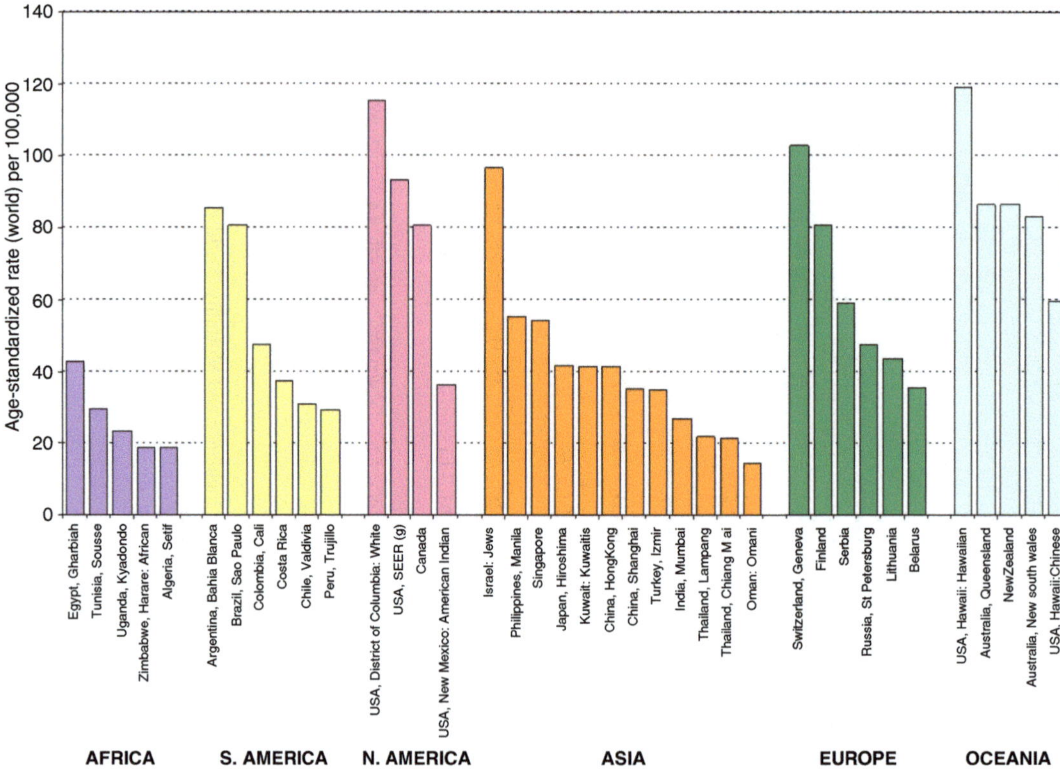

Fig. 1.1 Age-standardized incidence rates of female breast cancer in selected populations in different continents, 1998–2002 (created using data from Cancer Incidence in Five Continents, Vol. IX. IARC Scientific Publications No. 160. Lyon, IARC, 2007)

long-term high quality cancer data in many developing areas at the present time, where they are available, increases in breast cancer incidence and mortality are seen, an observation often more apparent within recent birth cohorts and a probable consequence of the adoption of western lifestyles. The trends in breast cancer incidence rates in selected populations in Africa, Asia, and Latin America are given in Figs. 1.2 and 1.3. The most rapid rises are seen in developing countries, where breast cancer risk has historically been low relative to industrialized countries [13–15]. In some Asian populations, rates are already the same as in Eastern Europe, and, in others, such as Manila, Philippines (58 per 100,000 women), and Singapore (57 per 100,000), rates are even higher (Fig. 1.1). Increasing trends in developing areas are considered the result of the "westernization" of lifestyles, an ill-defined surrogate for changes in factors such as childbearing, dietary habits, and exposure to exogenous estrogen, towards a distribution closer to that of women in industrialized countries [13–15]. The future worldwide breast cancer burden will be strongly influenced by large predicted rises in incidence throughout parts of Asia, due to an increasingly "westernized" lifestyle [16].

Only two decades ago, breast cancer was not on the public health agenda in many countries of Latin America, the Caribbean, and Asia. Epidemiological and demographic transitions, which have accelerated in these nations since the 1960s, have led to increased exposure to risk factors for breast cancer. Birth rates and infant mortality have decreased, leading to a proportionately higher population of adults and elders. Urbanization and other social changes, such as higher levels of education, physical inactivity, obesity, and the increasing employment and empowerment of women, have increased women's health

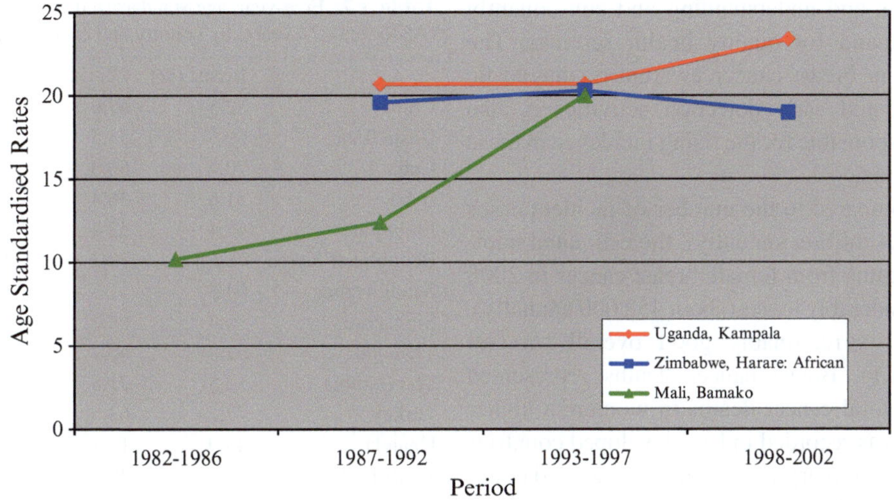

Fig. 1.2 Trends in age-standardized breast cancer incidence in selected African countries (created using data from Parkin et al. Cancer Incidence in Five Continents, Vol. I–VIII. IARC CancerBase No. 7. Lyon, 2005; and data from Curado et al. Cancer Incidence in Five Continents, Vol. IX. IARC Scientific Publications No. 160. Lyon, 2007)

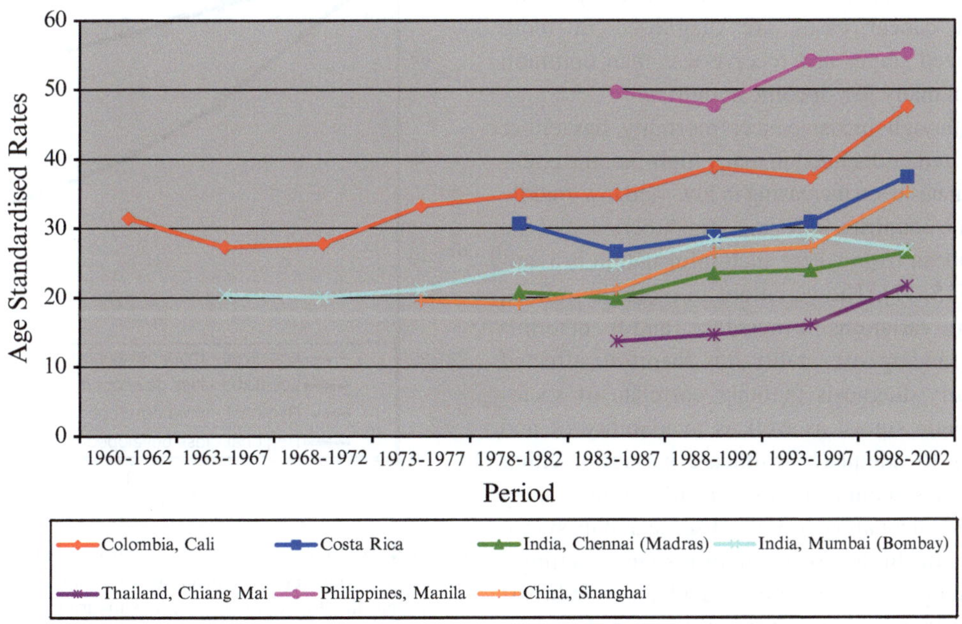

Fig. 1.3 Trends in age-standardized breast cancer incidence in selected countries in Asia and Latin America (created using data from Parkin et al. Cancer Incidence in Five Continents, Vol. I–VIII. IARC CancerBase No. 7. Lyon, 2005; and data from Curado et al. Cancer Incidence in Five Continents, Vol. IX. IARC Scientific Publications No. 160. Lyon, 2007)

awareness and understanding and consequently their demand for quality health services. The increase in breast cancer awareness, diagnostic imaging, and early detection activities is also partly responsible for the rising incidence in these populations.

As compared to the number of incident cases (about 1.4 million annually), the estimated number of deaths from female breast cancer in 2008 was considerably lower (about 458,000 annually), reflecting a reasonably good overall survival (Table 1.1). Breast cancer deaths represented 14 % of total cancer deaths in women; a higher number was recorded in less-developed countries (269,000 per year) than in more-developed countries (189,000 per year). Although the age-standardized death rates were lower in less-developed regions (15.5 per 100,000 women-years) than in more-developed countries (22.2 per 100,000), the mortality-to-incidence ratio was substantially higher in less-developed than in high-income countries. This is due to the fact that, in general, breast cancer cases are diagnosed in more advanced stages and receive less than optimum care in many low-income countries.

Although breast cancer mortality has either stabilized or declined in many high-income countries, it has been increasing in low- and low-middle income countries in Asia, Latin America, and the Caribbean from where such information is available [15–17]. The variations in mortality reflect, in part, variations in incidence (and its determinants) and by case fatality. It is, therefore, affected by early diagnosis (another correlate of socioeconomic status, as well as availability of and access to adequate healthcare services), either through screening or as a result of increasing individual awareness of the disease and its symptoms. In high- to medium-resource settings, mammographic screening and advances in breast cancer therapy in recent years have made a considerable contribution to improved survival and the subsequent reduction or stabilization of breast cancer death rates [13, 15, 16].

The population-based survival experience of breast cancer patients in selected less-developed countries is given in Table 1.2 [10, 11], where the 5-year survival ranged between 12 and 60 %. Comparison of the survival experience of localized and regionally spread breast cancer cases in better-developed health services in Singapore and Turkey with that of less-developed health services is shown in Fig. 1.4; survival of localized breast cancer cases in less-developed countries

Table 1.2 Five-year age-standardized relative survival (ASRs%; 0–74 years) by country and cancer site/type

	Breast (%)	Cervix (%)	Ovary (%)
China	82.5	67.0	56.1
Costa Rica	69.6	53.5	
Cuba	70.4	56.3	
India	51.6	46.4	25.4
Philippines	47.4	37.4	
Republic of Korea	78.6	79.2	58.8
Saudi Arabia	64.5		
Singapore	76.4	65.7	62.4
Thailand	62.8	60.7	47.5
The Gambia	12.5	21.8	
Turkey	77.2	63.5	59.7
Uganda	45.9	13.1	8.6
Zimbabwe	57.8	39.1	34.0

Created using data from Sankaranarayanan R et al. Cancer survival in Africa, Asia, the Caribbean and Central America (SurvCan). IARC Scientific Publications volume 162. Lyon, IARC, 2011

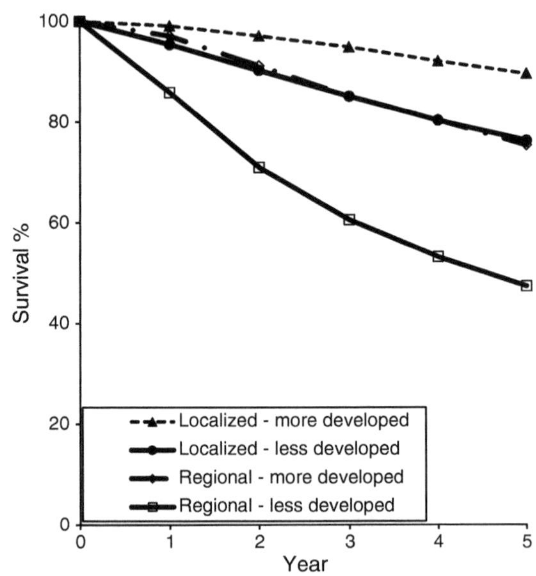

Fig. 1.4 Absolute survival of localized and regional extent of female breast cancer among more- and less-developed health services (from Sankaranarayanan R et al. Cancer survival in Africa, Asia, the Caribbean and Central America (SurvCan). IARC Scientific Publications volume 162. Lyon, IARC, 2011)

was similar to that of regionally spread breast cancer cases in more-developed health countries [10, 11], This indicates the enormous potential of early detection and appropriate medical care in improving survival and reducing mortality.

Breast cancer is the most prevalent cancer in the vast majority of countries globally [4]. The 5-year prevalence of breast cancer was 5.2 million women globally; this was 2.8 million and 2.4 million women, respectively, for more- and less-developed countries (Table 1.1). The 5-year prevalence rates reached 527 per 100,000 women in more-developed countries and 123 per 100,000 in less-developed countries [4].

The recent data pertaining to DALYs attributed to breast cancer in India and other less-developed countries are instructive. In India, of the estimated 3,403,176 DALYs contributed by all cancers in women in 2011, breast cancer contributed 1,088,642, of which 486,246 were due to YLL [6]. In a recent study, the total DALYs lost due to the 27 cancer sites in India and Uganda were 3,022 and 6,491 per 100,000 populations, respectively [7]. In India, lung, breast, cervical, and oral cancers were the main cause of loss in healthy years. In Uganda, HIV/AIDS defining cancers such as Kaposi sarcoma, non-Hodgkin lymphoma, and cervical cancers largely contributed to DALYs, in addition to esophageal and prostate cancer for men and breast cancer for women. In both countries, more than 90 % of DALYs lost were due to premature deaths from cancers.

The pattern, burden, and outcomes from breast cancer in less-developed countries call for urgent action to improve breast cancer control. Given the lack of effective and feasible primary prevention measures, early detection and adequate treatment are the only viable approaches for breast cancer control. High awareness and well-developed and accessible health services are essential prerequisites for an effective breast cancer control strategy based on early detection and treatment.

Given the low awareness, late stage presentation, inadequate treatment and follow-up care, low survival, and poorly developed health services, resources should be spent judiciously. It has been shown that detecting and treating stage I breast cancer patients resulted in 23.4, 12.3, and 19.3 DALYs averted per patient in Africa, North America, and Asia, respectively [18]. The corresponding average cost-effectiveness ratios (CERs) compared with no intervention were US$78, US$1,960, and US$62 per DALY averted. The number of DALYs averted per patient decreased with stage; the value was lowest for stage IV treatment (0.18–0.19), with average CERs of US$4,986 in Africa, US$70,380 in North America, and US$3,510 per DALY averted in Asia. An extensive breast cancer awareness program resulted in 16.1, 12.9, and 12.6 DALYs averted per patient and average CERs of US$75, US$915, and US$75 per DALY averted, respectively. These findings suggest that treating stage I disease and introducing an extensive breast cancer awareness program are the most cost-effective breast cancer interventions.

Early detection may be achieved by mammographic screening [19], clinical breast examination (CBE) [20, 21], and a high level of breast awareness among women and professional awareness. It is clear that mammographic screening is neither feasible nor cost effective in these countries [22, 23]. Mammographic screening of women aged 40–69 years in Ghana cost US$12,908 per DALY averted [22]. Cost-effectiveness studies in Ghana (US$1,299 per DALY averted) and India (US$1,341 for DALY averted) indicate biennial CBE screening, in combination with treatment of all stages, seem to be a cost-effective intervention for breast cancer control [22, 23]. However, it is not yet clear if systematic CBE screening can lead to significant reduction in breast cancer mortality and results from on-going randomized trials are awaited [20, 21]. Even CBE screening will require a certain level of health service organization and resources to ensure invitation, providing CBE, triage of CBE-positive women, and treatment of screen-detected women, which is not the case in many low-income countries as in sub-Saharan Africa. In order to be effective, it will require a high compliance at every level of the program for its effectiveness. Low awareness and poorly accessible and inadequately developed health services are major barriers for high compliance. Given the relatively low level of incidence, the yield of breast cancer cases per number of screened women is likely to be low. Given the lack of data about the effectiveness of CBE screening, any attempt to introduce it health services should be in phased manner, with careful monitoring of inputs and evaluation of outcomes. Moreover, their implementation is only meaningful if the capacity of basic cancer diagnosis, referral, and treatment and possibly palliative services is simultaneously improved.

Improving breast awareness among the general population, improving the skills of general practitioners in promptly identifying and referring women with breast lumps and other relevant symptoms, as well as providing adequate treatment and follow-up care seem to be the most universally applicable strategies to improve breast cancer survival and reduce mortality in less-developed countries. These have been shown to be cost-effective strategies for breast cancer control in a model-based study in Ghana (costing US$1,364 per DALY averted in Ghana) [22]. This fits well with the expectation that, if advanced cancers can be downstaged by early clinical diagnosis and adequately treated, many lives could be saved. Although it may be difficult to quantify the impact of breast awareness, the substantial gains in breast cancer survival and mortality, before widespread mammography screening, in high-income countries were due to increased general awareness and the improved provision of treatment in health services.

Burden and Control of Cancer of the Uterine Cervix

Cancer of the cervix is the third most common cancer among women worldwide and the second most in less-developed countries. However, it is the most common cancer among women in many low-income countries. It accounted for an estimated 530,000 new cases and 275,000 deaths annually around 2008 (Table 1.1). More than 80 % of the global burden is experienced in less-developed countries, where it accounts for nearly two-thirds of all gynecological cancer cases. Less-developed countries accounted for 453,000 new cases and 242,000 deaths annually around 2008. The age-standardized incidence rates in less-developed countries are twofold higher than in more-developed countries. It is more common than both breast and liver cancers together in areas with low human development index, which includes mostly low-income countries [24]. The high frequency of cervical cancer in these countries, despite the slowly declining incidence rates, is due to lack of or inefficient existing screening programs, combined with a high background prevalence of HPV infection [25–27]. It is the most common gynecological cancer, and more than four-fifths of cervical cancers are squamous cell carcinomas worldwide [8].

The lowest and highest age-standardized cervical cancer incidence rates observed in populations in the five continents, including rates from selected populations, are given in Fig. 1.5. There is a more than 20-fold variation in the incidence rates of cervical cancer worldwide, and the highest are observed in sub-Saharan Africa, Melanesia, Latin America, the Caribbean, South-Central Asia, South-East Asia, and Eastern Europe [8]. The age-standardized rates ranged from the lowest of 2.1 per 100,000 women in Gharbia, Egypt, to the highest of 47.3 per 100,000 African women in Harare, Zimbabwe [8]. The incidence is generally low in developed countries, with age-standardized incidence rates less than 10 per 100,000 women (Fig. 1.5). The incidence rates in developed countries in the 1950s and early 1960s were similar to those observed in less-developed countries today; however, widespread screening in developed countries has substantially reduced the burden over the last four decades [28]. Incidence rates lower than 7/100,000 women are observed in the Middle Eastern countries and China (Fig. 1.5) [8]. Trends in cervical cancer incidence rates in selected populations in Asia, Africa, and Latin America are shown in Figs. 1.6 and 1.7. Except in Uganda and Mali in Africa, cervical cancer incidence rates have been steadily and slowly declining in most populations due to changes in reproductive life styles, better education, empowerment of

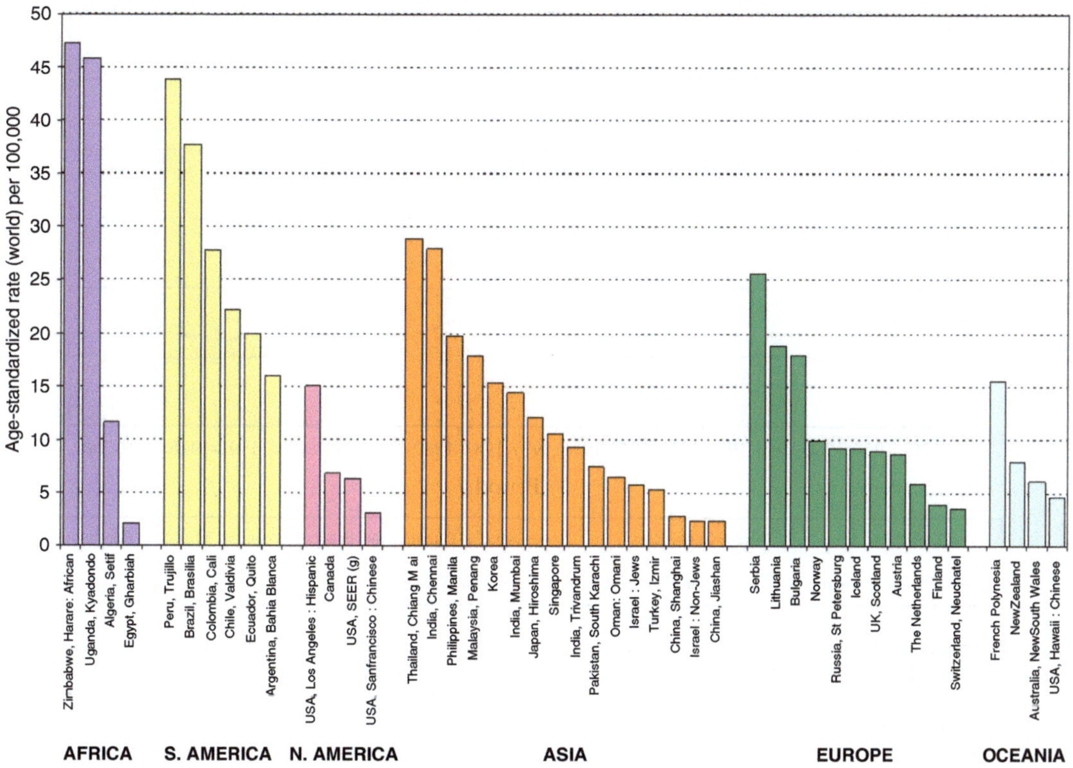

Fig. 1.5 Age-standardized incidence rates of cervix cancer in selected populations in different continents, 1998–2002 (created using data from Cancer Incidence in Five Continents, Vol. IX. IARC Scientific Publications No. 160. Lyon, IARC, 2007)

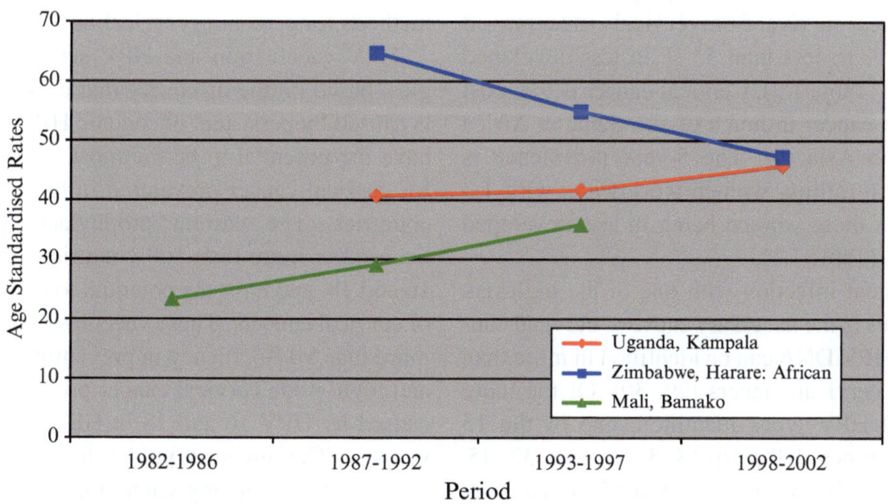

Fig. 1.6 Trends in age-standardized cervix cancer incidence in selected African countries (created using data from Parkin et al. Cancer Incidence in Five Continents, Vol. I–VIII. IARC CancerBase No. 7. Lyon, 2005; and data from Curado et al. Cancer Incidence in Five Continents, Vol. IX. IARC Scientific Publications No. 160. Lyon, 2007)

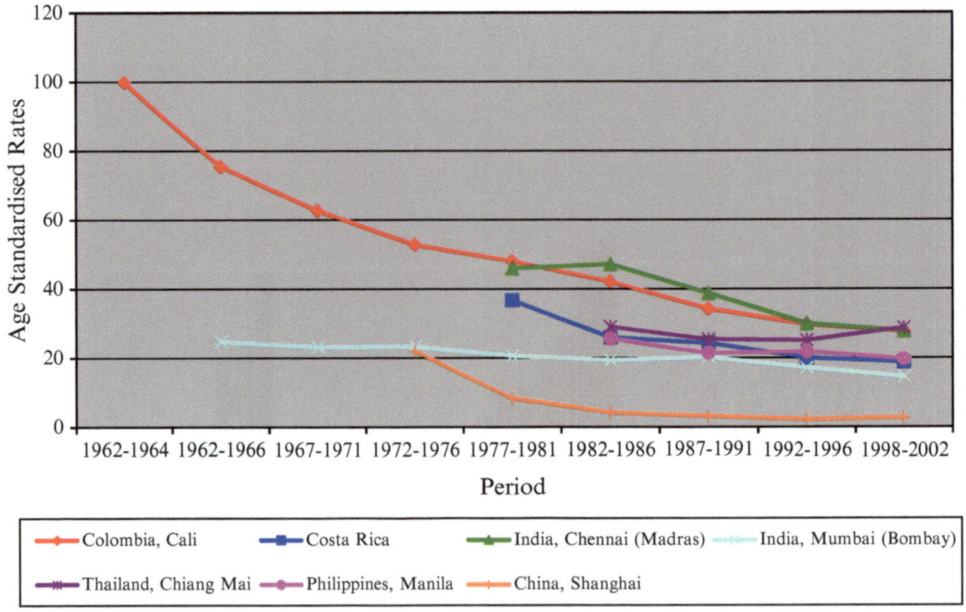

Fig. 1.7 Trends in age-standardized cervix cancer incidence in selected countries in Asia and Latin America (created using data from Parkin et al. Cancer Incidence in Five Continents, Vol. I–VIII. IARC CancerBase No. 7. Lyon, 2005; and data from Curado et al. Cancer Incidence in Five Continents, Vol. IX. IARC Scientific Publications No. 160. Lyon, 2007)

women, and improving socioeconomic conditions. However, in spite of the falling rates, cervical cancer still affects and kills substantial numbers of women in developing countries.

Five-year survival from cervical cancer ranged from 13 % to less than 55 % in less-developed countries (Table 1.2). Cervical cancer is the most prevalent cancer in much of sub-Saharan Africa and South Asia (4). The 5-year prevalence is around 1.6 million women worldwide, with 1.3 million of these women being in less-developed countries (Table 1.1).

Persistent infection with one of the high-risk HPV types is the necessary cause of cervical cancer, and HPV DNA can be identified in more than 95 % of cervical cancers [29, 30]. Of the more than 100 HPV types identified, one of the 15 high-risk types (HPV 16, 18, 31, 33, 35, 39, 45, 51, 52, 56, 58, 59, 68, 73, and 82) is causally associated with cervical neoplasia [29]. Most HPV infections are transient, and 80 % of them regress within 2 years; but some women who are infected with the high-risk types develop persistent infections. The knowledge that cervical cancer is caused by persistent high-risk HPV infection has led to the development of HPV vaccines to prevent cervical cancer and various HPV testing methods for screening cervical neoplasia.

HPV vaccination and HPV screening strategies, based on the discovery that cervical cancer is caused by persistent oncogenic HPV infection, have the potential to be the most effective tools for cervical cancer prevention in less-developed countries. The current prophylactic vaccines licensed in more than 100 countries target HPV 16 and 18, and have the potential to prevent 70 % of cervical cancers. These vaccines demonstrated more than 90 % efficacy in preventing infections and high-grade cervical cancer precursor lesions caused by HPV 16 and 18 in HPV naïve young women. The greatest public health benefit is derived by vaccinating young girls before sexual debut and exposure to HPV, particularly in low-resource countries [31, 32]. Thus, health planners should ensure that HPV vaccination is firmly in place for young adolescent girls between 9 and

13 years and concentrate on introducing affordable and effective screening approaches for cervical cancer prevention among women older than 30 years. Rwanda introduced a nationwide sensitization program followed by the first national HPV vaccination program in sub-Saharan Africa in 2011; it achieved 93.23 % coverage for three-dose course of vaccination among girls in grade 6, through school-based vaccination and community involvement in identifying girls absent from or not enrolled in school (33). Currently, the Global Alliance for Vaccines and Immunization (GAVI) has begun accepting applications to fund HPV vaccination in developing countries.

A number of field studies, including randomized trials and modeling studies, have demonstrated that the most efficient and cost-effective screening strategies in less-developed countries include visual inspection with acetic acid (VIA) and HPV testing, even if performed only once in a lifetime around 35 years [34–39]. A single round of VIA screening resulted in a 35 % reduction in cervical cancer mortality in South India [37]. A single HPV testing resulted in a 50 % reduction in the risk of developing advanced cancer and associated deaths [38]. Despite the fact that cervical cancer deaths almost equal those of maternal deaths and despite the availability of highly effective vaccination and screening strategies, cervical cancer control has not yet sufficiently seized the attention of governments and health authorities in most less-developed countries, including India which alone accounts for one-fifth of global burden. An integrated approach combining HPV vaccination and screening women at least once with HPV testing or visual screening can lead to a substantial reduction in the cervical cancer burden in underserved populations in less-developed countries.

Burden of Cancer of the Uterine Corpus (Endometrial Cancer)

Cancer of the uterine corpus, a cancer of postmenopausal women, accounted for an estimated 288,300 new cases and 73,800 deaths worldwide around 2008; there were 144,800 cases and 41,100 deaths in less-developed countries (Table 1.1). It is a much less common gynecological cancer in less-developed countries. Endometrial adenocarcinomas account for around 90 % of the uterine corpus cancers while papillary serous carcinoma, clear cell carcinomas, papillary endometrial carcinoma, and mucinous carcinoma account for the remaining cases (8).

More than 14-fold variation in the worldwide incidence has been observed during 1998–2002; ASRs exceeding 15 per 100,000 women are observed in Europe and North America, and rates are generally lower than 5 per 100,000 in populations in most developing countries [8] (Fig. 1.8). More than 90 % of the cases occur in women aged 50 years and over. An increased risk of endometrial cancer, associated with factors such as oral intake of estrogens (without progestin), early menarche, late menopause, low parity, extended periods of anovulation, and obesity can be related to long-term unopposed estrogenic stimulation, leading to proliferation and neoplastic transformation of endometrial cells. The association between long-term use of tamoxifen and endometrial cancer has been attributed to its estrogen agonist properties, and women receiving tamoxifen should be monitored carefully. Diabetes mellitus and hypertension are also associated with increased risk of endometrial cancer. A protective effect has been attributed to high parity, late age at last birth, long-term use of combined oral contraceptives, and physical activity. In pre- and perimenopausal women, endometrial cancer is relatively rare. Increasing trends in incidence among postmenopausal women have been observed in some countries such as India [40], whereas declining trends have been observed in China [41]. Cancer of uterine corpus has a much more favorable prognosis than those with ovarian and cervical cancer, with 5-year survival rates around 70 % in less-developed countries (Table 1.2). The 5-year prevalence is around 1.1 million women worldwide, 49 % of them estimated in less-developed countries (Table 1.1).

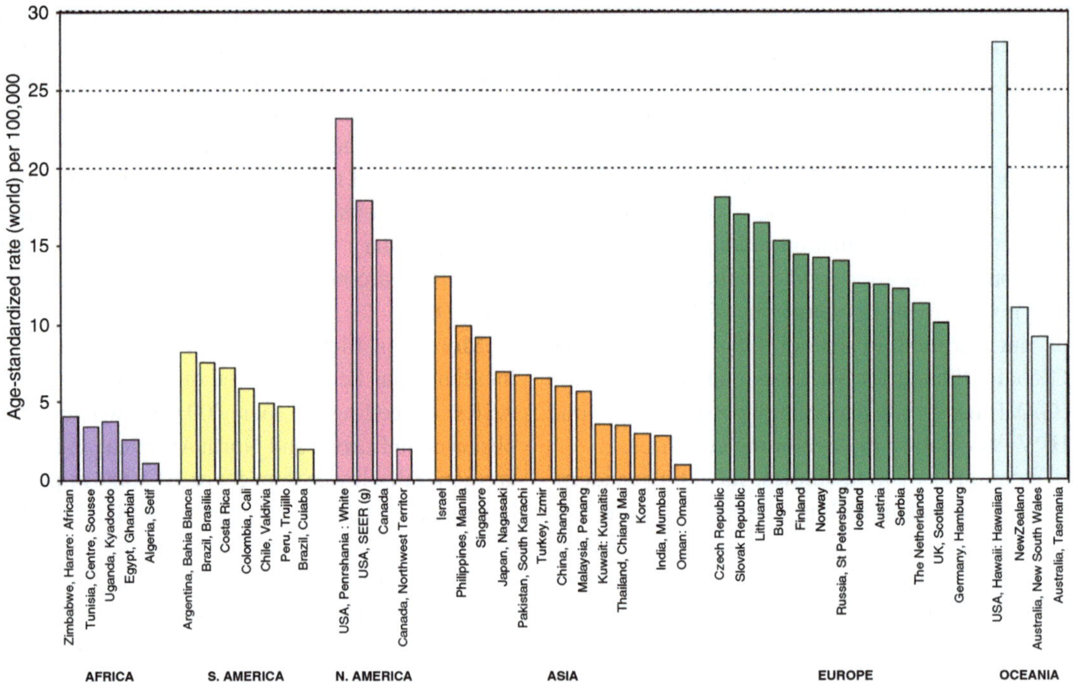

Fig. 1.8 Age-standardized incidence rates of corpus uteri cancer in selected populations in different continents, 1998–2002 (created using data from Curado et al. Cancer Incidence in Five Continents, Vol. IX. IARC Scientific Publications No. 160. Lyon, 2007)

Burden of Ovarian Cancer

Ovarian cancer ranks as the sixth most common cancer in women and accounted for 222,600 cases and 139,500 deaths worldwide around 2008 (Table 1.1). There were 125,200 incident cases and 75,700 deaths estimated in less-developed countries. The high proportion of deaths is due to the much less favorable prognosis of ovarian cancer, as compared to uterine corpus and cervical cancer. More than 80 % of ovarian cancers are epithelial in origin, the remaining constituted by germ cell tumors (10–15 %) in less-developed countries. The vast majority of epithelial ovarian cancers are diagnosed in postmenopausal women, whereas germ cell tumors occur in young women, with child bearing potential, in their twenties. Germ cell tumors account for 10–15 % of ovarian cancers in Asian and African populations. Dysgerminoma accounts for more than 70 % of germ cell tumors, whereas granulosa tumors constitute the most common sex cord-stromal tumor (8).

There is more than sevenfold variation in the worldwide occurrence of ovarian cancer, with the ASRs exceeding 8 per 100,000 women in Europe and North America [8] (Fig. 1.9). The rates vary between 4 and 8 per 100,000 women in Asia, Africa, and Latin America. Ovarian incidence rates have significantly increased in China and India over the last few decades [40–42].

The 5-year survival from ovarian cancer is less than 50 % in less-developed countries (Table 1.2); it varied between 9 % in Uganda and 47 % in Thailand. The 5-year prevalence is 549,900 women worldwide (Table 1.1). Most ovarian cancers are diagnosed in advanced clinical stages with poor prospects of long-term survival. The etiology and natural history of ovarian cancer is not well understood and thus the means of primary prevention are not clear. Less than 20 % of women with advanced stage disease survive long-term. When diagnosed in stage I, up to 90 % of patients can be cured with conventional surgery and chemotherapy.

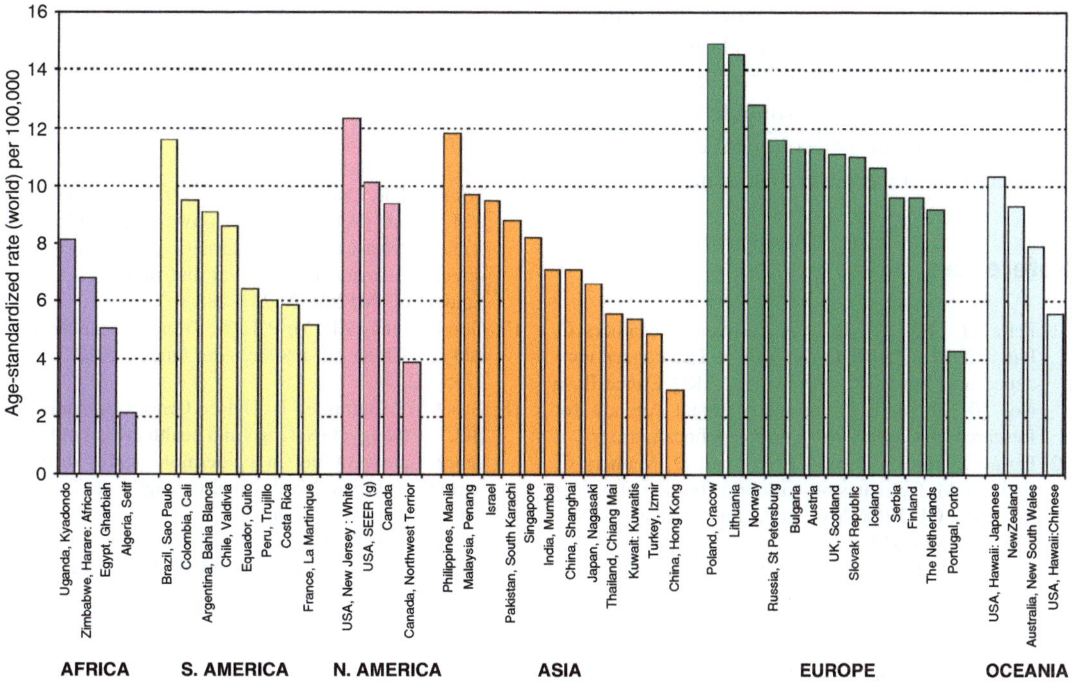

Fig. 1.9 Age-standardized incidence rates of ovarian cancer in selected populations in different continents, 1998–2002 (created using data from Cancer Incidence in Five Continents, Vol. IX. IARC Scientific Publications No. 160. Lyon, IARC, 2007)

Annual screening of asymptomatic post-menopausal women using a combination of transvaginal sonography and serum CA125 is being evaluated in clinical trials as a means to facilitate earlier detection of ovarian cancer. Current screening modalities are associated with high false-positive rates. There is currently no evidence that any test, including pelvic examination, CA125 or other biomarkers, ultrasound (including transvaginal ultrasound), or combination of tests, results in reduced mortality from ovarian cancer, and final results from on-going trials are awaited [43]. There is no evidence to support the use of any test, including pelvic examination, CA125 or other biomarkers, ultrasound (including transvaginal ultrasound), or combination of tests, for routine population-based screening for ovarian cancer. Early clinical diagnosis and treatment are currently the only means of controlling ovarian cancer.

Conclusion

The estimated global and regional data as well as data on incidence rates from population-based cancer registries indicate wide variations in the burden of breast and gynecological cancers, due to different levels of exposure to risk factors and to the striking disparity and inequity in health-care infrastructures and accessibility across the globe. Establishing and improving information systems, such as hospital medical records, hospital cancer registries, population-based cancer registries, and mortality registration systems in low-resource settings, will improve the accuracy and validity of data on global cancer burden and contribute to improving cancer control inputs. Advocacy and the political will to invest in creating awareness and in creating accessible as well as efficient health services hold the key to substantially reduce the burden and alleviate suffering from these major cancers in women in less-developed countries. A National Cancer Control Program (NCCP), as advocated by the WHO, provides the most suitable framework to improve breast and gynecological cancer control in the context of overall cancer control [44].

References

1. Ferlay J, Shin HR, Bray F, Forman D, Mathers C, Parkin DM. GLOBOCAN 2008 v 1.2, cancer incidence and mortality worldwide: IARC CancerBase No. 10 [internet]. Lyon: International Agency for Research on Cancer; 2010. http://globocan.iarc.fr.
2. Ferlay J, Shin HR, Bray F, Forman D, Mathers C, Parkin DM. Estimates of worldwide burden of cancer in 2008: GLOBOCAN 2008. Int J Cancer. 2010; 127(12):2893–917.
3. Parkin DM, Bray F, Ferlay J, Pisani P. Global cancer statistics, 2002. CA Cancer J Clin. 2005;55(2): 74–108.
4. Bray F, Ren JS, Masuyer E, Ferlay J. Global estimates of cancer prevalence for 27 sites in the adult population in 2008. Int J Cancer. 2013;132(5):1133–45. doi:10.1002/ijc.27711.
5. Murray CJ, Lopez AD. The incremental effect of age-weighting on YLLs, YLDs, and DALYs: a response. Bull World Health Organ. 1996;74(4):445–6.
6. Murthy NS, Nandakumar BS, Pruthvish S, George PS, Mathew A. Disability adjusted life years for cancer patients in India. Asian Pac J Cancer Prev. 2010;11(3):633–40.
7. Soerjomataram I, Lortet-Tieulent J, Ferlay J, Forman D, Mathers C, Parkin DM, et al. Estimating and validating disability-adjusted life years at the global level: a methodological framework for cancer. BMC Med Res Methodol. 2012;12(1):125.
8. Curado MP, Edwards B, Shin HR, Storm H, Ferlay J, Heanue M, et al. Cancer incidence in five continents, vol. IX. Lyon: International Agency for Research on Cancer; 2007.
9. World Health Organization (WHO) Databank. WHO statistical information system. Geneva: WHO; 2012. http://www.who.int/whosis.
10. Sankaranarayanan R, Swaminathan R, Brenner H, Chen K, Chia KS, Chen JG, et al. Cancer survival in Africa, Asia, and Central America: a population-based study. Lancet Oncol. 2010;11(2):165–73.
11. Sankaranarayanan R, Swaminathan R. Cancer survival in Africa, Asia, the Caribbean and Central America. IARC scientific publications No. 162. Lyon: International Agency for Research on Cancer; 2011.
12. United Nations. Population division. World Population Prospects, the 2008 revision. http://www.un.org
13. Bray F, McCarron P, Parkin DM. The changing global patterns of female breast cancer incidence and mortality. Breast Cancer Res. 2004;6(6):229–39.
14. Parkin DM, Nambooze S, Wabwire-Mangen F, Wabinga HR. Changing cancer incidence in Kampala, Uganda, 1991-2006. Int J Cancer. 2010;126(5): 1187–95.
15. Jemal A, Bray F, Center MM, Ferlay J, Ward E, Forman D. Global cancer statistics. CA Cancer J Clin. 2011;61(2):69–90.
16. Youlden DR, Cramb SM, Dunn NA, Muller JM, Pyke CM, Baade PD. The descriptive epidemiology of female breast cancer: an international comparison of screening, incidence, survival and mortality. Cancer Epidemiol. 2012;36(3):237–48.
17. Guo P, Huang ZL, Yu P, Li K. Trends in cancer mortality in China: an update. Ann Oncol. 2012;23(10): 2755–62.
18. Groot MT, Baltussen R, Uyl-de Groot CA, Anderson BO, Hortobagyi GN. Costs and health effects of breast cancer interventions in epidemiologically different regions of Africa, North America, and Asia. Breast J. 2006;12 Suppl 1:S81–90.
19. International Agency for Research on Cancer. IARC handbooks of cancer prevention, Breast cancer screening, vol. 7. Lyon: IARC Press; 2002.
20. Mittra I, Mishra GA, Singh S, Aranke S, Notani P, Badwe R, et al. A cluster randomized, controlled trial of breast and cervix cancer screening in Mumbai, India: methodology and interim results after three rounds of screening. Int J Cancer. 2010;126(4): 976–84.
21. Sankaranarayanan R, Ramadas K, Thara S, Muwonge R, Prabhakar J, Augustine P, et al. Clinical breast examination: preliminary results from a cluster randomized controlled trial in India. J Natl Cancer Inst. 2011;103(19):1476–80.
22. Zelle SG, Nyarko KM, Bosu WK, Aikins M, Niens LM, Lauer JA, et al. Costs, effects and cost-effectiveness of breast cancer control in Ghana. Trop Med Int Health. 2012;17(8):1031–43.
23. Okonkwo QL, Draisma G, der Kinderen A, Brown ML, de Koning HJ. Breast cancer screening policies in developing countries: a cost-effectiveness analysis for India. J Natl Cancer Inst. 2008;100(18): 1290–300.
24. Bray F, Jemal A, Grey N, Ferlay J, Forman D. Global cancer transitions according to the Human Development Index (2008-2030): a population-based study. Lancet Oncol. 2012;13(8):790–801.
25. Sankaranarayanan R, Budukh AM, Rajkumar R. Effective screening programmes for cervical cancer in low- and middle-income developing countries. Bull World Health Organ. 2001;79(10):954–62.
26. Bosch FX, de Sanjosé S. Chapter 1: Human papillomavirus and cervical cancer—burden and assessment of causality. J Natl Cancer Inst Monogr. 2003;31: 3–13.
27. International Agency for Research on Cancer. IARC handbooks of cancer prevention, Cervix cancer screening, vol. 10. Lyon: IARC Press; 2004.
28. Gustafsson L, Ponten J, Bergstrom R, Adami HO. International incidence rates of invasive cervical

cancer before cytological screening. Int J Cancer. 1997;71(2):159–65.
29. Munoz N, Bosch FX, de Sanjosé S, Herrero R, Castellsague X, Shah KV, et al. Epidemiologic classification of human papillomavirus types associated with cervical cancer. N Engl J Med. 2003; 348(6):518–27.
30. International Agency for Research on Cancer. IARC monographs on the evaluation of carcinogenic risks to humans, Human papillomaviruses, vol. 90. Lyon: International Agency for Research on Cancer; 2007.
31. Human papillomavirus vaccines. WHO position paper. Wkly Epidemiol Rec 2009;84(15):118–31.
32. Tsu V, Murray M, Franceschi S. Human papillomavirus vaccination in low-resource countries: lack of evidence to support vaccinating sexually active women. Br J Cancer. 2012;107(9):1445–50. doi:10.1038/bjc.2012.404.
33. Binagwaho A, Wagner CM, Gatera M, Karema C, Nutt CT, Ngabo F. Achieving high coverage in Rwanda's national human papillomavirus vaccination programme. Bull World Health Organ. 2012;90(8):623–8.
34. Goldie SJ, Gaffikin L, Goldhaber-Fiebert JD, Gordillo-Tobar A, Levin C, Mahe C, et al. Cost-effectiveness of cervical-cancer screening in five developing countries. N Engl J Med. 2005;353(20): 2158–68.
35. Denny L, Kuhn L, De SM, Pollack AE, Dupree W, Wright Jr TC. Screen-and-treat approaches for cervical cancer prevention in low-resource settings: a randomized controlled trial. JAMA. 2005;294(17):2173–81.
36. Denny L, Kuhn L, Hu CC, Tsai WY, Wright Jr TC. Human papillomavirus-based cervical cancer prevention: long-term results of a randomized screening trial. J Natl Cancer Inst. 2010;102(20):1557–67.
37. Sankaranarayanan R, Esmy PO, Rajkumar R, Muwonge R, Swaminathan R, Shanthakumari S, et al. Effect of visual screening on cervical cancer incidence and mortality in Tamil Nadu, India: a cluster-randomised trial. Lancet. 2007;370(9585):398–406.
38. Sankaranarayanan R, Nene BM, Shastri SS, Jayant K, Muwonge R, Budukh AM, et al. HPV screening for cervical cancer in rural India. N Engl J Med. 2009; 360(14):1385–94.
39. Ginsberg GM, Lauer JA, Zelle S, Baeten S, Baltussen R. Cost effectiveness of strategies to combat breast, cervical, and colorectal cancer in sub-Saharan Africa and South East Asia: mathematical modelling study. BMJ. 2012;344:e614.
40. Yeole BB. Trends in cancer incidence in female breast, cervix uteri, corpus uteri, and ovary in India. Asian Pac J Cancer Prev. 2008;9(1):119–22.
41. Song F, He M, Li H, Qian B, Wei Q, Zhang W, et al. A cancer incidence survey in Tianjin: the third largest city in China-between 1981 and 2000. Cancer Causes Control. 2008;19(5):443–50.
42. Wu QJ, Vogtmann E, Zhang W, Xie L, Yang WS, Tan YT, et al. Cancer incidence among adolescents and young adults in urban Shanghai, 1973-2005. PLoS One. 2012;7(8):e42607.
43. Gentry-Maharaj A, Menon U. Screening for ovarian cancer in the general population. Best Pract Res Clin Obstet Gynaecol. 2012;26(2):243–56.
44. World Health Organization. National cancer control programmes: policies and managerial guidelines. 2nd ed. Geneva: World Health Organization; 2002.

Breast Cancer: Pathology, Cytology, and Core Needle Biopsy Methods for Diagnosis

2

Yun Gong

Abstract

Successful cancer treatment relies on a combination of clinical examinations, imaging studies, and pathologic evaluations. Pathologic diagnosis should not be bypassed even when health care resources are very limited and clinical/radiologic findings are very suggestive of breast cancer. A timely and accurate pathologic diagnosis can be achieved by the use of appropriate tissue sampling techniques, optimal tissue processing, and competent interpretation of pathologic findings. Accurate preoperative pathologic diagnosis confirms the malignant nature of the lesion and documents baseline expression of prognostic and predictive biomarkers, thus enabling clinicians to make optimal therapeutic strategies such as planning the extent of the surgery. Methods of obtaining tissue samples and the cytohistological techniques and histopathological features of the spectrum of breast cancer pathology are discussed in detail.

Introduction

Breast cancer is the most common cancer in women in Western countries. Over the past decade, the incidence in many developing countries has been increasing at a more rapid rate than in developed countries, and breast cancer in these countries is often associated with poorer survival [1]. Of the breast cancer deaths around the world in 2002, more than 50% occurred in countries with limited resources [2]. This is largely due to late presentation of the disease, limited resources for the diagnosis, and treatment in these countries.

To improve breast cancer outcomes in these countries, it is important to increase breast cancer awareness and accurately recognize breast cancer, especially at an early stage, because early diagnosis is lifesaving and cost-effective and requires less aggressive therapy.

In 2005, the Breast Health Global Initiative stratified levels of resources in countries with limited resources (from lowest to highest) into basic, limited, enhanced, and maximal [3]. In these countries, the economic realities appear to

Y. Gong (✉)
Department of Pathology, University of Texas MD Anderson Cancer Center, 1515 Holcombe Boulevard, Unit 53, Houston, TX 77030, USA
e-mail: yungong@mdanderson.org

M.K. Shetty (ed.), *Breast and Gynecological Cancers: An Integrated Approach for Screening and Early Diagnosis in Developing Countries*, DOI 10.1007/978-1-4614-1876-4_2,

force physicians to support a paradigm shift away from sophisticated, expensive, and invasive modes of investigation in favor of cheaper, readily available, minimally invasive, yet reliable methods [4].

The commonly used sampling methods for preoperative pathologic diagnosis include fine-needle aspiration (FNA), core needle biopsy (CNB), and open surgical biopsy. Compared with open surgical biopsy, FNA and CNB are less invasive biopsy techniques in which the needle can be guided by palpation or imaging. For palpable lesions, the needle can be placed under the guidance of palpation; for nonpalpable mammographic abnormalities, the needle may be placed with image guidance.

FNA involves using a very small, thin needle to extract cells or fluid from the abnormal area. Since gaining its momentum in Europe in the 1950s, FNA has been adopted worldwide and has been proven to be safe, simple, fast, and cost-effective if properly performed [5–7] and if a quality cytopathology service is available. With FNA, it is possible to make "one-stop" diagnosis at outpatient clinics. A number of studies have demonstrated the reliability of FNA in the evaluation of breast lesions, with relatively high sensitivity and specificity, especially when combined with image guidance.

However, the success of FNA requires not only an excellent aspirator to obtain satisfactory aspirates but also breast cytopathologic expertise in interpreting the breast aspirates [8–10]. Recently, the popularity of FNA has been decreasing, which can be attributed in part to a shortage of training opportunities and paucity of well-trained or experienced cytopathologists at individual centers, leading to more diagnostic errors and higher rates of inadequate samples. Consequently, clinicians have become reluctant to rely on this technique for preoperative diagnosis. In addition, FNA has intrinsic limitations, largely because of the lack of reliable histologic architecture. Diagnostic difficulty may be encountered in certain lesions, even by experienced cytopathologists.

Nevertheless, FNA is considered suitable for low-resource settings particularly at the basic level. Currently, this technique continues to be used as first-line of pathologic investigation for breast lesions in some developed countries and in many developing countries [11–20].

Because of the limitations of FNA, many institutes in the developed countries have replaced FNA by other tissue-based diagnostic procedures such as CNB [8, 21–24]. Image-guided CNB encompasses ultrasound-guided CNB (USG-CNB) and mammographically guided vacuum-assisted core biopsy (VACB). Core tissue allows for histologic examination with which pathologists are familiar and thus is suitable in centers where experienced cytopathologists are not available. CNB provides a more definitive pathologic diagnosis than FNA for some lesions and also facilitates biomarker studies, similar to other surgical specimens. Although CNB is more invasive, time-consuming, and more expensive than FNA, it is less invasive and relatively more cost-effective than open surgical biopsy and is easily performed with minimal scarring [25].

Indications

The decision as to which method needs to be used depends on availability of technique and expertise, the lesion's nature (size, location, and consistency), the diagnostic performance, the physician's preference, and the patient's economic situation.

FNA

- For a newly identified, clinically and/or radiologically obvious malignancy of the breast, CNB is the sampling method usually preferred for histologic evaluation and biomarker studies. However, in countries with limited resources, FNA may be used as the sole sampling technique or as the first-line diagnostic tool for pathologic evaluation.
- When a major lesion of primary breast carcinoma is identified, it is important to know whether there is cancer elsewhere in the same quadrant (multifocal disease) or in different

quadrants (multicentric disease) before surgery is planned, especially when breast-conserving surgery is being considered. FNA is the preferred sampling method for assessing these satellite lesions.

- FNA can be reliably used for pathologic confirmation of an inoperable advanced-stage breast cancer before systemic therapy.
- During post-surgery follow-up of breast cancer patients, FNA is a preferred sampling method for newly developed chest wall lesions and for documentation of recurrence vs. reactive changes/fat necrosis.
- For breast lesions that appear radiologically benign or probably benign, FNA is preferred as the first-line sampling technique, and a benign diagnosis could save cost, time, and patient anxiety. Notably, benign breast lesions are far more common than breast cancer.
- For cystic lesions of the breast that are benign in the majority of cases, FNA is sufficient to obtain diagnostic tissue and sometimes even has served as a therapeutic procedure.
- Metastatic tumors of extramammary origin, although rare, can occur in the breast. FNA is usually sufficient for the diagnosis on the basis of cytologic features and/or immunoperoxidase findings [26, 27].
- Infectious diseases of the breast, including abscess, mastitis, and tuberculosis, can be reliably diagnosed by pathologic examination of FNA samples in conjunction with microorganism cultures of the aspirates [28, 29].
- Lymphoma of the breast can be sampled via FNA, and the aspirates are superior to core tissue for flow cytometric immunophenotyping [30, 31].
- Preoperative identification of metastatic disease of the local–regional lymph nodes (e.g., axillary, supraclavicular, infraclavicular, and internal mammary lymph nodes) has become an integral part of breast examination for patients with newly diagnosed breast cancer and is preferably conducted with FNA because it is the most accurate and cost-effective, yet safe, method. Axillary staging via FNA can spare sentinel node biopsy if axillary lymph node cytology is positive and can be followed by immediate axillary dissection or triage of advanced cases for adjuvant/neoadjuvant treatment [32].

CNB

- All the previously mentioned lesions, except for cyst contents, can be sampled by CNB. Nonpalpable and image-detected abnormalities, such as microcalcifications and architectural distortion, should be sampled by CNB [24, 25, 33]. VACB is more accurate for these lesions than USG-CNB [34–36].
- CNB may be used as a second-line diagnostic tool for lesions in which FNA fails to yield sufficient cells or in which FNA is unable to reach an unequivocal diagnosis [25, 37].
- CNB is the preferred diagnostic technique when determination of in situ carcinoma vs. invasive carcinoma/tumor subtyping is required, usually for newly identified, clinically, and/or radiologically apparent primary breast carcinoma, especially for patients who are candidates for neoadjuvant chemotherapy.

Limitations and Disadvantages

FNA

- FNA may yield low cellular aspirates and result in an unsatisfactory sample for lesions with abundant fibrotic or desmoplastic stroma, such as invasive lobular carcinoma.
- The intrinsic limitation of FNA is sampling error due to small sample size and the lack of reliable histologic architecture. Therefore, even when the aspirate is adequate in cellularity, a diagnosis may not be accurate. This does not necessarily reflect the inability of a pathologist to recognize a specific entity but is rather due to the inherent nature of the breast lesions. For example, in benign lesions, it may be difficult at times to distinguish between fibroadenoma and benign/low-grade phyllodes

tumor [38–41], fibroadenoma and fibrocystic change, and fibroadenoma and papillary lesions [42]. Occasionally, it may be challenging to distinguish myxoid fibroadenoma from colloid carcinoma [43–45] and to distinguish benign sclerosing lesions from low-grade carcinoma [46, 47]. In borderline or low-grade lesions, such as atypical ductal or lobular hyperplasia, papillary lesions, in situ low-grade ductal or lobular carcinoma, some tubular carcinomas, and invasive lobular carcinoma [48–51], it may be difficult to render a definitive diagnosis or distinguish one from the other. It has been reported that false-negative or equivocal cytologic diagnoses are associated with tubular carcinoma [52–58] and invasive lobular carcinoma [59–65] because their cytologic features may overlap with those of benign proliferative diseases. In malignant lesions, it may not be possible to distinguish invasive from in situ carcinoma [66–69] or to accurately specify tumor subtype in some cases. Previous studies reported cytologic features that can be used to predict invasion [66, 68–71]. These include malignant cell clusters forming tubular structures, single tumor cells with intracytoplasmic lumina, proliferation of fibroblasts and elastoid stromal fragments, and the infiltration of malignant cells into fibrofatty fragments. However, overlapping features can be seen in both invasive and in situ lesions. Over-relying on these criteria can lead to misdiagnosis.

CNB

- CNB has similar limitations to those of FNA such as sampling error due to the small amount of tissue obtained with CNB. Although less frequently than with FNA, misinterpretation can occasionally occur with CNB. For example, some phyllodes tumors on excision were initially diagnosed as fibroadenoma by CNB, in part due to intratumoral heterogeneity. Likewise, it may be problematic to distinguish benign papillary lesions from atypical or malignant ones, between atypical ductal hyperplasia and low-grade ductal carcinoma in situ, and between complex sclerosing lesion/radial scar and tubular carcinoma [72–74]. Approximately one-fifth of lesions diagnosed via CNB as ductal carcinoma in situ are associated with invasive component on excision [8, 75, 76].
- CNB requires local anesthesia, is unable to provide the on-site immediate assessment that FNA can provide, and takes longer to report results than FNA. Although touch imprints of CNB tissue may be evaluated during immediate assessment, the accuracy in predicting the histology of corresponding CNB is suboptimal [77].
- CNB is unable to aspirate fluid collections [78, 79].
- It may be difficult for CNB to sample some lesions that are close to the skin, near the chest wall, or in the axilla, as well as some types of calcifications [9, 74, 80].
- CNB, especially using a large bore needle, may be associated with histologic changes of the biopsy sites including hemosiderin deposition, fibrosis, foreign-body reaction, and infarction of some lesions such as papilloma [81].
- CNB may occasionally lead to reduction of tumor size, which can affect the decision for subsequent chemotherapy in tumors of borderline size [82]. Post-VACB ultrasonographic appearance mimicking malignancy has been reported [83].

Diagnostic Accuracy

FNA

The success of FNA depends on the nature of the lesion, the skill of the aspirator, and the experience of the interpreter. Availability of immediate assessment and feedback also affects the success rate.

A number of publications have demonstrated the high overall accuracy of FNA in the diagnosis of breast lesions. A large-scale study of 2,375 lesions from Thailand showed sensitivity, specificity, positive predictive value, and negative predictive values of 84.4%, 99.5%, 99.8%, and 84.3%, respectively; overall diagnostic accuracy of 91.3%; and false-positive and false-negative rates of 0.5% and 16.7%, respectively [11]. In a study from the United States that evaluated the utility of FNA in 1,158 clinically suspicious, palpable breast masses in women under and over the age of 40 years, the sensitivity, specificity, and positive predictive value in both groups were 97–99%, although the negative predictive value in women over age 40 years was 86%. The overall false-positive rate was <1% and false-negative rate was 9% [84].

Even for imaging-detected nonpalpable lesions, FNA cytologic evaluation is highly accurate when practiced in a multidisciplinary setting [85, 86]. In a study at The University of Texas MD Anderson Cancer Center evaluating nonpalpable, noncystic breast lesions sampled with ultrasound-guided FNA, the sensitivity and specificity in the diagnosis of cancer were 91% and 77%, respectively, and the false-positive and false-negative rates were 1% and 2%, respectively [79]. Combined with more recent studies, the overall sensitivity was 76–99%, specificity 60–100%, positive predictive value 94–100%, negative predictive value 67–96%, diagnostic accuracy 72–95%, false-positive rate 0–3%, and false-negative rate 3–18% [11–13, 17–19, 80, 84, 87].

False-positive results are uncommon and are usually due to interpretative error, and occasionally due to improper specimen preparation (e.g., distortion of the cells from vigorous smear spreading, air-drying artifact). False-negative diagnoses are more likely the effects of sampling error rather than interpretative problems.

CNB

As is the case for FNA, the success of CNB depends on the nature of the lesions, competence of the aspirator, and experience of the pathologist. A number of studies have reported very high sensitivity (91–99%), specificity (96–100%), positive predictive value (100%), and negative predictive value (100%), which are better than results for FNA for both palpable and nonpalpable lesions [88–91]. Also, the sensitivity of CNB increases with the number of cores taken (1 core, 76.2%; 2 cores, 80.9%; 3 cores, 89.2%; 4 cores, 95.2%) [92].

Sample Collection, Preparation, and Staining

FNA

It is controversial whether clinician or pathologist should perform the aspiration; however, practice makes perfect. Knowledge of the consistency of the lesion during physical examination or aspiration is helpful for predicting the nature of the lesion. For example, a hard lesion gritty to the needle is likely to be malignant, and a freely movable, well-defined, and rubbery mass is suggestive of a fibroadenoma.

Generally, for palpable breast masses, two to four needle passes are made. The needle gauge can be 22–25, depending on the quality of the lesion. The needle may be attached to a disposable syringe that is mounted to a pistol grip-like syringe holder to apply suction. A local anesthetic is usually not used, because the swelling that results can obscure the nodule. If a breast lesion is densely fibrous, a larger needle with suction is preferred, and, in this circumstance, local anesthesia may be advisable. One should release suction when blood or material is first seen in the hub of the needle. The needle is withdrawn from the lesion without any vacuum suction because the cells otherwise may end up in the syringe (rather than staying in the needle) and are difficult to expel onto slides. Fluid-filled cysts are the exception: if fluid is obtained, negative pressure should be maintained until the cyst is completely evacuated. Any residual mass requires re-aspiration of the solid component to avoid missing malignant cysts.

To prepare smears, the needle is removed from the syringe, which is filled with air. Pushing this air with the plunger of the syringe, a small drop of aspirated material is expressed onto each slide and smears prepared. After making direct smears, air-dried Diff-Quik-stained and alcohol- or Carnoy-fixed Papanicolaou-stained smears are routinely made. Diff-Quik staining preferably highlights cytoplasmic features and background material, whereas Papanicolaou staining is better for the evaluation of nuclear characteristics (i.e., nuclear membrane, chromatin, and nucleolus). In some laboratories, hematoxylin-eosin stain is used to stain the smears; in others laboratories, liquid-based preparations (e.g., ThinPrep, SurePath) may be made, either together with or to replace direct smears [93–96]. The advantages claimed for the liquid-based technique include better preservation of cellular morphology, and also the cytologic diagnosis can be made from one slide while the remaining material can be used for biomarkers. This technique, however, is not widely accepted since it results in shrinkage artifacts and a diminution in the background material that is often useful for diagnosis.

On-site immediate assessment for specimen adequacy is important to ensure high diagnostic accuracy and to reduce the incidence of unsatisfactory aspirates. Ideally, the immediate assessment should be performed by an experienced cytopathologist who should correlate the cytologic findings of direct smears available at the time of aspiration with the clinical and radiologic findings (triple test) to determine whether the FNA contains material representative of the target lesion. Mismatched triple test results require re-aspiration or concurrent CNB. There is no specific requirement for a minimum number of ductal cells to be present to fulfill adequacy of the aspirates of solid nodules [97]. An FNA is considered "inadequate" if the sample is nonrepresentative (such as scant cellularity incompatible with clinical and/or radiologic findings) or if the smears show significant distortion or artifacts and cannot be interpreted. Immediate assessment can also warrant a proper triage of material for cell block and/or ancillary studies. Cell block material should be collected for immediate assessment for cases in which architectural features might be crucial for making a definitive diagnosis because cell block material retains, at least partially, histologic architecture of the lesion. In addition, cell block is the preferred sample type for immunoperoxidase studies. A separate dedicated pass (if additional needle pass is deemed feasible by the aspirator) and needle rinse or tissue fragments scraped from a thick smear are all suitable for cell block. After centrifugation, the pellet is fixed in formalin, embedded in paraffin, and then sectioned and stained with hematoxylin-eosin, a process virtually identical to that used for surgical tissue specimens. Unstained cell block sections are used for immunoperoxidase studies. In cases where non-Hodgkin lymphoma is suspected based on immediate assessment, fresh cells should be collected as cell suspension for flow cytometric immunophenotyping. Likewise, in cases where an infectious process needs to be excluded, fresh samples should be collected for microorganism cultures.

CNB

CNB is usually conducted with image guidance. Both USG-CNB and VACB require local anesthesia. The former involves using a large-bore cutting needle (usually 14-gauge) and automated gun to remove one cylindrical core of breast tissue per insertion; three to four cores are routinely required to maximize the chance of definitive diagnosis. VACB is a semi-invasive, mini-resection biopsy procedure and involves using a vacuum-powered instrument (usually 9-gauge) to remove multiple pieces of breast tissue during one needle insertion. The tissue cores are fixed in formalin, embedded in paraffin, and then sectioned and stained with hematoxylin-eosin. Unstained sections are used for immunoperoxidase studies.

Complications

Complications in FNA are rare, and the most common ones are pain and bleeding [98–100]. The latter can be decreased by using a smaller bore needle and applying firm pressure after the needle exits the lesion. The other potential complications are vasovagal reactions, infection, and pneumothorax; infarction, epithelial displacement, and needle track malignant seeding are extremely rare and are attributed to the use of large-bore needles [20, 80, 101–104]. All theses complications can also occur with CNB, with discomfort and hematomas being the most common complications [79, 105].

Pathologic Report

Regardless of the type of sampling methods (FNA or CNB), the pathologic interpretation should be made on the basis of triple test whenever possible. Application of triple test can significantly reduce false-negative and false-positive interpretation in cytology diagnosis, with resulting false-negative rates of 0.4–1.7% [106]. When a discrepancy is encountered or a definitive diagnosis cannot be reached, a more invasive procedure (subsequent CNB or open surgical biopsy) should be considered for further evaluation. Cytologic examination should start with low magnification followed by high magnification. Features that need to be examined are listed next.

Low-Power Examination

- Background: necrotic debris, mucin, myxoid material, lipoproteinaceous material, inflammatory cells, blood elements, bipolar naked nuclei.
- Cellularity: high cellularity is often seen in neoplastic and proliferative disease.
- Cell arrangement: sizes and shapes of epithelial groups, monolayered cohesive sheet, three-dimensional cluster, papillary group, loosely cohesive or discohesive clusters, isolated cells.

High-Power Examination

- Cell type and proportion: epithelial cells, apocrine metaplastic cells, myoepithelial cells, mesenchymal cells, histiocytes.
- Size and shape of individual lesional cells.
- Cytoplasmic features: amount, granularity, vacuolization, intracytoplasmic lumina.
- Nuclear features: size and shape, nuclear/cytoplasmic ratio, location, pleomorphism, nuclear membrane irregularity, chromatin pattern, size of nucleolus, mitosis.

The National Cancer Institute has recommended five categories of diagnosis in breast aspiration cytology in order to bring a degree of uniformity to the diagnostic reporting [107]. These categories are unsatisfactory (C1); benign lesion (C2); atypical, probably benign (C3); suspicious, probably malignant (C4); and malignant (C5). For benign and malignant lesions, a general category of benign or malignant is better followed by a specific diagnosis whenever possible. For lesions with equivocal diagnosis, it is informative to include possible differential diagnosis and the likelihood of malignancy to allow clinicians to determine whether a close follow-up or histologic confirmation is appropriate [20, 108].

Unsatisfactory aspirate (C1) is often due to scant cellularity, poor preservation or distortion of the lesional cells, significant obscuring blood, or inflammatory components. The reported unsatisfactory rates are as high as 34% [11, 109]. This problem can be minimized by practicing aspiration skills, doing multiple needle passes for each lesion, and having a cytopathologist to perform on-site assessment. Studies have shown that the nondiagnostic rate was 20% without on-site assessment but was less than 1% with on-site assessment [11, 110]. In addition, FNA with ultrasound guidance should have a higher sensitivity than unguided FNA [85, 111].

Common Cytologic Features of Benign Lesions (Fig. 2.1)

- Variable cellularity
- Cohesive flat sheets of epithelial cells with honeycomb appearance; slight crowding when hyperplastic
- Small or slightly enlarged nuclei, evenly spaced from each other

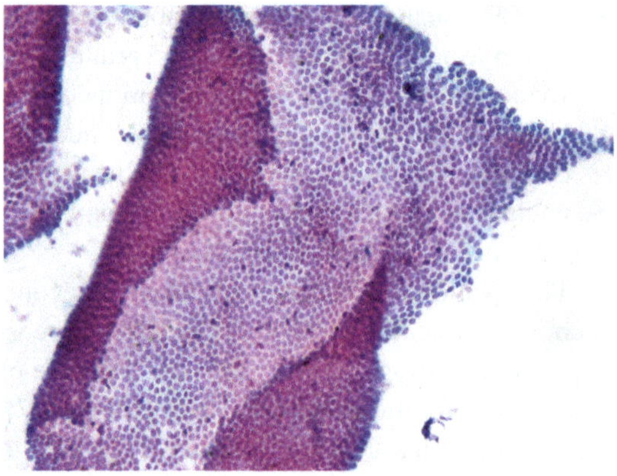

Fig. 2.1 Fine needle aspiration (FNA) smear of benign non-proliferative ductal epithelial cells, characterized by a cohesive flat sheet with honeycomb appearance. Interspersed within the monolayered ductal cells are myoepithelial cells with darker small individual nuclei (Papanicolaou stain)

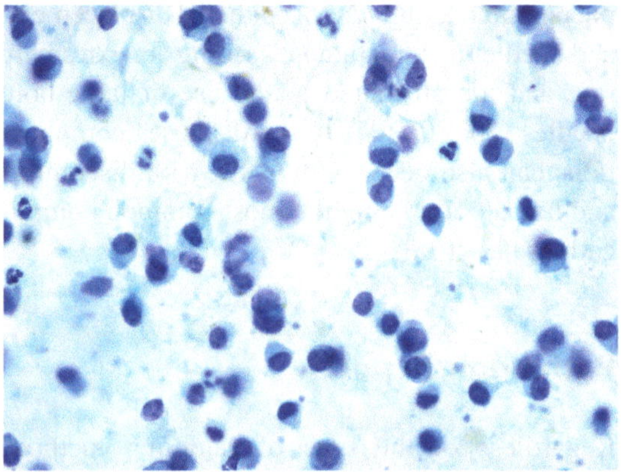

Fig. 2.2 FNA smear of a lobular carcinoma of the breast, characterized by eccentrically located nuclei with mild to moderate nuclear atypia and arranged in loosely cohesive clusters or single files (Papanicolaou stain)

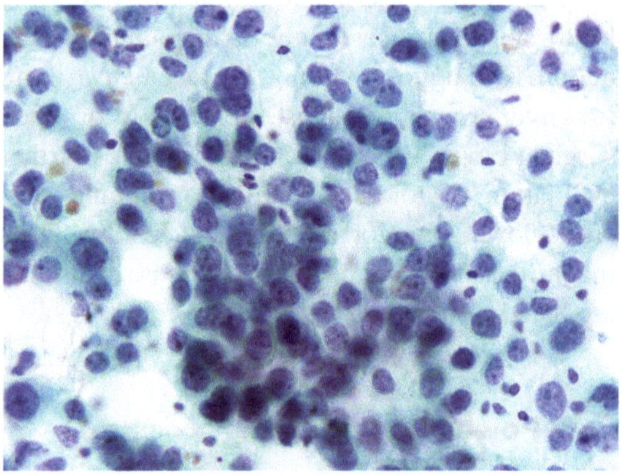

Fig. 2.3 FNA smear of a ductal carcinoma of the breast, characterized by hypercellular aspirate, pronounced nuclear atypia, and cellular pleomorphism (Papanicolaou stain)

- Smooth nuclear outline, fine chromatin, small to inconspicuous nucleoli
- Variable amounts of myoepithelial cells that appear as darker small individual nuclei within the epithelial fragments and in the background

Cytologic features of carcinomas vary significantly according to the histologic type, degree of differentiation, and the extent of stromal reaction. While some invasive ductal carcinoma (such as tubular carcinoma), lobular carcinoma, and mucinous carcinoma often show mild cytologic atypia and subtle malignant features (Fig. 2.2), the most commonly encountered ductal carcinomas show the following features (Fig. 2.3):

- Hypercellular aspirates
- Tumor cells forming three-dimensional, syncytial, or loosely cohesive clusters with numerous dispersed epithelial cells with intact cytoplasm
- Nuclear atypia encompassing enlarged, hyperchromatic, and pleomorphic nuclei, increased nuclear/cytoplasmic ratio, irregular nuclear membrane, coarse chromatin, presence of mitotic figures, and prominent nucleoli
- Absence of or rare myoepithelial cells
- Tumor necrosis

With a cytologic diagnosis of breast carcinoma, tumor typing and nuclear grading should be incorporated into the diagnosis whenever possible. Tumor typing is based on cellularity, arrangement of cell groups, cell morphology, nuclear size and pleomorphism, and background content [112]. Several scoring systems have been developed including Robinson's grading system, Mouriquand's grading system, and Fisher's modification of Black's nuclear grading method [113–116]. The Robinson's grading system has been reportedly the easier and better one due to its superior objectivity and reproducibility [117, 118].

Tumor type and grade determined on FNA samples correlate quite well with the corresponding histologic grade and may assist in clinical decision-making [112, 114, 116, 117, 119].

The equivocal categories of C3 and C4 account for 5–10% of breast aspiration cases. Of note, 20–50% of C3 cases (atypical, probably benign) and 80–95% of C4 cases (suspicious, probably malignant) turn out to be malignant in final diagnosis [14, 120–125]. Lesions with equivocal cytologic diagnosis require additional histologic confirmation for definitive diagnosis.

Owing to the lower diagnostic yield and accuracy rate of FNA in certain lesions, cost-effectiveness of FNA becomes a debatable issue. Although the cost for FNA as a single sampling procedure is cheaper than the cost for CNB, especially in cases where there is a palpable lesion and FNA is conducted without imaging guidance, the total cost for obtaining a reliable final diagnosis will be higher than for CNB alone for lesions that are initially sampled with FNA subsequently require histologic (CNB or open surgical biopsy) confirmation [126]. Therefore, it is important to select diagnostic modality based on clinical/radiologic indications.

Ancillary Studies

Ancillary studies used in breast lesions are mostly immunoperoxidase stains and occasionally special stains such as mucin or fungal staining. Both CNB and FNA samples can be used for the ancillary tests, with CNB being the preferred type. For FNA samples, cell block, direct smear, and liquid-based preparation are all suitable for ancillary studies, but cell block is optimal since it is analogous to surgical pathology material.

In cases in which a cell block is not available or contains insufficient cells, direct smear and liquid-based preparation can be tried for immunostains as long as the sample is reasonably cellular [127–129]. If the cells of interest are present on only a single or a few smears when a panel of immunostains is needed, a cell-transfer technique—in which the original smear material is divided into several pieces and then transferred onto multiple slides—may facilitate multiple immunomarker studies [130–133]. This technique can avoid a repeat biopsy solely for immunophenotyping of lesions.

There are several disadvantages of immunostaining on direct smear and liquid-based preparations:

1. Such sample types lack proper control tissue, which should be processed and fixed in the same way as the test specimen at each run of immunostaining
2. High background staining, which is usually associated with crowding of cells in a thick smear, or poor cytoplasmic preservation may lead to misinterpretation
3. Because of the lack of a reliable histologic architecture in the aspirated material, the mistaking of entrapped benign ductal cells, cells of ADH or DCIS for invasive tumor cells, can occur, leading to misinterpretation of biomarker results
4. Due to sampling error, tumor necrosis, or tumor fibrosis, it is a common limitation that only a small amount of cells are available for immunostaining, which may lead to a false-negative interpretation in tumors that express some markers only focally and heterogeneously

Therefore, caution should be exercised in the interpretation of immunostaining results on any samples that have limited lesional cells.

Prognostic and predictive factors most commonly tested in breast cancer samples are estrogen receptor (ER), progesterone receptor (PR), and human epidermal growth factor receptor 2 (HER2). Knowing the status of these biomarkers is crucial for the assessment of a patient's eligibility for endocrine therapy and anti-HER2-targeted therapies, respectively. Although the biomarkers are usually tested in surgically resected or CNB specimens of newly diagnosed primary breast carcinoma and require standardized fixation conditions (i.e., fixation in 10% neutral buffered formalin for 6–48 h for ER, PR, and HER2) [134–136], the markers are also frequently tested in cytologic specimens to determine their status in metastatic carcinoma, since metastatic tumors are often sampled via FNA.

Clinicians frequently request retesting of these markers in metastatic tumors even though the receptor status of the patient's primary tumor is known. It is believed that, due to tumor heterogeneity and possible clonal evolution during biologic progression of the tumor, metastatic deposits may show loss or gain of the expression of these receptors and demonstrate a receptor status different from the status in the corresponding primary tumors. Also, the receptor activity in metastatic breast cancer may be altered after intervening systemic therapy (chemotherapy or targeted therapy). Therefore, assessment of these markers in a metastatic setting has a direct effect on the management of metastatic disease. In some cases in which the primary origin of a metastatic tumor is uncertain, receptor status (especially ER) is performed on FNA material of a metastatic carcinoma to verify or rule out a breast origin. Rarely, an FNA sample of a primary breast carcinoma is used for testing these markers when cytologic samples are the only sample type available for biomarker study.

With decent cell block material, ER, PR, and HER2 can be tested using immunostaining; HER2 can also be tested via fluorescence in situ hybridization (FISH). Without cell block, direct smear or liquid-based preparation may be used. For ER and PR immunostaining, previous studies have shown that preprepared direct smears can be used [137–139]. However, preprepared smears should be made prospectively at the time of aspiration. In routine practice, a retrospective requisition for biomarker studies may be received after a cytologic diagnosis has been completed and cell block tissue or preprepared smears are not available. Under such circumstances, the existing Papanicolaou-stained smears that have been used for routine cytologic diagnosis may be used for ER and PR staining. A study at MD Anderson Cancer Center compared ER staining results between smears and corresponding tissue sections and reported that ER staining can be performed directly on previously Papanicolaou-stained smears (without destaining) and that antigen retrieval greatly improved ER detectability and staining intensity without causing false positivity [140]. This technique allows the use of archived slides for retrospective analysis of hormone receptor status, to visualize cytologic features and amounts of tumor cells on the slides prior to the tests, and thereby to enable selection of the "most representative" slide for staining (Figs. 2.4 and 2.5). In some centers, liquid-based monolayer preparation is used for ER and PR staining [141].

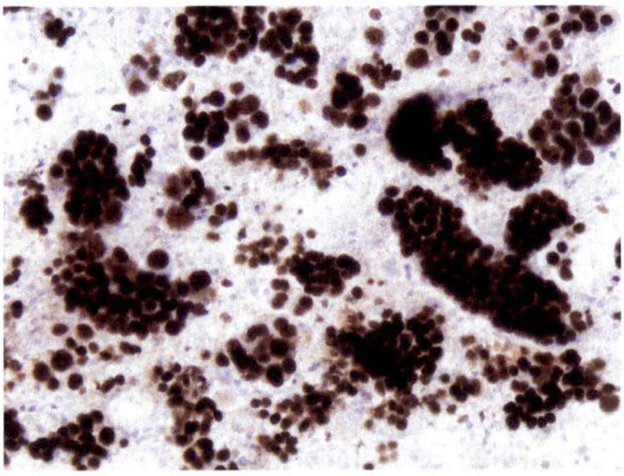

Fig. 2.4 Estrogen receptor was determined with immunocytochemical staining on a direct smear of a breast ductal carcinoma and was positive in approximately 95% tumor cells

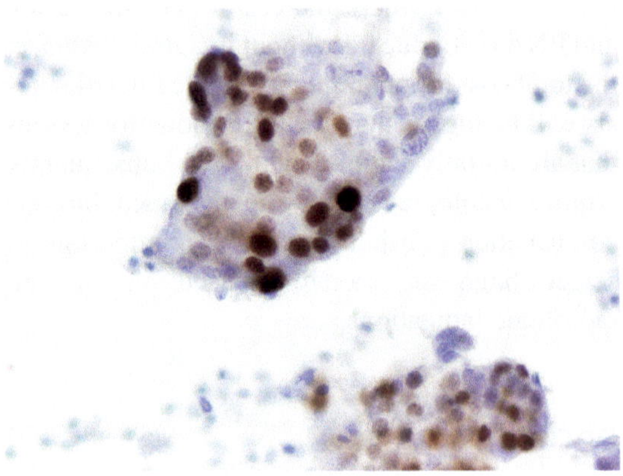

Fig. 2.5 Progesterone receptor was determined with immunocytochemical staining on a direct smear of a breast ductal carcinoma and was positive in approximately 40% tumor cells

For HER2, immunostaining of HER2 on direct smear or liquid-based preparation is not standardized and is insufficiently reliable for clinical use because it is associated with high variability in sample preparation, fixation, staining, and

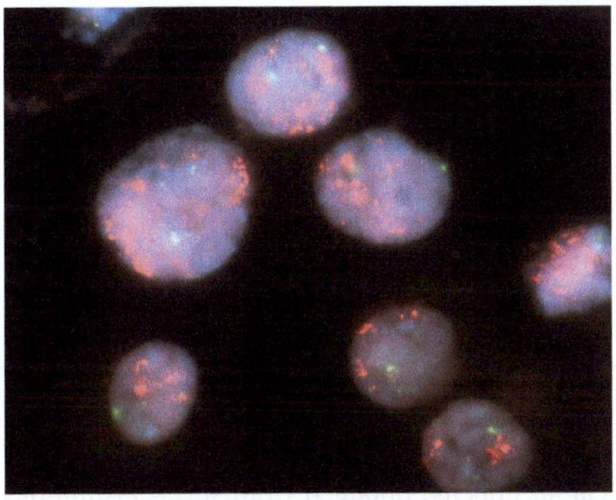

Fig. 2.6 HER2 testing using fluorescence in situ hybridization was performed on a direct smear of a breast ductal carcinoma and showed HER2 gene amplification

interpretation [142–144]. Therefore, the FISH method to detect HER2 gene amplification should be used instead. A number of studies have shown that HER2 status determined using FISH can be reliably evaluated in cytologic slides, with a concordance between cytologic samples and paired tissue sections of 91–100% [142, 145–148]. Compared with paraffin sections for FISH testing, the use of cytologic smears or touch imprint has the advantage of assessing monolayered tumor cells and enumerating all the HER2 signals within an entire nucleus without a truncating artifact (Fig. 2.6).

Chromogenic in situ hybridization is a bright field in situ hybridization method and is reportedly equally reliable to FISH in the determination of HER2 gene amplification [149–151]. This method detects HER2 copy number with a conventional peroxidase reaction and allows enumeration of gene copy number using a regular microscope along with histologic evaluation. Few studies have indicated that chromogenic in situ hybridization can potentially be performed on FNA material, including cell block sections, direct smears, or cytospins, and the reported sensitivity, specificity, and accuracy were 84.0%, 87.9%, and 86.2%, respectively [152, 153]. Utility of this technique for testing HER2 status on cytologic samples requires validation in large studies.

Overall, the decision to perform which test on which sample type should be made on the basis of sample type and expertise available at each institution. If a laboratory chooses to perform prognostic and predictive marker studies on cytology specimens, the reliability of preanalytic and analytic methods should be validated according to the current guidelines [135, 136]. For laboratories that do not have specific experience with smears and liquid-based preparations, an effort should be made to obtain cellular cell block tissue for these tests. Of note, ER, PR, and HER2 status should be assessed on the invasive component of the breast carcinoma. Because cytologic specimens cannot reliably discriminate invasive from in situ components, interpretation of ER, PR, and HER2 status in a primary setting should proceed cautiously, especially if the tumor is small.

Stability of Prognostic and Predictive Biomarkers

Evaluation of the stability of hormone receptor and HER2 status during disease progression or after intervening systemic endocrine therapy or chemotherapy is of clinical significance. Using validated methods for ER testing and FISH for HER2 testing in metastatic breast carcinoma (mostly on direct smears), researchers at MD Anderson Cancer Center compared the results with those of primary tumors and observed a high level of stability for both markers. The concordance rates between primary and paired metastatic breast carcinoma were 92.5% for ER and 97% for HER2 [154, 155]. When evaluating patients with HER2-positive primary breast carcinoma, these researchers found that a positive-to-negative conversion of HER2 status occurred in 15% of metastatic breast carcinoma; the loss of HER2 positivity in metastatic carcinoma occurred in similar rates in both trastuzumab-treated and trastuzumab-naïve control groups, indicating that the loss of HER2-positive status was probably unrelated to intervening trastuzumab-based therapy [156, 157]. Nevertheless, given the importance of these markers for clinical management, an effort should be made to retest their status in metastatic breast carcinoma.

Future Directions

To date, the common approach in identifying prognostic and predictive variables is to test one or a few markers in a cohort of patients, usually retrospectively. The resulting information may not fully capture the biologic heterogeneity in tumor growth, invasion, and metastasis and cannot accurately determine the risk of relapse for individual patients. Over the last decade, molecular testing, especially gene expression profiling microarray, has been used to identify more sophisticated prognostic and predictive factors for breast cancer patients. Gene combinations (i.e., gene signatures) seem more accurate than any single gene measurement alone.

It is reasonable to assume that CNB contains higher quality and amounts of RNA than does FNA for molecular testing. Several studies have demonstrated that both FNA and CNB samples yield adequate amounts of total RNA for microarray in experienced hands [158–160]. A learning curve has been observed during sample procurement via FNA. According to a study from MD Anderson Cancer Center, the success rate of gene expression profiling began at 70–75%, and then increased with practice to 97% [159]. It is not surprising that FNA and CNB show different cellular compositions, with a high proportion of carcinoma cells in FNA samples and more stromal cells and lymphocytes in CNB samples [158]. Selection of the preferred sample type for genomic studies should depend on whether the focus is on tumor cells only or on the tumor as well as its microenvironment (stroma).

Suitability of FNA samples for gene expression microarray has been shown in a number of studies that tried to identify prognostic and predictive variables, chemotherapy response predictor, and drug resistance mechanism [161–165]. During the course of systemic therapy, serial FNA may be an acceptable tool for tissue procurement in monitoring the response of tumor to the therapy and treatment-induced biomarker changes [166]. Investigators from multiple institutions assessed the ER and HER2 expression data derived from comprehensive expression microarray data and observed a significant correlation between mRNA expression of ER and HER2 and the routinely determined status via immunostaining and/or FISH, with overall accuracies around 90% [159]. In that study, mRNA cutoff values of ER and HER2 were defined using tumors sampled via FNA, and the performance of each cutoff was validated in two independent datasets (one FNA specimens and the other surgical specimens) obtained from seven institutions across five countries. These findings indicate that it is promising to generate ER and HER2 information from comprehensive microarray data; integration of ER and HER2 mRNA expression data with multigene signatures from the same microarray data may refine and improve their predictive power for tumor response to target therapies and therefore allow for optimizing clinical decision-making and tailoring of therapeutic regimens on an individual basis.

FNA of breast lesions preserved in PreservCyt medium seems an acceptable sample type for protein profiling evaluation by the surface-enhanced laser desorption–ionization time of flight (SELDI-TOF) methodology [167].

The application of promoter hypermethylation has been investigated in liquid-based aspiration specimens, and this technique has been shown to improve diagnostic accuracy of breast lesions in which cytological assessment is indeterminate or suspicious for malignancy. It therefore might be a valuable ancillary tool for cytology diagnosis of breast carcinoma [168, 169].

Breast Cancer Risk Assessment

Identification of women at high risk for developing breast cancer is an important step in cancer prevention because these women may benefit from preventive intervention such as anti-estrogen agents or surgery [170–172]. The risk stratification is assessed on the basis of the Gail risk score and pathologic findings. Nipple fluid aspiration, ductal lavage, random periareolar FNA (RPFNA), and CNB have been used for tissue acquisition [173]. Some researchers performed nipple aspiration followed by ductal lavage [174]; however, the latter two methods were both associated with low diagnostic yield and some discomfort. In addition, to date there are no data available regarding the efficacy or mortality reduction for ductal lavage used as a screening or diagnostic tool. RPFNA seems a better option for obtaining ductal and lobular cells and is the most accepted method by study participants [175–177]. The aspirated cells can be evaluated morphologically as well as for several biomarkers (epidermal growth factor receptor, ER, p53 protein, HER2, insulin-like growth factor 1, etc.) [176, 178]. A diagnosis of hyperplasia with atypia is associated with a high risk of developing breast cancer [173, 177]. Using FISH to screen for aneusomy in RPFNA samples, researchers at MD Anderson Cancer Center found that aberrations of chromosomal number were common in women at high risk for breast cancer; high-risk patients had significantly more monosomy of chromosomes 1, 11, and 17 and significantly more polysomy of chromosome 8 compared with low-risk patients [179].

Conclusions

Breast FNA and CNB are both useful for diagnosis, risk stratification, and biomarker testing.

Both procedures have their own specific advantages and limitations and can complement each other. While there is widespread preference for CNB in most developed countries, FNA is still a valuable initial procedure for evaluating palpable breast lesions in many developing countries in view of its ease, simplicity, affordability, safety, rapidity, low cost, and high degree of accuracy. There is no consensus as to which modality is preferable in breast lesion diagnosis. The option should be determined by several factors: availability of the necessary equipment and expertise, clinical/radiologic indications, the likelihood of achieving a definitive diagnosis, the need for biomarker studies, patient economic status, and the preferences of the managing clinician and the patient. On the public side, education on the availability of the affordable and less invasive diagnostic techniques may encourage women to seek care at earlier stages of the disease. In the future, genomic and proteomic techniques hold great promise to complement the existing diagnostic modalities for evaluating breast lesions.

References

1. Parkin DM, Bray F, Ferlay J, Pisani P. Global cancer statistics, 2002. CA Cancer J Clin. 2005;55(2):74–108.
2. Anderson BO, Jakesz R. Breast cancer issues in developing countries: an overview of the Breast Health Global Initiative. World J Surg. 2008; 32(12):2578–85.
3. Shyyan R, Masood S, Badwe RA, et al. Breast cancer in limited-resource countries: diagnosis and pathology. Breast J. 2006;12 Suppl 1:S27–37.
4. Vargas HI, Masood S. Implementation of a minimally invasive breast biopsy program in countries with limited resources. Breast J. 2003;9 Suppl 2:S81–5.
5. Lannin DR, Silverman JF, Walker C, Pories WJ. Cost-effectiveness of fine needle biopsy of the breast. Ann Surg. 1986;203(5):474–80.
6. Logan-Young W, Dawson AE, Wilbur DC, et al. The cost-effectiveness of fine-needle aspiration cytology and 14-gauge core needle biopsy compared with open surgical biopsy in the diagnosis of breast carcinoma. Cancer. 1998;82(10):1867–73.
7. Rimm DL, Stastny JF, Rimm EB, Ayer S, Frable WJ. Comparison of the costs of fine-needle aspiration and open surgical biopsy as methods for obtaining a pathologic diagnosis. Cancer. 1997;81(1):51–6.
8. Cobb CJ, Raza AS. Obituary: "alas poor FNA of breast—we knew thee well!". Diagn Cytopathol. 2005;32(1):1–4.
9. Feoli F, Paesmans M, Van Eeckhout P. Fine needle aspiration cytology of the breast: impact of experience on accuracy, using standardized cytologic criteria. Acta Cytol. 2008;52(2):145–51.
10. Howell LP. Equivocal diagnoses in breast aspiration biopsy cytology: sources of uncertainty and the role of "atypical/indeterminate" terminology. Diagn Cytopathol. 1999;21(3):217–22.
11. Chaiwun B, Settakorn J, Ya-In C, Wisedmongkol W, Rangdaeng S, Thorner P. Effectiveness of fine-needle aspiration cytology of breast: analysis of 2,375 cases from northern Thailand. Diagn Cytopathol. 2002; 26(3):201–5.
12. Hussain MT. Comparison of fine needle aspiration cytology with excision biopsy of breast lump. J Coll Physicians Surg Pak. 2005;15(4):211–4.
13. Medina-Franco H, Abarca-Perez L, Cortes-Gonzalez R, Soto-Germes S, Ulloa JA, Uribe N. [Fine needle

aspiration biopsy of breast lesions: institutional experience]. Rev Invest Clin. 2005;57(3):394–8.
14. Bulgaresi P, Cariaggi P, Ciatto S, Houssami N. Positive predictive value of breast fine needle aspiration cytology (FNAC) in combination with clinical and imaging findings: a series of 2334 subjects with abnormal cytology. Breast Cancer Res Treat. 2006; 97(3):319–21.
15. Orell SR, Miliauskas J. Fine needle biopsy cytology of breast lesions: a review of interpretative difficulties. Adv Anat Pathol. 2005;12(5):233–45.
16. Zagorianakou P, Fiaccavento S, Zagorianakou N, Makrydimas G, Stefanou D, Agnantis NJ. FNAC: its role, limitations and perspective in the preoperative diagnosis of breast cancer. Eur J Gynaecol Oncol. 2005;26(2):143–9.
17. Lau SK, McKee GT, Weir MM, Tambouret RH, Eichhorn JH, Pitman MB. The negative predicative value of breast fine-needle aspiration biopsy: the Massachusetts General Hospital experience. Breast J. 2004;10(6):487–91.
18. Mizuno S, Isaji S, Ogawa T, et al. Approach to fine-needle aspiration cytology-negative cases of breast cancer. Asian J Surg. 2005;28(1):13–7.
19. Tariq GR, Haleem A, Zaidi AH, Afzal M, Abbasi S. Role of FNA cytology in the management of carcinoma breast. J Coll Physicians Surg Pak. 2005; 15(4):207–10.
20. Das DK. Fine-needle aspiration cytology: its origin, development, and present status with special reference to a developing country, India. Diagn Cytopathol. 2003;28(6):345–51.
21. Britton PD, Flower CD, Freeman AH, et al. Changing to core biopsy in an NHS breast screening unit. Clin Radiol. 1997;52(10):764–7.
22. Gordon PB. Image-directed fine needle aspiration biopsy in nonpalpable breast lesions. Clin Lab Med. 2005;25(4):655–78, v.
23. Clarke D, Sudhakaran N, Gateley CA. Replace fine needle aspiration cytology with automated core biopsy in the triple assessment of breast cancer. Ann R Coll Surg Engl. 2001;83(2):110–2.
24. Meunier M, Clough K. Fine needle aspiration cytology versus percutaneous biopsy of nonpalpable breast lesions. Eur J Radiol. 2002;42(1):10–6.
25. Oyama T, Koibuchi Y, McKee G. Core needle biopsy (CNB) as a diagnostic method for breast lesions: comparison with fine needle aspiration cytology (FNA). Breast Cancer. 2004;11(4):339–42.
26. Shukla R, Pooja B, Radhika S, Nijhawan R, Rajwanshi A. Fine-needle aspiration cytology of extramammary neoplasms metastatic to the breast. Diagn Cytopathol. 2005;32(4):193–7.
27. Smymiotis V, Theodosopoulos T, Marinis A, Goula K, Psychogios J, Kondi-Pafiti A. Metastatic disease in the breast from nonmammary neoplasms. Eur J Gynaecol Oncol. 2005;26(5):547–50.
28. Berna-Serna JD, Madrigal M. Percutaneous management of breast abscesses. An experience of 39 cases. Ultrasound Med Biol. 2004;30(1):1–6.
29. Mehrotra R. Fine needle aspiration diagnosis of tuberculous mastitis. Indian J Pathol Microbiol. 2004;47(3):377–80.
30. Levine PH, Zamuco R, Yee HT. Role of fine-needle aspiration cytology in breast lymphoma. Diagn Cytopathol. 2004;30(5):332–40.
31. Geramizadeh B, Kaboli R, Vasei M. Fine needle aspiration cytology of Burkitt's lymphoma presenting as a breast mass. Acta Cytol. 2004;48(2):285–6.
32. Rao R, Lilley L, Andrews V, Radford L, Ulissey M. Axillary staging by percutaneous biopsy: sensitivity of fine-needle aspiration versus core needle biopsy. Ann Surg Oncol. 2009;16(5):1170–5.
33. Wallis M, Tardivon A, Helbich T, Schreer I. Guidelines from the European Society of Breast Imaging for diagnostic interventional breast procedures. Eur Radiol. 2007;17(2):581–8.
34. Costantini R, Sardellone A, Marino C, Giamberardino MA, Innocenti P, Napolitano AM. Vacuum-assisted core biopsy (Mammotome) for the diagnosis of non-palpable breast lesions: four-year experience in an Italian center. Tumori. 2005;91(4):351–4.
35. Dhillon MS, Bradley SA, England DW. Mammotome biopsy: impact on preoperative diagnosis rate. Clin Radiol. 2006;61(3):276–81.
36. Killebrew LK, Oneson RH. Comparison of the diagnostic accuracy of a vacuum-assisted percutaneous intact specimen sampling device to a vacuum-assisted core needle sampling device for breast biopsy: initial experience. Breast J. 2006;12(4):302–8.
37. Symmans WF, Weg N, Gross J, et al. A prospective comparison of stereotaxic fine-needle aspiration versus stereotaxic core needle biopsy for the diagnosis of mammographic abnormalities. Cancer. 1999; 85(5):1119–32.
38. Jayaram G, Sthaneshwar P. Fine-needle aspiration cytology of phyllodes tumors. Diagn Cytopathol. 2002;26(4):222–7.
39. Scolyer RA, McKenzie PR, Achmed D, Lee CS. Can phyllodes tumours of the breast be distinguished from fibroadenomas using fine needle aspiration cytology? Pathology. 2001;33(4):437–43.
40. Tse GM, Ma TK, Pang LM, Cheung H. Fine needle aspiration cytologic features of mammary phyllodes tumors. Acta Cytol. 2002;46(5):855–63.
41. Veneti S, Manek S. Benign phyllodes tumour vs fibroadenoma: FNA cytological differentiation. Cytopathology. 2001;12(5):321–8.
42. Simsir A, Waisman J, Thorner K, Cangiarella J. Mammary lesions diagnosed as "papillary" by aspiration biopsy: 70 cases with follow-up. Cancer. 2003;99(3):156–65.
43. Lopez-Ferrer P, Jimenez-Heffernan JA, Vicandi B, Ortega L, Viguer JM. Fine needle aspiration cytology of breast fibroadenoma. A cytohistologic correlation study of 405 cases. Acta Cytol. 1999;43(4): 579–86.
44. Simsir A, Tsang P, Greenebaum E. Additional mimics of mucinous mammary carcinoma: fibroepithelial lesions. Am J Clin Pathol. 1998;109(2):169–72.

45. Yeoh GP, Cheung PS, Chan KW. Fine-needle aspiration cytology of mucocelelike tumors of the breast. Am J Surg Pathol. 1999;23(5):552–9.
46. Kundu UR, Guo M, Landon G, Wu Y, Sneige N, Gong Y. Fine-needle aspiration cytology of sclerosing adenosis of the breast: a retrospective review of cytologic features in conjunction with corresponding histologic features and radiologic findings. Am J Clin Pathol. 2012;138(1):96–102.
47. Cho EY, Oh YL. Fine needle aspiration cytology of sclerosing adenosis of the breast. Acta Cytol. 2001;45(3):353–9.
48. Abendroth CS, Wang HH, Ducatman BS. Comparative features of carcinoma in situ and atypical ductal hyperplasia of the breast on fine-needle aspiration biopsy specimens. Am J Clin Pathol. 1991;96(5):654–9.
49. Lilleng R, Hagmar BM, Farrants G. Low-grade cribriform ductal carcinoma in situ of the breast. Fine needle aspiration cytology in three cases. Acta Cytol. 1992;36(1):48–54.
50. Venegas R, Rutgers JL, Cameron BL, Vargas H, Butler JA. Fine needle aspiration cytology of breast ductal carcinoma in situ. Acta Cytol. 1994;38(2):136–43.
51. Leifland K, Lundquist H, Mare K, Erhardt K, Fernstad R. Pre-operative simultaneous stereotactic core biopsy and fine-needle aspiration biopsy in the diagnosis of invasive lobular breast carcinoma. Acta Radiol. 2000;41(1):57–60.
52. Bondeson L, Lindholm K. Aspiration cytology of tubular breast carcinoma. Acta Cytol. 1990;34(1):15–20.
53. Cangiarella J, Waisman J, Shapiro RL, Simsir A. Cytologic features of tubular adenocarcinoma of the breast by aspiration biopsy. Diagn Cytopathol. 2001;25(5):311–5.
54. Dawson AE, Logan-Young W, Mulford DK. Aspiration cytology of tubular carcinoma. Diagnostic features with mammographic correlation. Am J Clin Pathol. 1994;101(4):488–92.
55. Dei Tos AP, Della Giustina D, De Martin V, Della Libera D, Bittesini L. Aspiration biopsy cytology of tubular carcinoma of the breast. Diagn Cytopathol. 1994;11(2):146–50.
56. Fischler DF, Sneige N, Ordonez NG, Fornage BD. Tubular carcinoma of the breast: cytologic features in fine-needle aspirations and application of monoclonal anti-alpha-smooth muscle actin in diagnosis. Diagn Cytopathol. 1994;10(2):120–5.
57. Gupta RK, Dowle CS. Fine needle aspiration cytology of tubular carcinoma of the breast. Acta Cytol. 1997;41(4):1139–43.
58. de la Torre M, Lindholm K, Lindgren A. Fine needle aspiration cytology of tubular breast carcinoma and radial scar. Acta Cytol. 1994;38(6):884–90.
59. Arisio R, Cuccorese C, Accinelli G, Mano MP, Bordon R, Fessia L. Role of fine-needle aspiration biopsy in breast lesions: analysis of a series of 4,110 cases. Diagn Cytopathol. 1998;18(6):462–7.
60. Greeley CF, Frost AR. Cytologic features of ductal and lobular carcinoma in fine needle aspirates of the breast. Acta Cytol. 1997;41(2):333–40.
61. Joshi A, Kumar N, Verma K. Diagnostic challenge of lobular carcinoma on aspiration cytology. Diagn Cytopathol. 1998;18(3):179–83.
62. Leach C, Howell LP. Cytodiagnosis of classic lobular carcinoma and its variants. Acta Cytol. 1992;36(2):199–202.
63. Lerma E, Fumanal V, Carreras A, Esteva E, Prat J. Undetected invasive lobular carcinoma of the breast: review of false-negative smears. Diagn Cytopathol. 2000;23(5):303–7.
64. Rajesh L, Dey P, Joshi K. Fine needle aspiration cytology of lobular breast carcinoma. Comparison with other breast lesions. Acta Cytol. 2003;47(2):177–82.
65. Sadler GP, McGee S, Dallimore NS, et al. Role of fine-needle aspiration cytology and needle-core biopsy in the diagnosis of lobular carcinoma of the breast. Br J Surg. 1994;81(9):1315–7.
66. Bondeson L, Lindholm K. Prediction of invasiveness by aspiration cytology applied to nonpalpable breast carcinoma and tested in 300 cases. Diagn Cytopathol. 1997;17(5):315–20.
67. Maygarden SJ, Brock MS, Novotny DB. Are epithelial cells in fat or connective tissue a reliable indicator of tumor invasion in fine-needle aspiration of the breast? Diagn Cytopathol. 1997;16(2):137–42.
68. McKee GT, Tambouret RH, Finkelstein D. Fine-needle aspiration cytology of the breast: invasive vs. in situ carcinoma. Diagn Cytopathol. 2001;25(1):73–7.
69. Shin HJ, Sneige N. Is a diagnosis of infiltrating versus in situ ductal carcinoma of the breast possible in fine-needle aspiration specimens? Cancer. 1998;84(3):186–91.
70. Sauer T, Garred O, Lomo J, Naess O. Assessing invasion criteria in fine needle aspirates from breast carcinoma diagnosed as DICS or invasive carcinoma: can we identify an invasive component in addition to DCIS? Acta Cytol. 2006;50(3):263–70.
71. Bofin AM, Lydersen S, Hagmar BM. Cytological criteria for the diagnosis of intraductal hyperplasia, ductal carcinoma in situ, and invasive carcinoma of the breast. Diagn Cytopathol. 2004;31(4):207–15.
72. Masood S, Loya A, Khalbuss W. Is core needle biopsy superior to fine-needle aspiration biopsy in the diagnosis of papillary breast lesions? Diagn Cytopathol. 2003;28(6):329–34.
73. Hoda SA, Rosen PP. Practical considerations in the pathologic diagnosis of needle core biopsies of breast. Am J Clin Pathol. 2002;118(1):101–8.
74. Masood S. Core needle biopsy versus fine needle aspiration biopsy: are there similar sampling and diagnostic issues? Clin Lab Med. 2005;25(4):679–88, vi.
75. Dillon MF, McDermott EW, Quinn CM, O'Doherty A, O'Higgins N, Hill AD. Predictors of invasive disease in breast cancer when core biopsy demonstrates DCIS only. J Surg Oncol. 2006;93(7):559–63.

76. Meijnen P, Oldenburg HS, Loo CE, Nieweg OE, Peterse JL, Rutgers EJ. Risk of invasion and axillary lymph node metastasis in ductal carcinoma in situ diagnosed by core-needle biopsy. Br J Surg. 2007; 94(8):952–6.
77. Farshid G, Pieterse S. Core imprint cytology of screen-detected breast lesions is predictive of the histologic results. Cancer. 2006;108(3):150–6.
78. Ballo MS, Sneige N. Can core needle biopsy replace fine-needle aspiration cytology in the diagnosis of palpable breast carcinoma. A comparative study of 124 women. Cancer. 1996;78(4):773–7.
79. Fornage BD. Sonographically guided needle biopsy of nonpalpable breast lesions. J Clin Ultrasound. 1999;27(7):385–98.
80. He Q, Fan X, Yuan T, et al. Eleven years of experience reveals that fine-needle aspiration cytology is still a useful method for preoperative diagnosis of breast carcinoma. Breast. 2007;16(3):303–6.
81. Bonneau C, Lebas P, Michenet P. [Histologic changes after stereotactic 11-gauge directional vacuum assisted breast biopsy for mammary calcification: experience in 31 surgical specimens]. Ann Pathol. 2002;22(6):441–7.
82. Yang JH, Lee WS, Kim SW, Woo SU, Kim JH, Nam SJ. Effect of core-needle biopsy vs fine-needle aspiration on pathologic measurement of tumor size in breast cancer. Arch Surg. 2005;140(2):125–8.
83. Docktor BJ, MacGregor JH, Burrowes PW. Ultrasonographic findings 6 months after 11-gauge vacuum-assisted large-core breast biopsy. Can Assoc Radiol J. 2004;55(3):151–6.
84. Ariga R, Bloom K, Reddy VB, et al. Fine-needle aspiration of clinically suspicious palpable breast masses with histopathologic correlation. Am J Surg. 2002;184(5):410–3.
85. Liao J, Davey DD, Warren G, Davis J, Moore AR, Samayoa LM. Ultrasound-guided fine-needle aspiration biopsy remains a valid approach in the evaluation of nonpalpable breast lesions. Diagn Cytopathol. 2004;30(5):325–31.
86. Zardawi IM, Hearnden F, Meyer P, Trevan B. Ultrasound-guided fine needle aspiration cytology of impalpable breast lesions in a rural setting. Comparison of cytology with imaging and final outcome. Acta Cytol. 1999;43(2):163–8.
87. Mansoor I, Jamal AA. Role of fine needle aspiration in diagnosing breast lesions. Saudi Med J. 2002; 23(8):915–20.
88. Homesh NA, Issa MA, El-Sofiani HA. The diagnostic accuracy of fine needle aspiration cytology versus core needle biopsy for palpable breast lump(s). Saudi Med J. 2005;26(1):42–6.
89. Usami S, Moriya T, Kasajima A, et al. Pathological aspects of core needle biopsy for non-palpable breast lesions. Breast Cancer. 2005;12(4):272–8.
90. Verkooijen HM. Diagnostic accuracy of stereotactic large-core needle biopsy for nonpalpable breast disease: results of a multicenter prospective study with 95% surgical confirmation. Int J Cancer. 2002; 99(6):853–9.
91. Westenend PJ, Sever AR, Beekman-De Volder HJ, Liem SJ. A comparison of aspiration cytology and core needle biopsy in the evaluation of breast lesions. Cancer. 2001;93(2):146–50.
92. Dennison G, Anand R, Makar SH, Pain JA. A prospective study of the use of fine-needle aspiration cytology and core biopsy in the diagnosis of breast cancer. Breast J. 2003;9(6):491–3.
93. Veneti S, Daskalopoulou D, Zervoudis S, Papasotiriou E, Ioannidou-Mouzaka L. Liquid-based cytology in breast fine needle aspiration. Comparison with the conventional smear. Acta Cytol. 2003; 47(2):188–92.
94. Kontzoglou K, Moulakakis KG, Konofaos P, Kyriazi M, Kyroudes A, Karakitsos P. The role of liquid-based cytology in the investigation of breast lesions using fine-needle aspiration: a cytohistopathological evaluation. J Surg Oncol. 2005;89(2):75–8.
95. Biscotti CV, Shorie JH, Gramlich TL, Easley KA. ThinPrep vs. conventional smear cytologic preparations in analyzing fine-needle aspiration specimens from palpable breast masses. Diagn Cytopathol. 1999;21(2):137–41.
96. Joseph L, Edwards JM, Nicholson CM, Pitt MA, Howat AJ. An audit of the accuracy of fine needle aspiration using a liquid-based cytology system in the setting of a rapid access breast clinic. Cytopathology. 2002;13(6):343–9.
97. Howell LP, Gandour-Edwards R, Folkins K, Davis R, Yasmeen S, Afify A. Adequacy evaluation of fine-needle aspiration biopsy in the breast health clinic setting. Cancer. 2004;102(5):295–301.
98. Daltrey IR, Kissin MW. Randomized clinical trial of the effect of needle gauge and local anaesthetic on the pain of breast fine-needle aspiration cytology. Br J Surg. 2000;87(6):777–9.
99. Satchithananda K, Fernando RA, Ralleigh G, et al. An audit of pain/discomfort experienced during image-guided breast biopsy procedures. Breast J. 2005;11(6):398–402.
100. Zagouri F, Sergentanis TN, Gounaris A, et al. Pain in different methods of breast biopsy: emphasis on vacuum-assisted breast biopsy. Breast. 2008; 17(1):71–5.
101. Bates T, Davidson T, Mansel RE. Litigation for pneumothorax as a complication of fine-needle aspiration of the breast. Br J Surg. 2002;89(2):134–7.
102. Kaufman Z, Shpitz B, Shapiro M, Dinbar A. Pneumothorax. A complication of fine needle aspiration of breast tumors. Acta Cytol. 1994; 38(5):737–8.
103. Lee KC, Chan JK, Ho LC. Histologic changes in the breast after fine-needle aspiration. Am J Surg Pathol. 1994;18(10):1039–47.
104. Pinto RG, Couto F, Mandreker S. Infarction after fine needle aspiration. A report of four cases. Acta Cytol. 1996;40(4):739–41.

105. Florentine BD, Cobb CJ, Frankel K, Greaves T, Martin SE. Core needle biopsy. A useful adjunct to fine-needle aspiration in select patients with palpable breast lesions. Cancer. 1997;81(1):33–9.
106. Abati A. Uniform approach to breast aspirates: the quest becomes reality. Diagn Cytopathol. 1996; 15(1):vii–viii.
107. National Cancer Institute Fine-Needle Aspiration of Breast Workshop Subcommittees. The uniform approach to breast fine-needle aspiration biopsy. Diagn Cytopathol. 1997;16(4):295–311.
108. Ozkara SK, Ustun MO, Paksoy N. The gray zone in breast fine needle aspiration cytology. How to report on it? Acta Cytol. 2002;46(3):513–8.
109. Pisano ED, Fajardo LL, Tsimikas J, et al. Rate of insufficient samples for fine-needle aspiration for nonpalpable breast lesions in a multicenter clinical trial: The Radiologic Diagnostic Oncology Group 5 Study. The RDOG5 investigators. Cancer. 1998; 82(4):679–88.
110. Nasuti JF, Gupta PK, Baloch ZW. Diagnostic value and cost-effectiveness of on-site evaluation of fine-needle aspiration specimens: review of 5,688 cases. Diagn Cytopathol. 2002;27(1):1–4.
111. Houssami N, Ciatto S, Ambrogetti D, et al. Florence-Sydney Breast Biopsy Study: sensitivity of ultrasound-guided versus freehand fine needle biopsy of palpable breast cancer. Breast Cancer Res Treat. 2005;89(1):55–9.
112. Robinson IA, McKee G, Kissin MW. Typing and grading breast carcinoma on fine-needle aspiration: is this clinically useful information? Diagn Cytopathol. 1995;13(3):260–5.
113. Mouriquand J, Pasquier D. Fine needle aspiration of breast carcinoma: a preliminary cytoprognostic study. Acta Cytol. 1980;24(2):153–9.
114. Robinson IA, McKee G, Nicholson A, et al. Prognostic value of cytological grading of fine-needle aspirates from breast carcinomas. Lancet. 1994;343(8903):947–9.
115. Fisher ER, Redmond C, Fisher B. Histologic grading of breast cancer. Pathol Annu. 1980;15(Pt 1): 239–51.
116. Zoppi JA, Pellicer EM, Sundblad AS. Cytohistologic correlation of nuclear grade in breast carcinoma. Acta Cytol. 1997;41(3):701–4.
117. Wani FA, Bhardwaj S, Kumar D, Katoch P. Cytological grading of breast cancers and comparative evaluation of two grading systems. J Cytol. 2010;27(2):55–8.
118. Robles-Frias A, Gonzalez-Campora R, Martinez-Parra D, et al. Robinson cytologic grading of invasive ductal breast carcinoma: correlation with histologic grading and regional lymph node metastasis. Acta Cytol. 2005;49(2):149–53.
119. Zafar N, Jamal S, Mamoon N, Luqman M, Anwar M. Typing and grading of cytological category C5 breast lesions. J Coll Physicians Surg Pak. 2005; 15(4):221–4.
120. Chaiwun B, Sukhamwang N, Lekawanvijit S, et al. Atypical and suspicious categories in fine needle aspiration cytology of the breast: histological and mammographical correlation and clinical significance. Singapore Med J. 2005;46(12):706–9.
121. Bak M, Szabo E, Mandoky L. [The "gray zone" in fine needle aspiration cytology of the breast]. Magy Seb. 2005;58(1):3–7.
122. Mander BJ, Beresford PA, Tildsley G, Qureshi T, Wishart GC. Management of patients with intermediate (C3) cytology and a solitary breast lump. Breast. 2001;10(2):163–5.
123. Boerner S, Fornage BD, Singletary E, Sneige N. Ultrasound-guided fine-needle aspiration (FNA) of nonpalpable breast lesions: a review of 1885 FNA cases using the National Cancer Institute-supported recommendations on the uniform approach to breast FNA. Cancer. 1999;87(1):19–24.
124. Deb RA, Matthews P, Elston CW, Ellis IO, Pinder SE. An audit of "equivocal" (C3) and "suspicious" (C4) categories in fine needle aspiration cytology of the breast. Cytopathology. 2001;12(4):219–26.
125. Kanhoush R, Jorda M, Gomez-Fernandez C, et al. 'Atypical' and 'suspicious' diagnoses in breast aspiration cytology. Cancer. 2004;102(3):164–7.
126. Hukkinen K, Kivisaari L, Heikkila PS, Von Smitten K, Leidenius M. Unsuccessful preoperative biopsies, fine needle aspiration cytology or core needle biopsy, lead to increased costs in the diagnostic workup in breast cancer. Acta Oncol. 2008;47(6): 1037–45.
127. Dabbs DJ, Abendroth CS, Grenko RT, Wang X, Radcliffe GE. Immunocytochemistry on the Thinprep processor. Diagn Cytopathol. 1997;17(5):388–92.
128. Guiter GE, Gatscha RM, Zakowski MF. ThinPrep vs. conventional smears in fine-needle aspirations of sarcomas: a morphological and immunocytochemical study. Diagn Cytopathol. 1999;21(5):351–4.
129. Leung SW, Bedard YC. Immunocytochemical staining on ThinPrep processed smears. Mod Pathol. 1996;9(3):304–6.
130. Gong Y, Joseph T, Sneige N. Validation of commonly used immunostains on cell-transferred cytologic specimens. Cancer. 2005;105(3):158–64.
131. Mehta P, Battifora H. How to do multiple immunostains when only one tissue slide is available. The "peel and stick" method. Appl Immunohistochem. 1993;1:297–8.
132. Miller RT, Kubier P. Immunohistochemistry on cytologic specimens and previously stained slides (when no paraffin block is available). J Histotechnol. 2002;25(4):251–7.
133. Sherman ME, Jimenez-Joseph D, Gangi MD, Rojas-Corona RR. Immunostaining of small cytologic specimens. Facilitation with cell transfer. Acta Cytol. 1994;38(1):18–22.
134. Goldstein NS, Ferkowicz M, Odish E, Mani A, Hastah F. Minimum formalin fixation time for consistent estrogen receptor immunohistochemical

staining of invasive breast carcinoma. Am J Clin Pathol. 2003;120(1):86–92.
135. Hammond ME, Hayes DF, Dowsett M, et al. American Society of Clinical Oncology/College of American Pathologists guideline recommendations for immunohistochemical testing of estrogen and progesterone receptors in breast cancer. Arch Pathol Lab Med. 2010;134(6):907–22.
136. Wolff AC, Hammond ME, Schwartz JN, et al. American Society of Clinical Oncology/College of American Pathologists guideline recommendations for human epidermal growth factor receptor 2 testing in breast cancer. J Clin Oncol. 2007;25(1):118–45.
137. Confortini M, Carozzi F, Bozzola L, et al. Interlaboratory reproducibility of the immunocytochemical assessment of oestrogen and progesterone receptors and proliferative activity in fine needle aspiration of breast cancer. Cytopathology. 2002;13(2):92–100.
138. Masood S. Estrogen and progesterone receptors in cytology: a comprehensive review. Diagn Cytopathol. 1992;8(5):475–91.
139. Jayaram G, Elsayed EM. Cytologic evaluation of prognostic markers in breast carcinoma. Acta Cytol. 2005;49(6):605–10.
140. Gong Y, Symmans WF, Krishnamurthy S, Patel S, Sneige N. Optimal fixation conditions for immunocytochemical analysis of estrogen receptor in cytologic specimens of breast carcinoma. Cancer. 2004;102(1):34–40.
141. Petroff BK, Clark JL, Metheny T, Xue Q, Kimler BF, Fabian CJ. Optimization of estrogen receptor analysis by immunocytochemistry in random periareolar fine-needle aspiration samples of breast tissue processed as thin-layer preparations. Appl Immunohistochem Mol Morphol. 2006;14(3):360–4.
142. Beatty BG, Bryant R, Wang W, et al. HER-2/neu detection in fine-needle aspirates of breast cancer: fluorescence in situ hybridization and immunocytochemical analysis. Am J Clin Pathol. 2004;122(2):246–55.
143. Nizzoli R, Bozzetti C, Crafa P, et al. Immunocytochemical evaluation of HER-2/neu on fine-needle aspirates from primary breast carcinomas. Diagn Cytopathol. 2003;28(3):142–6.
144. Kocjan G, Bourgain C, Fassina A, et al. The role of breast FNAC in diagnosis and clinical management: a survey of current practice. Cytopathology. 2008;19(5):271–8.
145. Gu M, Ghafari S, Zhao M. Fluorescence in situ hybridization for HER-2/neu amplification of breast carcinoma in archival fine needle aspiration biopsy specimens. Acta Cytol. 2005;49(5):471–6.
146. Moore JG, To V, Patel SJ, Sneige N. HER-2/neu gene amplification in breast imprint cytology analyzed by fluorescence in situ hybridization: direct comparison with companion tissue sections. Diagn Cytopathol. 2000;23(5):299–302.
147. Nizzoli R, Guazzi A, Naldi N, Fraciosi V, Bozzetti C. HER-2/neu evaluation by fluorescence in situ hybridization on destained cytologic smears from primary and metastatic breast cancer. Acta Cytol. 2005;49(1):27–30.
148. Tomas AR, Praca MJ, Fonseca R, Andre S, Mendonca E. Assessing HER-2 status in fresh frozen and archival cytological samples obtained by fine needle aspiration cytology. Cytopathology. 2004;15(6):311–4.
149. Gong Y, Gilcrease M, Sneige N. Reliability of chromogenic in situ hybridization for detecting HER-2 gene status in breast cancer: comparison with fluorescence in situ hybridization and assessment of interobserver reproducibility. Mod Pathol. 2005;18(8):1015–21.
150. Gong Y, Sweet W, Duh YJ, et al. Chromogenic in situ hybridization is a reliable method for detecting HER2 gene status in breast cancer: a multicenter study using conventional scoring criteria and the new ASCO/CAP recommendations. Am J Clin Pathol. 2009;131(4):490–7.
151. Gong Y, Sweet W, Duh YJ, et al. Performance of chromogenic in situ hybridization on testing HER2 status in breast carcinomas with chromosome 17 polysomy and equivocal (2+) herceptest results: a study of two institutions using the conventional and new ASCO/CAP scoring criteria. Am J Clin Pathol. 2009;132(2):228–36.
152. Lin F, Shen T, Prichard JW. Detection of Her-2/neu oncogene in breast carcinoma by chromogenic in situ hybridization in cytologic specimens. Diagn Cytopathol. 2005;33(6):376–80.
153. Sumiyoshi K, Shibayama Y, Akashi S, et al. Detection of human epidermal growth factor receptor 2 protein and gene in fine needle aspiration cytology specimens and tissue sections from invasive breast cancer: can cytology specimens take the place of tissue sections? Oncol Rep. 2006;15(4):803–8.
154. Gong Y, Booser DJ, Sneige N. Comparison of HER-2 status determined by fluorescence in situ hybridization in primary and metastatic breast carcinoma. Cancer. 2005;103(9):1763–9.
155. Gong Y, Han EY, Guo M, Pusztai L, Sneige N. Stability of estrogen receptor status in breast carcinoma: a comparison between primary and metastatic tumors with regard to disease course and intervening systemic therapy. Cancer. 2011;117(4):705–13.
156. Xiao C, Gong Y, Han EY, Gonzalez-Angulo AM, Sneige N. Stability of HER2-positive status in breast carcinoma: a comparison between primary and paired metastatic tumors with regard to the possible impact of intervening trastuzumab treatment. Ann Oncol. 2011;22(7):1547–53.
157. Niikura N, Liu J, Hayashi N, et al. Loss of human epidermal growth factor receptor 2 (HER2) expression in metastatic sites of HER2-overexpressing primary breast tumors. J Clin Oncol. 2012;30(6):593–9.
158. Symmans WF, Ayers M, Clark EA, et al. Total RNA yield and microarray gene expression profiles from

fine-needle aspiration biopsy and core-needle biopsy samples of breast carcinoma. Cancer. 2003;97(12):2960–71.
159. Gong Y, Yan K, Lin F, et al. Determination of oestrogen-receptor status and ERBB2 status of breast carcinoma: a gene-expression profiling study. Lancet Oncol. 2007;8(3):203–11.
160. Assersohn L, Gangi L, Zhao Y, et al. The feasibility of using fine needle aspiration from primary breast cancers for cDNA microarray analyses. Clin Cancer Res. 2002;8(3):794–801.
161. Pusztai L, Ayers M, Stec J, et al. Gene expression profiles obtained from fine-needle aspirations of breast cancer reliably identify routine prognostic markers and reveal large-scale molecular differences between estrogen-negative and estrogen-positive tumors. Clin Cancer Res. 2003;9(7):2406–15.
162. Sotiriou C, Powles TJ, Dowsett M, et al. Gene expression profiles derived from fine needle aspiration correlate with response to systemic chemotherapy in breast cancer. Breast Cancer Res. 2002; 4(3):R3.
163. Tabchy A, Valero V, Vidaurre T, et al. Evaluation of a 30-gene paclitaxel, fluorouracil, doxorubicin, and cyclophosphamide chemotherapy response predictor in a multicenter randomized trial in breast cancer. Clin Cancer Res. 2010;16(21):5351–61.
164. Anderson K, Hess KR, Kapoor M, et al. Reproducibility of gene expression signature-based predictions in replicate experiments. Clin Cancer Res. 2006;12(6):1721–7.
165. Hess KR, Anderson K, Symmans WF, et al. Pharmacogenomic predictor of sensitivity to preoperative chemotherapy with paclitaxel and fluorouracil, doxorubicin, and cyclophosphamide in breast cancer. J Clin Oncol. 2006;24(26):4236–44.
166. Boeddinghaus I, Johnson SR. Serial biopsies/fine-needle aspirates and their assessment. Methods Mol Med. 2006;120:29–41.
167. Fowler LJ, Lovell MO, Izbicka E. Fine-needle aspiration in PreservCyt: a novel and reproducible method for possible ancillary proteomic pattern expression of breast neoplasms by SELDI-TOF. Mod Pathol. 2004;17(8):1012–20.
168. Jeronimo C, Monteiro P, Henrique R, et al. Quantitative hypermethylation of a small panel of genes augments the diagnostic accuracy in fine-needle aspirate washings of breast lesions. Breast Cancer Res Treat. 2008;109(1):27–34.
169. Pu RT, Laitala LE, Alli PM, Fackler MJ, Sukumar S, Clark DP. Methylation profiling of benign and malignant breast lesions and its application to cytopathology. Mod Pathol. 2003;16(11):1095–101.
170. Fisher B, Costantino JP, Wickerham DL, et al. Tamoxifen for prevention of breast cancer: report of the National Surgical Adjuvant Breast and Bowel Project P-1 Study. J Natl Cancer Inst. 1998;90(18):1371–88.
171. Hartmann LC, Schaid DJ, Woods JE, et al. Efficacy of bilateral prophylactic mastectomy in women with a family history of breast cancer. N Engl J Med. 1999;340(2):77–84.
172. Rebbeck TR, Levin AM, Eisen A, et al. Breast cancer risk after bilateral prophylactic oophorectomy in BRCA1 mutation carriers. J Natl Cancer Inst. 1999; 91(17):1475–9.
173. Masood S. Cytomorphology as a risk predictor: experience with fine needle aspiration biopsy, nipple fluid aspiration, and ductal lavage. Clin Lab Med. 2005;25(4):827–43, viii–ix.
174. Dooley WC, Ljung BM, Veronesi U, et al. Ductal lavage for detection of cellular atypia in women at high risk for breast cancer. J Natl Cancer Inst. 2001;93(21):1624–32.
175. Arun B, Valero V, Logan C, et al. Comparison of ductal lavage and random periareolar fine needle aspiration as tissue acquisition methods in early breast cancer prevention trials. Clin Cancer Res. 2007;13(16):4943–8.
176. Fabian CJ, Kimler BF, Zalles CM, et al. Short-term breast cancer prediction by random periareolar fine-needle aspiration cytology and the Gail risk model. J Natl Cancer Inst. 2000;92(15):1217–27.
177. Zalles CM, Kimler BF, Simonsen M, Clark JL, Metheny T, Fabian CJ. Comparison of cytomorphology in specimens obtained by random periareolar fine needle aspiration and ductal lavage from women at high risk for development of breast cancer. Breast Cancer Res Treat. 2006;97(2):191–7.
178. Arun B, Valero V, Liu D, et al. Short-term biomarker modulation prevention study of anastrozole in women at increased risk for second primary breast cancer. Cancer Prev Res (Phila). 2012;5(2):276–82.
179. Sneige N, Liu B, Yin G, Gong Y, Arun BK. Correlation of cytologic findings and chromosomal instability detected by fluorescence in situ hybridization in breast fine-needle aspiration specimens from women at high risk for breast cancer. Mod Pathol. 2006;19(5):622–9.

3 Gynecological Cancers: Pathology and Cytological Methods for Diagnosis of Gynecological Cancers

Nalini Gupta and Arvind Rajwanshi

Abstract

Gynecological cancers represent cancers arising from the female genital tract. The most common cancer in female genital tract is carcinoma cervix. Carcinoma cervix is preceded by precancerous lesions, which can be detected by screening tests such as cervical Pap smear and HPV detection. Endometrial carcinoma is usually detected on endometrial curettings or biopsy, as endometrial aspiration cytology is not reliable. Cervical smear may occasionally represent cells arising from endometrial carcinoma. Majority of ovarian tumors are epithelial tumors, papillary serous carcinoma being the most common. Although FNAC in ovarian neoplasms is not a preferred technique, the same may be performed in young females as initial work-up, in advanced ovarian malignancies, and in the follow-up of patients after chemotherapy or radiotherapy. This chapter includes pathology of gynecological cancers and cytological evaluation of the same such as cervical Pap test for cervical carcinomas and fine needle aspiration cytology mainly for ovarian tumors.

Abbreviations

AGCT	Adult granulosa cell tumor
AIS	Adenocarcinoma in situ
CCC	Clear cell carcinoma
CEA	Carcinoembryonic antigen
CIN	Cervical intraepithelial neoplasia
CIS	Carcinoma in-situ
CK	Cytokeratin
ESS	Endometrial stromal sarcoma
FDA	Food and drug administration
FNAC	Fine needle aspiration cytology
H&E	Hematoxylin and Eosin stain
HPV	Human papilloma virus
HSIL	High grade squamous intraepithelial lesions
JGCT	Juvenile granulosa cell tumor
LBC	Liquid based cytology
LMS	Leiomyosarcoma
LSIL	Low-grade squamous intraepithelial lesions

N. Gupta • A. Rajwanshi (✉)
Department of Cytology and Gynaecological Pathology, Postgraduate Institute of Medical Education and Research, Chandigarh 160 012, India
e-mail: rajwanshiarvind@gmail.com

M.K. Shetty (ed.), *Breast and Gynecological Cancers: An Integrated Approach for Screening and Early Diagnosis in Developing Countries*, DOI 10.1007/978-1-4614-1876-4_3,

MGG	May Grünwald Geimsa stain
MMMT	Malignant mixed müllerian tumor
Pap	Papanicolaou stain
PAS	Periodic acid-Schiff's stain
PCR	Polymerase chain reaction
SCC	Squamous cell carcinoma
SIL	Squamous intraepithelial lesions
STIC	Serous tubal intra-epithelial carcinoma
TBS	The Bethesda System
VIA	Visual inspection using acetic acid
VILI	Visual inspection using Lugol's iodine

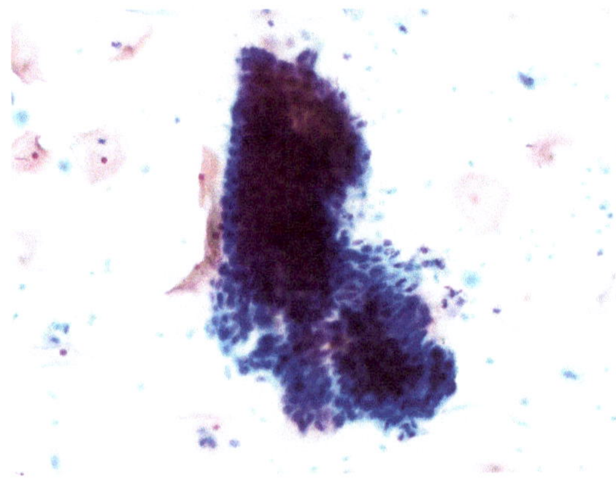

Fig. 3.1 SurePath™ (BD Worldwide, Franklin Lakes, NJ) LBC cervical sample showing a hyperchromatic crowded cell group (HCCG) representing severe dysplasia/HSIL (Pap x100X)

Introduction

Gynecological cancers represent cancers arising from female genital tract, which consists of the uterus and cervix, vagina, vulva, bilateral fallopian tubes, and ovaries. Among the gynecological cancers, cervical carcinoma is the most common cancer and the second most common cancer among women worldwide, with an estimated 529,000 new cases and 274,000 deaths annually as per GLOBOCAN 2008 [1]. About 80% of the cervical cancer cases occur in developing countries. Endometrial cancer is the second most common gynecological cancer, followed by ovarian carcinoma. In general, epithelial tumors are the more common; however, sarcomas can occur in cervix, uterus, vagina, and vulva. Rarely melanoma, lymphoma, and metastatic tumors can involve female genital tract. In addition to epithelial tumors, germ cell tumors and sex cord stromal tumors are known to arise from the ovaries. Peritoneal fluid cytology is done for staging of gynecological cancers, especially for ovarian and endometrial cancers.

Carcinoma of the Uterine Cervix

Cervical cancer is the most or second most common cancer among women in developing countries. The age-standardized rate for incidence is 15.2/100,000 women and for mortality is 7.8/100,000 women. The incidence of cervical cancer in India varies from 16.3 to 30.6 per lakh [2]. Cervical cancer has marked differences in incidence according to demographic variables (age, social class, marital status, ethnicity, religion, and occupation). The majority of cervical cancer is squamous cell carcinoma (SCC), and human papilloma virus (HPV) has been strongly associated with cervical carcinoma, especially HPV 16 and HPV 18. Cervical cancer is unique as it is preceded by precancerous lesions, which can be detected by screening methods and treated.

Cervical Intraepithelial/Precancerous Lesions

Persistent HPV infection of cervical squamous epithelium can lead to squamous intraepithelial lesions (SIL), which can be low-grade (LSIL) and high-grade SIL. According to The Bethesda System (TBS) 2001, LSIL includes koilocytosis and CIN1, and HSIL includes moderate dysplasia (CIN2), severe dysplasia (CIN3) (Figs. 3.1 and 3.2), and carcinoma in situ (CIS). About 60% of CIN1 lesions regress, 30% persist, 10% progress to CIN3, and 1% to invasive SCC. CIN2 lesions regress in 40% of the cases, 40% persist, 20% progress to CIN3, and 5% progress to SCC (Figs. 3.3 and 3.4). The likelihood of CIN3 regressing is 33%, and the likelihood of progressing to SCC is more than 12% [3, 4].

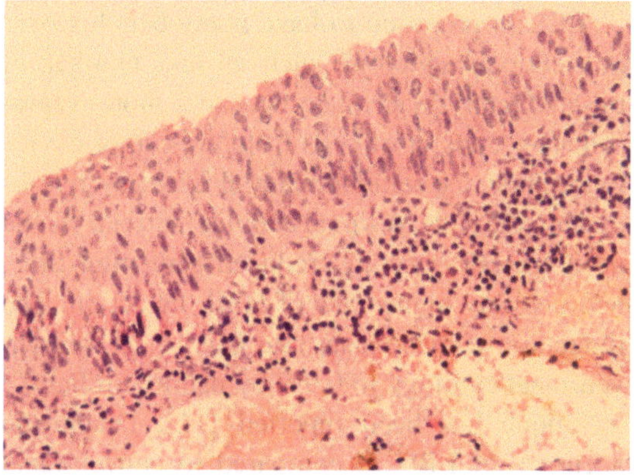

Fig. 3.2 Cervical biopsy showing CIN 3 (cervical intraepithelial neoplasia) changes (H&E x40X)

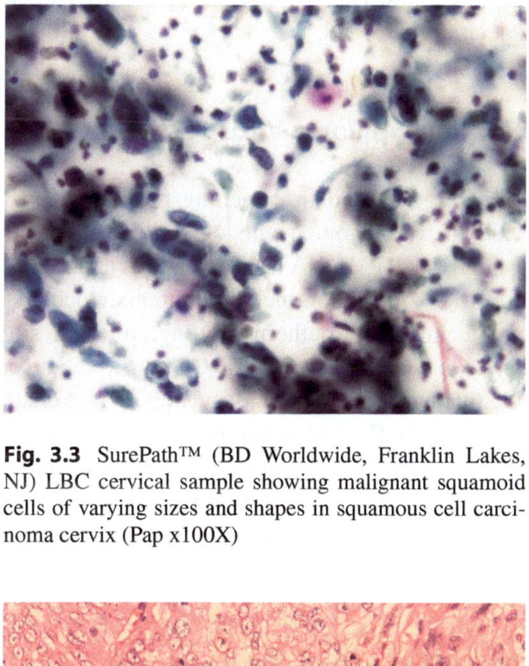

Fig. 3.3 SurePath™ (BD Worldwide, Franklin Lakes, NJ) LBC cervical sample showing malignant squamoid cells of varying sizes and shapes in squamous cell carcinoma cervix (Pap x100X)

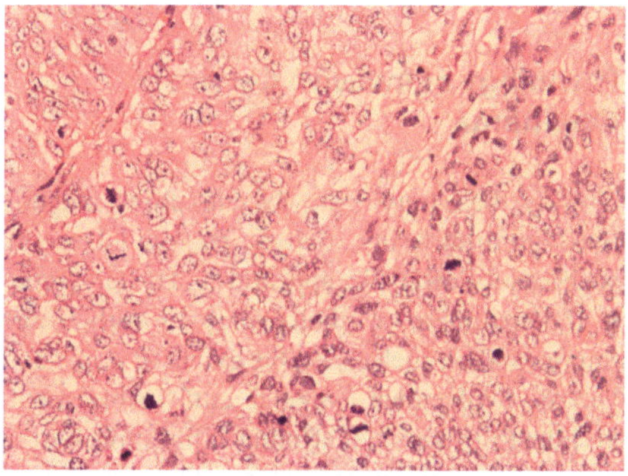

Fig. 3.4 Cervical biopsy showing squamous cell carcinoma cervix (H&E x40X)

Adenocarcinoma in situ (AIS) is a preinvasive glandular lesion of uterine cervix. Nearly two-thirds of cases of AIS have associated preinvasive squamous lesions or invasive SCC [5, 6], and risk factors for AIS are similar to that of preinvasive squamous lesions [7].

Screening for Cervical Precancerous Lesions

The objective of cervical cancer screening programs is to reduce the incidence of the disease and mortality from the disease by identifying women in precancerous stage or early invasive cancers and treating these women appropriately. The conventional screening modality for cervical pre-cancer is the cytological Pap smear test. Cervical Pap cytology by conventional method has worked efficiently for the last 50 years, with more than 80% potential decrease in mortality from cervical cancer in developed countries. This test was first introduced by Papanicolaou and Babes in 1920, and, since then, despite the proven effectiveness of conventional Pap smear, the accuracy of conventional smear has been questioned. Liquid-based cytology (LBC) and HPV testing are another two relatively new technologies in the field of cervical cancer screening. LBC technique was introduced in the mid-1990s to improve the performance of Pap test. LBC improves specimen adequacy and reduces screening time as compared to conventional cytology. Other methods for cervical screening include unaided visual inspection of cervix, visual inspection using acetic acid (VIA), visual inspection using Lugol's iodine (VILI), and colposcopic examination. Computer-assisted cytological interpretation of cervical smears, use of physical real time devices, and detection of molecular surrogate markers of cervical cancer—such as ProEx™ C, p16^{INK4A}, pRb, p27, p53, MCM5 and CDC6, Ki-67, etc.—have also been evaluated [8, 9]. Dual immunostaining for p16^{INK4a} and Ki-67 on cervical smears has been evaluated, and kits are commercially available for the same [9, 10]. Among these, cervical cytology is still the mainstay of cervical cancer prevention programs.

Cervical Cytology

Two techniques available for cervical cytology are (1) conventional method and (2) liquid-based cervical cytology. Conventional Pap smear involves collection of exfoliated cells from the cervix, especially the transformation zone, by a spatula/collection device, and the sample is smeared on the glass slide and stained with Papanicolaou stain. These can result in false negative diagnoses either due to sampling or screening errors. Sampling errors can occur when abnormal cells are not scraped off, abnormal cells stick on the wooden spatula resulting in cell loss, or the cells transferred to the slide may not be representative of an abnormality. Screening error can occur if the smears are too thick with numerous polymorphs, mucus, or blood obscuring the abnormal cells.

Liquid-based cytology includes a number of different LBC techniques, such as ThinPrep™ (Hologic Inc., Bedford, MA), SurePath™ (BD Worldwide, Franklin Lakes, NJ), Cytoeasy, Cytoscreen, PapSpin, etc. The US Food and Drug Administration (FDA) approved two liquid-based tests for cervical screening, namely the ThinPrep™ in 1996 and the SurePath™ in 1999. Pap test by LBC involves the use of Cervex-Brush® (Rovers Medical Devices, Oss, The Netherlands) or a combination of a plastic spatula and endocervical brush to collect cervical sample from transformation zone. The head of the spatula/brush is either kept in the vial containing preservative by detaching the head of the brush (SurePath™ samples) or removed after rinsing the spatula/brush in the preservative vial (ThinPrep™ samples). In ThinPrep™, clumps of cells and mucus are broken by mechanical agitation, and then this solution is filtered to allow inflammatory cells and red blood cells to pass through and epithelial cells are retained. These epithelial cells are then passed on to the glass slide and stained. In SurePath™ LBC method, the cellular clumps are broken, and the cells are separated with the help of density gradient centrifugation. The epithelial cell pellet is resuspended and transferred to the glass slide. The diameter of the circle for ThinPrep™ sample is 22 and 18 mm for SurPath™ sample.

LBC is proposed to have many benefits over conventional cytology such as less number of unsatisfactory/inadequate smears, more representative transfer of cells from collecting device to the slide, the cellular material is evenly distributed on the slide, residual cellular material can be used for HPV testing, reduced screening time, and possibly higher rate of HSIL detection. The reduction of inadequate rate from 9.1% in conventional cytology to 0.9% by using SurePath™ technique has been reported [11]. Diagnostic accuracy of LBC as compared to conventional cytology is a matter of great debate, as several studies have shown increased sensitivity of LBC over conventional method [12–14], whereas others have shown decreased or equal sensitivity and specificity [15, 16].

Human Papilloma Virus Testing

Another test used in screening programs especially to triage women with low-grade SIL lesions is high risk HPV DNA testing. Various techniques for hrHPV detection include immunocytochemical techniques, southern blotting, filter in situ hybridization, Digene Hybrid Capture™ (Digene, Gaithersburg, MD) HCII assay, Polymerase chain reaction (PCR), and genotyping methods [8, 17, 18]. FDA approved Qiagen's (Hilden, Germany) "hybrid-capture" test for detection of HPV infection in 2003. Polymerase chain reaction has also been used for viral load determination [19].

Pathology of Invasive Cervical Carcinoma

Grossly, these tumors may be endophytic and diffusely infiltrative or exophytic polypoidal tumors with a cauliflower-like appearance. Hysterectomy is the treatment of choice only in early stage tumors and, in such cases, the extent of upper and lateral involvement, vaginal cuff involvement, and depth of cervical stromal infiltration by the tumor are important to evaluate. On microscopy, the most common carcinoma is SCC (Fig. 3.4), followed by an endocervical adenocarcinoma

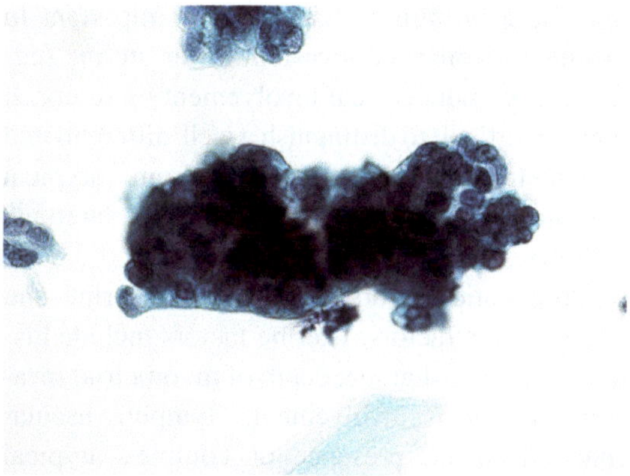

Fig. 3.5 SurePath™ (BD Worldwide, Franklin Lakes, NJ) LBC cervical sample showing a cluster of atypical cells representing an endocervical adenocarcinoma (Pap x100X)

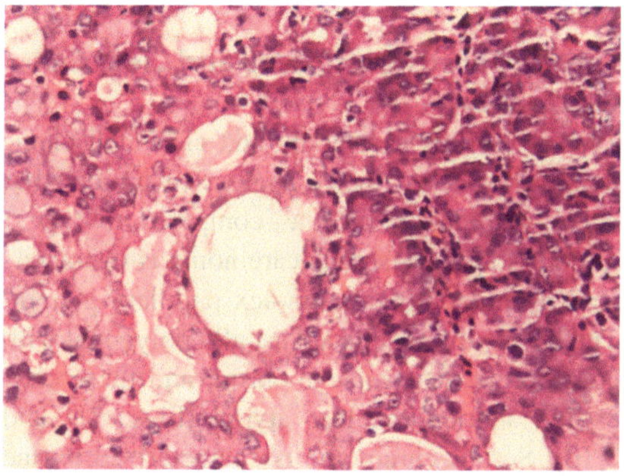

Fig. 3.6 Cervical biopsy showing an endocervical adenocarcinoma (H&E x40X)

(Figs. 3.5 and 3.6). Other uncommon types include adenosquamous, verrucous, warty, glassy cell, clear cell adenosquamous, neuroendocrine, adenoid-cystic, Mucoepidermoid, and small cell carcinoma. Adenocarcinoma of the cervix can be minimal deviation adenocarcinoma, mucinous adenocarcinoma, endometrioid adenocarcinoma, and clear cell adenocarcinoma.

Secondary Tumors

Cervix can be involved by direct extension from endometrial, rectal, or urinary bladder tumors. Metastases to the cervix are rare, the most common sites being the gastrointestinal tract, the ovary, the breast, lung, kidney, and, rarely, melanoma. The tumor cells from cervical metastatic lesions may get sampled in Pap smears and rarely are the first indication of the tumor [20].

Malignant Tumors of the Uterus

Malignant tumors of the uterus include endometrial carcinoma, endometrial stromal sarcoma, and malignant mixed müllerian tumor (MMMT). Malignant tumor arising from the smooth muscle of the myometrium is leiomyosarcoma.

Endometrial Carcinoma

Endometrial carcinoma is divided into two forms: type I tumors (endometrioid carcinoma) account for 70–80% of cases and are estrogen related, whereas the type II tumors (papillary serous or clear cell tumors) account for about 20% of cases, are unrelated to estrogen stimulation, and have an aggressive clinical behavior [21]. This dualistic model of endometrial tumorigenesis was proposed by Bokhman in 1983. Obesity, nulliparity, hypertension, and diabetes are risk factors for type I carcinomas, and these often develop in a background of endometrial hyperplasia. Other predisposing factors include dysfunctional uterine bleeding, estrogen replacement therapy, polycystic ovarian disease, and tamoxifen use. Most serous (type II) cancers have p53 mutations [22], and endometrioid (type I) adenocarcinoma demonstrates larger numbers of genetic changes including microsatellite instability (MSI), or specific mutation of PTEN, K-ras, and β-catenin genes [23, 24].

Cytologic screening of endometrial cancer is possible by direct endometrial sampling or cervical Pap sample. However, these are difficult to interpret and are only of moderate reliability. Endometrial biopsy or curettage is usually performed to detect any endometrial pathology. 1–11% of the cases with the presence of endometrial cells on Pap smear may be associated with endometrial adenocarcinoma (Fig. 3.7) [25, 26].

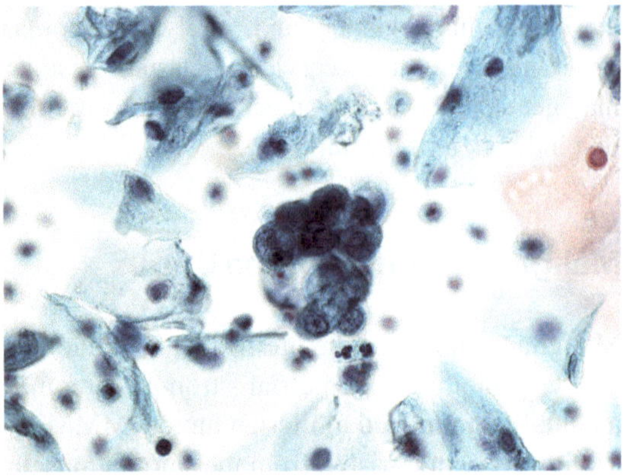

Fig. 3.7 SurePath™ (BD Worldwide, Franklin Lakes, NJ) LBC cervical sample showing a three dimensional cluster of atypical cells representing endometrioid type of endometrial adenocarcinoma (Pap x100X)

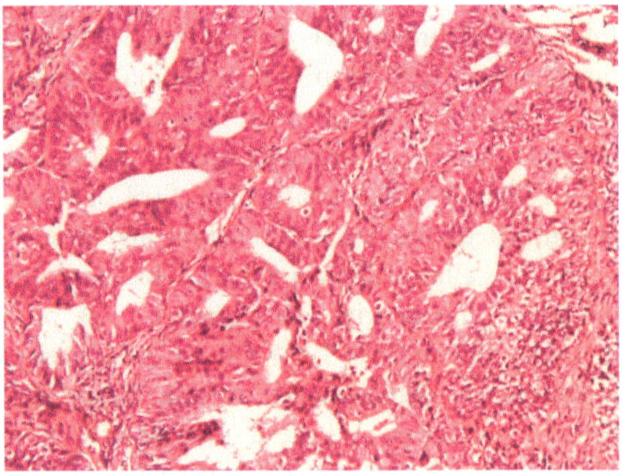

Fig. 3.8 Endometrial curettings showing a well-differentiated endometrioid adenocarcinoma (H&E x40X)

Type I: Endometrioid Adenocarcinoma

Type I: endometrioid adenocarcinoma accounts for almost 70–80% of all endometrial carcinomas. The majority of females are postmenopausal, and only 1–8% of endometrial carcinomas occur in women under 40 years of age [27]. The most common clinical presentation is abnormal vaginal bleeding. The gross appearance in this tumor may vary from shaggy endometrial surface to exophytic polypoidal growth arising from endometrium and infiltrating the myometrium. On microscopy, these tumors comprise of complex glandular pattern (Fig. 3.8) and can have solid to villoglandular appearance. These are divided into three grades using both architectural and nuclear criteria. Squamous differentiation may be a prominent feature. It is important to evaluate myometrial invasion, lower uterine segment, and endocervical involvement by tumor. It may be difficult to distinguish a well-differentiated endometrioid adenocarcinoma from atypical complex endometrial hyperplasia in curettage samples.

Prognostic factors include both uterine and extra-uterine factors. Uterine factors include histologic type and grade, depth of myometrial invasion, cervical involvement, lympho-vascular space invasion, presence of complex atypical hyperplasia, and hormone receptor status. Extra-uterine factors include adnexal involvement, intra-peritoneal metastasis, positive peritoneal cytology, and pelvic and para-aortic lymph node metastasis.

Type II: Serous Carcinoma and Clear Cell Carcinoma

Type II: serous carcinoma and clear cell carcinoma present as highly aggressive tumors that occur in older women as compared to type I tumors. Papillary serous carcinoma is characterized by predominant complex papillary pattern. The lining tumor cells are usually polygonal with eosinophilic to clear cytoplasm, and these cells exhibit marked nuclear atypia (Figs. 3.9 and 3.10). Serous carcinoma is characterized by the discordance between its architectural pattern and nuclear morphology. These tumors usually show strong nuclear immunopositivity for p53.

Clear cell carcinoma usually exhibits solid, tubular, papillary, or cystic patterns. The tumor cells are usually clear to eosinophilic and show prominent "hobnail" pattern. Nuclear atypia may be marked, and PAS positive, diastase-resistant intracellular as well as extracellular hyaline globules may be noted. This tumor is usually a high grade, deeply invasive tumor, and the prognosis is poor.

Malignant Mixed Müllerian Tumor (Carcinosarcoma)

MMMT accounts for less than 5% of malignant uterine tumors. It is a biphasic tumor composed

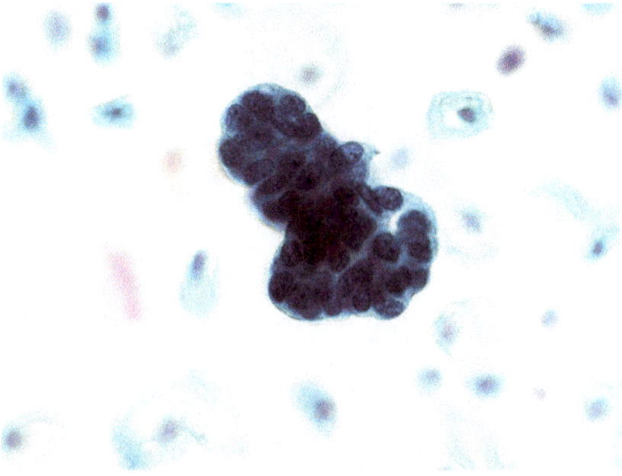

Fig. 3.9 SurePath™ (BD Worldwide, Franklin Lakes, NJ) LBC cervical sample showing a papillary cluster of atypical cells representing papillary serous type of endometrial adenocarcinoma (Pap x100X)

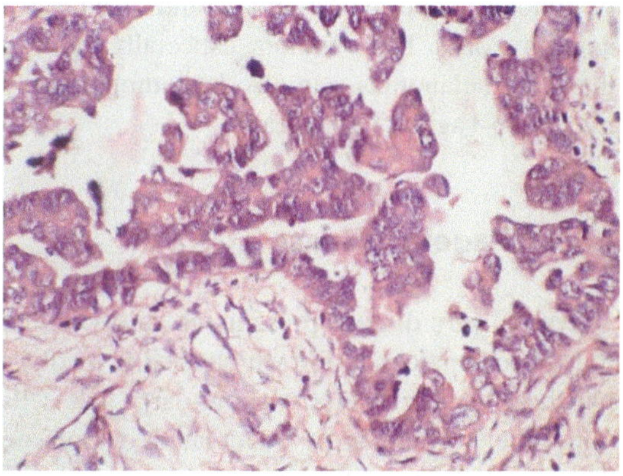

Fig. 3.10 Endometrial curettings showing a papillary serous type of endometrial adenocarcinoma (H&E x40X)

of malignant epithelial as well as sarcomatous components. Majority of the women are postmenopausal and present with postmenopausal bleeding. Grossly, MMMTs are usually polypoidal tumors that fill whole of the uterine cavity, often protruding through the cervical os. Microscopically, these are divided into homologous type and heterologous type. The most common type of epithelial component is endometrioid adenocarcinoma. Serous, clear cell, mucinous, squamous carcinoma can occur. Mesenchymal component is usually endometrial stromal sarcoma or fibrosarcoma and rarely leiomyosarcoma. When heterologous component is present, rhabdomyosarcoma and chondrosarcoma are the most common types identified. These tumors may metastasize to pelvic and para-aortic lymph nodes, pelvis, vagina, peritoneal surfaces of abdomen, and lungs.

Endometrial Stromal Sarcoma

Endometrial stromal sarcoma (ESS) is a tumor of endometrial stromal cells that invades the myometrium. ESS is divided into low-grade ESS and high-grade ESS. These occur in the fourth and fifth decades of life, and usually patients are premenopausal. Abnormal vaginal bleeding, cyclical menorrhagia, and abdominal pain are the frequent presenting symptoms. Grossly, the myometrium may be diffusely thickened or a nodular tumor may be evident in the endometrial cavity. The tumor permeates the myometrium and may be seen as poorly demarcated yellowish tiny nodules or cords in dilated channels. On microscopy, most ESS are of low grade type with relatively uniform appearing small oval tumor cells, which resemble stromal cells. Numerous small blood vessels and arterioles may be noted throughout the tumor resembling spiral arterioles. The individual tumor cells are enveloped by reticulin fibers. The nests, trabeculae, and cords of tumor cells invade the myometrium by invasion of lympho-vascular channels, which is a characteristic feature of this tumor. Areas of hyaline fibrosis may be noted. The tumor cells in ESS stain positive for CD10 antigen and are negative for Caldesmon. Smooth muscle actin and desmin are also usually negative, and therefore these stains may be of help in differentiating ESS from leiomyosarcoma. This tumor rarely is subjected to fine needle aspiration cytology (FNAC). On FNAC, the tumor cells are usually present in loose clusters and singly. The nuclei are plump, oval, and moderately pleomorphic. The chromatin is usually bland, and one or two small nucleoli may be noted [28]. High-grade ESS is defined as a sarcoma without specific features or heterologous elements but with an infiltrative pattern suggestive of an origin from endometrial stromal cells [29].

Müllerian Adenosarcoma

Müllerian adenosarcoma is a biphasic tumor composed of benign epithelial component and a sarcomatous stroma. Grossly, it is usually a polypoid tumor growing in the endometrial cavity. On microscopy, the fibrous/stromal papillary structures are lined by bland-appearing epithelium, and tubular and cleft-like structures are seen within the stroma. The mesenchymal component can be homologous or heterologous type. Müllerian adenosarcoma with a sarcomatous overgrowth (MASO) is an aggressive variant of this tumor.

Leiomyosarcoma

Leiomyosarcoma (LMS) accounts for about 1.3% of the uterine malignancies and about one-third of uterine sarcomas. It usually affects women in their sixth decade of life. The common symptoms are abnormal vaginal bleeding, lower abdominal pain/distension, or awareness of abdominal mass. Grossly, majority of LMS are solitary intramural masses. The cut surface is soft or fleshy, and areas of hemorrhage and necrosis may be seen. Irregular infiltrative margins may or may not be identifiable grossly. On microscopy, the tumor is highly cellular composed of fascicles of cigar-shaped to spindle cells showing nuclear atypia. Tumor cell necrosis is usually prominent but need not be present. Mitoses are numerous (>10/10 high power fields). These tumors should be distinguished from atypical and mitotically active leiomyoma. Epithelioid and myxoid variants of LMS are known. Myxoid variant is of particular importance as the mitotic index and cellularity may not be high, but tumor size of more than 5 cm is significant. These tumors are rarely subjected to FNAC or any other cytological techniques for diagnosis.

Tumors of Vagina and Vulva

SCC accounts for more than 80% of all malignancies (Fig. 3.11). Other malignancies include clear cell adenocarcinoma, embryonal rhabdomyosarcoma (sarcoma botryoid), malignant melanoma, lymphoma, leiomyosarcoma, and aggressive angiomyxoma. These tumors, especially carcinomas and melanomas, can also be sampled rarely in cervico-vaginal Pap smears.

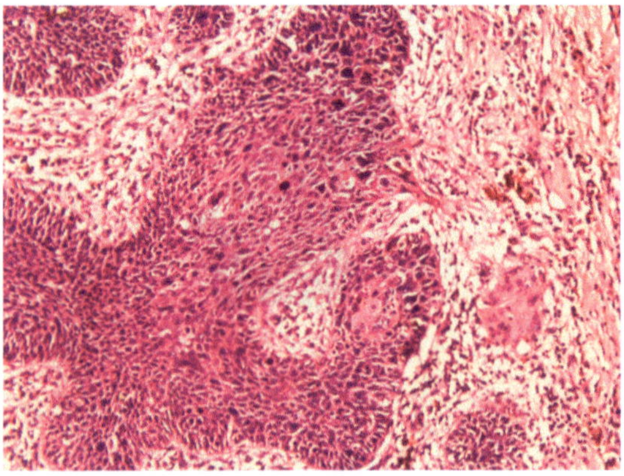

Fig. 3.11 Vulval biopsy showing a superficially invasive squamous cell carcinoma (H&E x40X)

Vulval Paget's Disease

Vulval Paget's disease presents as an erythematous or eczematous lesion which usually involves hair-bearing skin. A biopsy shows large pale cells with finely granular to vacuolated cytoplasm. These cells form nests or a layer along the basement membrane and are positive for mucin and MUC1and MUC5AC. The incidence of an underlying carcinoma varies from 0 to 30% in vulval Paget's disease. This can also be detected by scrape cytology and smears show pale, large vacuolated cells demonstrating nuclear pleomorphism with or without associated inflammation.

Ovarian Tumors

Ovarian cancers are the fifth most common cause of mortality from all cancers in women in the developed world [30]. The proportion of ovarian cancer varies from 1.7 to 8.7% of all female cancers in various urban and rural population-based registries operating under the network of the National Cancer Registry program (NCRP) of

Indian Council Medical Research (ICMR) [31]. Ovarian cancer rates increase with rising age. Hereditary ovarian cancer occurring in approximately 10% cases is mainly due to mutations in BRCA1 or BRCA2 tumor suppressor genes. An effective screening test is not possible for the general population because ovarian cancer is uncommon and the ovaries are not easy to access. High risk females can be screened by serial ultrasonography with/without serum CA125 levels. Ovarian cancer can spread locally to contra-lateral ovary, peritoneum, and para-aortic and pelvic lymph nodes. Patient may present with ascites. Despite controversial views regarding FNAC in ovarian lesions, it can be useful in initial workups of primary ovarian neoplasms, biopsy of superficial masses in patients with known prior disease, and follow-up of patients undergoing chemotherapy/radiotherapy [32].

Classification of Ovarian Tumors

Ovarian tumors are classified based on the cell of origin:

1. Surface epithelial tumors account for about 90–95% of ovarian malignancies. These are further divided into serous, mucinous, endometrioid, transitional, mixed tumors, and malignant mixed Müllerian tumor (MMMT).
2. Germ cell tumors account for about 15–20% of all ovarian neoplasms and are divided into:
   (a) Dysgerminoma
   (b) Teratoma: mature and immature
   (c) Endodermal sinus tumor (Yolk sac tumor)
   (d) Embryonal carcinoma
   (e) Choriocarcinoma
   (f) Mixed germ cell tumor
3. Sex cord-stromal tumors: account for about 5–10% of all ovarian neoplasms and are categorized into:
   (a) Granulosa cell tumor: adult and Juvenile type
   (b) Fibroma-thecoma
   (c) Sertoli leydig cell tumor
   (d) Leydig cell tumor
   (e) Others
4. Metastatic tumors account for about 5% of ovarian malignancies, and usually arise from breast, colon, endometrium, stomach, gall bladder, and cervical cancers.
5. Other rare tumors arise from ovarian soft tissue, etc.

Ovarian Surface Epithelial Tumors

Pathogenesis of Ovarian Surface Epithelial Tumors

According to the most recent findings, the majority of "ovarian" carcinomas arise outside the ovary from the fimbrial end of the fallopian tube. A dualistic model has been proposed which divided ovarian carcinomas into type I and type II [33]. Type I tumors are generally low-grade indolent tumors and are usually confined to the ovary. These exhibit a shared lineage between benign cystic tumors and the corresponding carcinomas, often through an intermediate (borderline tumor) step, supporting the morphologic continuum of tumor progression. These are characterized by specific mutations including KRAS, BRAF, ERBB2, CTNNB1, and PTEN. Type II tumors are aggressive and present in advanced stage. These tumors are genetically unstable and show TP53 mutations in more than 80% cases [33].

Serous Carcinoma/Papillary Serous Cystadenocarcinoma

Serous carcinoma is the most common type of ovarian cancer accounting for approximately 50% of all malignant ovarian tumors. The peak age is in the fifth and sixth decades, and approximately two-thirds of cases involve both ovaries. Serum CA125 levels are elevated in about 90% of the cases, and about 70–84% cases present in advanced stage with disseminated disease involving abdominal and pelvic cavities [34].

Grossly, these tumors can have wide variation in size and are typically multilocular and cystic with soft friable papillae filling the cysts containing serous or bloody fluid. There are solid areas which can have variegated appearance due to hemorrhage and necrosis. On microscopy, serous carcinoma typically displays a complex papillary pattern with solid areas. The papillae are lined by cuboidal to low columnar epithelium which

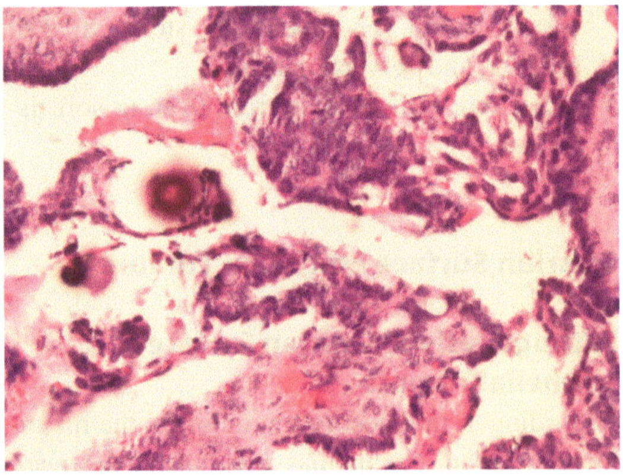

Fig. 3.12 Papillary serous adenocarcinoma of the ovary with psammoma bodies (H&E x40X)

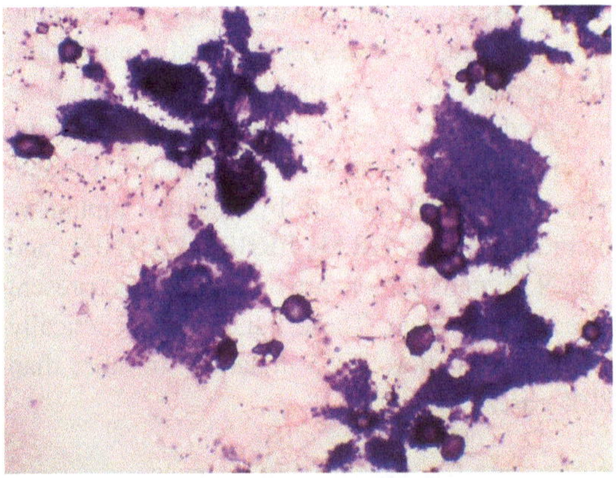

Fig. 3.13 FNAC of papillary serous adenocarcinoma of the ovary with psammoma bodies (H&E x20X)

shows nuclear pleomorphism, atypia, and pseudostratification. Psammoma bodies are seen in about 25% cases (Fig. 3.12). Serous tumors are positive for epithelial membrane antigen, Cytokeratin 7, and CA125. CK20 is negative in a majority of serous ovarian carcinomas.

FNAC is usually performed in advanced stage tumors for tissue diagnosis. Usually the smears are highly cellular and show papillary clusters and dispersed population of malignant cells exhibiting nuclear atypia (Fig. 3.13). Psammoma bodies may or may not be seen. The differential diagnosis on cytology includes reactive mesothelial proliferation, endometrioid carcinoma, and metastatic carcinoma.

Mucinous Carcinoma/Mucinous Cystadenocarcinoma

These comprise approximately 11% of all ovarian carcinomas and are bilateral in about 10–12% cases. These tumors generally present as a large abdomino-pelvic mass due to their large size. About 63% of patients have FIGO stage I disease. Ascites may occur, but pseudomyxoma peritonei is associated with mucinous tumors of appendix and not with ovarian mucinous tumors. Grossly, these are usually large, multiloculated cystic tumors with solid areas and intracystic nodules. The cysts contain thick viscous mucinous material. On microscopy, the cystic areas are lined by tall columnar mucinous lining epithelium which can be endocervical or intestinal type. Papillae project into cystic spaces and the spaces contain eosinophilic mucinous material. Stromal invasion, architectural complexity, and nuclear stratification and atypia are the characteristic features. Pools of mucin may be seen in adjacent ovarian stroma leading to inflammatory reaction. Mucinous carcinomas are positive for carcinoembryonic antigen (CEA), CK7 and about 70% cases are positive for CK20. Majority of these tumors are CDX2 negative. The main differential diagnosis includes metastatic colorectal carcinoma, which is CK7+ and CK20+ and also CDX2 positive.

FNAC usually yields thick highly viscous mucinous material. Single cells, irregular clusters, and syncytial groups of atypical cells are seen in smears. The cells usually show nuclear atypia, which is not as prominent as seen in serous carcinomas.

Endometrioid Adenocarcinoma

Endometrioid adenocarcinoma comprises of approximately 17.5% of ovarian carcinomas. Co-existent endometriosis may be demonstrated in 15–20% cases. Synchronous endometrioid tumors of the uterus may be seen in about 10–30% cases. Grossly, the tumors have a smooth outer surface, and the cut section is usually solid and cystic with cysts containing soft friable masses and hemorrhagic fluid. On microscopy, the tumor is typically characterized by a complex glandular proliferation with back-to-back arrangement and

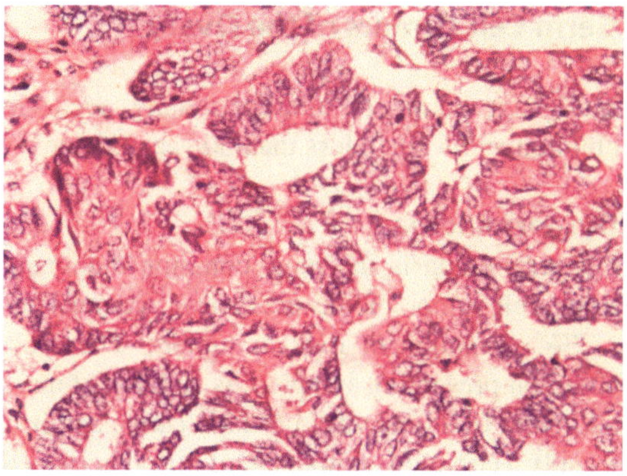

Fig. 3.14 Endometrioid adenocarcinoma of the ovary with focal squamous differentiation (H&E x40X)

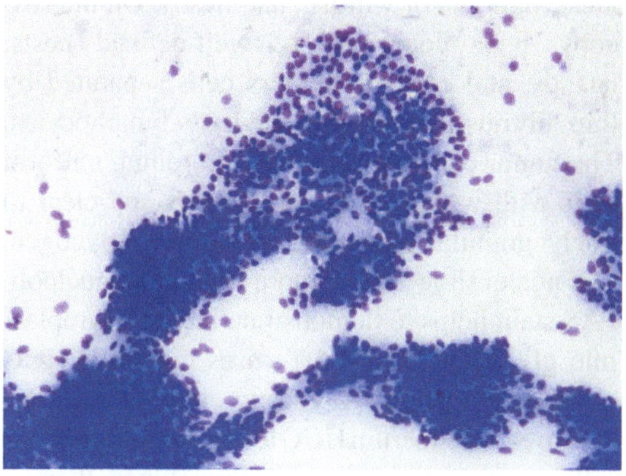

Fig. 3.15 FNAC of endometrioid adenocarcinoma of the ovary (MGG x40X)

stromal invasion. Confluent or cribriform proliferation of glands and solid areas may be seen. The cystic spaces are lined by tall columnar epithelium. Squamous differentiation may be noted in up to 50% cases (Fig. 3.14). About one-third of cases may exhibit endometrioid component mixed with other epithelial components such as clear cell or papillary serous component. These tumors are CK7 positive and CK20 negative.

On FNAC, the malignant cells may resemble cells of serous carcinoma. Micro-acini and tall columnar cells with granular cytoplasm favor endometrioid carcinoma (Fig. 3.15).

Clear Cell Carcinoma

Clear cell carcinoma (CCC) comprises about 7.4% of ovarian carcinomas. The average age at

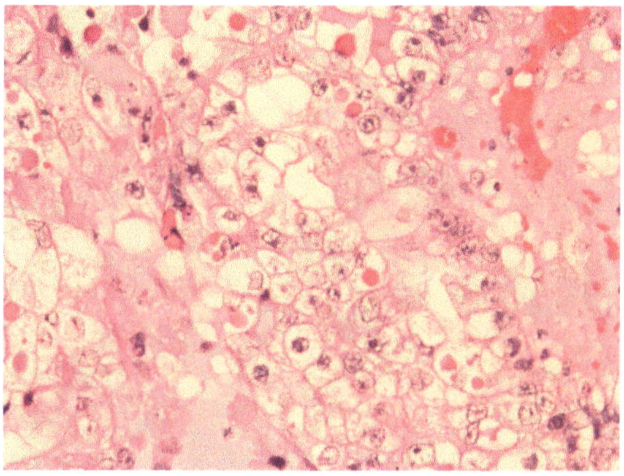

Fig. 3.16 Clear cell carcinoma of the ovary with hyaline globules (H&E x40X)

the time of diagnosis ranges from 48 to 58 years. This tumor has been associated with paraneoplastic hypercalcemia. Twenty-four to fifty percent of the patients are known to have associated pelvic endometriosis [35]. According to Yoshikawa and colleagues, the order of the prevalence of endometriosis in each histologic type is clear cell (39.2%) > endometrioid (21.2%) > serous (3.3%) > mucinous type (3.0%) [36]. Grossly, the tumor shows honeycomb cut surface or a thick-walled cyst with fleshy nodules. On microscopy, this tumor displays several different patterns such as solid, tubulo-papillary, papillary, and tubule-cystic. The solid pattern has sheets of polyhedral cells having abundant clear cytoplasm, which may exhibit PAS positive hyaline globules (Fig. 3.16). These cells are separated by delicate fibrovascular sepate. The cores of papillae often exhibit prominent hyalinization. The tumor cells are usually large, pleomorphic, and have prominent cell borders and prominent nucleoli. Nuclei may protrude into the cystic lumina giving a "hobnail" appearance. The main differential diagnosis includes yolk sac tumor and dysgerminoma. IHC panel comprising of CK7, EMA, CD15 (Leu M1), and alpha fetoprotein (αFP) is recommended to differentiate between yolk sac tumor and clear cell carcinoma of the ovary [37]. The tumor cells in CCC are positive for CK7, EMA, and CD15 and negative for αFP.

On FNAC, CCC is characterized by cells with abundant clear to pale, vacuolated cytoplasm

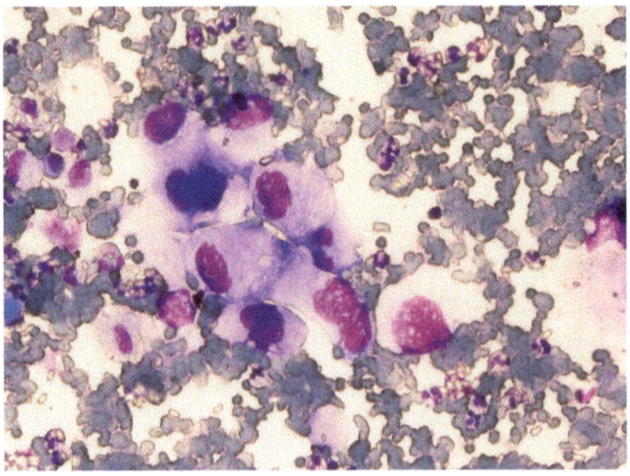

Fig. 3.17 FNAC of clear cell carcinoma of the ovary (MGG x40X)

(Fig. 3.17). The nuclear pleomorphism may be evident with prominent nucleoli. The tumor should be differentiated from metastatic renal cell carcinoma.

Malignant Transitional Cell Tumor

Some investigators have divided malignant transitional cell tumor into malignant Brenner tumor, in which a benign or atypical proliferative Brenner component is identified, and a transitional cell carcinoma, in which these components are not identified. On microscopy, thick, blunt papillary folds with fibrovascular folds are noted, and these are lined by transitional epithelium as seen in urothelial carcinomas.

Small Cell Carcinoma

Small cell carcinoma is a rare, aggressive tumor with a dimorphic population of large and small malignant cells. This tumor is often associated with paraneoplastic hypercalcemia [38].

Malignant Mixed Müllerian Tumor (Carcinosarcoma)

MMMT comprises less than 1% of ovarian neoplasms and resembles its uterine counterpart. It is characterized by an intimate admixture of malignant epithelial and sarcomatous components; these tumors can be of the homologous or heterologous type. Only epithelial or sarcomatous components may be represented on FNAC.

Germ Cell Tumors of the Ovary

Malignant germ cell tumors mainly occur in children and women less than 30 years of age.

Dysgerminoma

Dysgerminoma is the most common malignant germ cell tumor of the ovary and accounts for 1–2% of malignant ovarian tumors. The most common presenting symptom is abdominal mass and pain. It is bilateral in 5–10% cases, and it is usually a common component of mixed germ cell tumor. Grossly, dysgerminoma is usually a firm large solid tumor with smooth nodular external surface. The cut surface is homogenous, lobulated, light tan or whitish, and fleshy. On microscopy, it is composed of well-defined nests, islands, and cords of tumors cells separated by thin fibrous septae infiltrated by lymphocytes. The tumor cells are large, oval to round, uniform cells with well-defined cell borders and clear to finely granular cytoplasm containing glycogen. The nuclei show one or more prominent nucleoli. PAS stain helps to demonstrate the intracytoplasmic glycogen. About 5% cases can have HCG positive syncytiotrophoblastic cells, which may lead to elevated serum HCG levels. Granulomatous inflammation may be noted. Sometimes, there is marked anaplasia of the tumor cells, and the tumor is designated as anaplastic dysgerminoma. Dysgerminoma is placental specific alkaline phosphatase (PLAP) and CD117 (C-kit).

On FNAC, the smears are usually cellular and show predominantly dispersed population of large round fragile tumor cells with clear to vacuolated cytoplasm, central round nuclei, pale chromatin, and one or more prominent nucleoli. Another characteristic feature is tigroid background of the smear due to the glycogen, which is better appreciable in MGG-stained smears. Background shows lymphocytes and plasma cells. Differential diagnosis on cytology includes poorly differentiated carcinoma, large cell lymphoma, and malignant melanoma.

Immature Teratoma

Immature teratoma is a malignant teratoma comprising of an admixture of mature and immature/

embryonal tissues derived from all the three germ layers: ectoderm, mesoderm, and endoderm. It accounts for less than 1% of teratomas of the ovary, the majority being dermoid cysts and mature cystic teratomas. It occurs predominantly in children and young adults. Patients usually present with abdominal mass and pain. Rarely, patients have acute abdominal symptoms due to torsion or rupture of the tumor. Grossly, it is usually unilateral and can co-exist with a mature teratoma in the contra-lateral ovary. The tumor is large and firm, and the cut surface is both solid and cystic. Solid areas can be fleshy or hard and gritty. The cystic areas may show hair follicles or tooth as seen in mature cystic teratoma. It is important to sample various areas of the tumor in order to demonstrate various components of immature teratoma. On microscopy, in addition to mature component derived from ectodermal, mesodermal, and endodermal layers, immature components are seen. Primitive neuroepithelium and neuroblasts are seen along with immature embryonal stroma and cartilage. Immature teratoma should be graded, as the prognosis depends upon the grade and stage of the tumor. The most widely used grading system divides immature teratoma into three grades, from grade 1 for a tumor showing limited amount of immature tissue (not >1 low power field/slide) to grade 3 for a tumor with abundant immature tissue (≥4 low power fields/slide). Immature teratoma may have areas of hyalinization and necrosis, leftover predominant mature elements, or maturation of immature components after chemotherapy.

Carcinoid Tumor

Carcinoid Tumor is an uncommon tumor and is usually a part of a teratoma. Ovarian carcinoids are found mainly in peri- or postmenopausal women. About one-third are associated with carcinoid syndrome. On gross examination, the tumor has a smooth surface, and the cut surface is solid, tan to yellow, and homogeneous. Microscopically, the morphology is as seen in carcinoid tumors elsewhere with organoid trabecular, insular, or solid patterns. The tumor cells are uniform with fine speckled chromatin and inconspicuous nucleoli. Strümal carcinoid shows a combination of carcinoid tumor with Strüma ovarii.

Yolk Sac Tumor (Endodermal Sinus Tumor)

Yolk Sac Tumor is a neoplasm of children, adolescents, and young adults. Elevated serum αFP (alpha fetoprotein) is almost always demonstrable in these tumors. Grossly, the tumors are unilateral and large, and on the cut surface they are solid and are cystic with areas of hemorrhage and necrosis. On microscopy, the majority of the tumors show a combination of different patterns, most common being the reticular or microcystic pattern. Other patterns include festoon or pseudo-papillary pattern; alveolar–glandular, myxomatous, macrocystic, hepatic, polyvesicular vitelline pattern; and solid pattern. Schiller–Duval bodies are a characteristic feature. PAS positive diastase-resistant intracytoplasmic hyaline globules are seen.

On FNAC, the smears show irregular, large, three-dimensional papillary or ball-like clusters of malignant cells with irregular coarse chromatin and prominent nucleoli. These clusters are usually seen associated with brightly eosinophilic extracellular matrix material. Hyaline globules and Schiller–Duval bodies may be seen. It is important to evaluate if this is a component of mixed germ cell tumor; therefore, FNAC should be attempted from different areas of the tumor.

Embryonal Carcinoma

Embryonal carcinoma is uncommon in the ovary as compared to testis, and it is usually a component of mixed germ cell tumor. Presenting symptoms include abdominal pain and hormone-related symptoms such as menstrual irregularity or precocious pseudopuberty. Serum β-HCG levels are usually elevated along with αFP levels. These tend to be large, solid, and fleshy tumors grossly. On microscopy, the tumor cells are markedly pleomorphic and are arranged in cords, glands, and papillae (Fig. 3.18). Syncytiotrophoblastic cells are usually present along with cellular stromal tissue.

Choriocarcinoma

Pure primary ovarian choriocarcinoma is extremely rare.

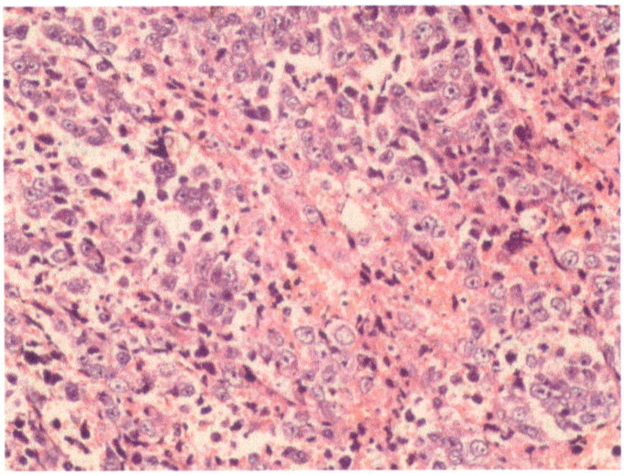

Fig. 3.18 Embryonal carcinoma of the ovary with markedly pleomorphic tumor cells (H&E x40X)

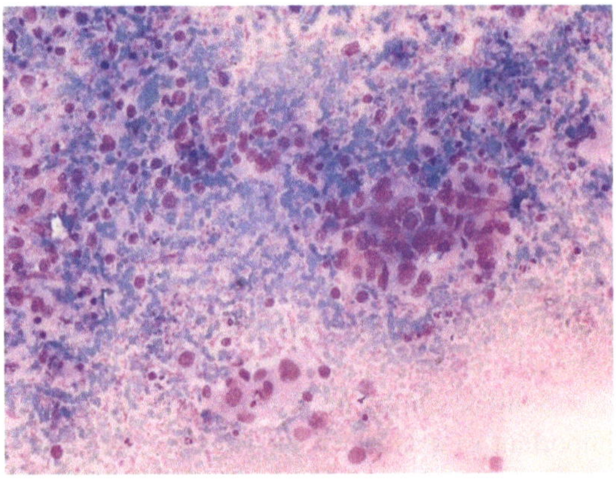

Fig. 3.19 FNAC of mixed germ cell tumor representing embryonal carcinoma component (MGG x40X)

Malignant Mixed Germ Cell Tumor

Malignant mixed germ cell tumors contain a mixture of malignant germ cell elements, the most common being a combination of dysgerminoma and yolk sac tumor (Fig. 3.19). Embryonal carcinoma, choriocarcinoma, and polyembryoma are rare.

Sex Cord-Stromal Tumors

These account for about 5–10% of all ovarian neoplasms.

Granulosa Cell Tumor

Adult Granulosa Cell Tumor

Adult granulosa cell tumor (AGCT) accounts for about 1–2% of all ovarian tumors and more than 90% of all granulosa cell tumors. AGCT mainly occurs in peri- or postmenopausal women. These are the most common estrogenic ovarian tumors clinically, and about 5–10% patients have endometrial carcinoma. The most common presenting symptom is postmenopausal bleeding. Rarely, these tumors are androgenic or hormonally inactive. Serum inhibin is a useful marker. Grossly, these may vary in size and are encapsulated with a smooth-lobulated outline. The cut surface may be solid or predominantly cystic. On microscopy, the variety of patterns can be seen, such as micro and macrofollicular, trabecular, water-silked, insular, solid- tubular, gyriform, or sarcomatoid (Fig. 3.20). Call–Exner bodies are a characteristic feature, and the tumor cells have angulated nuclei and nuclear grooves resulting in a "coffee-bean" appearance. The presence of theca cells in varying quantities may be seen. FNAC is rarely attempted and may show small sized tumor cells with eosinophilic round bodies (Fig. 3.21).

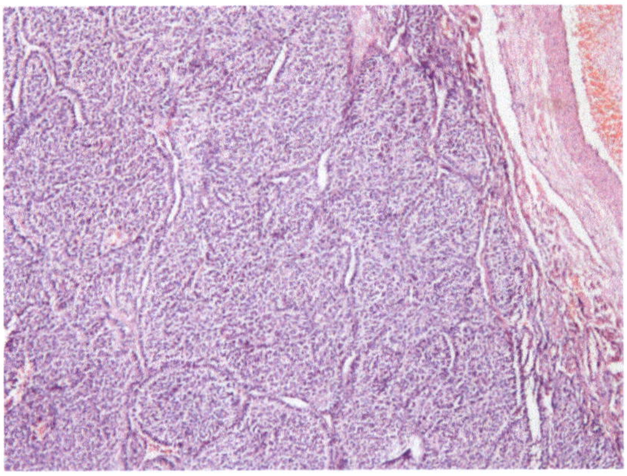

Fig. 3.20 Solid pattern in a case of adult granulosa cell tumor (H&E x40X)

Juvenile Granulosa Cell Tumor

The majority of juvenile granulosa cell tumor (JGCT) occurs in the first three decades of life. Most common presentation is pseudo-precocity. Grossly, these tumors are similar to AGCT and are usually solid as well as cystic masses. On microscopy, there is a diffuse solid or macrofollicular growth pattern with follicular lumina filled with eosinophilic or basophilic secretions. The tumor cells generally have round, hyperchromatic

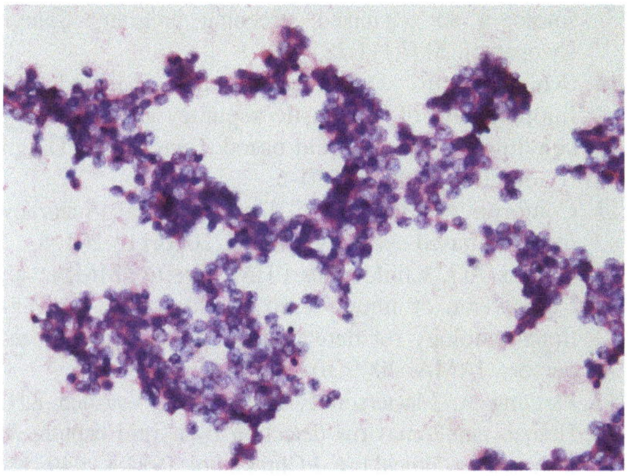

Fig. 3.21 FNAC in a case of adult granulosa cell tumor (H&E x40X)

nuclei which lack nuclear grooves. Foci containing theca cells are seen.

Both AGCT and JGCT show immuno-positivity for CD99, inhibin, and calretinin.

Thecoma

Thecoma occurs over a wide age range, but most patients are peri- or postmenopausal. These can be small tumors to large solid masses with a well-defined capsule. The cut section is typically yellowish with foci of hemorrhage and necrosis. On microscopy, these are usually cellular tumors composed of fascicles of plump spindle cells. The tumor cells have fusiform nuclei, bland chromatin, and abundant intracytoplasmic fat, the last being positive with oil-red O. Hyaline plaque are often conspicuous. On reticulin staining, the reticulum fibers typically surround individual tumor cells, which is a helpful feature to differentiate it from AGCT.

Fibroma

Fibroma is the most common sex cord-stromal tumor. It is a benign tumor which accounts for 1–5% of all ovarian tumors. The clinical symptoms can be nonspecific and rarely are associated with Meigs' syndrome. Grossly, these vary from small in size to very large in size. On cut section, these are solid, hard tumors with a whorled appearance. Microscopically, they are composed of closely packed spindle cells associated with varying amounts of hyalinization and collagenization.

Sertoli-Leydig Cell Tumor

The Sertoli-Leydig cell tumor is a rare tumor. Most occur in young women, and about 50% of these tumors are hormonally active. The most common presentation includes signs of virilization, which develop in about one-third of the cases. Grossly, these are usually solid neoplasms with yellow to tan on the cut surface. Cystic components can be variable. On microscopy, these have been divided into six subtypes: well-differentiated, intermediate differentiation, poorly differentiated, tumors with heterologous elements, retiform, and mixed. Well-differentiated tumors usually have well-defined tubules and trabeculae composed of columnar sertoli cells. Leydig cells are large polygonal cells with eosinophilic cytoplasm. The prognosis of this tumor is usually good and depends upon the stage and the degree of differentiation of the tumor.

Rarely, lymphoma or soft tissue tumors may be seen involving the ovaries.

Metastatic Tumors

The most common primary sites for metastatic tumors are the breast, uterus, stomach, colon, and gallbladder. Krukenberg tumor is an ovarian neoplasm, which is characterized by bilateral nodular ovarian enlargement and shows sheets of signet-ring cells on microscopy.

Carcinoma of Fallopian Tube

Fallopian tubal malignancies account for about 1% of all genital tract malignancies.

It is recently established that tubal fimbria is the main site for serous carcinogenesis. Tubal fimbrial end shows foci of strong p53 immunostaining, termed as "p53 signature" in benign appearing mucosa, and serous tubal intra-epithelial carcinoma (STIC) lesions, which are supposed to be the site of origin for high-grade pelvic serous carcinoma (high grade ovarian serous carcinoma). The majority of patients are postmenopausal and present with vaginal bleeding, vaginal discharge, pelvic pain, or a pelvic mass. Grossly, the tube is swollen due to a papillary or solid growth filling the tubal lumen. The fimbriated end is closed in about 50% cases. On microscopy, the most common type is papillary serous type, others being endometrioid, clear cell, squamous, small cell, lymphoepithelial-like, or transitional type. The prognosis mainly depends upon the stage of the tumor.

References

1. Ferlay J, Shin H-R, Bray F, Forman D, et al. Estimates of worldwide burden of cancer in 2008: GLOBOCAN 2008. Int J Cancer. 2010;127:2893–917.
2. Arulponni TR, Janaki MG, Nirmala S, Ramesh BS, Rishi KS, Kirthi K. Carcinoma cervix treated with radiotherapy—our experience with emphasis on our concern. J Obstet Gynaecol India. 2010;60:61–5.
3. Ostor AG. Natural history of cervical intraepithelial neoplasia: a critical review. Int J Gynecol Pathol. 1993;12:186–92.
4. Holowaty P, Miller AB, Rohan T, et al. Natural history of dysplasia of the uterine cervix. J Natl Cancer Inst. 1999;91:252.
5. Colgan TJ, Lickrish GM. The topography and invasive potential of cervical adenocarcinoma in situ, with and without associated squamous dysplasia. Gynecol Oncol. 1990;36:246–9.
6. Denehy TR, Gregori CA, Breen JL. Endocervical curettage, cane margins, and residual adenocarcinoma in situ of the cervix. Obstet Gynecol. 1997;90:1–6.
7. Ursin G, Pike MC, Preston-Martin S, et al. Sexual, reproductive, and other risk factors for adenocarcinoma of the cervix, results from a population based case– control study. Cancer Causes Control. 1996;7:391–401.
8. Gupta N, Srinivasan R, Rajwanshi A. Functional biomarkers in cervical precancer: an overview. Diagn Cytopathol. 2010;38:618–23.
9. Gupta N, Desai M. New technologies in cervical cancer screening. BIDA AGM. 2011;18:5–6.
10. Ridder R, Luyten A, Scherbring S, Reinecke-Luettge A, Schmidt D, Petry KU. Triaging PAP negative, HPV positive cervical cancer screening test results by p16/Ki67 dual stained cytology. Acta Cytol. 2010; 54(3):404–5.
11. National Institute for Clinical Excellence (NICE). NHS Technology Appraisal Guidance 69. Guidance on the use of liquid-based cytology (LBC) for cervical screening. London: National Institute for Clinical Excellence; 2003.
12. Utagawa ML, Pereira SM, Makabe S, et al. Pap test in a high risk population comparison of conventional and liquid-based cytology. Diagn Cytopathol. 2004; 31:169–72.
13. Strander B, Andersson-Ellstrom A, Milsom I, et al. Liquid-based cytology versus conventional papanicolaou smear in an organized screening program. Cancer Cytopathol. 2007;111:285–91.
14. Schledermann D, Ejersbo D, Hoelund B. Improvement of diagnostic accuracy and screening conditions with liquid-based cytology. Diagn Cytopathol. 2006;34:780–5.
15. Confortini M, Bergeron C, Desai M, et al. Accuracy of liquid-based cytology. Cancer. 2010;118:203–8.
16. Siebers AG, Klinkhamer PJJM, Grefte JMM, et al. Comparison of liquid-based cytology with conventional cytology for detection of cervical cancer precursors. JAMA. 2009;302:1757–64.
17. Farthing A, Masterson P, Mason WP, Vousden KH. Human papillomavirus detection by hybrid capture & it's possible clinical use. J Clin Pathol. 1994;47:649–52.
18. Ergünay K. Detection and typing of human Papilloma virus by polymerase chain reaction and hybridization assay in cervical samples with cytological abnormalities. Mikrobiyol Bull. 2008;42:273–82.
19. Hubbard RA. Human papillomavirus testing methods. Arch Pathol Lab Med. 2003;127:940–5.
20. Gupta N, Dudding N, Smith JHF. Cytomorphological features of extra-genital metastases in SurePath™ cervical liquid-based cytology: a series of eight cases. Cytopathology 2012; doi: 10.1111/j.1365-2303.2011.00945.x.
21. Liu FS. Molecular carcinogenesis of endometrial cancer. Taiwan J Obstet Gynecol. 2007;46:26–32.
22. Sherman ME, Bur ME, Kurman RJ. p53 in endometrial cancer and its putative precursors: Evidence for diverse pathways of tumorigenesis. Hum Pathol. 1995;26:1268–74.
23. Mutter GL. PTEN, a protean tumor suppressor. Am J Pathol. 2001;158:1895–8.
24. Matias-Guiu X, Catasus L, Bussaglia E, et al. Molecular pathology of endometrial hyperplasia and carcinoma. Hum Pathol. 2001;32:569–77.
25. Cherkis RC, Patten Jr SF, Andrews TJ, Dickinson JC, Patten FW. Significance of normal endometrial cells detected by cervical cytology. Obstet Gynecol. 1988;71:242–4.
26. DuBeshter B, Warshol DP, Angel C, Dvoretsky PM, Lin JY, Raubertas RF. Endometrial carcinoma: the relevance of cervical cytology. Obstet Gynecol. 1991;77:458–62.
27. Ronneett BM, Zaino RJ, Ellenson LH, Kurman RJ. Endometrial carcinoma. In: Kurman RJ, editor. Blaustein's pathology of the female genital tract. 5th ed. New Delhi: Springer; 2004. p. 501–59.
28. Gupta N, Awasthi A, Rajwanshi A, Malhotra S. Fine needle aspiration cytology of low grade endometrial stromal sarcoma—a case report. Acta Cytol. 2007;51(3):461–3.
29. Scully RE, Bonfiglio TA, Kurman RJ, Silverberg SG, Wilkinson EJ. World Health Organization international histological classification of tumors: histological typing of female genital tract tumors. 2nd ed. Berlin: Springer; 1994.
30. Auersperg N. Origin of ovarian carcinomas: a unifying hypothesis. Int J Gynaecol Pathol. 2010;30: 12–21.

31. Murthy NS, Shalini S, Suman G. Changing trends in incidence of ovarian cancer—the Indian scenario. Asian Pac J Cancer Prev. 2009;10:1025–30.
32. Layfield LJ, Berek JS. Fine-needle aspiration cytology in the management of gynecologic oncology patients. Cancer Treat Res. 1994;70:1–13.
33. Kurman RJ, Shih IeM. The origin and pathogenesis of epithelial ovarian cancer—a proposed unifying theory. Am J Surg Pathol. 2010;34:433–43.
34. Partridge EE, Phillips JL, Menck HR. The National Cancer Data Base report on ovarian cancer treatment in United States hospitals. Cancer. 1996;78:2236–46.
35. Komiyama S, Aoki D, Tominaga E, Susumu N, Udagawa Y, Nozawa S. Prognosis of Japanese patients with ovarian clear cell carcinoma associated with pelvic endometriosis: clinicopathologic evaluation. Gynecol Oncol. 1999;72:342–6.
36. Yoshikawa H, Jimbo H, Okada S, Matsumoto K, Onda T, Yasugi T, Taketani Y. Prevalence of endometriosis in ovarian cancer. Gynecol Obstet Invest. 2000;50:11–7.
37. Ramalingam P, Malpica A, Silva EG, Gershenson DM, Liu JL, Deavers MT. The use of cytokeratin 7 and EMA in differentiating ovarian yolk sac tumors from endometrioid and clear cell carcinomas. Am J Surg Pathol. 2004;28:1499–505.
38. Dharan M. Intra-operative cytology of small cell carcinoma of the ovary with hypercalcemia: a case report. Acta Cytol. 1993;37:61–6.

Screening and Early Diagnosis of Breast Cancer: Proven Methodology and an Optimized Strategy for Developing Countries

4

Mahesh K. Shetty

Abstract

Breast cancer is emerging as a major health care challenge in developing countries. Most recent data show that breast cancer is the most frequently diagnosed cancer in women and the leading cause of mortality from cancer. Breast cancer incidence in developing countries accounts for 51 % of the worldwide incidence. Younger women, i.e., between the ages of 15 and 49, are diagnosed with breast cancer in developing countries in a higher proportion than in developed countries (23 % to 10 %). Cost-effective health care interventions are urgently needed to reduce the increasing mortality rate from breast cancer. This chapter provides an overview of methods that have been extensively studied and whose benefits have been validated to screen for breast cancer in developed countries. Screening mammography is discussed in detail, and its benefits and potential harms are presented with an outline of the challenges of implementation and extensive resources that an organized or an opportunistic program involves. Potential low cost alternatives that may be more relevant in low resource settings such as clinical breast examination (CBE) and breast self-examination are presented. Finally, an optimal strategy for screening for breast cancer is described. This involves improved awareness of breast health among women through education and self-awareness, and periodic screening CBE performed by a trained health care professional combined with a focused sonographic evaluation of screen positive women. A detailed discussion of the use of ultrasound in characterizing palpable abnormalities in the breast and its role in optimally triaging patients who need diagnostic tissue sampling, thereby minimizing false positives, is presented. Finally, the pros and cons of fine needle aspiration biopsy and large core needle biopsy in the assessment of palpable solid masses that need tissue diagnosis are discussed.

M.K. Shetty, (✉)
Woman's Center for Breast Care and MRI,
Woman's Hospital of Texas,
Houston, TX 77054, USA
e-mail: mshetty@womens-radiology.com

M.K. Shetty (ed.), *Breast and Gynecological Cancers: An Integrated Approach for Screening and Early Diagnosis in Developing Countries*, DOI 10.1007/978-1-4614-1876-4_4,

Introduction to Breast Cancer Screening

Screening is defined as the presumptive identification of unrecognized disease by means of tests, examinations, or other procedures that can be applied rapidly. The World Health Organization outlines a number of important prerequisites to justify implementation of an effective screening program [1]:

- Target cancer should have a high prevalence and be associated with a high mortality and morbidity.
- The screening test has to be safe, effective, and acceptable.
- The compliance of the target population in attending initial screening, diagnosis, and follow-up visits has to be high.
- Effective treatment should be available to be delivered to screen positive cases.

An ideal screening test is one that detects a high percentage of cancers (sensitivity) and has a low false-positive rate so that disease-free women are not subjected to unnecessary diagnostic tests. A high prevalence of cancer in the target population being screened is an important prerequisite since even the best screening test will be ineffective when deployed in a population with a low prevalence of cancer. National and/or professional or regulatory body guidelines in individual countries for cancer screening should be based on cancer incidence and prevalence statistics. These need to address at what age and how frequently screening needs to be performed. Additional influencing factors to be taken into consideration will also include cost effectiveness of screening strategy. Quality control and assurance of effectiveness, accuracy, and consistency has to be applied to and monitored in health care personnel performing and interpreting these tests as well as in the equipment used for this purpose. An effective and robust referral system for women testing positive for cancers needs to be in place. An information system that can send out invitations for initial screening, for follow-up visits, and repeat screening at predetermined intervals is a must to ensure success [1].

Global incidence of breast cancer increased from 641,000 in 1980 to 1.64 million in 2010. Breast cancer has killed 425,000 women, of whom 68,000 were women younger than 49 in developing countries [2]. Breast cancer is now the leading cause of cancer in women and the leading cause of cancer mortality. Fifty-one percent of breast cancer cases occur in developing countries [2], which have a higher mortality rate for breast cancer than developed countries due to diagnosis at a late stage as well as due to lack of availability of effective treatment. Screening for breast cancer is justified considering the fact this cancer has a documented preclinical stage that can be diagnosed. Early diagnosis has a better prognosis, requiring less treatment with consequent benefit to the individual and the society. Numerous clinical trials have been undertaken in developed countries over the last several decades to test the efficacy of breast cancer screening in reducing breast cancer mortality. It remains to be seen whether these results can be reproduced in developing countries or if it is feasible to implement an organized, robust program on a large scale in developing countries [3]. Screening for breast cancer can be either population-based, organized screening as is in place in some European countries, or it can be opportunistic screening as is in place in the USA. An organized screening program is very resource intensive and rarely justified in a country where the prevalence rates are not high. Opportunistic screening refers to screening tests, usually a mammogram outside of a national or regional screening program. Here, the patient and the referring doctor assume responsibility for further testing if screening results are positive. Such screening programs require enormous financial and human resources, involving: a massive information campaign that effectively reaches out to the target population; building a health care infrastructure to provide screening, diagnosis, and treatment of cancers; and creating a continuous supply of trained health care professionals, specifically mammography technologists, nurses, pathologists, and radiologists. Many of the developing countries do not offer training to radiologists in breast imaging. Breast cancer screening implementation has several competing health care priorities that can be tackled at much lower cost. An organized mammographic screening program is not feasible in the foreseeable future in developing countries.

Early detection is distinct from screening and is more practical for developing countries. The aim of such an approach is to identify cancer at a relatively early stage, with the potential of curing with the least physical effects. In a typical scenario, a woman presents with a symptom and is assessed appropriately by a health care professional. Early diagnosis, however, requires education of women so that they understand the signs and symptoms and seek care; it also requires trained health care workers, particularly in rural settings, who appropriately evaluate women presenting with breast symptoms. Breast cancer may be diagnosed at an earlier stage, possibly Stage II or lower, with a prognosis significantly better than the currently prevailing situation of presentation of a large number of women at Stage III and Stage IV of the disease. Such an approach requires only limited resources and is an appropriate first step. This has been outlined in the Breast Health Global Initiative Guidelines as an option when level of resources are basic, and it includes breast health awareness consisting of educating women, self-examination, and clinical breast examination (CBE). The evaluation goal is for a baseline assessment and repeated survey [4]. Three of the most commonly studied methods for breast cancer screening, i.e., screening mammography, clinical breast exam, and breast self-examination, are discussed next in this chapter, followed by a suggested strategy optimal for developing countries.

Screening Mammography

Randomized clinical trials (RCTs) study the efficacy of a screening methodology; efficacy is thus measured in experimental studies. The effectiveness of a screening modality, on the other hand, is defined as the extent to which a specific intervention when deployed in routine circumstances does what it is supposed to do, in a specific population [5]. The role of mammography in reducing breast cancer mortality has been demonstrated in multiple RCTs as well as in organized mammography screening services. The first randomized controlled study to demonstrate a significant benefit of screening mammography was the Swedish Two-County Trial. A total of 77,080 women aged 40–74 years were randomized in geographical clusters and invited to be screened; 55,985 women were assigned to a no-invitation group. A single view mammogram was performed every 33 months in women in age group 50–74 years and every 24 months in the age group 40–49 years. In this trial, a 30 % mortality reduction was achieved when those women who were invited to be screened were compared to those who were not invited to be screened [6]. In the same study, when those women who actually attended screening were compared to those who did not, a still higher mortality reduction of 42 % was observed [6, 7].

A meta-analysis of all the RCTs testing the efficacy of screening mammography to date demonstrated a significant reduction in breast cancer mortality of 20–35 % in women in age group 50–69 years [8]. How do the results of these RCTs translate into clinical practice, i.e., service screening, i.e., effectiveness vs. efficacy? This has been studied by Tabar et al. In the age group of women between 20 and 69 years, there were 6,807 women who were diagnosed with breast cancer over a 29-year period in two counties in Sweden, and there were 1,863 breast cancer deaths. These investigators reported a 63 % mortality reduction in mortality from incident breast carcinoma in women ages 40–69 during the service screening period of 1988–1996 compared with breast cancer mortality during the time period when no screening was available (1968–1977). The reduction in mortality observed during the service screening period when adjusted for selection bias was 48 %. The reason for a more significant mortality reduction in service screening compared to RCTs can be attributed to a number of logical factors. These include significant improvements in mammographic techniques since the randomized trial era, and the inherent limitations of RCTs in quantifying mortality reduction due to compliance and contamination rates, and prevalence screen. The number of screening rounds, length of follow-up, and length of screening intervals, which in the Swedish two-county trial was 33 months for women aged 50–74, are additional factors that lead to better results in service screening [9]. In a review of seven population-based community screening programs in the USA that included 463,372 women, the sensitivity of mammography was 75 % and the specificity was 92.3 %. Sensitivity was similar to what was shown in RCTs. Breast density contributes to the overall sensitivity, with only 63 % sensitivity noted in women with dense breasts and 87 % in women with entirely fatty breasts [10].

The literature supporting the benefits of screening mammography in reducing mortality from breast cancer is extensive, and the overwhelming body of evidence is strongly in favor of offering this service to women in countries with a high prevalence of breast cancer. The controversy regarding benefits of screening mammography and the debate as to when breast cancer screening should commence, how often to screen, and when to stop screening rage on. The Council of the European Union and the International Agency for Research on Cancer Expert Working Group have recommended use of bi-annual mammography for women age 50–69 [11]. In the USA, the Society of Breast Imaging and the Breast Imaging Commission of the American College of Radiology recommend an annual screening mammography for women of average risk starting at age 40 [12].

Limitations of and Potential Harm from Screening Mammography

There are some who question the benefit of screening mammography. Controversies regarding the false positives resulting from mammography, the benefit of performing screening in women in their 40s, and whether mammography over-diagnoses cancer, leading to unneeded treatment interventions, comprise some of the issues. Approximately 95 % of women with abnormalities on the screening mammogram do not have breast cancer [13]. In a review commissioned by the US Preventive Services Task Force, the sensitivity of mammography for a 1-year screening interval was found to be 71–96 % and substantially lower for women in their 40s. The specificity was 94–97 %; it has to be borne in mind that false positive meant recall of the patient for additional views and resolution of the abnormality, in most instances without the need for a biopsy or surgical intervention. The positive predictive value of one-time mammography ranged from 2 to 12 % for abnormal results requiring further evaluation and from 12 to 78 % for abnormal results requiring biopsy. There is continued increase in predictive value with age [14].

Screening Women in Their 40s

Women in their 40s have denser breast and a lower incidence of breast cancer accounting for decreased sensitivity of mammography; nevertheless, in this age group, women tend to have faster growing cancers [13]. The evidence of reduction of mortality for women between 40 and 49 years is lower yet significant. A study that looked at the data from all four Swedish trials for women in this age group reported a 23 % mortality reduction at randomization achieved from a median trial time of 7 years, median follow up of 12.8 years, and a screening interval of 18–24 months [15]. About 18 % of cancers, both in-situ and malignant, are reported in women between the ages of 40–49 in the USA. A longitudinal cohort study in 1977 of women in this age group who had primary breast cancer was undertaken over an 18 year period. A significant increase in the percentage of mammography-detected cancer was seen over time (28–58 %), and a concurrent decline in patient- and physician-detected breast cancer (73–42 %) was seen over time, with a consequent increase in lower stage disease detection and decrease in higher stage disease [16]. A study of 31,814 average risk women reported that the positive predictive value for further evaluation was 1–4 % for women ages 40–49, 4–9 % for women ages 50–59, 10–19 % for women ages 60–69, and 18–20 % for women ages 70 or older [17].

Harms of Mammography Screening

Overdiagnosis refers to diagnosis of cancers, particularly DCIS which may have never progressed to an invasive stage and resulted in death. Such patients would have undergone surgery, chemotherapy, and/or radiotherapy along with their consequent harm [18]. The presumptive evidence for "over-diagnosis" is suggested by the fact that breast cancer diagnosis in the screened group remained persistently higher even after many years when compared to the control group of non-screened women in large RCTs. This assertion is contentious because diagnosing more breast cancer cases cannot be somehow construed to be a bad thing. It has been shown without question that mortality rate reduction should be the one and only benchmark of success of screening mammography. Despite the criticism that mammography may find, DCIS that may never become invasive is a moot point since the same detractors of screening have no answer for the fact that we do not know which ones proceed to invasive stage and which ones do not.

Two observational studies of women who underwent the current standard technique of a two view mammography and included millions of person years of observation reported a much stronger mortality reduction than has been shown in RCTs of 30–40 % for women in their 40s. In fact, RCTs tend to underestimate the benefit of screening mammography because it includes all women in the screened group who are invited to be screened including those who do not actually end up getting a mammogram and it does not exclude women in the control group who may end up getting a mammogram outside the trial. As has been previously pointed out, in several RCTs the mammographic quality was not comparable to the current standards and a one view mammogram only was obtained which limits the cancer detection rate [19].

Mammographic Interpretation and Quality Assurance in Mammography, Medical Audit, and Benchmarks

Interpretive accuracy varies among radiologists, especially in mammography. A study that examined the relationship between radiologists' confidence in their assessments and their accuracy in interpreting mammograms found that confidence in mammography assessments was associated with better accuracy, especially for low-volume readers. Asking for a second opinion when confidence in an assessment is low may increase accuracy [20]. The other significant potential harm resulting from screening mammography is from false-positive results that lead to unnecessary patient anxiety and unneeded breast biopsies. Although this is a shortcoming of mammography, it is a given that any screening modality is bound to have some false positive as no test is perfect. However, much can be done to minimize the false positives, and we next address ways of achieving this objective.

The US Congress enacted the Mammography Quality Standards Act (MQSA) to ensure that all women have access to quality mammography for the detection of breast cancer in its earliest, most treatable stages, and it charged the Federal Drug Administration with developing and implementing the MQSA regulations [21]. The scope of the act included establishing minimum national quality standards for mammography facilities to ensure safe, reliable, and accurate mammography. All facilities had to undergo periodic certification by accredited bodies to ensure compliance with federal standards. This included adequate training of both radiologists and technologists. European guidelines for quality control and quality assurance in breast cancer screening and diagnosis were developed. The purpose of such a rigorous quality assurance program in breast cancer screening was to diminish the potential harm that can result from mammography such as unnecessary anxiety and morbidity, inappropriate economic cost, and the use of ionizing radiation [11]. A screening program should strive to reduce and avoid unnecessary work up of clearly benign abnormalities, to reduce anxiety, and to maintain a cost-effective program. Somewhat similar to the mandated requirements in the USA, the European guidelines for quality assurance recommended the need for QA on all mammography units, implementation of a robust accreditation of all screening programs, and emphasized the need for all staff to hold professional qualifications to perform and interpret mammograms and to undertake specialist training and participate in CME, updates, and external quality assessment schemes. Each screening unit should have a lead professional to oversee overall quality assurance and performance of the screening mammography program. Strict adherence to such national and regional guidelines are critical for a successful screening program, and many countries where screening programs are in place or are being implemented adopt similar measures to ensure quality.

Mammography Interpretation Benchmarks

A screening program must have benchmarks to serve as minimally acceptable criteria for interpretive performance. This was recently studied by Carney et al. [22]. The study was aimed to identify minimally acceptable performance standards for interpreting screening mammograms. They reported that a sensitivity of less than 75 %, specificity less than 88 % or greater than 95 %, recall rate less than 5 % and greater than 12 %, PPV 2 of less than 20 % or greater than 40 %, and cancer detection rate of 2.5 per 1,000 interpretations indicate low performance [22]. If underperforming physicians moved into the acceptable range by additional training, detection of an additional 14 cancers per 100,000 women screened and a reduction in the number of false positive examinations by 880 per 100,000 women screened would be expected [22]. Radiologists interpreting moderate (1,001–2,000) and those with high volume (>2,000) had a higher sensitivity [22]. It is of interest to note that the recall rate in the USA is twice the recall rate in the United Kingdom (e.g., 12.5–14.4 % vs. 7.6 %), with no difference in cancer detection rate [23]. This may have to do at least in part to the practice of defensive medicine in the USA rather than interpretive skills since failure to diagnose breast cancer is the leading cause of malpractice litigation in the USA. Among other things, MQSA mandated implementation of the American College of Radiology BIRADS™ (Breast Imaging Reporting and Data System, ACR, Reston, VA) recommendations for mammogram interpretation and final assessment categories have helped to standardize mammographic reporting in the USA [24]. Per the BIRADS reporting system, a standard mammogram report should include a description of the breast composition, i.e., breast composition is almost entirely fat (<25 % glandular), there are scattered fibroglandular densities (25–50 % glandular), breast tissue is heterogeneously dense (51–75 % glandular), and breast tissue is extremely dense (>75 % glandular) [24]. This is important since it gives an idea about the volume of attenuating tissue in the breast and hence an idea of the relative sensitivity of the examination. The next step in the interpretation of a mammogram is a description of significant findings such as a mass (size, morphology), calcifications (morphology and distribution), architectural distortion, and special cases (dilated ducts, intramammary lymph nodes, global and focal asymmetry) [24]. Both category 1 and 2 indicate absence of mammographic evidence of malignancy. The BIRADS™ three probably benign category is used when there is a finding that has a less than 2 % risk of malignancy. Most mammographers follow a sequence of 6, 12, 24, and 36 months of mammographic surveillance for women in this assessment category. During mammographic reading, understanding the normal variation in the mammographic patterns as well as identifying the subtle signs of malignancy are equally important. The subtle signs are often faint microcalcifications and indirect signs of malignancy such as areas of architectural distortion, focal asymmetry, solitary dilated duct, and small developing densities. Increasing the true positives is more important than reducing false positives. An important goal of the mammographer should also be to increase cancer detection rate. The importance of comparison with prior mammograms is very important. An analysis of 48,281 consecutive mammography examinations for which previous mammography (9,825 diagnostic, 38,456 screening) had been performed between 1997 and 2001 reported that, for screening mammography, comparison with previous examinations significantly decreases false positive and permits detection of cancers at an earlier stage. For diagnostic mammography, comparison with previous examinations increases true-positive findings. In the diagnostic setting, comparison with previous examinations increases the biopsy yield from 38 to 51 % and the overall cancer detection rate from 11/1,000 to 39/1,000. A significant decrease in the frequency of axillary node metastasis and the cancer stage for screening mammography was observed [25, 26].

The National Cancer Institute outlines a "discovery-development-delivery" approach to cancer research [27]:

> Discovery is the process of generating new information about fundamental cancer processes from the genetic to the population level. Development is the process of creating and evaluating tools and interventions that are valuable in detecting, diagnosing, predicting, treating, and preventing cancer. Delivery involves promoting and facilitating the application of evidence-based cancer interventions [27].

The Breast Cancer Surveillance Consortium was established by the NCI in 1994. The benefits of screening mammography have been well established in large RCTs; however, the effectiveness of screening mammography had to be studied in routine clinical practice. It was also recognized that useful information could only be obtained by linking screening patterns and performance parameters as outlined by national bodies and professional societies such as the American College of Radiology with cancer outcomes. At the present time, seven data collection and research centers and the statistical coordinating center comprise the BCSC. A key program of NCI's Division of Cancer Control and Population Sciences focuses on the delivery component, and its research wing aims to promote adoption of proven intervention methods in clinical and public health practice. The BCSC links surveillance data on breast screening practices with data from population-based cancer registries. Most recent data which includes data on screening mammography performed from 2002 to 2006 and analyzed in 2009 show a cancer detection rate of 4.6 per 1,000 women amongst 1,960,500 mammograms performed. Sensitivity and specificity for 2,264,089 screening mammography examinations from 2002 to 2006, based on BCSC data as of 2009, was as follows: sensitivity: 84.1 %; specificity: 90.4 %. The recall rate was 10 %. PPV 2 was 23.6 % (cases where biopsy was recommended) and PPV 3 was 28.9 % (cases where biopsy was performed within 1 year) [27]. An analysis of the results of 47,798 screening and 13,286 diagnostic mammograms found that radiologists that are specialized in breast imaging detected more cancers and more early stage cancers, recommended more biopsies, and had lower recall rates than did the general radiologists. Cancer detection rate of specialists was 6 % compared to 3.4 % for generalists. A database of such large samples of screened population allows the Consortium to study and publish several key features of community based breast cancer screening programs such as characteristics of women that affect the performance of screening mammography, characteristics of radiologists, radiology facility, or mammographic technologists affecting performance of screening mammography, and characteristics of mammography equipment that affects the performance of screening mammography. The low-contrast detectability was studied using a full-field digital mammography system and was compared with results obtained from an optimized screen-film system. Results showed that using a softer X-ray beam for thin breasts and a harder X-ray beam for thick breasts improved digital mammography's ability to detect low-contrast lesions when the average glandular dose was kept constant. Under this constraint, optimum low-contrast lesion detection with digital mammography was superior to that of conventional screen-film mammography (SFM) for all but the thinnest breasts.

Recall rate of women undergoing mammography is one of the audit benchmarks, since performing additional imaging to rule out cancer increases false-positive rates. False-positive mammograms also lead to anxiety, excess costs, and morbidity from subsequent biopsies, many of which result in a benign diagnosis. The false-positive rate for screening mammography is higher in the USA than in European countries. In a study that looked at three groups of radiologists interpreting mammograms; the sensitivity in the group considered high volume readers, which included those who read >301 mammograms each month, was significantly higher than in those who read <100 or those who read between 100 and 300 mammograms. The specificity was also better among high volume readers although was not statistically significant. In the USA, the minimum number of mammograms required is 480/year compared to 5,000/year required in the UK [28, 29]. Others have also shown that increasing minimum interpretive volume requirements in the USA while adding a minimal requirement for diagnostic interpretation could reduce the number of false-positive work-ups without hindering cancer detection [30].

About two-thirds of all mammography equipment in the USA is digital, predominantly full-field digital systems. A study of total of 49,528 asymptomatic women presenting for screening mammography at 33 sites in the USA and Canada underwent both digital and film mammography [31]. The overall diagnostic accuracy of full-field digital mammography (FFDM) and SFM as a means of screening for breast cancer was found to be similar, but digital mammography was found to be more accurate in women under the age of 50 years, women with radiographically dense breasts, and premenopausal or perimenopausal women [31]. Another study that compared the miss rate of breast cancer found no difference in those who underwent SFM from those who underwent FFDM. The missed cancers in the SFM group of 52,444 women had microcalcifications on the prior mammograms in 34 % compared to 18 % in the FFDM group of 35,127 women; focal asymmetry at the site of cancer was seen more frequently at the site of missed cancers in women who underwent FFDM, 27 % compared to 10 % in those who underwent SFM [32].

Screening by Clinical Breast Exam

Most professional societies that issue recommendations for screening mammography also recommend physician or health care worker perform periodic CBE. CBE in such a setting plays a complementary role. The number of women in the USA undergoing mammography has increased steadily since 1990, especially in women with limited access to health care [33]. In 1997, 71 % of women in the USA older than 41 years reported having undergone mammography in the previous 2 years compared to 54 % in 1989. Women and their physicians are making decisions about screening; they need information about the underlying risk of the condition being screened for, the effectiveness of the procedure in preventing an untoward outcome such as death, and the potential ill effects of screening, such as false-positive tests. For policymakers and payers, cost effectiveness is an important factor in decisions about the allocation of finite resources [8].

CBE has been studied as a low cost alternative to mammographic surveillance to reduce mortality by early detection of breast cancer. CBE identifies about 60 % of cancers that are detected by mammography and a few that are not seen on mammography. There has been no RCT undertaken to evaluate the efficacy of CBE in the early diagnosis of breast cancer by comparing women who received CBE and those who did not. An estimate based on all RCTs reported sensitivity of CBE for detection of breast cancer at 54 % and specificity at 94 %. Indirect evidence of its value comes from the Canadian National Breast Screening Study, where women were divided into two groups, one that received screening with physician performed CBE alone and a second group that received both CBE and screening mammography. There were 39,405 women enrolled in this clinical trial. These investigators found that in the two groups breast cancer mortality and nodal involvement was similar [13, 34–36]. The sensitivity of CBE in clinical practice has been reported to be considerably lower compared to the Canadian National Breast Cancer Screening Study: a sensitivity of 28–36 % only in clinical practice compared to 63 % achieved with CNBCSS [13].

A cost effectiveness analysis of screening mammography and CBE in India reported that a single CBE at age 50 lead to a 2 % decrease in breast cancer mortality rate and had an estimated cost effectiveness ratio of Int.$793 per life year gained; a 16.3 % mortality rate reduction was possible with biennial CBE at a cost effectiveness ratio of Int.$1,341. CBE performed annually from ages of 40–60 years was estimated to be as effective as screening mammography for reducing breast cancer mortality at a fraction of the cost [37]. It has been pointed out that health policy makers are critical of BSE and CBE and more tolerant towards inconsistent and negative findings of mammographic screening [38]. CBE may find tumors that are not seen on mammography or in breast tissue that is not imaged at mammography, such as in the axilla or the chest wall above the breast, an area that may not show up well or get excluded on routine mammographic views. The value of CBE, which requires no special equipment, should not be discredited, particularly in developing countries. Failure to demonstrate efficacy in controlled clinical trials may not mean that an intervention is not effective, particularly when can be implemented at a low cost. It is, however, imperative that primary care providers and health care workers be well versed in the method of CBE, so that women who present with a complaint or in whom a lump is discovered are then offered appropriate further imaging with ultrasound.

Screening by Breast Self-Examination

Breast self-examination has the advantage of being patient centered and noninvasive, and can be carried out by women in the comfort of their home. If the challenges of educating women on breast self-awareness and of training to perform structured BSE are overcome, it makes sense to implement this method as part of a breast cancer screening strategy. Compliance will be the greatest challenge, and even in the USA only one-third of women perform regular BSE; the reported sensitivity is also low (20–30 %), and the prospects in developing countries may be even more challenging [39]. A large randomized controlled trial in Shanghai, China, that included 266,064 women who worked in textile factories provided half of the women with intensive initial instruction that included practice with breast models, regular reminders, and practice examinations under supervision biannually for 5 years. There was no change in breast cancer mortality in the intervention group at 10 years of follow-up. There was a significantly higher rate of biopsy due to false-positive findings (1.8 % in the instruction group compared to 1 % in the control group). However, these findings have to be interpreted with caution, since the study group had a high percentage of young women (40 % in their 30s); in this age group, no method of screening has ever been shown to be effective in reducing mortality, and also a higher false-positive rate is to be expected due to the hormonally induced cyclical changes in the breast tissue. The time to measure mortality change in this large clinical trial may have been too short [40]. The first large scale clinical trial conducted in Russia also did not show any benefit in reducing breast cancer mortality in women undergoing BSE. This trial has been criticized for not having practiced BSE well and for the lack of critical analysis of cluster randomization data [41, 42]. A case–control study within the CNBSS women showed that in those with a higher score there was a lower score of being diagnosed with advanced breast cancer and thereby lower odds of death from breast cancer [43]. A similar benefit was seen in a cohort of nearly 30,000 women in Finland, where a relative risk of 0.75 for breast cancer mortality relative to that expected from the general population was found [44]. This study suggested that a well performed BSE combined with a physician visit to act on the findings of BSE was critical in providing this benefit [44].

Optimal Strategy for Breast Cancer Screening in Developing Countries

The fundamental prerequisite when formulating a strategy to implement programs aiming to diagnose breast cancer at an early stage with an aim to improve mortality is to have data on the prevalence of breast cancer in the target population. The existing cancer burden is taken into account while crafting the most cost-effective strategy that would be appropriate for the resources of the country and relevant to the cancer burden of the target population. Effective strategy will have to be tailored to a country or region based on prevalence of cancer and resources available in that particular country: there can be no one-size-fits-all developing country strategy. Breast cancer statistics in developing countries are sketchy, incomplete, and may not be accurate. A starting point in the breast cancer-control strategy would require developing countries to assess the existing cancer burden by setting up accurate statistics to determine the breast cancer incidence and mortality [45]. The strengths and limitations of the existing health care systems will have to be assessed, and a cancer-control strategy has to be put in place once both system inefficiencies and patient barriers are identified. The release of the Cancer Atlas of India is an example of one such effort at establishing a cancer registry [46]. Cancer statistics and data in developing countries are sparse, but a definite upward trend is apparent particularly in urban areas where a more westernized lifestyle has led to an increase in the incidence of breast cancer [47]. In Mumbai, India, over a 30 year period, the incidence of age standardized rate of breast cancer increased 1.1 % per year in women in age group 30–64 years, similar to that in Shanghai, China, and other urban areas in mid and low resource countries. The rate is still about one-third of those seen in Caucasian women in the USA. In Mumbai, India, breast cancer represented 32 % of cancer burden in women in the 2001–2005 period, compared to 18 % for cervical cancer which has decreased in incidence over the years and ovarian cancer which has remained steady and accounted for 7 % of the cancer burden [47, 48]. The changing pattern reflects adoption of a more sedentary life style, dietary changes of increased consumption of alcohol and meat combined with fertility pattern changes of delayed age of first child birth, fewer children, and shortened breast feeding time [47, 48]. In a mid resource setting, the screening strategy adopted in an urban setting with a more affluent population may have to be different than one adopted in the rural population. In rural areas, the degree of existing breast health awareness as well as expected compliance with a newly initiated screening program will be more challenging than in an urban area. The infrastructure and health care expertise available in urban areas such as Mumbai, Shanghai, or Manila may allow setting up of comprehensive screening and diagnostic breast centers similar to those that exist in developed nations. Opportunistic screening using mammography and work up of abnormalities utilizing diagnostic mammography and sonography may be feasible in urban areas. Funding mechanism in these sprawling urban areas is largely expected to be one involving a combination of government supported and individually supplemented. The strategy described next, on the other hand, is one that will be suited to the low resource countries and the rural population that is government funded, keeping in mind the limited resources available [47, 48].

The age distribution of breast cancer is reportedly lower in low resource countries than in high resource countries. A recent publication of global breast and gynecological cancer data reported that 23 % of breast cancer cases occurred in age group 15–49 in developing countries compared to 10 % in developed countries [2]. Increased incidence of breast cancer in younger women has been attributed by some to the average lower age of women in the population rather than to a higher age-specific incidence [45]. It may still be advisable to start screening at an earlier age in these settings. The target population to be screened should probably include women in the age group 40–69 years. The proposed methodology would include an annual CBE followed by focused diagnostic breast sonographic evaluation of screen positive women. Those women in whom a palpable solid mass is seen and determined to be suspicious based on ultrasound morphologic features undergo ultrasound-guided biopsy for optimal sampling [48–50]. Tissue sampling can be achieved using fine needle aspiration biopsy or large core needle biopsy. The rationale of this suggested methodology is explained next. Following a screening CBE, further assessment of screen positive cases is most optimally carried out by diagnostic sonography rather than by diagnostic mammography for many reasons [48–50] (Tables 4.1 and 4.2). Mammography has limitations in the evaluation of the symptomatic woman, particularly in those with dense breasts.

Table 4.1 Limitations of mammography as a screening modality in developing countries

Resource-intense modality, expensive to set up and maintain
Poor sensitivity in women with dense breasts
Screen detected abnormalities may require additional evaluation with sonography
Substantial recall rate would mean repeat clinic visit
Discomfort from breast compression may affect patient compliance
Screen-film mammography is not optimal for telemedicine reads or consultation
Image-guided biopsy of mammographic abnormalities is cumbersome and requires additional investment in stereotactic biopsy units

Table 4.2 Advantages of sonography in breast cancer screening and diagnosis

Several large clinical studies such as the ACRIN 6666 have shown that US can detect small cancers not seen on mammography due to dense breast tissue
Cost-effective modality: initial capital expenditure and operational expense are considerably lower than mammography
Ultrasound can be used for screening and diagnosis of other cancers in women
Telemedicine feasible modality
Portable equipment easy to transport and for use in mobile clinics
No need to recall for additional imaging evaluation as in mammography
Sonographic examination of the breast is better tolerated by women due to lack of the need for breast compression
Fine needle aspiration biopsy feasible: procedure is cytology based and similar to PAP smears. US is used as the imaging guide to obtain the sample

A false-negative rate of 16.5 % has been reported for mammography in patients with a palpable breast abnormality (Fig. 4.1a, b) [51]. Mammographic abnormalities identified in a symptomatic woman usually require additional diagnostic ultrasound work up, and, in those with a suspicious palpable solid mass seen on a mammogram and a sonogram, the latter is a better modality for tissue sampling (Fig. 4.4c). Overall, diagnostic ultrasound is superior and a cost-effective alternative to diagnostic mammography for the assessment of the symptomatic patient in a LRC. Ultrasound is a safe, well-tolerated, relatively inexpensive modality that can be readily used in the evaluation of a palpable lump in a woman where a positive physical finding was detected during the course of a screening CBE. Ultrasound has also the added potential of being used to stage breast cancer [49, 50].

The recommendations for triple assessment of symptomatic women at a breast clinic traditionally consisted of physical assessment, diagnostic mammography, and Fine Needle Aspiration Biopsy (FNAB) [52–56]. As stated previously, substituting diagnostic mammography with diagnostic ultrasound is particularly suitable in low resource settings. There are data to support the fact that findings of cytology are best considered in combination with imaging morphology and characterization of solid masses. Such an approach will improve the PPV, thereby allowing for optimal management of symptomatic women with suspicious findings at imaging and cytology. In a consecutive series of 2,334 women, PPV for cytology findings of atypical, suspicious, and malignant was 55, 95.9, and 99.4 %, respectively. However, when an atypical finding at cytology is seen in combination with a suspicious finding on imaging, the PPV improved to 83.3 % and PPV for suspicious lesions increased to 98.5–98.7 %, potentially allowing for management decisions of open biopsy and/or planning surgery [57]. Core needle biopsies have been reported to be more accurate than FNAB [54]; in a LRC, the latter may be preferred as a less invasive and a more cost-effective alternative. FNAB has the advantages of being a minimally invasive procedure, well tolerated with minimal complications and patient discomfort and providing rapid results. FNABs are usually performed using a 21–25-gauge needle and a 10-mL syringe mounted on an aspiration device. However, as stated next, FNAB requires an experienced cytologist for interpretation. This proposed strategy is discussed in greater detail, including the role of ultrasound in women with a palpable abnormality of the breast and the biopsy of those palpable masses that are deemed to be suspicious.

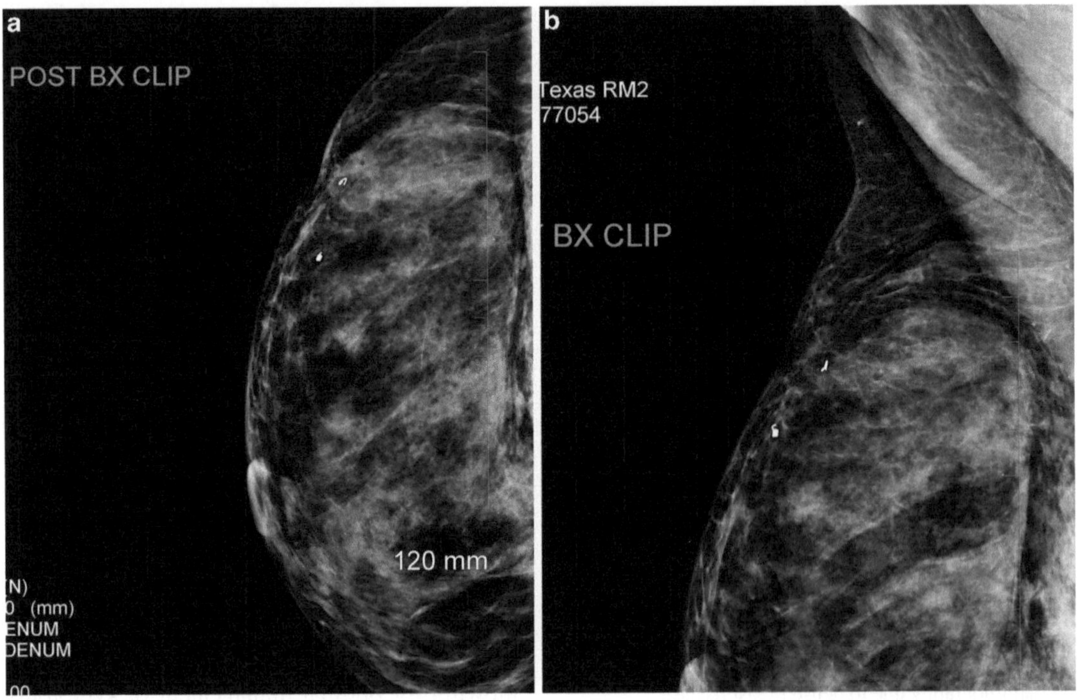

Fig. 4.1 False-negative mammogram in a patient with a palpable cancer (ultrasound image of the palpable mass is shown in Fig. 4.4c). (**a**) Craniocaudal view demonstrating no mammographic evidence of malignancy. Post ultrasound biopsy clips are seen at the site of solid palpable mass proven to be an invasive ductal cancer. (**b**) Mediolateral oblique view also showing no abnormal finding at the site of biopsy proven palpable cancer

Sonographic Evaluation of Palpable Breast Masses

Palpable abnormalities of the breast have a predominantly benign etiology, particularly in young women. Malignancy has been reported in 3.4–6 % of cases [58, 59]. In one series of 605 women under the age of 40, a cancer rate of 5 % was reported [60]. Imaging is critical to avoid unnecessary intervention and to improve accuracy of diagnosis. Focused sonography is quick, cost effective, and accurate in the assessment of a palpable abnormality. It is ideally combined with physical examination and provides a benign diagnosis with no further intervention needed in most instances [61]. Benign etiologies that are readily identified under ultrasound include cysts (Fig. 4.2a), benign lymph nodes (Fig. 4.2b), dermal lesions such as an infected epidermal cyst (Fig. 4.2c), fat lobules, palpable ridge of normal tissue [62], as well as the rare entity of Mondor's disease (Fig. 4.2d) where patient presents with a painful palpable cord. Sonographic diagnosis of superficial thrombophlebitis is diagnosed using real-time and color Doppler assessment of the palpable finding [63]. We have reported these characteristic findings in a small series of five patients. A majority of palpable lumps represent cysts, 25 % in a series of 300 [64]. In a series of women presenting with a palpable abnormality that we have published, 36.7 % (151/411) of palpable abnormalities were proven to be cysts, with a benign diagnosis provided by sonography in 39.4 % of cases precluding any further intervention [58]. In the same series, 168 palpable lumps had negative findings on sonography (45.1 %). Overall, only 14.6 % of women with a palpable abnormality had a solid mass to account for the palpable finding, excluding nearly 85 % of women from further intervention, demonstrating the value of ultrasound in the management of a woman presenting with a palpable lump [58].

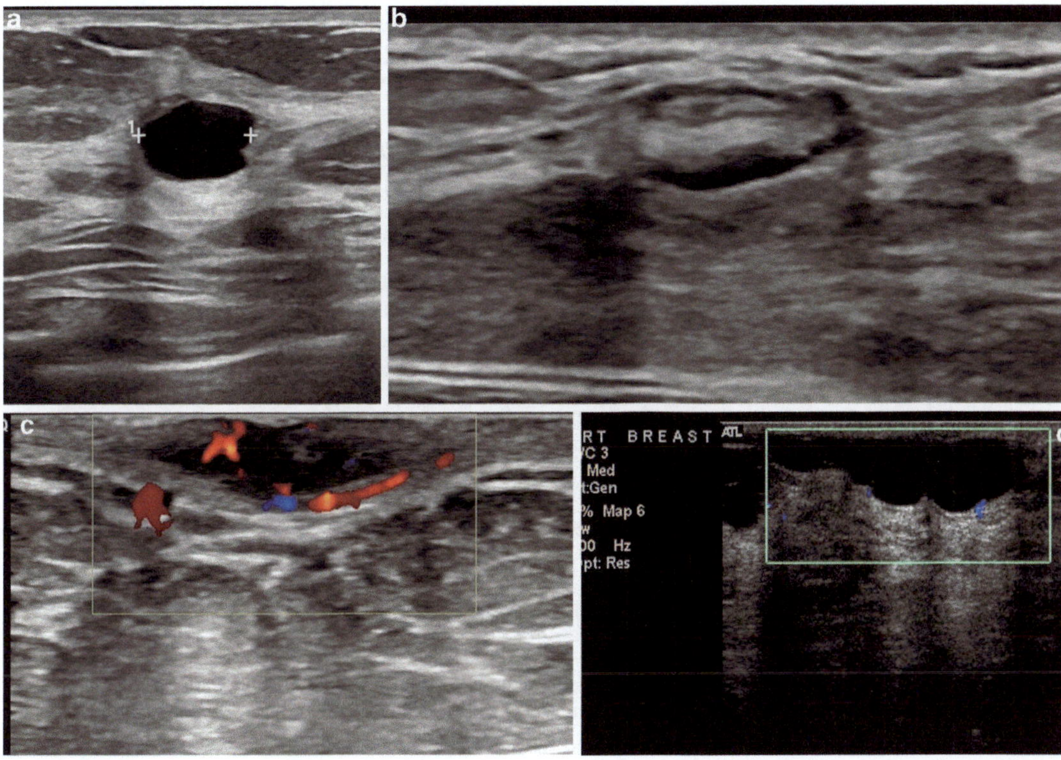

Fig. 4.2 Benign causes for palpable lumps diagnosed by sonography, no further work up is needed. (**a**) Cyst. (**b**) Lymph node. (**c**) Infected epidermal cyst. (**d**) Thrombosed superficial vein in Mondor's disease of the breast

When a palpable solid mass is seen, characterization based on previously published reports allows a mass to be categorized in one of three groups: benign, probably malignant, or indeterminate. For a mass to be considered benign, one of three groups of findings have to be present: intense uniform hyperechogenicity, ellipsoid shape with a thin echogenic capsule, two to three gentle lobulations with a thin echogenic capsule (Fig. 4.3a–c). The negative predictive value of intense uniform hyperechogenicity was 100 %, a thin echogenic pseudo capsule was 99.2 %, ellipsoid shape was 99.1 %, and four or fewer gentle lobulations was 98.8 % [62].

There are nine malignant features described by these investigators. These included the following (positive predictive value for each of the malignant feature is within parenthesis):

Spiculation (91.8 %)

A solid mass that is taller than it is wide (81.2 %)

A mass with angular margins (67.5 %)

One that demonstrates posterior acoustic shadowing (64.9 %)

A mass that demonstrates a branching pattern [61]

Hypoechogenicity (60.1 %)

Calcifications (59.6 %)

Duct extension (50.8 %)

Microlobulations (48.2 %)

A solid mass is initially interrogated for presence of malignant features (Fig. 4.4a–f), and, when absent, these described benign features are sought. If benign characteristics are seen, a solid mass is classified as being benign. Solid masses which do not demonstrate malignant or specific benign features are then classified as indeterminate with a recommendation for tissue diagnosis (Fig. 4.5) [62].

Description of Benign Features [62]

Intense and uniform *hyperechogenicity* (Fig. 4.3a) refers to markedly hyperechoic tissue compared to the echogenicity of fat. Hyperechogenicity should be uniform and usually corresponds to

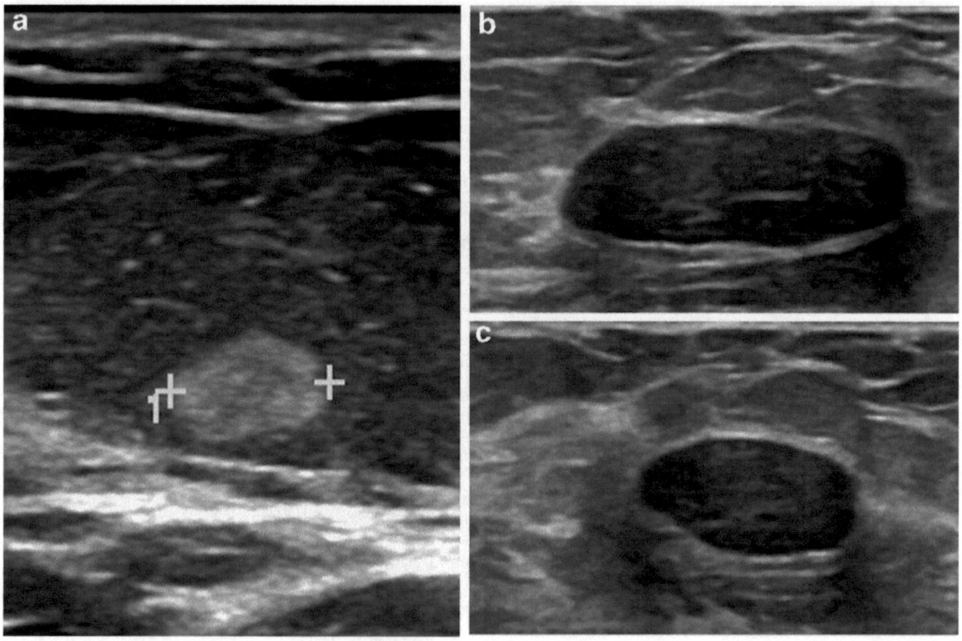

Fig. 4.3 Palpable solid masses demonstrating benign sonographic features. (**a**) Circumscribed uniformly hyperechoic mass. (**b**) Ellipsoid shaped solid mass with benign features. (**c**) Ellipsoid shaped solid mass with benign features

fibrous tissue; this criterion cannot be applied to masses that have areas of decreased echogenicity within other than fat lobules or ducts, or terminal lobular ductal units that are larger than 4 mm.

An *ellipsoid shape* (Fig. 4.3b) or a mass that is taller than wider refers to a sagittal and transverse diameter that is greater than the aneroposterior dimensions. A *thin echogenic capsule* (Fig. 4.3b) indicates a slow growing lesion; in order to demonstrate this finding in its entire extent, the transducer will have to be angled and studied in real time in multiple planes. *Gentle lobulations* are gently curving, smooth, and few in number (3 or less) as opposed to microlobulations that are features of a malignant mass. Since some purely intraductal cancers may have a thin echogenic capsule and a few malignant ellipsoid masses with gentle lobulations do not have a thin echogenic capsule, using these criteria in combination improves the accuracy of characterizing breast masses [5].

Description of Malignant Features [62]

Spiculation (Fig. 4.4f) is seen as alternating hyperechoic and hypoechoic lines that radiate from the surface of a mass. The appearance of these spicules is modified depending on whether hyperechoic tissue surrounds the mass. A mass that is *taller than wide* (Fig. 4.4b) is when any part of a mass is greater in its aneroposterior dimension than in its sagittal or transverse dimension, indicating that the tumor is aggressive and transgressing the normal tissue planes of the breast. *Angular margins* refer to the junction between the hypoechoic central portion of the solid mass and the surrounding tissue; this interface may be acute, obtuse, or 90°. *Branching pattern* (Fig. 4.4a) in a solid mass is akin to duct extension and refers to presence of multiple broad based projections extending from the surface of the mass. *Marked hypoechogenicity* (Fig. 4.4c) is a finding described in comparison to the surrounding tissue. *Duct extension* (Fig. 4.4d) is said to be present when there is radial extension of the tumor either within or along a duct coursing in the direction of the areola. *Posterior acoustic shadowing* (Fig. 4.4e) is considered present even when mild or present behind a small portion of the mass. *Calcifications* refer to punctate calcifications seen in a mass; these are more suggestive of a malignant process. Calcifications are more apparent when a mass is

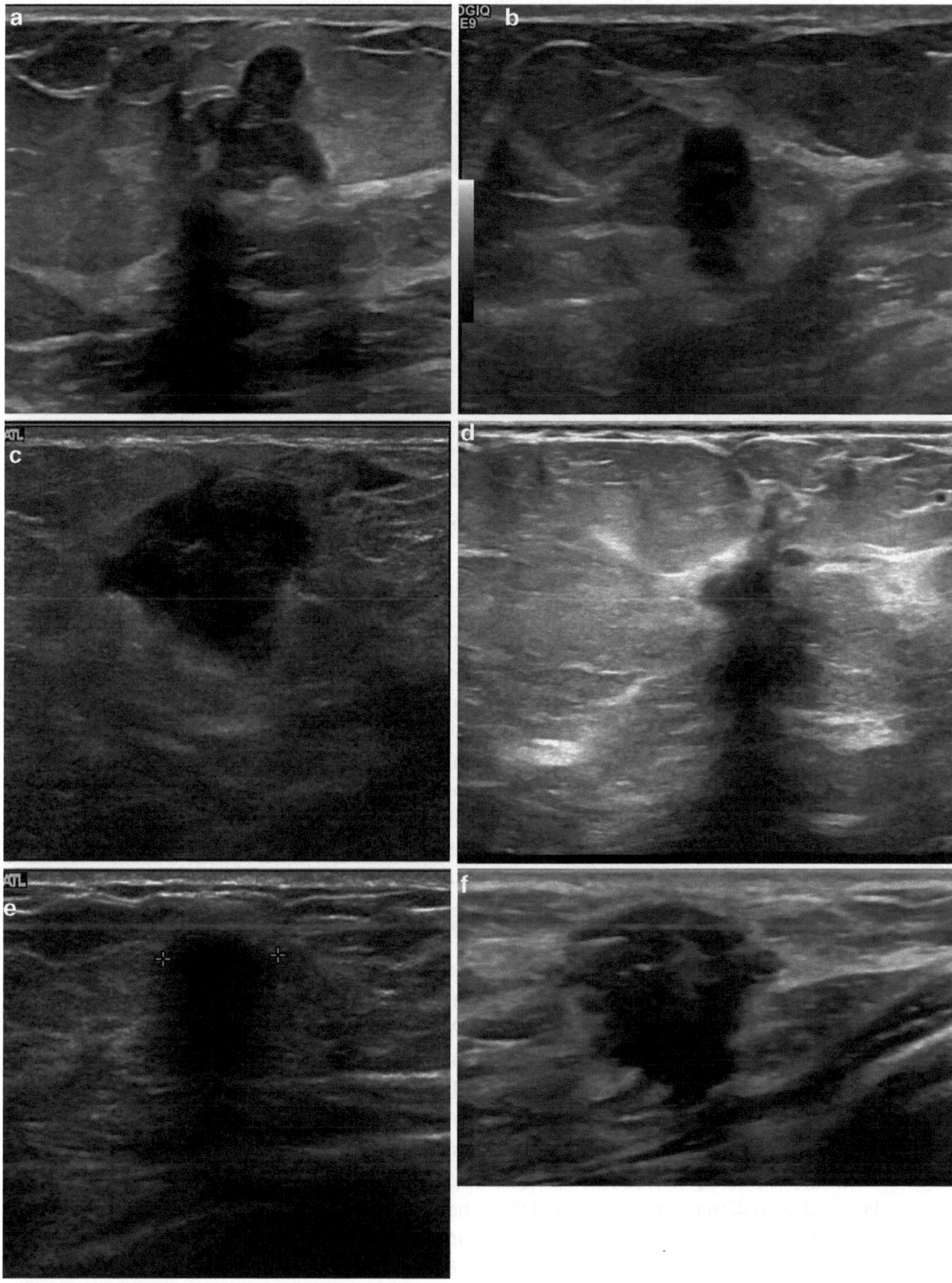

Fig. 4.4 Palpable solid masses demonstrating malignant morphological features and histologically proven to be invasive cancers at core needle biopsy. (**a**) Solid mass with a branching pattern. (**b**) Solid hypoechogenic mass that is taller than wide. (**c**) Intensely hypoechogenic mass. (**d**) A palpable mass with intraductal extension. (**e**) A solid mass with posterior acoustic shadowing. (**f**) A palpable solid mass with a spiculated margin

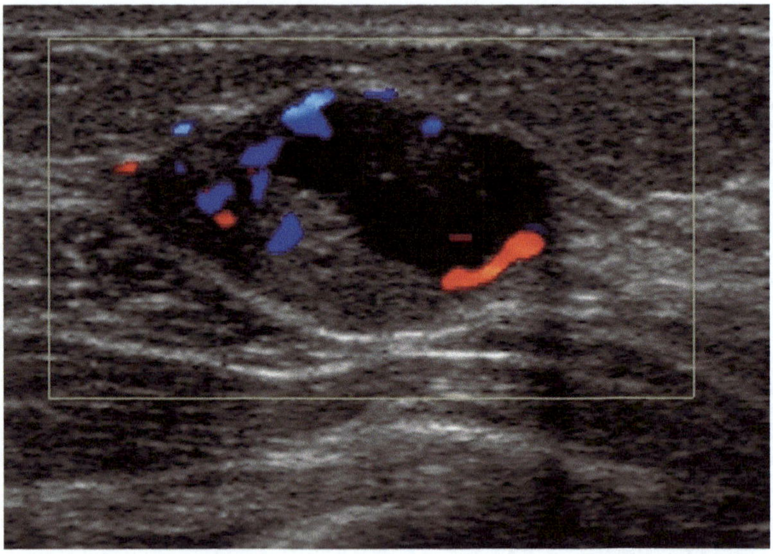

Fig. 4.5 Palpable right breast mass showing indeterminate sonographic features. US-guided core biopsy confirmed a fibroadenoma

intensely hypoechogenicity. *Microlobulations* refer to presence of 1–2 mm lobulations on the surface of a solid mass.

Using this criteria, Stavros and others, in a series of 750 solid masses, characterized 625 masses as benign (83 %) and 125 as malignant. Mammography did poorly compared with sonography in characterizing a malignant mass. Mammography did not identify 24/125 malignant masses that were correctly characterized by sonography; an additional five malignant masses were classified as probably benign based on mammographic features [62]. The high negative predictive value of sonography in excluding malignancy in a solid mass was proven in this study where only two (0.5 %) of the 426 solid masses that were characterized as benign were malignant, one of which was a metastasis from lung cancer [62]. The malignancy rate amongst masses classified as malignant was 73 %, and the cancer rate in the group considered as indeterminate was 12.3 % [62]. Others have studied the accuracy of ultrasound in being able to distinguish benign from malignant masses with similar results [65–67]. The value of sonography in diagnosing malignant palpable masses was reported in a multi institutional study of palpable masses undergoing sonography; all 293 of 616 palpable masses were correctly characterized as probably malignant by sonography [65]. In a retrospective series of 162 masses undergoing biopsy, three most reliable discriminatory features of a benign mass were round or oval shape (67/71, 94 % benign), circumscribed margins (95/104, 91 % benign), and a width to aneroposterior dimensions >1.4 (82/92, 89 %) [66]. Morphological features most suggestive of a malignant mass were an irregular shape (19/31, 61 %), width to aneroposterior ratio of <1.4 (28/70, 40 %), microlobulations (4/6, 67 %), and spiculation (2/3, 67 %). Like others, these investigators found that internal echotexture of a mass and presence of posterior acoustic enhancement does not help in the distinction between a benign or malignant mass. Uniform hyperechogenicity, although a very useful feature in characterizing a mass as benign, is not very helpful since it is a finding uncommonly encountered in a mass [66]. Some of the descriptors of a mass, such as a thin echogenic capsule, are a finding that may be subject to considerable interobserver variability [66, 67]. If the three most useful sonographic features of a benign solid mass were strictly applied, the positive biopsy ratio would potentially increase from

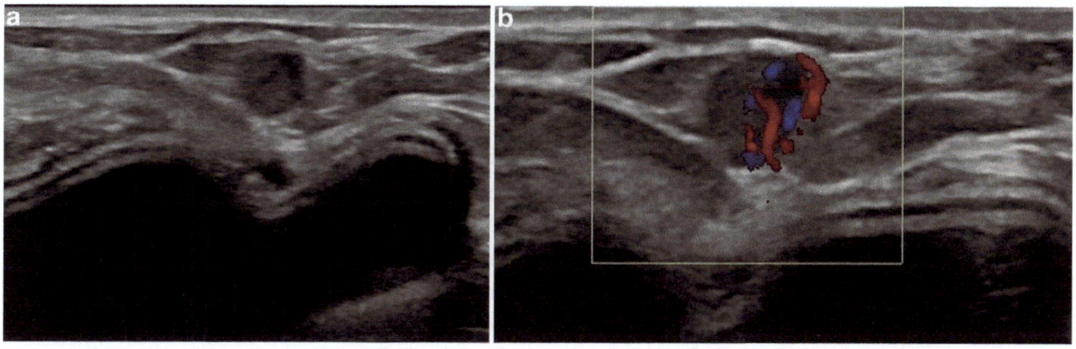

Fig. 4.6 Color Doppler imaging. (**a**) Solid palpable round mass with indeterminate morphological features in a patient with an implant. (**b**) Color Doppler imaging demonstrated rich vascularity. US-guided core biopsy confirmed an invasive ducta

23 to 39 % [66]. Using benign mass criteria of an oval or lobulated shape, circumscribed margins, internal echogenicity of isoechoic, mildly hypoechoic or hyperechoic, a mass that was wider than tall, and a non-shadowing mass or one with increased posterior echoes, 144 of 844 solid masses were categorized as benign; there was only one malignant mass in this group, indicating that biopsy avoidance is a feasible alternative when clearly benign sonographic features are demonstrated in a solid mass [66, 67].

Supplemental Tools to Real-Time Sonography to Characterize Solid Palpable Masses

Color Doppler

Neovascularization is a feature of malignant tumors, and hence color and power Doppler imaging has been proposed as a complementary tool in the evaluation of a solid breast mass [68–72].

Color Doppler imaging reflects the mean intravascular frequency shift caused by the Doppler effects of flowing red blood cells, whereas the power Doppler represents the intensities of the Doppler signals within a time period. On ultrasound images, hypervascularity (92.9 %) and presence of irregular vessels (73.2 %) are features of malignant tumors (Fig. 4.6a, b). Other associated features in a malignant mass indicative of a malignant mass are presence of rich vascularization (vessel mass ratio >10 % in 54.2 % of cases) and more than one vascular pole [69]. Typical color Doppler signs of malignancy are intratumoral vessels that are central (86 % in malignancy vs. 51 % in benignity), penetrating (65 % vs. 34 %), branching (56 % vs. 22 %), and disordered (42 % vs. 8 %). Power Doppler imaging can be used to depict a significant intratumoral increase in blood flow ($P \leq 0.0001$) compared with the flow in normal breast tissue [72]; an increased vascularity on power Doppler images in the area of a possible isoechoic nodule in fat increases confidence that the finding indicates an abnormality [73]. However, such a finding is not useful until the presence of a focal isoechoic mass is suspected. False-negative findings at B-mode US screening of the breast are not improved by using Doppler imaging [69]. Isoechoic lesions surrounded by fat can result in false-negative interpretations and a delayed diagnosis of breast cancer. Color and power Doppler imaging in combination with spatial compound imaging, tissue harmonic imaging, elastography power Doppler fremitus imaging, and contrast agent enhancement have been proposed as supplemental techniques to aid in identification of such isoechoic masses [73].

Elastography

Sonoelastography is a method that attempts to distinguish benign from malignant masses [74–76]. Tissue compression results in tissue deformation;

the extent of this deformation is measured. It is based on the premise that elasticity of a malignant tissue is harder than benign masses. Hence, malignant masses will have a greater elasticity coefficient. The color map of tissue elasticity is superimposed on the real-time greyscale ultrasound image, with each color representing a certain level of elasticity. The more commonly studied method utilizes an elasticity score that is categorized from 1 to 5; softer lesions that are likely benign have a score of 1–3, and harder masses that are more likely malignant [75]. The value of elastography is dubious, and biopsy avoidance based on findings of elastography is unlikely to be widely accepted in clinical practice. As Dempsey points out in an editorial opinion:

> We cannot, therefore, afford to continue to function in a mindset where we try at all cost to avoid doing a simple, rapid, and accurate needle biopsy by which a definite histologic diagnosis can be made. We must not attempt to substitute one or more time-consuming, physician-inefficient, costly, and often inaccurate imaging studies that, based on data currently available, accomplish nothing more than producing a needless procrastination in a timeline that should be efficiently targeted to quickly establishing a firm diagnosis from which proper patient management can be promptly initiated [77].

Follow Up of Sonographically Identified Solid Masses

To improve specificity of sonographic evaluation of solid palpable breast masses, it is imperative to characterize masses that have predominantly benign features as benign and to adopt a surveillance strategy; this is particularly important in a screening program in developing countries. The number of false-positive biopsies in such settings has to get as low as reasonably possible. In these situations where compliance is a challenge to begin with, the perception that attending such screening clinics results in excessive and/or unnecessary biopsies may threaten the success of a breast cancer screening program. However, unlike in mammography where studies have established criteria for follow up of certain findings such as circumscribed masses, grouped punctuate microcalcifications, and focal asymmetry [78], similar large prospective studies other than the one published by Stavros have not been carried out for sonographic findings. Interobserver variability has also been an issue with specific sonographic morphologic features as pointed out previously; nevertheless, several retrospective studies have established the value of utilizing sonographic morphology in classifying solid masses as benign and thereby avoiding biopsy [62, 66, 67, 79, 80]. A mass that is oval or macrolobulated, demonstrates circumscribed margins of the entire circumference, has width greater than height, and is isoechoic or mildly hypoechoic fulfills the criteria of a benign mass. Using these criteria, 445 solid, non-palpable masses were classified as probably benign and followed 2–5 years; the first follow-up was at 6 months. There was only one cancer in this group, resulting in a negative predictive value of 99.8 % [79]. A retrospective study of palpable masses also had comparable results [80]. These investigators used the criteria of round, oval, lobular masses with circumscribed margins, homogenous echo texture, and no malignant features. There were 372 solid palpable masses identified by sonography. Follow up was either clinical or imaging; an advantage of palpable masses is that they can be followed up for interval enlargement by clinical examination. There was only one cancer in the 375 solid palpable mass that was recommended for follow-up; in a 2.5 mm round hypoechoic mass that was considered a cyst or a solid mass, a 1.5 mm focus of DCIS was found surrounded by fibrocystic change. Therefore, one single false negative was likely an incidental focus of intraductal cancer. The cancer incidence, even taking into account this single case, was 0.3 % [80].

Breast Cancer Staging with Ultrasound

Breast ultrasound is a useful tool not only to diagnose breast cancer but can also be used to stage the cancer and hence can play an important role in the management of a patient diagnosed with breast cancer. Local and regional staging of breast cancer involves documentation of primary tumor size, identifying multifocality and multicentricity, and assessing regional nodal status. Multifocal disease is diagnosed when there are two cancers in one quadrant of the breast, and multicentricity is when there are two or more cancers in different quadrants of the breast [81].

Multicentricity precludes breast conservation surgery and results in mastectomy. Lymph node status is the single most important prognostic factor in a breast cancer patient and is very easily and accurately assessed by sonography. Axillary ultrasound and sonographic-guided fine needle aspiration biopsy of abnormal lymph nodes allow one to diagnose axillary nodal metastasis; in positive cases, a sentinel node biopsy is not needed and patients undergo axillary lymph node dissection. Mammography, on the other hand, images the axilla incompletely. Routine sonographic assessment of ipsilateral axillary, infraclavicular, internal mammary, and supraclavicular nodal basins is recommended [81–86].

Ultrasound-Guided Biopsy of Solid Palpable Masses

Large Core Needle Biopsy

Percutaneous biopsy under imaging guidance has nearly replaced open surgical biopsy for nonpalpable as well as palpable lesions identified during screening mammography or diagnostic sonography. This has served to minimize the harm resulting from the often touted false positive surgical procedures resulting from screening women with mammography. Presurgical localization is now performed for selected indications, such as in those patients with a biopsy proven cancer, in those who have imaging pathological discordance at core needle biopsy, in those with high risk lesions such as atypical ductal hyperplasia, radial scar, papillary lesions diagnosed at percutaneous biopsy, or where core needle biopsy is not an option or fails to provide a definitive histological diagnosis [87]. The malignant open biopsy rate has decreased from 2.04 per 1,000 women in 1996/1997 to 0.40 per 1,000 women in 2008/2009, as the nonoperative diagnosis rate for cancers has increased from 63 % to a substantial 95 % [88, 89]. Percutaneous image-guided large core needle biopsy is preferably performed under ultrasound guidance. Mammographic guidance requires a stereotactic biopsy system which can be an add-on device to existing mammography equipment. This is obviously not an option when mammography services are unavailable or limited in availability in developing countries. Apart from this reason, ultrasound-guided biopsy is quicker, is better tolerated, and is a natural choice for all abnormalities seen on a breast ultrasound examination. We recommend sonography as the preferred modality for assessing palpable abnormalities of the breast whether discovered during BSE or during CBE. For this reason, it is the optimal imaging modality for guidance. The recognized gold standard in developed countries is use of 14-guage needle with a throw or excursion of at least 2.2 cm. There have been encouraging results with use of smaller gauge needles, which may represent better choices in developing countries [90–92].

A consecutive series of US-guided core needle biopsies in 1,532 lesions had discordance in only 62 lesions; there were seven malignancies in 55 of those lesions that underwent vacuum-assisted percutaneous biopsy with larger needles. There were 12 cancers diagnosed at repeat biopsy confirmed at surgery [90]. In a consecutive series of 1,069 lesions biopsied using a 16-guage needle under ultrasound guidance, there were only 28 lesions with discordance, only six lesions were malignant, and all were diagnosed at repeat biopsy using a large 10-guage needle and using vacuum-assisted biopsy [91]. In one series of 235 lesions where a routine postfire needle tip position was confirmed in the orthogonal plane to confirm satisfactory sampling, the sensitivity of US-guided core needle biopsy using an 18-guage needle for breast cancer was 96 % (199/207 lesions) [92].

Fine Needle Aspiration Biopsy

Fine needle aspiration biopsy has been well established in the diagnosis of breast lesions. Its advantage is that it is quick, inexpensive, has minimal to no complications, and is well tolerated by patients. Its usefulness has been documented in several studies [93, 94]. Fine needle aspiration cytology (FNAC) is an established and accurate method for diagnosing breast lesions. In recent years, there has been increased use of core needle biopsy [94]. The challenges for routine use of fine needle aspiration biopsy are lack of experienced cytopathologist, availability during the procedure to check adequacy of sampling so that repeat sampling can be performed, reliable distinction of invasive from in-situ cancer, and difficulty in equating cytomorphologic features in aspirates with histologic classification system especially for benign lesions [94]. A study that looked at 4,367 FNABs for which histologic correlates were available for 1,275 lesions reported that the false positive and false negative for FNAB was 1.7 % (7/404) and 7.1 % (45/635), respectively, compared to 0 and 5.7 % for core needle biopsy. Inadequate sampling was seen in 15.1 % of lesions undergoing FNAB and was attributed to presence of collagenous lesions and to physicians inexperienced in performing FNAB [94]. Core needle biopsy is the preferred method when FNAB provides inadequate specimen for fibrotic or collagenous lesions such as lobular cancer or radial scar [94]. A meta-analysis of 46 studies was performed to assess the value of FNAB [93]. FNAB is quicker, better tolerated, and cheaper to perform than a core needle biopsy, and its results can be obtained within hours, a potentially great advantage in developing countries, particularly in rural settings or where a woman has traveled a distance to participate in a screening program. In situations where compliance may suffer if multiple clinic visits are needed, same visit results seem to be inherently advantageous. However, core needle biopsy is more robust, accurate, and reliable when compared to FNAB; the false-negative rate and the rate of insufficient samples are significantly lower. Advantages of FNAB over CNB are a lower complication rate, lower incidence of hematoma, and the rare pneumothorax. Many institutes in the USA, UK, and Canada now prefer CNB to FNAB; however, the latter still retains its use in parts of Europe and Asia [93].

The National Cancer Institute recommendation for the diagnosis of breast aspiration cytology is:

C1 = unsatisfactory
C2 = cells present all benign; no suspicious features
C3 = cells suspicious but probably benign
C4 = cells suspicious but probably malignant
C5 = definitely malignant

C3 and C4 require further testing for confirmation, and C5 can undergo surgery based on the cytology findings. The meta-analysis included 29 studies from Asia and 17 from North America and Europe. When C1 (unsatisfactory samples) was excluded, the sensitivity was 92.7 % and the specificity was 94.8 %. Unsatisfactory sample was treated as positive so that a potential breast cancer diagnosis was not delayed [93]. Underestimation rate in the unsatisfactory sample group was 27.5 %. Therefore, it is strongly recommended that unsatisfactory samples undergo either CNB or open surgical biopsy [94]. Vacuum-assisted biopsy is routinely used in the USA for stereotactic and MRI-guided breast biopsy. However, it is not widely used to biopsy lesions seen under ultrasound. All lesions that are seen under ultrasound are best biopsied under ultrasound guidance; the advantages are cost, patient comfort, procedure time, and no ionizing radiation. MRI-guided biopsy is expensive and time consuming, and is reserved for abnormalities that are identified only on MRI; a second look ultrasound is routinely performed for MRI-detected abnormalities in an attempt to substitute a preferred modality for guidance to MRI. The added sensitivity of using vacuum-assisted device is minimal and comes with significant added cost and a higher complication rate; in any case, it is not a sensible option in low resource settings. Postfire needle position verification is important and increases the yield of adequate samples during US-guided percutaneous breast biopsy. Postfire needle position is confirmed in an orthogonal plane [95]. The reported complication rate of VAB ranges from 0 to 9 % with a mean of 2.5 % [95]. The complication rate reported for core needle biopsy is as low as 0.2 % [95].

Lastly it is important to be aware of some abnormalities that are suggested based on morphological

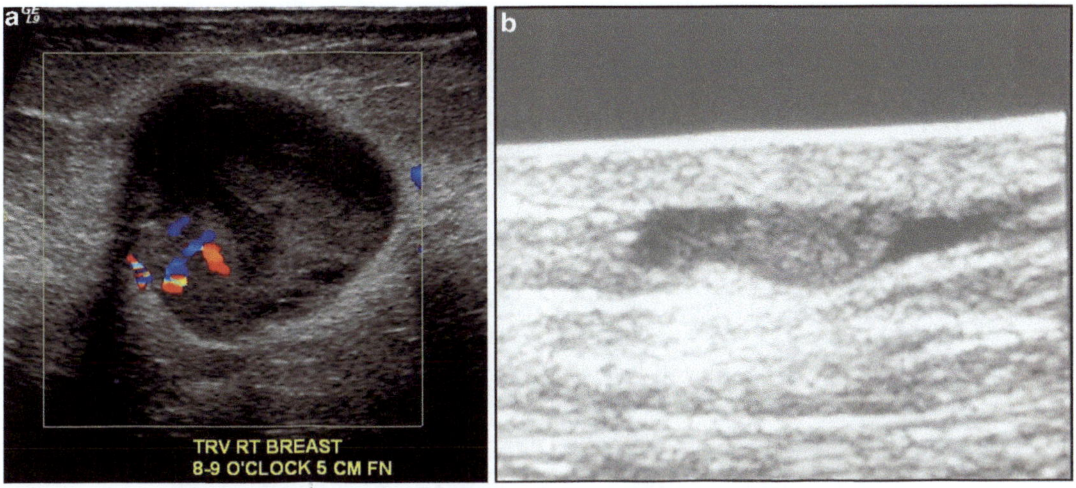

Fig. 4.7 Palpable abnormalities that are best excised surgically without percutaneous biopsy. (**a**) A cyst with a large irregular vascular mural nodule histologically proven at open surgical biopsy to be a low grade intracystic papillary cancer. (**b**) An intraductal mass histologically confirmed to be an intraductal papilloma with DCIS at open surgical biopsy. Patient presented with bloody nipple discharge

appearance that should prompt a recommendation for open surgical biopsy, bypassing core needle or fine needle aspiration biopsy (Fig. 4.7a, b). These include intraductal masses (Fig. 4.7b), intracystic masses (Fig. 4.7a) that require excision due to association of invasive cancer and a risk of underestimation of disease when sampled by needle techniques, and large tumors that may have to be excised for symptomatic relief and/or due to a risk of Phylloides tumor. In these circumstances, referral to a regional facility for surgical management is most appropriate.

Summary

In the face of increasing incidence and mortality from breast cancer, implementation of health care interventions aimed at early diagnosis are critical to reduce the disparity in mortality rates that currently exist between developed and developing countries. Screening mammography has proven benefits as shown in multiple clinical trials in reducing mortality from breast cancer. An organized screening mammography program, however, is not a feasible or cost-effective strategy in developing countries for many reasons, most importantly because of the prohibitive cost and the resources needed to set up such a program (Table 4.1). A well-organized screening mammography program requires the manpower resources of physicians skilled in reading mammography, technologists competent in obtaining satisfactory images, patient tolerance of a somewhat uncomfortable exam, relatively costly initial equipment costs, and maintenance costs for equipment. Regulatory body oversight to ensure quality in the performance and interpretation of screening studies are additional challenges in low- to mid-resource countries that are simultaneously facing competing health care priorities such as malnutrition and communicable diseases. A set up for opportunistic screening mammography with availability of diagnostic mammography, diagnostic sonography, and image-guided percutaneous biopsy including stereotactic biopsy for abnormalities such as microcalcifications or other findings that are only visible at mammography may be an option in urban areas of mid resource countries.

The aim of a breast cancer screening program will be to find a high percentage of the cancers that exist in the target population and finding these cancers while keeping false positives as low as possible. The goal should also be to find small and preferably node negative cancers (Fig. 4.8a–c),

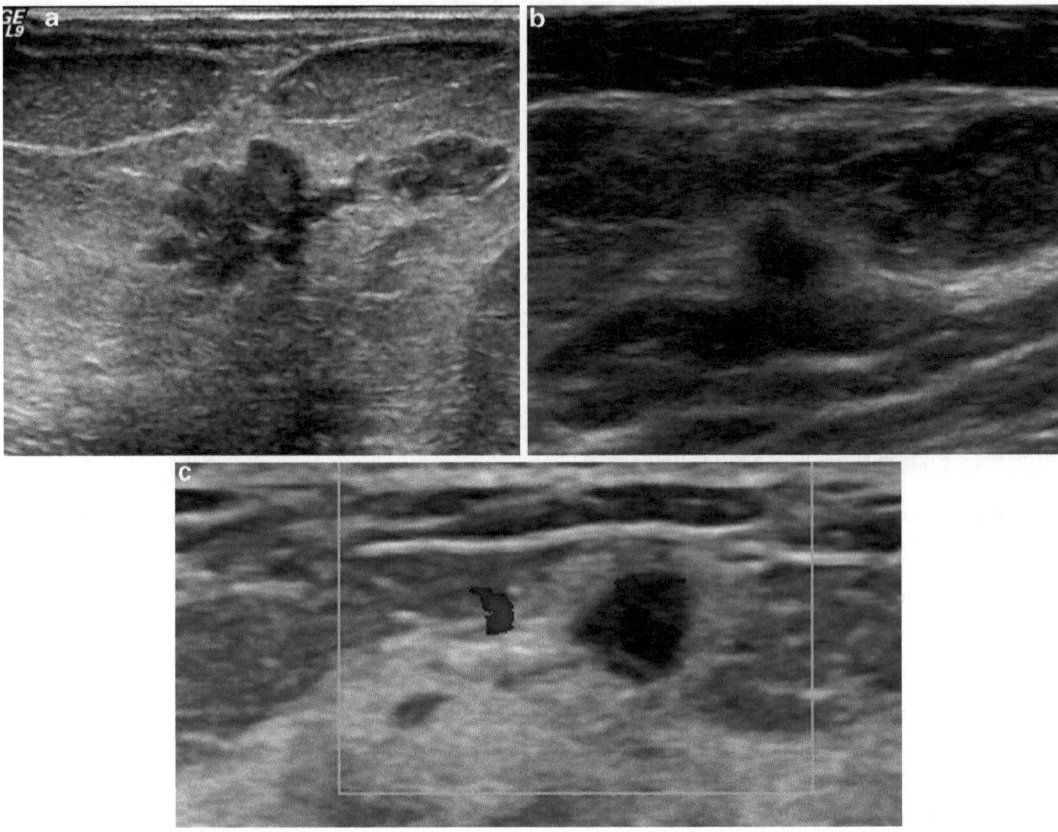

Fig. 4.8 Examples of small node negative early stage palpable breast cancers identified on ultrasound. (**a**) Intraductal mass seen on ultrasound of a palpable mass histologically proven to be DCIS. (**b**) Small irregular mass with malignant sonographic features histologically confirmed to be an invasive ductal cancer. (**c**) Small spiculated mass with malignant features confirmed to be an invasive cancer by a US-guided core needle biopsy

although, without use of high quality mammography and skilled mammography physicians, this may be a difficult goal; downstaging cancers from the now prevalent Stage 3 and Stage 4 to a Stage 1B to Stage 2 cancers may be feasible. This by itself is expected to make a significant difference in mortality and morbidity.

For the majority of women in developing countries, particularly those residing in rural areas, and for programs that are government funded, a modified triple assessment approach as outlined (Fig. 4.9) consisting of a high quality CBE by health care workers who have received formal training in performing breast examination; this is most practical. Such a screening examination in women aged 40–64 years performed on an annual basis is recommended. In those with a palpable abnormality, a focused breast ultrasound should be performed. Diagnostic mammography is not a feasible method of evaluating a palpable abnormality in low resource settings for many reasons described earlier. Substituting ultrasound has several advantages including less cost, better triaging of palpable abnormalities to determine the need for tissue sampling, and a superior method of guidance for biopsy of solid palpable masses. Core needle biopsy of such masses during a single visit ensures better patient compliance. Ultrasound is helpful in significantly reducing the need to biopsy of a significant number of benign abnormalities that account for palpable lumps. Judicious use of ultrasound has a potential to have an acceptable positive biopsy rate. Comprehensive training of physicians and health care workers performing

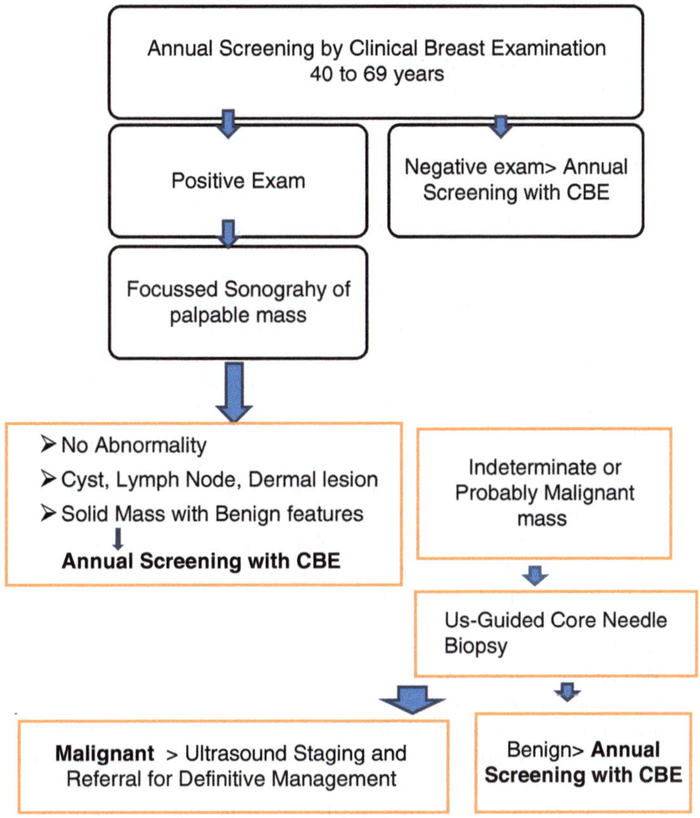

Fig. 4.9 Algorithm of proposed breast cancer screening strategy

this ultrasound and providing telemedicine support as needed will be key to the success of this modified triple assessment approach. Such an approach will, however, have to be validated through rigorous large observational studies; RCTs, although ideal to prove benefit of mortality reduction, may not be feasible. RCTs have been traditionally considered the gold standard; observational studies have also been shown to perform well in testing efficacy of a certain intervention in a population [96].

References

1. World Health Organization. Screening for various cancers. http://www.who.int/cancer/detection/variouscancer/en/index.html.
2. Forouzanfar MH, Foreman KJ, Delossantos AM, Lozano R, Lopez AD, Murray CJ, et al. Breast and cervical cancer in 187 countries between 1980 and 2010: a systematic analysis. Lancet. 2011;378(9801):1461–84.
3. Panieri E. Breast cancer screening in developing countries. Best Pract Res Clin Obstet Gynaecol. 2012;26(2):283–90.
4. The Breast Health Global Initiative (BHGI) resource stratified matrix guidelines. Breast J. 2006;12 (Suppl 1):S117–20.
5. Last JM. A dictionary of epidemiology. New York, NY: Oxford University Press; 1995. p. 52.
6. Tabár L, Fagerberg CJG, Gad A, et al. Reduction in mortality from breast cancer after mass screening with mammography: randomized trial from the breast cancer screening working group of the Swedish national board of health and welfare. Lancet. 1985;1:829–32.
7. Tabar L, Fagerberg G, Chen HH, et al. Efficacy of breast cancer screening by age. New results from the Swedish two county trials. Cancer. 1995;75:2507–17.
8. Fletcher SW, Elmore JG. Clinical practice: mammographic screening for breast cancer. N Engl J Med. 2003;348:1672–80.
9. Tabar L, Vitak B, Chen H-H, Yen MF, Duffy SW, Smith RA. Beyond randomized controlled trials: organized mammographic screening substantially reduces breast carcinoma mortality. Cancer. 2001;91(9):1724–31.
10. Carney PA, Miglioretti DL, Yankaskas BC, et al. Individual and combined effects of age, breast density, and hormone replacement therapy use on the

accuracy of mammography. Ann Intern Med. 2003;138:168–75.
11. Perry N, Broeders M, Wolf CD, Tornberg S, Holland R, Karsa LV. European guidelines for quality assurance in breast cancer screening and diagnosis. Fourth edition-summary document. Ann Oncol. 2008;19:614–22.
12. Lee CH, Dershaw DD, Kopans D, Evans P, Monsees B, Monticciolo D, et al. Breast cancer screening with imaging: recommendations from the society of breast imaging and the ACR on the use of mammography, breast MRI, breast ultrasound, and other technologies for the detection of clinically occult breast cancer. J Am Coll Radiol. 2010;7:18–27.
13. Elmore JG, Armstrong K, Lehman CD, Fletcher SW. Screening for breast cancer. JAMA. 2005;293(10):1245–56.
14. Humphrey LL, Helfand M, Chan BKS, Woolf SH. Breast cancer screening: a summary of the evidence. Ann Intern Med. 2002;137:347–60.
15. Larsson LG, Andersson I, Bjurstam N, Fagerberg G, Frisell J, Tabár L, et al. Updated overview of the Swedish randomized trials on breast cancer screening with mammography: age group 40–49 at randomization. J Natl Cancer Inst Monogr. 1997;22:57–61.
16. Malmgren J, Parikh JA, Atwood MK, Kaplan HJ. Impact of mammography detection on the course of breast cancer in women aged 40–49 years. Radiology. 2012;262(3):797–806.
17. Kerlikowske K, Grady D, Barclay J, Sickles EA, Eaton A, Ernster V. Positive predictive value of screening mammography by age and family history of breast cancer. JAMA. 1993;270(20):2444–50.
18. Woloshin S, Schwartz LM. The benefits and harms of mammography screening. Understanding the trade-offs. JAMA. 2010;303(2):164–5.
19. Berg WA. Benefits of screening mammography. JAMA. 2010;303(2):168–9.
20. Geller BM, Bogart A, Carney PA, Elmore JG, Monsees BS, Miglioretti DL. Is confidence of mammographic assessment a good predictor of accuracy? AJR Am J Roentgenol. 2012;199(1):W134–41.
21. Mammography Quality Standards Act of 1992. Mammography facilities requirement for accrediting bodies, and quality standards and certifying requirements: interim rules (21 CFR 900). December 21 1993; 58:57558–72. http://www.fda.gov/Radiation-Emitting Products/MammographyQualityStandards ActandProgram/Regulations/ucm110906.htm.
22. Carney PA, Sickles EA, Monsees BA, Bassett LA, et al. Identifying minimally acceptable interpretive performance criteria for screening mammography. Radiology. 2010;255(2):354–61.
23. Smith-Bindman R, Chu PW, Miglioretti DL, et al. Comparison of screening mammography in the United States and the United Kingdom. JAMA. 2003;290:2129–37.
24. D'Orsi CJ, Bassett LW, Feig SA, et al. Breast imaging reporting and data system. 3rd ed. Reston, VA: American College of Radiology; 1998.
25. Burnside ES, Sickles EA, Sohlich RE, Dee KE. Differential value of comparison with previous examination in diagnostic versus screening mammography. AJR Am J Roentgenol. 2002;179(5):1173–7.
26. Sickles EA, Wolverton DE, Dee KE. Performance parameters for screening and diagnostic mammography: specialist and general radiologists. Radiology. 2002;224(3):861–9.
27. National Cancer Institute. Breast Cancer Surveillance Consortium: evaluating screening performance in practice. NIH Publication No. 04-5490. Bethesda, MD: National Cancer Institute, National Institutes of Health, U.S. Department of Health and Human Services, April 2004. Available at http://breastscreening.cancer.gov/espp.pdf.
28. Esserman L, Cowley H, Eberle C, Kirkpatrick A, Chang S, Berbaum K, et al. Improving the accuracy of mammography: volume and outcome relationships. J Natl Cancer Inst. 2002;94(5):369–75.
29. Elmore JG, Carney PA. Does practice make perfect when interpreting mammography? J Natl Cancer Inst. 2002;94(5):321–3.
30. Buist DS, Anderson ML, Haneuse SJ, et al. Influence of annual interpretive volume on screening mammography performance in the United States. Radiology. 2011;259(1):72–84.
31. Pisano ED, Gatsonis C, Hendrick E, et al. Diagnostic performance of digital versus film mammography for breast-cancer screening. N Engl J Med. 2005;353(17):1773–83.
32. Hoff SR, Abrahamsen A-L, Samset JH, Vigeland E, Klepp O, Hofvind S. Breast cancer: missed interval and screening-detected cancer at full-field digital mammography and screen-film mammography—results from a retrospective review. Radiology. 2012;264:378–86.
33. Meissner HI, Breen N, Yabroff KR. Whatever happened to clinical breast examination. Am J Prev Med. 2003;25(3):259–63.
34. Weiss NS. Breast cancer mortality in relation to clinical breast examination and breast self examination. Breast J. 2003;9 Suppl 2:S86–9.
35. Barton MB, Harris R, Fletcher SW. Does this patient have breast cancer? The screening clinical breast examination: should it be done? How? JAMA. 1999;282:1270–80.
36. Miller AB, To T, Baines CJ, Wall C. Canadian National Breast Screening Study-2: 13-year results of a randomized trial in women aged 50–59 years. J Natl Cancer Inst. 2000;92:1490–9.
37. Okonkwo QL, Draisma G, Kinderen AD, et al. Breast cancer screening policies in developing countries: a cost effectiveness analysis for India. J Natl Cancer Inst. 2008;100:1290–300.
38. Kearney AJ, Murray M. Breast cancer screening recommendations: is mammography the only answer? J Midwifery Womens Health. 2009;54:393–400.
39. O'Malley MS, Fletcher SW. US Preventive Services Task Force. Screening for breast cancer with breast

self-examination: a critical review. JAMA. 1987;257: 2196–203.
40. Thomas DB, Gao DL, Ray RM, et al. Randomized trial of breast self-examination in Shanghai: final results. J Natl Cancer Inst. 2002;94:1445–57.
41. Semiglazov VF, et al. Study of the role of breast self-examination in the reduction of mortality from breast cancer. Eur J Cancer. 1993;29A:2039–46.
42. Miller AB, Bianes CJ. The role of clinical breast examination and breast self-examination. Prev Med. 2011;53:118–20.
43. Harvey BJ, et al. Effect of breast self-examination techniques on the risk of death from breast cancer. CMAJ. 1997;157(9):1205–12.
44. Gastrin G, et al. Incidence and mortality from breast cancer in the Mama program for breast screening in Finland, 1973–1986. Cancer. 1994;73:2168–74.c. J. 157, 1205–12.
45. Harford JB, Otero IV, Anderson BO, Cazap E, et al. Problem solving for breast health care delivery in low and middle resource countries (LMCs): consensus statement from the Breast Health Global Initiative. Breast. 2011;20 Suppl 2:S20–9.
46. Nandakumar A, Gupta PC, Gangadhara P, et al. Geographic pathology revisited: development of an atlas of cancer in India. Int J Cancer. 2005;116:740–54.
47. Dhillon PK, Yeole BB, Dikshit R, Kurkure AP, Bray F. Trends in breast, ovarian and cervical cancer incidence in Mumbai, India over a 30-year period, 1976–2005: an age–period–cohort analysis. Br J Cancer. 2011;105:723–30.
48. Anderson BO, Cazap E, El Saghir NS, et al. Optimization of breast cancer management in low-resource and middle-resource countries: executive summary of the Breast Health Global Initiative consensus, 2010. Lancet Oncol. 2011;12(4):387–98.
49. Shetty MK. Screening and diagnosis of breast cancer in low-resource countries: what is state of the art? Semin Ultrasound CT MR. 2011;32(4):300–5.
50. Shetty MK, Longatto-Filho A. Early detection of breast, cervical, ovarian and endometrial cancers in low resource countries: an integrated approach. Indian J Surg Oncol. 2011;2(3):165–71.
51. Coveney EC, Geraghty JG, O'Laoide R, Hourihane JB, O'Higgins NJ. Reasons underlying negative mammography in patients with palpable breast cancer. Clin Radiol. 1994;49:123–5.
52. Blamey RW. The British Association of Surgical Oncology Guidelines for surgeons in the management of symptomatic breast disease in the UK (1998 revision). BASO Breast Specialty Group. Eur J Surg Oncol. 1998;24(6):464–76.
53. Cytology Sub-group of the National Co-ordinating Committee for breast screening pathology. Guidelines for cytology procedures and reporting in breast cancer screening. NHSBSP 1993;No 22.
54. Chuo CB, Corder AP. Core biopsy vs fine needle aspiration cytology in a symptomatic breast clinic. Eur J Surg Oncol. 2003;29(4):374–8.
55. Marilin M, Mohammadi A, Masood S. The value of fine needle aspiration biopsy in the diagnosis and prognostic assessment of palpable breast lesions. Diagn Cytopathol. 2012;40(1):26–34.
56. Ariga R, Bloom K, Reddy VB, Kluskens L, et al. Fine needle aspiration of clinically suspicious palpable breast masses with histopathologic correlation. Am J Surg. 2002;184(5):410–3.
57. Bulgaresi P, Cariaggi P, Ciatto S, Houssami N. Positive predictive value of breast fine needle aspiration cytology (FNAC) in combination with clinical and imaging findings: a series of 2334 subjects with abnormal cytology. Breast Cancer Res Treat. 2006; 97:319–21.
58. Shetty MK, Shah YP, Sharman RS. Prospective evaluation of the value of combined mammographic and sonographic assessment in patients with palpable abnormalities of the breast. J Ultrasound Med. 2003; 22(3):263–8.
59. Barton MB, Elmore JG, Fletcher SW. Breast symptoms among women enrolled in a health maintenance organization: frequency, evaluation, and outcome. Ann Intern Med. 1999;130:651–7.
60. Morrow M, Wong S, Venta L. The evaluation of breast masses in women younger than forty years of age. Surgery. 1998;124:634–40.
61. Harvey JA. Sonography of palpable breast masses. Semin Ultrasound CT MR. 2006;27:284–97.
62. Stavros AT, Thickman D, Rapp CL, Dennis MA, Parker H, Sisney GA. Solid breast nodules: use of sonography to distinguish between benign and malignant lesions. Radiology. 1995;196:123–34.
63. Shetty MK, Watson AW. Mondor's disease of the breast: sonographic and mammographic findings. AJR Am J Roentgenol. 2001;177(4):893–6.
64. Hilton SW, Leopold GR, Olson LK, Wilson SA. Real-time breast sonography: application in 300 consecutive patients. AJR Am J Roentgenol. 1986;147: 479–86.
65. Georgian-Smith D, Taylor KJW, Madjar H, et al. Sonography of palpable breast cancer. J Clin Ultrasound. 2000;28:211–6.
66. Mainiero MB, Goldkamp A, Lazarus E. Characterization of breast masses with sonography can biopsy of some solid masses be deferred? J Ultrasound Med. 2005;24(2):161–7.
67. Rahbar G, Sie AC, Hansen GC, et al. Benign versus malignant solid breast masses: US differentiation. Radiology. 1999;213:889–94.
68. Srivastava A, Hughes LE, Woodcock JP, Laidler P. Vascularity in cutaneous melanoma detected by Doppler sonography and histology: correlation with tumour behaviour. Br J Cancer. 1989;59(1):89–91.
69. Schroeder RJ, Bostanjoglo M, Rademaker J, Maeurer J, Felix R. Role of power Doppler techniques and ultrasound contrast enhancement in the differential diagnosis of focal breast lesions. Eur Radiol. 2003;13(1):68–79.
70. Giuseppetti GM, Baldassarre S, Marconi E. Color Doppler sonography. Eur J Radiol. 1998;27 Suppl 2:S254–8.
71. Kook SH, Park HW, Lee YR, Lee YU, Pae WK, Park YL. Evaluation of solid breast lesions with

power Doppler sonography. J Clin Ultrasound. 1999;27(5):231–7.
72. Milz P, Lienemann A, Kessler M, Reiser M. Evaluation of breast lesions by power Doppler sonography. Eur Radiol. 2001;11(4):547–54.
73. Kim MJ, Kim JY, Yoon JH, Youk JH, Moon HJ, Son EJ, et al. How to find an isoechoic lesion with breast US. Radiographics. 2011;31(3):663–76.
74. Zhao QL, Ruan LT, Zhang H, Yin YM, Duan SX. Diagnosis of solid breast lesions by elastography 5-point score and strain ratio method. Eur J Radiol. 2012;81(11):3245–9.
75. Thitaikumar A, Ophir J. Effect of lesion boundary conditions on axial strain pp elastograms: a parametric study. Ultrasound Med Biol. 2007;33(9):1463–7.
76. Itoh A, Ueno E, Tohno E, et al. Breast disease: clinical application of US elastography for diagnosis. Radiology. 2006;239(2):341–50.
77. Dempsey PJ. New ultrasound-based imaging technologies are claimed to avoid unnecessary breast biopsies, but what is an "unnecessary" image-guided needle biopsy of the breast? J Clin Ultrasound. 2010;38(3):111–2.
78. Sickles EA. Periodic mammographic follow-up of probably benign lesions: results in 3184 consecutive cases. Radiology. 1991;179:463–8.
79. Graf O, Helbich TH, Hopf G, Graf C, Sickles EA. Probably benign breast masses at US: is follow-up an acceptable alternative to biopsy? Radiology. 2007; 244(1):87–93.
80. Harvey JA, Nicholson BT, Lorusso AP, Cohen MA, Bovbjerg VE. Short-term follow-up of palpable breast lesions with benign imaging features: evaluation of 375 lesions in 320 women. AJR Am J Roentgenol. 2009;193:1723–30.
81. Yang WT. Staging of breast cancer with ultrasound. Semin Ultrasound CT MR. 2011;32:331–41.
82. Fisher B. Sounding board. Breast-cancer management: alternatives to radical mastectomy. N Engl J Med. 1979;301:326–8.
83. Holland R, Veling SH, Mravunac M, et al. Histologic multifocality of Tis, T1-2 breast carcinomas. Implications for clinical trials of breastconserving surgery. Cancer. 1985;56:979–90.
84. Lagios MD, Westdahl PR, Rose MR. The concept and implications of multicentricity in breast carcinoma. Pathol Annu. 1981;16:83–102.
85. Berg WA, Gilbreath PL. Multicentric and multifocal cancer: wholebreast US in preoperative evaluation. Radiology. 2000;214:59–66.
86. Shen J, Hunt KK, Mirza NQ, et al. Intramammary lymph node metastases are an independent predictor of poor outcome in patients with breast carcinoma. Cancer. 2004;101:1330–7.
87. Shetty MK. Presurgical localization of breast abnormalities: an overview and analysis of 202 cases. Indian J Surg Oncol. 2010;1(4):278–83.
88. O'Flynn EA, Wilson AR, Michell MJ. Image-guided breast biopsy: state-of-the-art. Clin Radiol. 2010;65: 259–70.
89. NHS. http://www.cancerscreening.nhs.uk/breastscreen/publications/baso2008-2009.pdf. Accessed 3 July 2012.
90. Wang ZL, Liu G, Li JL, Su L, Liu XJ, Wang W, et al. Breast lesions with imaging-histologic discordance during 16-gauge core needle biopsy system: would vacuum-assisted removal get significantly more definitive histologic diagnosis than vacuum-assisted biopsy? Breast J. 2011;17(5):456–61.
91. Li JL, Wang ZL, Su L, Liu XJ, Tang J. Breast lesions with ultrasound imaging-histologic discordance at 16-gauge core needle biopsy: can re-biopsy with 10-gauge vacuum-assisted system get definitive diagnosis? Breast. 2010;19(6):446–9.
92. Uematsu T, Kasami M, Uchida Y, et al. Ultrasonographically guided 18-gauge automated core needle breast biopsy with post-fire needle position verification (PNPV). Breast Cancer. 2007;14(2): 219–28.
93. Yu Y-H, Wei W, Liu JL. Diagnostic value of fine-needle aspiration biopsy for breast mass: a systematic review and meta-analysis. BMC Cancer. 2012;12(4): 1–14.
94. Berner A, Davidson B, Sigstad E, Risberg B. Fine-needle aspiration cytology vs. core biopsy in the diagnosis of breast lesions. Diagn Cytopathol. 2003;29(6): 344–8.
95. Uematsu T. How to choose needles and probes for ultrasonographically guided percutaneous breast biopsy: a systematic approach. Breast Cancer. 2012; 19:238–41.
96. Concato J, Shah N, Horwitz RI. Randomized, controlled trials, observational studies, and the hierarchy of research designs. N Engl J Med. 2000;342(25): 1887–92.

HPV and Cervical Cancer

5

Laura Sichero and Luisa Lina Villa

Abstract

About 15% of all human cancers are caused by viruses; human papillomaviruses (HPV) only are responsible for at least 5% of tumors worldwide. All cervical cancers can be linked to high-risk HPV infections which accounts for about 10% of female cancers in developing countries. Moreover a significant proportion of cancers arising in other anatomical locations are attributed to HPV. The transformation mechanism of certain HPVs is attributed to the pleiotropic effects of two viral oncoproteins, E6 and E7, the continuous expression of which is required for cell transformation. These proteins prevent keratinocytes senescence and can extend their life span and block terminal differentiation promoting the accumulation of mitotic defects, genomic instability, and neoplasia. Tumors arise several years after exposure to the virus which is a clear indication that other factors operate during different stages of tumor development, which include in large proportion the immune responses affecting both the virus and the infected individual. The very high negative predictive value of HPV testing speaks in favor of its use in screening of cervical cancer to reduce the mortality related to this neoplasia particularly in developing countries.

Abbreviations

BPV	Bovine papillomavirus
CIN	Cervical intraepithelial neoplasia
DNA	Deoxyribonucleic acid
EGFR	Epidermal growth factor receptor
HDAC	Histone deacetylase
HPV	Human papillomavirus
LCR	Long control region
MHC	Major histocompatibility complex

L. Sichero (✉) • L.L. Villa
Molecular Biology Laboratory, Center for Translational Oncology, Cancer Institute of São Paulo, Av Dr Arnaldo, 251, andar 8, São Paulo 01246-090, Brazil
e-mail: laura.sichero@icesp.org.br; llvilla@incthpv.org.br

M.K. Shetty (ed.), *Breast and Gynecological Cancers: An Integrated Approach for Screening and Early Diagnosis in Developing Countries*, DOI 10.1007/978-1-4614-1876-4_5,

mRNA	Messenger ribonucleic acid
PV	Papillomavirus
VLP	Virus-like particles
WHO	World Health Organization

Introduction

Cervical cancer is the second most common cancer among women worldwide. According to the World Health Organization (WHO) statistics, there are approximately 500,000 new cases registered each year out of which 250,000 cases are fatal. Cervical cancer remains a significant problem particularly in underdeveloped and developing countries in which about 80% of the cases occur. The highest rates of incidence of this neoplasia are observed in South America, Africa, and South Asia [1]. On the other hand, screening programs have significantly reduced the incidence of disease in developed countries over the past 50 years [2].

According to a recent meta-analysis that included data from more than 1,000,000 women worldwide, genital HPV prevalence among cytologically normal cervical smears is about 10%, ranging from 1.6 to 41.9% [3]. In addition, among women diagnosed with cervical intraepithelial neoplasia (CIN), HPV prevalence varies from 50 to 90% and from 80 to 99% among those with cervical tumors [4, 5]. Overall, higher HPV prevalence is observed in Africa and South America and is lowest in Europe and intermediate in Asia. Concerning female age-specific prevalence of HPV, several studies reported a peak at younger ages (25 years) shortly after sexual initiation for most women, generally attributed to higher levels of sexual activity with multiple partners and low viral immunity [6, 7]. In some populations, age-specific prevalence declines sharply and achieves very small levels at older ages. In other populations such as those in India and sub-Saharan Africa, HPV prevalence remains almost unaltered across ages [8]. Additionally, in the Americas, Africa, and Europe, an apparent second peak of HPV infection among women aged 45 years and older is observed, which could possibly be attributed to hormonal changes preceding menopause, changes in male/female sexual behavior, or even higher rates of HPV persistence at older ages [3, 9].

The relative risk of developing cervical cancer in patients with high-risk HPV persistent infection is on average 50-fold higher as compared to HPV negative women [10]. Among all HPV types that infect the anogenital tract, HPV-16 is the most prevalent worldwide [11]. HPV-16 occurs in 30% of cytologically normal HPV-positive samples and in 50–90% of HPV-positive tumors [12]. The detection of HPV-18 ranges from 10 to 20% of cervical cancers samples. On the other hand, there is wide variation in the prevalence of the lesser prevalent HPV types throughout the world [6]. Types 6, 11, 59, 68, 73, and 82 are consistently rare across cervical cancer studies [13]. The incidence of high-risk HPV infections is higher comparing to low-risk types [14, 15].

Variation of HPV prevalence within each histological category may be an effect of different methodologies used for detecting and typing viral DNA, including the use of different primers in PCR reactions and cohort effects, in addition to cytological misclassification and/or errors during collection of cervical specimens. Nevertheless, studies conducted in different countries but using identical methodologies pointed out variations in HPV infection prevalence, suggesting that this discrepancy can be further influenced by the sexual behavior intrinsic of each population [16]. For instance, the prevalence of HPV DNA in men and women was shown to be five times higher in Colombia than in Spain, consistent with the incidence of cervical cancer in these countries [17].

Papillomavirus (PV) represents a heterogeneous group of viruses. To date, over 150 different HPV types have been described, of which about 40 infect the anogenital region [18]. Viral types associated with the development of malignant lesions are classified as high risk or oncogenic. Since 1995, the International Agency for Cancer Research of the WHO concluded that there is sufficient biological and epidemiological evidence to classify HPVs 16 and 18 as carcinogens type I, i.e., carcinogenic in humans. More recently, HPVs 31, 33, 35, 39, 45, 51, 52, 56, 58, 59, and 66 were further included in this group [10].

Cervical Cancer Etiology

Since the early 1970s, a link between HPV infection and the development of neoplastic lesions was observed [19]. In humans, papillomavirus infections cause several benign proliferations including warts or papillomas, intraepithelial lesions in the anogenital area, and papillomas and carcinomas in diverse head and neck anatomical subsites.

Several observations pointed to the etiological involvement of HPV in the development of cervical carcinoma:

1. Constitutive expression of E6 and E7 viral oncoproteins is detected in malignant cells
2. E6 and E7 expression stimulates cellular immortalization, uncontrolled cell proliferation, and chromosomal instability
3. Inhibition of E6 and E7 expression in cervical carcinoma cell lines induces cell proliferation arrest, following reversal of the malignant phenotype
4. Virtually all cervical cancers test positive for HPV DNA

Altogether, high-risk HPVs are classified as type I carcinogens: the attributable risk of HPV for cervical cancer is much higher than smoking is for lung cancer [20].

Epidemiological and case–control studies further pointed towards the strong association between infection by some HPV types and the development of genital warts and cervical cancer. The importance of this observation is highlighted by the 2008 Nobel Prize awarded to Prof. Harald zur Hausen for his discovery that high-risk HPVs are the causative agents of cervical cancer. Currently, the WHO considers that there is sufficient experimental and epidemiological evidence to consider 13 HPV types as the main etiological agents of cervical cancer. HPVs affecting the anogenital region are derived from five species:

- α-5 (HPVs 26, 51, 69, and 82)
- α-6 (HPVs 53, 30, and 56)
- α-7 (HPVs 18, 39, 45, 59, 68, and 70)
- α-9 (HPVs 16, 31, 33, 35, 52, 58, and 67)
- α-10 (HPVs 6, 11, 13, 44, and 74) [18]

Low-risk HPV types are strongly associated with benign proliferations such as common warts and condilomas, while high-risk HPV types are strongly associated with the development of high-grade intraepithelial lesions and cervical carcinoma [5, 6, 21]. The prevalence of each type differs with the severity of the injury; for example, the incidence of HPVs 16 and 18 gradually increases with the progression to invasive carcinoma [6].

HPV Transmission

Infection with genital HPV types is considered the most commonly diagnosed sexually transmitted disease [17, 22]. Most individuals (~75%) who engage in sexual activity will become infected with HPV at least once during their lifetime [23].

Anogenital HPV infections are primarily transmitted by sexual contact in both genders [24]. It is believed that HPV infections are easily transmitted through microscopic traumas in the mucosa or skin occurring during sexual intercourse. Therefore, markers of sexual activity such as age at first debut and high number of recent/lifetime sexual partners are strongly associated with sexual behavior of affected individuals [25]. In addition to peno-vaginal contact, HPV is also transmitted by other sexual practices, including peno-anal intercourse, oral sex, and digital-vaginal sex [26]. HPV DNA is rarely detected among adolescents without sexual experience. Presence of preexisting HPV infection(s) is also associated with higher risk of acquiring another HPV type [27] in addition to multiparity, extensive use of oral contraceptive, tobacco use, and history of having sexually transmitted diseases [28]. Male partner sexual behavior significantly increases the risk, whereas circumcision was related to reduction in risk of HPV infection [29]. It was further shown that condom use is not fully protective against the transference of HPV infection. Some studies found high agreement of type-specific concordance between genital HPV infections in heterosexual couples; however, most verified a comparatively poor correlation between HPV-positivity and types among cervical and penile samples [17, 30].

The nonsexual mode of transmission of genital HPVs is also observed, although at lower rates. Vertical transmission resulting in juvenile respiratory papillomatosis [31] and horizontal transmission of low-risk HPV to the vulva and vagina using fingers [10], tampons, and non-penetrative intercourse have been described. It was observed that the risk of infection by high-risk HPVs is associated with sexual variables, whereas risk of infection by low-risk HPVs types is predominantly associated with sociodemographic and hygiene variables [32].

Natural History of HPV Infections

Most HPV infections do not lead to the development of cervical lesions and may be eliminated by the immune system in a short period of time, usually within 6 months. Clearance of an HPV type leaves the individual partially immune to that genotype [33]. Severe alterations in the immune system result in higher prevalence of clinically apparent HPV infections [34]. In fact, HIV-induced immunosuppression impairs cell-mediated immune control of HPV infections [35].

Cervical cancer arises following distinct and sequential steps: acute infection with high-risk HPV type(s), followed by detectable viral persistence (rather than clearance) linked to the development of cervical precancerous lesions, and eventually invasion. Most HPV infections are transient, and viral clearance occurs spontaneously without ever causing lesions. However, a small proportion of HPV infections, particularly with high-risk HPV types, may take longer, between 12 and 24 months, to clear [2]. Nevertheless, a small number of women develop persistent HPV infections and these can last for years. Although there is no consensus concerning the length of time that implies persistence, this is usually defined as the detection of the same HPV type (or, with a higher degree of assurance, the same intratypic variant) two or more times over a certain period of time. Persistence is more prevalent among women over 30 years and among women infected with high-risk HPV [10, 36]. Data from cohort studies indicate that the mean length of infection is between 4 and 20 months, with HR-HPV types lasting longer than LR-HPV infections [15, 36, 37].

Women persistently infected are at greater risk of developing cervical cancer compared to individuals with transient infection and women without infection [37–39]. Viral persistence thus presents as a decisive event in HPV-induced cervical carcinogenesis, and diverse studies confirm that risk of CIN and invasive cervical cancer is strongly associated with continuous detection of HPV DNA.

About half of the women infected with HPV do not develop detectable antibodies in the serum and harbor risk of reinfection with the same HPV type. Failure of the immune system to clear persistent HPV infections can lead to the development of cervical cancer after several decades [10]. Further, regarding HPV natural history, the extent to which viral infections are cleared remains a major unresolved question [40]. Although the term "clearance" is applied when an HPV infection is undetectable using sensitive test methods, HPV may not be completely eliminated [41].

HPV natural history studies have shown that time between high-risk oncogenic HPV infection and the development of CIN, carcinoma in situ, and invasive cancer is relatively long [42]. CIN has a peak incidence between 25 and 35 years of age, whereas the incidence of cervical cancer occurs between 55 and 65 years. This observation points towards a latency period of several years between initial infection and the development of CIN and progression to invasive cancer.

The natural history of HPV-related disease starts with an acute infection resulting in the development of either a subclinical or a clinically apparent infection. Subclinical infections usually clear without symptoms. However, after a persistent infection has been established, the process of carcinogenesis takes place with disruption of the normal maturation of the transformation zone cervical epithelium. These alterations result in pre-invasive lesions (dysplasias) that are commonly asymptomatic and only detected by cytological procedures. If the resulting low- and high-grade lesions are left untreated, these may grow and eventually become invasive. Nevertheless, until invasion occurs, the entire stepwise precancerous lesion process is reversible. Actually, most HPV infected women will clear infection, and precancerous lesions will regress.

However, a portion of low- and high-grade lesions will progress to become invasive if untreated [10]. The interval from first infection to high-grade CIN is usually less than the time from high-grade CIN to cancer, which has been estimated to be about 7–10 years. It was originally believed that there was a natural and organized progression of cervical disease from CIN1 to CIN2 to CIN3 and then the development of invasive cervical cancer [43]. However, high-grade changes were observed to occur from persistent HPV infection without necessarily progressing through lower-grade appearing abnormalities [44, 45].

The high prevalence of HPV infections in the general female population and the relative low rate of cervical cancer indicates that both exogenous and inherent factors of the virus and the host can impact HPV infections' fate: a benign proliferative lesion or a tumor prone to malignant transformation during the course of several years, or simply elimination of infected cells [46]. The ability to evade the immune system is one of the key factors in virus prevalence and persistence. In the case of HPV infection, the low level of viral gene expression in the basal cells, together with the absence of inflammation and cell lysis, limits the effective antigen presentation of viral products to the immune system. Besides, it has been observed that these viruses restrict the efficacy antigen presentation through different mechanisms [47]. Altogether, these mechanisms contribute to delay the elimination of infected cells, which might explain the unusual persistence of HPV infection in immune competent individuals.

Virus-related factors have also been implicated in HPV-induced carcinogenesis. For instance, for HPV-16 (and other carcinogenic types) intratypic variants are relevant to the natural history of cervical neoplasia [48]. Viral loads were also clearly associated with concurrent disease and risk of neoplasia [49]. Additionally, susceptibility to or protection from cervical carcinoma and precursor lesions has been associated with MHC (major histocompatibility complex) class I and II alleles and haplotypes [50, 51]. For cervical carcinogenesis, steroid hormones (estrogens and progesterone) can also make women more prone in the initiation and successful development of progression of the disease in combination with HPV infection [52]. Finally, the association between HPV and other sexually transmitted agents such as herpes simplex, HIV, *Trichomonas*, *Chlamydia*, cytomegalovirus, *Treponema*, and *Gardnerella* in the development of cervical neoplasia has been addressed [10].

Organization of HPV Genome

HPV consists of a non-enveloped capsid of approximately 50 nm in diameter that encloses a single circular double-stranded DNA molecule with about 8,000 bp associated with cellular histones [10]. Overall, the diverse HPV types present a well-conserved genomic organization. The viral genome is divided into three functional regions: a regulatory region (LCR or long control region), the early (E) region, and late (L) region (Fig. 5.1). Seven or eight genes are arranged within the early region and two in the late region. All genes are transcribed from a single DNA strand in a polycistronic mRNA [53]. Genes of the early region, designated *E1*, *E2*, …, *E8*, are

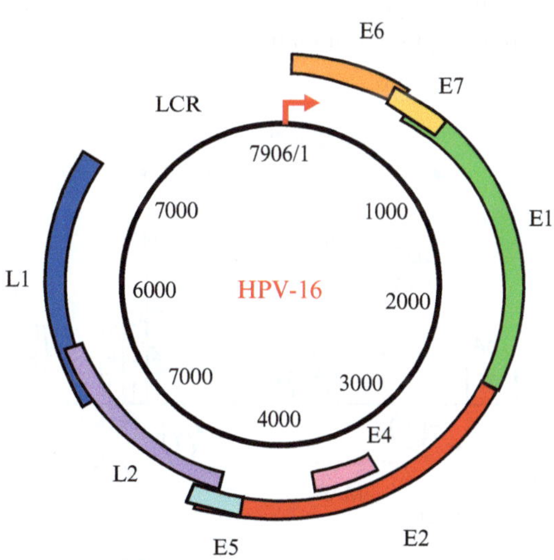

Fig. 5.1 Physical map of the HPV-16 genome. The viral genome is divided into three functional regions: a regulatory region (*LCR* or long control region), and the early (*E*) and late (*L*) regions

involved in replication and transcription control (*E1*, *E2*) and in cell transformation (*E5*, *E6*, and *E7*). *L1* and *L2* late genes encode the major and minor proteins of the capsid, respectively.

Regulation of HPV Expression

The LCR comprises approximately 10% of the viral genome in a region between *L1* and *E6* genes [54]. The regulation of HPV expression is controlled by diverse viral and cellular transcription factors that bind to specific *cis*-elements within the LCR. The nucleotide sequence of this noncoding segment of the viral genome diverges largely among different HPV types. In high-risk oncogenic HPVs, transcription starts from two major viral promoters, one of which initiates transcription of viral early genes upstream from the *E6* gene. HPV-16 early promoter is known as P97. HPV LCR is active exclusively in epithelial cells, the natural host of these infections.

Intra-genome HPV transcriptional regulation is mediated by the E2 viral protein [55]. Within the LCR, four E2 conserved binding sites are observed in most HPV types infecting the anogenital mucosa. The LCR is functionally divided into three segments: 5′ distal, central, and the 3′ end (Fig. 5.2). The 5′ distal segment encloses sites for transcription termination and polyadenylation of the polycistronic transcript. The central segment of the LCR surrounds an epithelial specific transcription enhancer region and is flanked by two E2 binding sites [56]. Most cellular transcription factors bind to *cis*-elements within this region, regulating transcription of the early viral genes from the promoter located at the 3′ end of the LCR [57]. These include AP1, NFI, TEF1, OCT1, YY1, BRN-3a, NF-IL6, KRF-1, NFκB, FOXA1, and GATA3, among others [54, 58]. Additionally, the enhancer of many genital HPV types is activated by glucocorticoid and progesterone receptors increasing *E6* and *E7* expression [59]. The polycistronic transcript starting at E6 is differentially edited, thus encoding all viral genes. The 3′ end region further contains a single E1 binding site that defines the origin of replication.

HPV Proteins

E1 and E2 Early Proteins

The E1 protein interacts with the cellular polymerase α [60] and binds to the viral origin within the LCR in complex with the E2. This genome region needs to be unrolled for viral replication to occur. E1 has an ATP-dependent helicase activity essential for viral replication [61]. Additionally, both E1 and E2 interact with topoisomerase I.

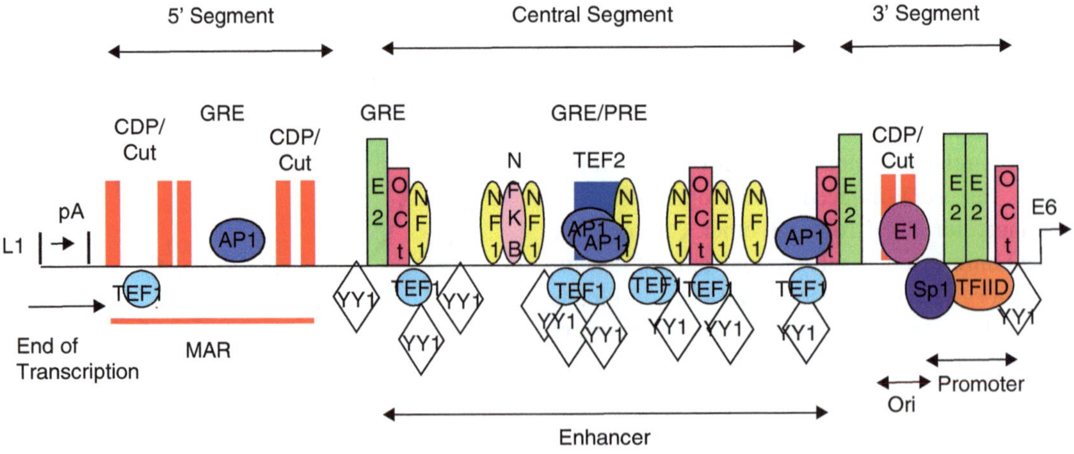

Fig. 5.2 Schematic representation of the HPV-16 LCR: the four E2 protein-binding sites are conserved among the LCRs of all genital HPVs. E2 binding sites from the 5′ end divide the LCR into three functionally distinct segments

The E2 protein is composed by an amino-terminal transactivation domain, a carboxy-terminal DNA binding domain, and a central hinge region. This protein is the main regulator of viral gene transcription and affects viral expression by forming dimers that bind to specific binding sites within the LCR [55]. Additionally, E2 is involved in viral DNA replication and interacts with and recruits E1 to the origin [62]. E2 is also important to ensure an even distribution of viral genomes among daughter cells during mitosis [63].

E4 Early Protein

The involvement of the E4 protein in HPV life cycle is still unclear. This protein is incorrectly classified as early since it was detected only in the more differentiated epithelial layers associated with the keratin cytoskeleton. This protein is not required for transformation or viral persistence. E4 also seems to be involved in the maturation and release of viral particles into the extracellular environment [64].

E5 Early Protein

The E5 protein is hydrophobic and predominantly localized to the endoplasmic reticulum [65]. E5 is the major transforming protein for BPV-1 (bovine papillomavirus); in contrast to its human counterpart, HPV E5 has weak transforming activity. In HPV infected cells, E5 protein amplifies the mitogenic signal of the epidermal growth factor receptor (EGFR) [66], possibly by binding to the vacuolar ATPase and thus altering the endosomal pH and EGFR turnover [67]. Through the activation of EGFR, E5 can interfere with several signal transduction pathways, including the mitogen-activated protein (MAP) kinase pathway [68]. In tissue culture assays, HPV E5 can enhance the transforming activity of E6 and E7 [69], suggesting a supportive role of this protein in tumor progression. E5 also reduces the surface levels of MHC class I proteins [70].

E6 Early Protein

The E6 protein of HPV infecting the anogenital region is generally well conserved (45–70% homologous to HPV-16 E6). This protein contains 151 amino acids and presents four Cys-XX-Cys motifs essential for zinc binding, since it results in the formation of two zinc finger structures spaced apart by 29 amino acids. These motifs are central for transcriptional activation, transformation, immortalization, and association with some cellular proteins [71].

The best known property of high-risk HPV E6 protein is the binding to cellular TP53 tumor suppressor protein as part of a trimeric complex with the cellular protein E6AP ubiquitin ligase, and the consequent TP53 degradation via the ubiquitin-dependent proteolysis pathway [72]. High-risk HPV E6 also interacts with PDZ proteins, which play an important role in signal transduction. Proteins of this family such as MUPP-1, hSCRIB, and hDlg are degraded after binding to the carboxy-terminus of E6 [73, 74]. Another cellular protein termed E6BP (E6 binding protein) further interacts with high-risk HPV and BPV-1 E6. This protein is identical to a calcium binding protein, ERC-55, although the importance of this interaction is unknown as yet. Additionally, other cellular proteins have been identified which bind to E6 from high-risk HPV types, including the transcriptional co-activator p300/CBP [75], and paxillin, which is involved in signal transduction from the plasma membrane to the actin cytoskeleton [76]. Furthermore, it was shown that the HPV-16 E6 induces telomerase activity in human keratinocytes at early stages of infection, increasing the life span of infected cells [77]. E6 activates hTERT transcription through the combined action of MYC and SP1 [78].

E7 Early Protein

E7 is a phosphoprotein of 98 amino acids harboring two Cys-XX-Cys motifs similar to the E6 protein, suggesting an evolutionary relationship between these proteins. The E7 amino-terminal region encloses two domains that correspond partly and completely to conserved regions 1 and 2 (CR-1 and CR-2) of the adenovirus E1A protein, respectively. Both regions of adenovirus E1A protein are associated with cell transformation [71].

Similarly to E1A, high-risk HPV E7 interacts with hypophosphorylated pRb, the product of the retinoblastoma tumor suppressor gene, and degrades pRB through ubiquitination-dependent proteolysis [79]. Accordingly, negative cell cycle regulation by pRb is lost releasing E2F transcription factor family members associated before in complexes with pRb. High-risk HPV E7 binds to pRb with greater affinity than low-risk HPV E7. This difference seems to result from a single amino acid change at position 21 that also influences the ability of E7 to cooperate with activated RAS in the transformation of mouse liver cells. E7 protein also impairs cell cycle regulation through interactions with histone deacetylases (HDAC) [71]. Indeed, high-risk HPV E7 was also shown to associate with pRb-related proteins such as P107 and P130, apart from inhibiting cyclin-dependent kinases p27 and p21 [80]. Additionally, E7 expression leads to cyclins A and E constitutive expression [81]. E7 expression also induces an abnormal number of centrosomes in primary human keratinocytes, leading to aneuploidy and genomic instability of infected cells [82]. The expression of E7 promotes the accumulation of p16INK4a whose expression is repressed by pRb. For this reason, p16 expression has been proposed as a biomarker for identifying epithelial dysplasia among cervical biopsies [83].

L1 and L2 Late Proteins

The L1 late protein is the major constituent of the viral capsid, representing about 80% of total viral proteins. This protein harbors type-specific epitopes and is highly immunogenic [64]. The L2 protein is less conserved and abundant than L1. It is the minor component of the viral capsid, but it has an important role in the incorporation of the viral DNA within the virion and in the interaction of the mature virion with the cell surface [10].

L1 and L2 expression in heterologous systems has made it possible to obtain empty virus-like particles (VLP). Still, it was demonstrated that L1 alone is sufficient for the formation of these particles [84]. These are relatively resistant to heat and organic solvents, and have proved to be an important source of viral antigens for serological tests and the development of HPV prophylactic vaccines [85].

HPV Taxonomy

First evidence of HPV genome diversity dates to the early 1970s and relies on the observation that mRNA prepared from plantar warts hybridized with DNA from other plantar warts but not with DNA obtained from other anatomical sites [19]. Genetic heterogeneity of HPV DNA was further corroborated based on differences in restriction enzyme cleavage patterns [86].

HPV belongs to the *Papillomaviridae* family [18]. *L1* is the most conserved gene within the genome and has therefore been used for the identification of new papillomavirus types over the past 15 years. Based on the complete *L1* nucleotide sequence, PVs were grouped in a phylogenetic tree wherein higher-order clusters comprise different genus that are identified by Greek letters (Fig. 5.3). Different genera share less than 60% of nucleotide sequence identity in the *L1* gene. In addition, lower-order clusters consist of species, numbered sequentially, and members within each species share between 60 and 70% nucleotide identity in *L1* region. The majority of HPV types are grouped into three different genera:

- *α-papillomavirus*, encloses HPV types predominantly isolated from genital lesions
- *β-papillomavirus* referred as HPV related to *Epidermodysplasia verruciformis*
- *γ-papillomavirus β-* and *γ-papillomavirus* were mainly isolated from cutaneous lesions [18]

HPV types comprise genotypes once these are defined as a viral genome with an *L1* late gene complete sequence that is at least 10% dissimilar from that of any other type [10]. About 40 HPV types infect the anogenital region among the

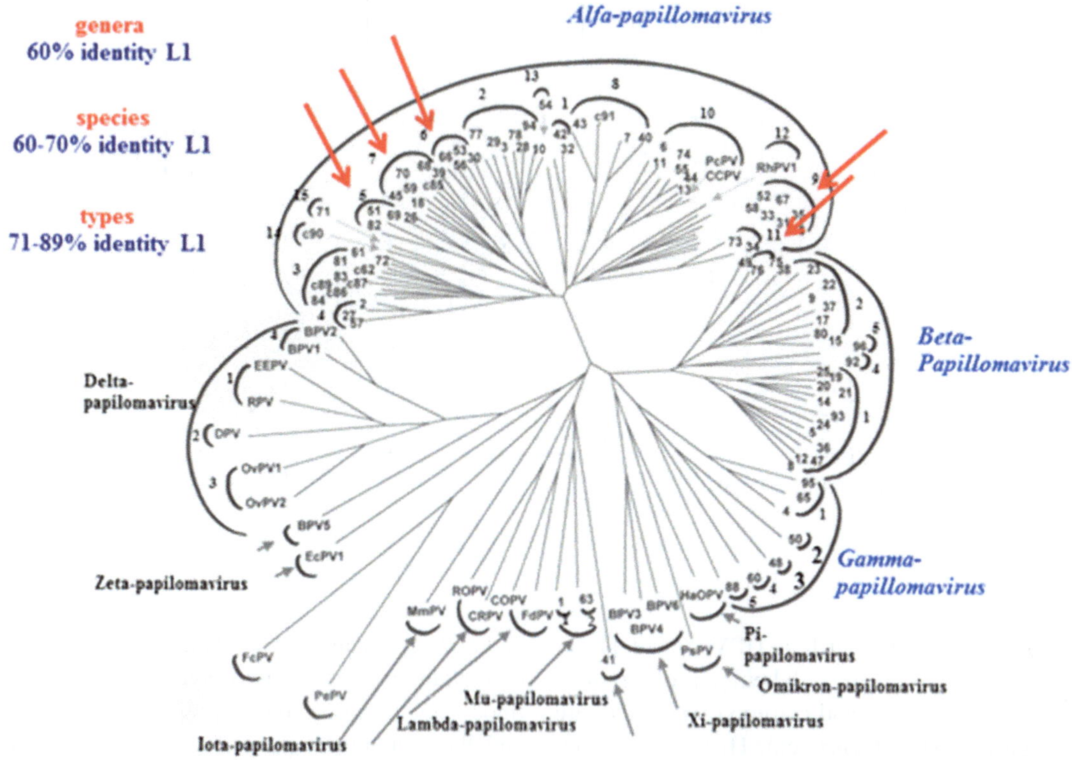

Fig. 5.3 Phylogenetic tree of papillomavirus based on L1 nucleotide sequence alignment. The majority of HPV types are grouped into three different genera: *α-papillomavirus*; *β-papillomavirus*; and *γ-papillomavirus*. *Red arrows* indicates species containing high-risk oncogenic HPVs. (Modified with permission of Elsevier from de Villiers EM, Fauquet C, Broker TR, Bernard HU, zur Hausen H. Classification of papillomaviruses. Virology 2004 Jun 20;324(1):17–27)

more than 150 HPV types described to date [18]. Many of these HPV types have been shown to be ubiquitous and are distributed globally. Sequence comparison of isolates from the same HPV type revealed some intratypic nucleotide heterogeneity. As a result, the Papillomavirus Nomenclature Committee has established that HPV genomes are classified into molecular variants when they present more than 98% of identity to the prototype sequence in the *L1* gene [87].

Analysis of the complete genome of 12 HPV-16 isolates further revealed that 4% of the full viral sequence is variable within the eight viral genes and that amino acid positions are 9.9% variable [88]. This study also showed that *E4* and *E5* genes are more variable than the LCR, which was previously shown to be as high as 5% dissimilar among molecular variants [89]. Due to the high prevalence of these viral types worldwide, the most extensive studies concerning HPV intratypic nucleotide heterogeneity have been conducted for HPV-16 [88–90], followed by HPVs 18 and 45 [91], HPVs 6 and 11 [92, 93], HPVs 5 and 8 [94], and, more recently, HPVs 53 [95], 31, 33, 35, and 52 [96]. Comparative nucleotide sequence analysis of these viruses suggests that HPV-16 evolved separately over a long period in Africa and Eurasia. The dispersion and the low rate of evolution documented imply that HPV co-evolved with their natural hosts over a period of a few million years [91]. It is estimated that the diversity observed between HPVs 16, 18, and probably other types represents more than 200,000 years of evolution from a precursor genome probably originated in Africa.

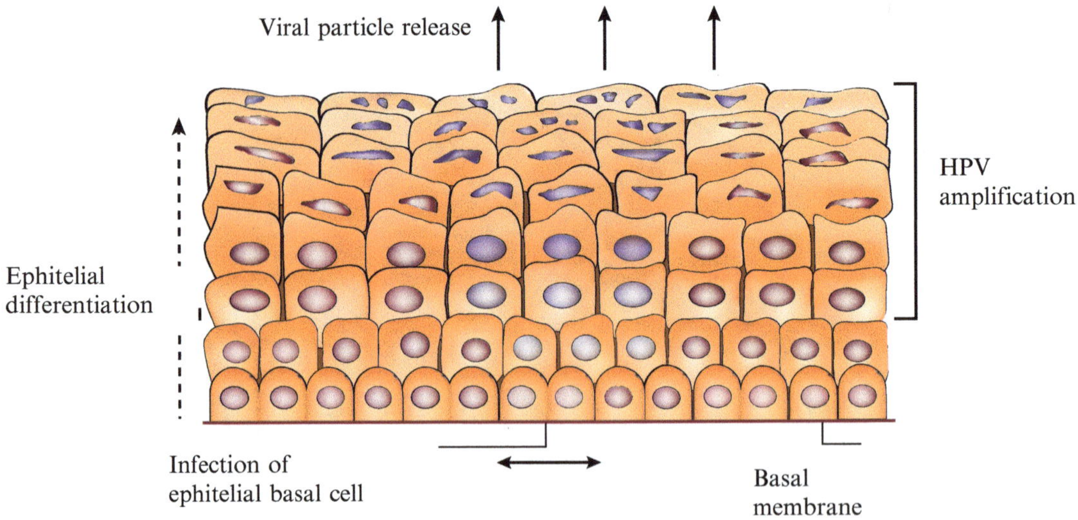

Fig. 5.4 HPV life cycle

Some viral types such as HPVs 6 and 11 are associated exclusively with benign proliferations such as condilomas and common warts, and are designated low-risk oncogenic HPV. On the other hand, high-risk oncogenic HPVs are considered the causative agents of most cervical cancers, with over 99% of cervical lesions containing any of these viral sequences (i.e., HPVs 16, 18, 31, and 33, etc.) [97]. HPV-16 is undoubtedly the most carcinogenic viral type as measured by numbers of cases of cervical cancer and its immediate precursor, CIN grade 3 (CIN3) [11].

HPV Life Cycle

All HPV-associated lesions are of epithelial origin, including the columnar epithelium of the uterine endocervix, the stratified squamous epithelium of the ectocervix, and the squamous epithelium of the skin. The diverse HPV types infect the epithelia of different anatomical sites; however, functional differences, yet unknown, constrain viral infection by specific HPV types to restricted epithelium types.

Cervical cancers arise mostly at the cervical transformation zone. In this region, the stratified squamous epithelium of the vagina gathers and substitutes the glandular epithelium of the endocervical canal. The stratified squamous epithelium encloses various layers of cells (keratinocytes): the basal, spinous, and granular layers, and the stratum corneum (Fig. 5.4). The basal layer is composed of proliferating cells which may remain dividing within this layer, or may well migrate to the suprabasal layers (spinous and granular) and enter into an ordered pattern of differentiation. The stratum corneum is the most superficial layer of the epidermis and is composed of cells that do not undergo metabolic processes. These are flattened cells, with a cellular skeleton filled with keratin, which protect the epidermis. Cells from the basal layer are responsible for the maintenance and regeneration of the tissue, and, in order to preserve the thickness of the epithelium, the rate basal cell proliferation must be equivalent to the stratum corneum cell loss.

Initial infection by HPV localizes to cells of the basal layers of the stratified epithelium that become exposed as a result of small traumas occurring, for instance, during sexual intercourse. Experimental evidence indicates that HPV virion initially binds to heparan sulfate proteoglycans on the basement membrane [98] where it undergoes a conformational change that allows the cleavage by a furin and exhibition of a L2 N-terminal region. HPV virions are further shifted to a receptor on the basal epithelial cell

[99]. It is probable that L1 binds to this second receptor once the initial internalization steps of L1-only VLPs and infectious L1/L2 capsids are indistinguishable [100].

After infection of basal epithelial cells, HPV genomes are established as episomes in the cell nucleus. This is usually associated with low viral copy numbers, no cytological abnormality, and early genes are expressed preferentially although at low levels [99]. Viral genome replication and protein expression occur only in differentiated epithelial layers. HPV promoters are active in spinous and granular suprabasal layers, suggesting that the synchronization of the viral life cycle to the epithelial differentiation program may be due in part to the binding in the LCR of cellular transcription factors differentially expressed in various layers of the epithelium. In suprabasal cells, E1 and E2 viral proteins are expressed, HPV replication takes place, and viral load is increased to about 50–100 copies per cell. During the division of infected cells, one of the daughter cells continues to divide in the basal layer serving as a reservoir of viral DNA [10].

HPV-positive suprabasal cells fail to withdraw from the cell cycle and continue to support DNA synthesis and express cell proliferation markers [101]. HPV-16 E7 has been shown to be necessary and sufficient to induce DNA synthesis in suprabasal cells [101] by interacting with members of the retinoblastoma (Rb) family (p105 (pRB), P107, and P130). E6 and E7 expression is also important for the maintenance of viral episomes in undifferentiated epithelial layers, although the mechanism by which this occurs has not yet been completely elucidated. Mature viral particles are released by the desquamating superficial keratinocytes [64].

Since HPV requires differentiation of the squamous epithelium in order to complete its life cycle, the development of an in vitro system able to keep replication of this virus was a challenge for many years. Today, the most used method to study viral life cycle is epithelia organotypic culture. Histologically, these cultures resemble the epithelium from which they are derived once all of the epithelial layers can be seen in these cultures. Immortalized HPV 16 or 18 keratinocytes were further used for the establishment of organotypic cultures, and these clearly were abnormal epithelium and looked like squamous intraepithelial neoplasia in vivo, i.e., showed disorganized tissue architecture and mitotic cells in all living epithelial layers [102]. Additionally, the organotypic cultures derived from HPV immortalized cells could be distinguished from normal keratinocytes by the pattern of PCNA expression through all epithelial layers, indicating maintenance of a proliferative state. Increasing degrees of dysplasia were also associated with decreased expression of differentiation markers such as cytokeratin 10 and profilaggrin [64].

HPV Oncogenic Potential

HPV DNA often integrates into the cell genome; this event is more commonly observed in malignant lesions such as CIN3, carcinoma in situ, and invasive cancer, as compared to CIN grades 1/2 (CIN 1 and 2) and benign lesions. Integration of the virus is randomly distributed over the whole genome, although some clear predilection for fragile sites was observed [103]. Whether viral integration alters cellular gene expression in any biologically relevant manner remains unclear. On the other hand, interruption of the viral genome usually occurs between the 3′ end of the *E1* gene and the 5′ end of *E2* gene, and results in constitutive E6 and E7 expression [71]. It was observed that *E6* and *E7* mRNAs expressed from integrated copies show increased stability and that integration confers a selective growth advantage over cells with only episomal viral DNA [104]. The continuous synthesis of E6 and E7 oncoproteins is an essential step towards the development of malignant tumors.

The biological activity of E6 and E7 proteins depends on the host cell infected with the virus or transfected with selected HPV genes. Both E6 and E7 proteins independently cooperate with activated RAS oncogene in immortalization and transformation of mouse and rat liver primary cells. E6 or E7 expression is also sufficient to transform rodent immortalized cells [105, 106]. Furthermore, regardless of RAS or E7, E6 is able to transform NIH3T3 cells [107], immortalize human mammary epithelial cells, and human liver cells [108].

Once squamous epithelial cells are the natural HPV host, genital human keratinocyte cultures have been extensively used to study E6 and E7 functions. It was shown that both proteins cooperate in the immortalization of primary human keratinocytes [109, 110], and in the inhibition of terminal differentiation of these cells induced by serum and calcium [111]. Although they have altered growth and differentiation, HPV immortalized cells are unable to grow independent of anchorage and induce tumors in athymic mice. Additional genetic changes seem to be necessary for malignant progression [9].

The molecular interaction between HPV and cellular proteins has been the subject of numerous studies over the past 20 years. As described, high-risk HPVs E6 and E7 stimulate cell proliferation by interacting with and suppressing the function of cellular proteins involved in cell cycle regulation. Many proteins have been identified that bind to high-risk oncogenic HPV E6 and E7 and probably many remain to be described. These proteins are located in different cellular compartments and may differently contribute to the transforming activity of HPV. TP53 and pRB proteins are well-characterized targets of the high-risk HPV oncoproteins, but recent studies have shown that interference in additional pathways is equally important for transformation to occur. Different studies suggest that binding of HPV E6 protein to PDZ protein family members and activation of hTERT is necessary for cell immortalization, while high-risk E6 TP53 HPV-mediated degradation is important for cell transformation. However, immortalization of these cells further requires the inactivation of the pRb pathway through mutation in this gene or interaction with viral E7 oncoprotein. The interaction of high-risk HPV E7 with the HDAC has proven crucial for immortalization of primary human keratinocytes and for maintenance of the episomes.

Most HPV-associated tumors have numerous chromosomal imbalances, including whole chromosomes gains or losses and chromosomal rearrangements that may be observed in premalignant HPV-associated cervical lesions. For this reason, genetic instability is believed to be an early event in HPV-induced carcinogenesis, occurring before integration of the virus into the host chromosomes [112].

Concluding Remarks

High-risk HPV types are the causative agents of cervical cancers as well as of tumors in the anogenital and oropharyngeal areas of both women and men. Knowledge about HPV oncogenes and their transformation abilities led to the recognition of the viral origin of cervical premalignant and malignant lesions. The implications for cervical cancer prevention and control are inestimable: screening with HPV testing has proven to be more sensitive than Pap testing while allowing for a proper monitoring of HPV diseases after the introduction of prophylactic vaccines. The advent of highly efficacious HPV vaccines against HPVs 16 and 18 shows promise in contributing to the reduction of a considerable proportion of tumors that, without intervention, will continue to increase in number.

References

1. Pisani P. The cancer burden and cancer control in developing countries. Environ Health. 2011;10 Suppl 1:S2.
2. Parkin DM, Bray F. Chapter 2: The burden of HPV-related cancers. Vaccine. 2006;24 Suppl 3: S3/11–25.
3. Bruni L, Diaz M, Castellsagué X, Ferrer E, Bosch FX, de Sanjosé S. Cervical human papillomavirus prevalence in 5 continents: meta-analysis of 1 million women with normal cytological findings. J Infect Dis. 2010;202(12):1789–99.
4. Bosch FX, Manos MM, Muñoz N, Sherman M, Jansen AM, Peto J, et al. Prevalence of human papillomavirus in cervical cancer: a worldwide perspective. International biological study on cervical cancer (IBSCC) Study Group. J Natl Cancer Inst. 1995;87(11):796–802.
5. Walboomers JM, Jacobs MV, Manos MM, Bosch FX, Kummer JA, Shah KV, et al. Human papillomavirus is a necessary cause of invasive cervical cancer worldwide. J Pathol. 1999;189(1):12–9.
6. Guan P, Howell-Jones R, Li N, Bruni L, de Sanjosé S, Franceschi S, et al. Human papillomavirus types in 115,789 HPV-positive women: a meta-analysis

from cervical infection to cancer. Int J Cancer. 2012;131(10):2349–59.
7. Smith JS, Melendy A, Rana RK, Pimenta JM. Age-specific prevalence of infection with human papillomavirus in females: a global review. J Adolesc Health. 2008;43(4 Suppl):S5–25; S25.e1–41.
8. Thomas JO, Herrero R, Omigbodun AA, Ojemakinde K, Ajayi IO, Fawole A, et al. Prevalence of papillomavirus infection in women in Ibadan, Nigeria: a population-based study. Br J Cancer. 2004; 90(3):638–45.
9. Herrero R, Castle PE, Schiffman M, et al. Epidemiologic profile of type-specific human papillomavirus infection and cervical neoplasia in Guanacaste, Costa Rica. J Infect Dis. 2005; 191(11):1796–807.
10. IARC Monographs on the Evaluation of Carcinogenic Risks to Humans, Lyon, Inc. 2007;90:689.
11. Van der Marel J, Quint WG, Schiffman M, van de Sandt MM, Zuna RE, Terence Dunn S, et al. Molecular mapping of high-grade cervical intraepithelial neoplasia shows etiological dominance of HPV16. Int J Cancer. 2012;131(6):E946–53.
12. Bauer HM, Ting Y, Greer CE, Chambers JC, Tashiro CJ, Chimera J, et al. Genital human papillomavirus infection in female university students as determined by a PCR-based method. JAMA. 1991;265(4):472–7.
13. Tota JE, Chevarie-Davis M, Richardson LA, Devries M, Franco EL. Epidemiology and burden of HPV infection and related diseases: implications for prevention strategies. Prev Med. 2011;53 Suppl 1:S12–21.
14. Muñoz N, Bosch FX, Castellsagué X, Díaz M, de Sanjose S, Hammouda D, et al. Against which human papillomavirus types shall we vaccinate and screen? The international perspective. Int J Cancer. 2004; 111(2):278–85.
15. Richardson H, Kelsall G, Tellier P, Voyer H, Abrahamowicz M, Ferenczy A, et al. The natural history of type-specific human papillomavirus infections in female university students. Cancer Epidemiol Biomarkers Prev. 2003;12(6):485–90.
16. Bosch FX, Muñoz N, de Sanjosé S, Guerrerro E, Gaffari AM, Kaldor J, et al. Importance of human papillomavirus endemicity in the incidence of cervical cancer: an extension of the hypothesis on sexual behavior. Cancer Epidemiol Biomarkers Prev. 1994;3(5):375–9.
17. Castellsagué X, Gaffari A, Daniel RW, Bosch FX, Muñoz N, Shah KV. Prevalence of penile human papillomavirus DNA in husbands of women with and without cervical neoplasia: a study in Spain and Colombia. J Infect Dis. 1997;176(2):353–61.
18. de Villiers EM, Fauquet C, Broker TR, Bernard HU, zur Hausen H. Classification of papillomaviruses. Virology. 2004;324(1):17–27.
19. zur Hausen H, Meinhof W, Scheiber W, Bornkamm GW. Attempts to detect virus-secific DNA in human tumors. I. Nucleic acid hybridizations with complementary RNA of human wart virus. Int J Cancer. 1974;13(5):650–6.
20. Franco EL, Harper DM. Vaccination against human papillomavirus infection: a new paradigm in cervical cancer control. Vaccine. 2005;23(17–18):2388–94.
21. Schiffman MH, Bauer HM, Hoover RN, Glass AG, Cadell DM, Rush BB, et al. Epidemiologic evidence showing that human papillomavirus infection causes most cervical intraepithelial neoplasia. J Natl Cancer Inst. 1993;85(12):958–64.
22. Franco EL, Villa LL, Ruiz A, Costa MC. Transmission of cervical human papillomavirus infection by sexual activity: differences between low and high oncogenic risk types. J Infect Dis. 1995;172(3):756–63.
23. Baseman JG, Koutsky LA. The epidemiology of human papillomavirus infections. J Clin Virol. 2005;32 Suppl 1:S16–24.
24. Burchell AN, Richardson H, Mahmud SM, et al. Modeling the sexual transmissibility of human papillomavirus infection using stochastic computer simulation and empirical data from a cohort study of young women in Montreal, Canada. Am J Epidemiol. 2006;163(6):534–43.
25. Moscicki AB, Hills N, Shiboski S, et al. Risks for incident human papillomavirus infection and low-grade squamous intraepithelial lesion development in young females. JAMA. 2001; 285(23):2995–3002.
26. Hernandez BY, Wilkens LR, Zhu X, et al. Transmission of human papillomavirus in heterosexual couples. Emerg Infect Dis. 2008;14(6):888–94.
27. Rousseau MC, Pereira JS, Prado JC, Villa LL, Rohan TE, Franco EL. Cervical coinfection with human papillomavirus (HPV) types as a predictor of acquisition and persistence of HPV infection. J Infect Dis. 2001;184(12):1508–17.
28. Schiffman M, Kjaer SK. Chapter 2: Natural history of anogenital human papillomavirus infection and neoplasia. J Natl Cancer Inst Monogr. 2003; 31:14–9.
29. Castellsagué X, Bosch FX, Muñoz N, Meijer CJ, Shah KV, de Sanjose S, et al. Male circumcision, penile human papillomavirus infection, and cervical cancer in female partners. N Engl J Med. 2002; 346(15):1105–12.
30. Baken LA, Koutsky LA, Kuypers J, Kosorok MR, Lee SK, Kiviat NB, et al. Genital human papillomavirus infection among male and female sex partners: prevalence and type-specific concordance. J Infect Dis. 1995;171(2):429–32.
31. Shah K, Kashima H, Polk BF, Shah F, Abbey H, Abramson A. Rarity of cesarean delivery in cases of juvenile-onset respiratory papillomatosis. Obstet Gynecol. 1986;68(6):795–9.
32. Rousseau MC, Franco EL, Villa LL, Sobrinho JP, Termini L, Prado JM, et al. A cumulative case–control study of risk factor profiles for oncogenic and nononcogenic cervical human papillomavirus infections. Cancer Epidemiol Biomarkers Prev. 2000;9(5):469–76.

33. Schiffman M, Castle PE, Jeronimo J, Rodriguez AC, Wacholder S. Human papillomavirus and cervical cancer. Lancet. 2007;370(9590):890–907.
34. Vuyst HD, Ndirangu G, Moodley M, Tenet V, Estambale B, Meijer CJ, et al. Prevalence of human papillomavirus in women with invasive cervical carcinoma by HIV status in Kenya and South Africa. Int J Cancer. 2012;131(4):949–55.
35. Palefsky J. Human papillomavirus-related disease in people with HIV. Curr Opin HIV AIDS. 2009;4(1): 52–6.
36. Hildesheim A, Schiffman MH, Gravitt PE, Glass AG, Greer CE, Zhang T, et al. Persistence of type-specific human papillomavirus infection among cytologically normal women. J Infect Dis. 1994;169(2):235–40.
37. Franco EL, Villa LL, Sobrinho JP, Prado JM, Rousseau MC, Désy M, et al. Epidemiology of acquisition and clearance of cervical human papillomavirus infection in women from a high-risk area for cervical cancer. J Infect Dis. 1999;180(5):1415–23.
38. Evander M, Edlund K, Gustafsson A, Jonsson M, Karlsson R, Rylander E, et al. Human papillomavirus infection is transient in young women: a population-based cohort study. J Infect Dis. 1995; 171(4):1026–30.
39. Ho GY, Burk RD, Klein S, Kadish AS, Chang CJ, Palan P, et al. Persistent genital human papillomavirus infection as a risk factor for persistent cervical dysplasia. J Natl Cancer Inst. 1995;87(18):1365–71.
40. Gravitt PE. The known unknowns of HPV natural history. J Clin Invest. 2011;121(12):4593–9.
41. Schiffman M, Rodriguez AC, Chen Z, Wacholder S, Herrero R, Hildesheim A, et al. A population-based prospective study of carcinogenic human papillomavirus variant lineages, viral persistence, and cervical neoplasia. Cancer Res. 2010;70(8):3159–69.
42. Nobbenhuis MA, Walboomers JM, Helmerhorst TJ, Rozendaal L, Remmink AJ, Risse EK, et al. Relation of human papillomavirus status to cervical lesions and consequences for cervical-cancer screening: a prospective study. Lancet. 1999;354(9172):20–5.
43. Richart RM. A theory of cervical carcinogenesis. Obstet Gynecol Surv. 1969;24(7 Pt 2):874–9.
44. Cuzick J, Szarewski A, Terry G, Ho L, Hanby A, Maddox P, et al. Human papillomavirus testing in primary cervical screening. Lancet. 1995;345(8964): 1533–6.
45. Koutsky LA, Holmes KK, Critchlow CW, Stevens CE, Paavonen J, Beckmann AM, et al. A cohort study of the risk of cervical intraepithelial neoplasia grade 2 or 3 in relation to papillomavirus infection. N Engl J Med. 1992;327(18):1272–8.
46. Wang SS, Hildesheim A. Chapter 5: Viral and host factors in human papillomavirus persistence and progression. J Natl Cancer Inst Monogr. 2003;31: 35–40.
47. Stanley M. Immune responses to human papillomavirus. Vaccine. 2006;24 Suppl 1:S16–22.
48. Sichero L, Ferreira S, Trottier H, Duarte-Franco E, Ferenczy A, Franco EL, et al. High grade cervical lesions are caused preferentially by non-European variants of HPVs 16 and 18. Int J Cancer. 2007;120(8):1763–8.
49. Schlecht NF, Trevisan A, Duarte-Franco E, Rohan TE, Ferenczy A, Villa LL, et al. Viral load as a predictor of the risk of cervical intraepithelial neoplasia. Int J Cancer. 2003;103(4):519–24.
50. Apple RJ, Erlich HA, Klitz W, Manos MM, Becker TM, Wheeler CM. HLA DR-DQ associations with cervical carcinoma show papillomavirus-type specificity. Nat Genet. 1994;6(2):157–62.
51. Maciag PC, Schlecht NF, Souza PS, Franco EL, Villa LL, Petzl-Erler ML. Major histocompatibility complex class II polymorphisms and risk of cervical cancer and human papillomavirus infection in Brazilian women. Cancer Epidemiol Biomarkers Prev. 2000;9(11):1183–91.
52. de Villiers EM. Relationship between steroid hormone contraceptives and HPV, cervical intraepithelial neoplasia and cervical carcinoma. Int J Cancer. 2003;103(6):705–8.
53. Chen EY, Howley PM, Levinson AD, Seeburg PH. The primary structure and genetic organization of the bovine papillomavirus type 1 genome. Nature. 1982;299(5883):529–34.
54. O'Connor M, Chan SY, Bernard HU. Transcription factor binding sites in the LCR of genital HPVs. In: Myers G et al., editors. Human papillomaviruses. A compilation and analysis of nucleic acid and amino-acid sequences, III. Los Alamos: Los Alamos National Laboratory; 1995. p. 21–41.
55. Thierry F, Yaniv M. The BPV1-E2 trans-acting protein can be either an activator or a repressor of the HPV18 regulatory region. EMBO J. 1987;6(11):3391–7.
56. Gloss B, Bernard HU, Seedorf K, Klock G. The upstream regulatory region of the human papilloma virus-16 contains an E2 protein-independent enhancer which is specific for cervical carcinoma cells and regulated by glucocorticoid hormones. EMBO J. 1987;6(12):3735–43.
57. Thierry F, Spyrou G, Yaniv M, Howley P. Two AP1 sites binding JunB are essential for human papillomavirus type 18 transcription in keratinocytes. J Virol. 1992;66(6):3740–8.
58. Sichero L, Sobrinho JS, Villa LL. Identification of novel cellular transcription factors that regulate HPVs 18 and 16 early promoters. J Infect Dis. 2012;206(6):867–74.
59. Chan WK, Klock G, Bernard HU. Progesterone and glucocorticoid response elements occur in the long control regions of several human papillomaviruses involved in anogenital neoplasia. J Virol. 1989;63(8):3261–9.
60. Bonne-Andrea C, Santucci S, Clertant P, Tillier F. Bovine papillomavirus E1 protein binds specifically DNA polymerase alpha but not replication protein A. J Virol. 1995;69(4):2341–50.

61. Wilson VG, West M, Woytek K, Rangasamy D. Papillomavirus E1 proteins: form, function, and features. Virus Genes. 2002;24(3):275–90.
62. Chiang CM, Ustav M, Stenlund A, Ho TF, Broker TR, Chow LT. Viral E1 and E2 proteins support replication of homologous and heterologous papillomaviral origins. Proc Natl Acad Sci U S A. 1992;89(13):5799–803.
63. van Tine BA, Dao LD, Wu SY, Sonbuchner TM, Lin BY, Zou N, et al. Human papillomavirus (HPV) origin-binding protein associates with mitotic spindles to enable viral DNA partitioning. Proc Natl Acad Sci U S A. 2004;101(12):4030–5.
64. zur Hausen H. Papillomaviruses and cancer: from basic studies to clinical application. Nat Rev Cancer. 2002;2(5):342–50.
65. DiMaio D, Mattoon D. Mechanisms of cell transformation by papillomavirus E5 proteins. Oncogene. 2001;20(54):7866–73.
66. Leechanachai P, Banks L, Moreau F, Matlashewski G. The E5 gene from human papillomavirus type 16 is an oncogene which enhances growth factor-mediated signal transduction to the nucleus. Oncogene. 1992;7(1):19–25.
67. Conrad M, Bubb VJ, Schlegel R. The human papillomavirus type 6 and 16 E5 proteins are membrane-associated proteins which associate with the 16-kilodalton pore-forming protein. J Virol. 1993; 67(10):6170–8.
68. Crusius K, Rodriguez I, Alonso A. The human papillomavirus type 16 E5 protein modulates ERK1/2 and p38 MAP kinase activation by an EGFR-independent process in stressed human keratinocytes. Virus Genes. 2000;20(1):65–9.
69. Stöppler MC, Straight SW, Tsao G, Schlegel R, McCance DJ. The E5 gene of HPV-16 enhances keratinocyte immortalization by full-length DNA. Virology. 1996;223(1):251–4.
70. Ashrafi GH, Brown DR, Fife KH, Campo MS. Down-regulation of MHC class I is a property common to papillomavirus E5 proteins. Virus Res. 2006;120(1–2):208–11.
71. Longworth MS, Laimins LA. Pathogenesis of human papillomaviruses in differentiating epithelia. Microbiol Mol Biol Rev. 2004;68(2):362–72.
72. Huibregtse JM, Scheffner M, Howley PM. Localization of the E6-AP regions that direct human papillomavirus E6 binding, association with p53, and ubiquitination of associated proteins. Mol Cell Biol. 1993;13(8):4918–27.
73. Kiyono T, Hiraiwa A, Fujita M, Hayashi Y, Akiyama T, Ishibashi M. Binding of high-risk human papillomavirus E6 oncoproteins to the human homologue of the Drosophila discs large tumor suppressor protein. Proc Natl Acad Sci U S A. 1997;94(21):11612–6.
74. Pim D, Banks L. Interaction of viral oncoproteins with cellular target molecules: infection with high-risk vs low-risk human papillomaviruses. APMIS. 2010;118(6–7):471–93.
75. Patel D, Huang SM, Baglia LA, McCance DJ. The E6 protein of human papillomavirus type 16 binds to and inhibits co-activation by CBP and p300. EMBO J. 1999;18(18):5061–72.
76. Tong X, Howley PM. The bovine papillomavirus E6 oncoprotein interacts with paxillin and disrupts the actin cytoskeleton. Proc Natl Acad Sci U S A. 1997;94(9):4412–7.
77. Klingelhutz AJ, Foster SA, McDougall JK. Telomerase activation by the E6 gene product of human papillomavirus type 16. Nature. 1996;380(6569):79–82.
78. Oh ST, Kyo S, Laimins LA. Telomerase activation by human papillomavirus type 16 E6 protein: induction of human telomerase reverse transcriptase expression through Myc and GC-rich Sp1 binding sites. J Virol. 2001;75(12):5559–66.
79. Dyson N, Guida P, Münger K, Harlow E. Homologous sequences in adenovirus E1A and human papillomavirus E7 proteins mediate interaction with the same set of cellular proteins. J Virol. 1992; 66(12):6893–902.
80. Münger K, Howley PM. Human papillomavirus immortalization and transformation functions. Virus Res. 2002;89(2):213–28.
81. Zerfass K, Schulze A, Spitkovsky D, Friedman V, Henglein B, Jansen-Dürr P. Sequential activation of cyclin E and cyclin A gene expression by human papillomavirus type 16 E7 through sequences necessary for transformation. J Virol. 1995; 69(10):6389–99.
82. Duensing S, Duensing A, Flores ER, Do A, Lambert PF, Münger K. Centrosome abnormalities and genomic instability by episomal expression of human papillomavirus type 16 in raft cultures of human keratinocytes. J Virol. 2001;75(16):7712–6.
83. Klaes R, Friedrich T, Spitkovsky D, Ridder R, Rudy W, Petry U, et al. Overexpression of p16(INK4A) as a specific marker for dysplastic and neoplastic epithelial cells of the cervix uteri. Int J Cancer. 2001;92(2):276–84.
84. Kirnbauer R, Taub J, Greenstone H, Roden R, Dürst M, Gissmann L, et al. Efficient self-assembly of human papillomavirus type 16 L1 and L1-L2 into virus-like particles. J Virol. 1993;67(12):6929–36.
85. Galloway DA. Papillomavirus vaccines in clinical trials. Lancet Infect Dis. 2003;3(8):469–75.
86. Gissman L, zur Hausen. Human papillomaviruses: physical mapping and genetic heterogeneity. Proc Natl Acad Sci U S A. 1976;73:1310–3.
87. Bernard HU. The clinical importance of the nomenclature, evolution and taxonomy of human papillomaviruses. J Clin Virol. 2005;32 Suppl 1:S1–6.
88. Chen Z, Terai M, Fu L, Herrero R, DeSalle R, Burk RD. Diversifying selection in human papillomavirus type 16 lineages based on complete genome analyses. J Virol. 2005;79(11):7014–23.
89. Ho L, Chan SY, Burk RD, Das BC, Fujinaga K, Icenogle JP, et al. The genetic drift of human papillomavirus type 16 is a means of reconstructing

prehistoric viral spread and the movement of ancient human populations. J Virol. 1993;67(11):6413–23.
90. Smith B, Chen Z, Reimers L, van Doorslaer K, Schiffman M, Desalle R, et al. Sequence imputation of HPV16 genomes for genetic association studies. PLoS One. 2011;6(6):e21375.
91. Ong CK, Chan SY, Campo MS, Fujinaga K, Mavromara-Nazos P, Labropoulou V, et al. Evolution of human papillomavirus type 18: an ancient phylogenetic root in Africa and intratype diversity reflect coevolution with human ethnic groups. J Virol. 1993;67(11):6424–31.
92. Heinzel PA, Chan SY, Ho L, O'Connor M, Balaram P, Campo MS, et al. Variation of human papillomavirus type 6 (HPV-6) and HPV-11 genomes sampled throughout the world. J Clin Microbiol. 1995; 33(7):1746–54.
93. Burk RD, Chen Z, Harari A, Smith BC, Kocjan BJ, Maver PJ, et al. Classification and nomenclature system for human Alphapapillomavirus variants: general features, nucleotide landmarks and assignment of HPV6 and HPV11 isolates to variant lineages. Acta Dermatovenerol Alp Panonica Adriat. 2011;20(3):113–23.
94. Deau MC, Favre M, Orth G. Genetic heterogeneity among human papillomaviruses (HPV) associated with epidermodysplasia verruciformis: evidence for multiple allelic forms of HPV5 and HPV8 E6 genes. Virology. 1991;184(2):492–503.
95. Prado JC, Calleja-Macias IE, Bernard HU, Kalantari M, Macay SA, Allan B, et al. Worldwide genomic diversity of the human papillomaviruses-53, 56, and 66, a group of high-risk HPVs unrelated to HPV-16 and HPV-18. Virology. 2005;340(1):95–104.
96. Calleja-Macias IE, Kalantari M, Huh J, Ortiz-Lopez R, Rojas-Martinez A, Gonzalez-Guerrero JF, et al. Genomic diversity of human papillomavirus-16, 18, 31, and 35 isolates in a Mexican population and relationship to European, African, and Native American variants. Virology. 2004;319(2):315–23.
97. Schiffman M, Clifford G, Buonaguro FM. Classification of weakly carcinogenic human papillomavirus types: addressing the limits of epidemiology at the borderline. Infect Agent Cancer. 2009;4:8.
98. Schiller JT, Day PM, Kines RC. Current understanding of the mechanism of HPV infection. Gynecol Oncol. 2010;118(1 Suppl):S12–7.
99. Kines RC, Thompson CD, Lowy DR, Schiller JT, Day PM. The initial steps leading to papillomavirus infection occur on the basement membrane prior to cell surface binding. Proc Natl Acad Sci U S A. 2009;106(48):20458–63.
100. Day PM, Gambhira R, Roden RB, Lowy DR, Schiller JT. Mechanisms of human papillomavirus type 16 neutralization by 12 cross-neutralizing and 11 type-specific antibodies. J Virol. 2008;82(9):4638–46.
101. Flores ER, Allen-Hoffmann BL, Lee D, Sattler CA, Lambert PF. Establishment of the human papillomavirus type 16 (HPV-16) life cycle in an immortalized human foreskin keratinocyte cell line. Virology. 1999;262(2):344–54.
102. Delvenne P, Hubert P, Jacobs N, Giannini SL, Havard L, Renard I, et al. The organotypic culture of HPV-transformed keratinocytes: an effective in vitro model for the development of new immunotherapeutic approaches for mucosal (pre)neoplastic lesions. Vaccine. 2001;19(17–19):2557–64.
103. Wentzensen N, Wilz B, Findeisen P, Wagner R, Dippold W, von Knebel Doeberitz M, et al. Identification of differentially expressed genes in colorectal adenoma compared to normal tissue by suppression subtractive hybridization. Int J Oncol. 2004;24(4):987–94.
104. Jeon S, Lambert PF. Integration of human papillomavirus type 16 DNA into the human genome leads to increased stability of E6 and E7 mRNAs: implications for cervical carcinogenesis. Proc Natl Acad Sci U S A. 1995;92(5):1654–8.
105. Kanda T, Furuno A, Yoshiike K. Human papillomavirus type 16 open reading frame E7 encodes a transforming gene for rat 3Y1 cells. J Virol. 1988;62(2):610–3.
106. Storey A, Pim D, Murray A, Osborn K, Banks L, Crawford L. Comparison of the in vitro transforming activities of human papillomavirus types. EMBO J. 1988;7(6):1815–20.
107. Sedman SA, Barbosa MS, Vass WC, Hubbert NL, Haas JA, Lowy DR, et al. The full-length E6 protein of human papillomavirus type 16 has transforming and trans-activating activities and cooperates with E7 to immortalize keratinocytes in culture. J Virol. 1991;65(9):4860–6.
108. Band V, De Caprio JA, Delmolino L, Kulesa V, Sager R. Loss of p53 protein in human papillomavirus type 16 E6-immortalized human mammary epithelial cells. J Virol. 1991;65(12):6671–6.
109. Barbosa MS, Schlegel R. The E6 and E7 genes of HPV-18 are sufficient for inducing two-stage in vitro transformation of human keratinocytes. Oncogene. 1989;4(12):1529–32.
110. Hawley-Nelson P, Vousden KH, Hubbert NL, Lowy DR, Schiller JT. HPV16 E6 and E7 proteins cooperate to immortalize human foreskin keratinocytes. EMBO J. 1989;8(12):3905–10.
111. Münger K, Phelps WC, Bubb V, Howley PM, Schlegel R. The E6 and E7 genes of the human papillomavirus type 16 together are necessary and sufficient for transformation of primary human keratinocytes. J Virol. 1989;63(10):4417–21.
112. Korzeniewski N, Spardy N, Duensing A, Duensing S. Genomic instability and cancer: lessons learned from human papillomaviruses. Cancer Lett. 2011;305(2):113–22.

Screening for Cervical Cancer in Low-Resource Countries

6

Laurie Elit

Abstract

The World Health Organization (WHO) has outlined prerequisites necessary to determine if a mass screening programme should be developed. This chapter reviews the evidence for each of these prerequisites as they pertain to cervical cancer, with particular attention to low-resource settings. The evidence for cervical screening to prevent cervical cancer is based on a review of literature published between 2000 and 2011. The level of evidence supporting the use of three types of screening tests (cervical cytology, visual inspection, HPV testing), diagnosis (with colposcopy and biopsy), and treatment (with cryotherapy, laser, LEEP, cold-knife cone biopsy, or hysterectomy) is examined as a means of preventing cervical cancer or downstaging the disease. The benefits of a population-based programme are described and supported by examples of such programmes of in low-resource countries. In those jurisdictions where cervical cancer is a major cause of cancer incidence and mortality, the optimal approach is an organized screening programme. For low-resource settings, a "see-and-treat" approach with either VIA or careHPV™ followed by cryotherapy is the most cost-effective strategy.

Dedicated to John Sellors 1946–2011: John Sellors and I were to co-author this chapter. Unfortunately, Dr. Sellors died on December 31, 2011. He spent the later decades of his life introducing, assessing, and implementing many of the screening methods described in this chapter in low-resource settings.

It is for man to tame the chaos; on every side, whilst he lives, to scatter the seeds of science and of song, that climate, corn, animals, men, may be milder, and the germs of love and benefit may be multiplied.

Ralph Waldo Emerson, Uses of Great Men: http://www.bartleby.com/109/9.html. Accessed 28 Dec 2011.

L. Elit (✉)
Department of Obstetrics and Gynecology, Hamilton Health Sciences Centre, Hamilton, ON, Canada L8V 5C2
e-mail: laurie.elit@jcc.hhsc.ca

M.K. Shetty (ed.), *Breast and Gynecological Cancers: An Integrated Approach for Screening and Early Diagnosis in Developing Countries*, DOI 10.1007/978-1-4614-1876-4_6,

Introduction

The WHO has outlined prerequisites necessary to determine if a mass screening programme should be developed [1]. These prerequisites include:

1. The disease must be common enough to justify mass screening
2. It must be associated with significant mortality
3. Effective treatment is available for pre-invasive or early invasive disease
4. Detection and treatment of a presymptomatic state result in benefits beyond those obtained through treatment of symptomatic disease

In this chapter, we will review the evidence available for each of these prerequisites as they pertain to cervical cancer [2].

Magnitude of the Problem

Globally, cervical cancer accounts for 10 % of all female cancers, making it the third leading cause of cancer and the fourth leading cause of cancer death in women [3]. Annually, 530,232 women are affected with cervical cancer (ASR 15.2), and 275,008 women die of their disease (ASR 7.8). The mortality to incidence ratio is 52 %. Eighty-five percent of cervical cancer cases occur in low-resource countries, and 85 % of these women die of their disease [4–8]. In low-resource settings, cervical cancer is the second leading cause of cancer and death compared to high-resource settings, where it is the tenth leading cause of cancer [3]. Age-standardized incidence rates are highest in Africa (i.e. ASR 69 per 100,000 in Tanzania), Central America (i.e. ASR 55 per 100,000 in Bolivia), south central and eastern Asia (i.e. ASR 24.6 per 100,000) and South America (i.e. ASR 23.9 per 100,000) [9]. These rates are astronomical when compared to rates of less than 6 per 100,000 in Australia/New Zealand, Europe, and North America [10]. These disparities in part are based on whether there is access to an organized screening programme [11]. Thus, in low-resource settings where such programmes are non-existent, women with cervical cancer often present to hospital with symptoms such as bleeding and foul smelling discharge, which reflect advanced/metastatic disease [12]. Thus, globally, cervical cancer is a common and deadly disease fulfilling the first and second prerequisites put forward by the WHO to justify mass screening.

Process of Cervical Cancer Development

Cervical cancer arises in the transformation zone of the uterine cervix. This area undergoes dynamic change especially at puberty where squamous epithelium impinges upon the glandular epithelium in a process known as metaplasia. The human papilloma viral infection is a very common sexually acquired infection that is introduced with the onset of sexual activity. In most cases, the viral infection is resolved by the woman's own immune system. However, if there is a persistent infection, especially with the oncogenic types of HPV (i.e. 16, 18, 31, 33, 35, 39, 45, 51, 52, 56, 57, 58, 68, etc.), the viral oncoproteins produce loss of the cell cycle controls. The cells reflect this with a change in nuclear to cytoplasmic ration, loss of nuclear regularity, and chromatin clumping. These cytologic changes are known as dysplasia or, following a more contemporary nomenclature using the Bethesda terminology, squamous and/or adeno intraepithelial lesion (SIL) (see ref. [20]). The degree of cellular and architectural changes in the cervical biopsy is classified in terms of levels of cervical intraepithelial neoplasia (CIN). In the mildest form, CIN 1, the HPV infection causes changes in the lowest one-third of the epithelium. Often (80 %), a CIN 1 lesion will resolve over 12–24 months, especially in young women. However, in the most severe form, CIN 3, the cellular changes affect the whole epithelium above the basement membrane. The risk of a CIN 3 lesion progression to cancer is estimated to be 31.3 % (95 % CI 22.7–42.3) if the lesion is not detected and treated [13]. The peak incidence of an HPV infection occurs when a women is in her 20s. The peak incidence of CIN 3 is seen in her 30s [13, 14]. The peak incidence of cervical cancer is in the mid-40s [15]. This transition from infection to dysplasia (SIL or CIN) to cancer takes several years, thus allowing the opportunity for detection by a screening test.

In the case of cervical cancer, there is a presymptomatic/precancerous disease state that spans a significant period of time during which, if identified, there is the potential to remove the disease. This meets prerequisite 4 of the WHO criteria justifying mass screening (Table 6.1).

Prevention as a Component of the Disease Continuum (Framework)

Cervical Screening should be part of a woman's regular health journey, where asymptomatic women are assessed with a test to determine if a precancerous lesion is present. Then, if found, *Cervical Diagnosis* becomes part of the cervical cancer journey, where women with a positive screening test are sent for further diagnostic test(s). Further along that path, *Cervical Treatment* involves removing the disease to prevent the occurrence of cancer or identifying and treating asymptomatic early stage cancer (Fig. 6.1).

Table 6.1 Comparing Classification Systems for Squamous Lesions.

Dysplasia (cytology)	CIN (histology)	Bethesda (cytology)
Normal	Normal	Normal
Atypia	Atypia	ASCUS
HPV effect	HPV effect	LSIL
Mild dysplasia	CIN 1	
Moderate dysplasia	CIN 2	HSIL
Severe dysplasia	CIN 3	
Carcinoma in Situ (CIS)		
Cancer	Cancer	Cancer

Definition of Low-, Medium-, and High-Resource Countries

There are many ways of defining "developing" or "low-resource countries." Some agencies use a definition based on rate of literacy or life expectancy [16]. For this chapter, we will use the classification put forward by the World Bank. The Gross National Income per capita is divided into three strata: low-resource countries (US$ 1,005 or less), middle-resource (low-middle is US$ 1,006–3,975; upper-middle US$ 3,976–12,275), and high-resource countries (US$ 12,276 or more) [17].

The remainder of this chapter will focus in more detail on the WHO prerequisites 3 and 4 as they pertain to cervical cancer prevention.

Methods

For this chapter, we reviewed the literature on the screening modalities for cervical cancer in low-resource settings, and we included MEDLINE,

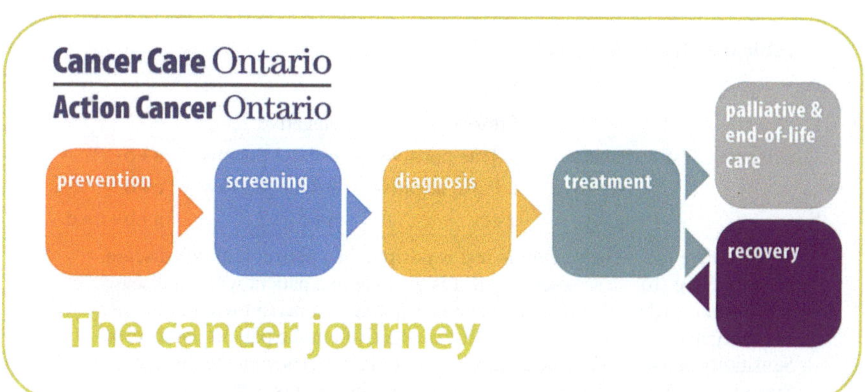

Fig. 6.1 Prevention as part of the disease continuum. (Courtesy of Cancer Care Ontario, Toronto, Ontario, Canada)

CINAHL, EMBASE, GOOGLE, and the Cochrane library from 2000 to December 2011. Bibliographies of relevant review articles and included studies were scanned for additional relevant publications. Included in the literature search strategy were terms such as "cervical cancer," "cervical neoplasm," "utero-cervical neoplasm," "screening," "developing country," "low-resource country," "cervical cytology," and "VIA testing" and "HPV testing." We excluded non-English publications.

Screening Tests

What Makes a Good Screening Test?

For a screening test to be clinically useful, it must be simple, inexpensive, accurate, and acceptable by the patient. In this section, we will review the available screening tests, their efficacy, advantages, and limitations. There are three screening tests which will be reviewed: cervical cytology, visual inspection, and oncogenic HPV assessment. The best way to think about screening is as a therapeutic intervention. In this chapter, randomized trials examine the effect of screening on patient important outcomes. The outcomes of interest are that cervical cancer screening will (1) reduce the *incidence* of cervical cancer through detection and removal of precancerous lesions and (2) reduce disease progression through detection of invasive cancers in the early stages, thereby improving the chance for cure and reducing *mortality* [18]. See Table 6.2.

The possible consequences of screening are that some women will have a true-positive result (a) (i.e. HSIL) with clinically significant disease (CIN 3), and they will benefit from treatment. However there are some patients with inconsequential disease (ASCUS), and they may experience the consequences of labelling, investigation, and treatment for disease (HPV infection) which may never affect their lives. Women with a false-positive result (b) may be adversely affected by the risks associated with investigation (i.e. colposcopically directed biopsy). False Negative (c) involves women who, for example, have a normal Pap test when they actually have disease; this result delays investigations. Patients with a true negative (d) experience the benefit associated with accurate reassurance of being disease free, but they may have experienced inconvenience, cost, and anxiety associated with screening [19].

Cervical Cytology (Otherwise Known as the Pap Test or Pap Smear)

In 1940, George Papanicolaou discovered that cells retrieved from the apex of the vagina could reflect changes in the cervix that over time led to cervical cancer. Today, cervical cytology is obtained usually by a physician. After the woman is counselled about the purpose of the test and gives permission to have the test, she is examined

Table 6.2 Test parameters

		Disease		
		Present	Negative	
Screening Test	Positive	a-True positive	b-False positive	a+b
	Negative	c-False negative	d-True negative	c+d
		a+c	b+d	a+b+c+d

True positive (a)—The screening test is positive in a patient with the disease
False positive (b)—The screening test is positive in a patient without disease
True negative (d)—The screening test is negative in a patient without disease
False negative (c)—The screening test is negative but the patient has disease
Sensitivity: a/a+c—The rate of test positivity in patients with the disease
Specificity: d/b+d—The rate of test negativity in patients without the disease
Positive predictive value: a/a+b—Rate of disease in patients with a positive test
Negative predictive value: d/c+d—Rate of no disease in patients with a negative test

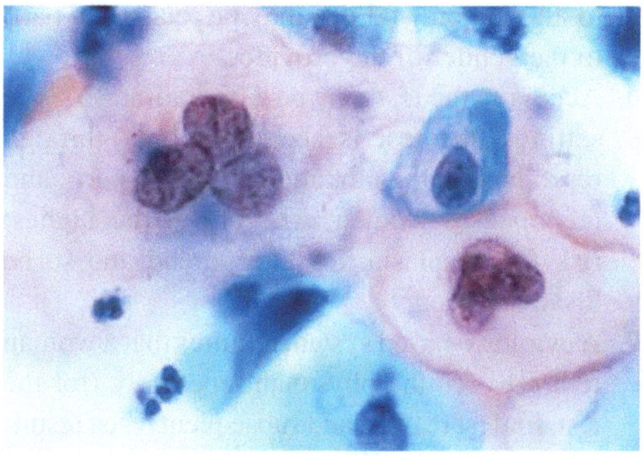

Fig. 6.2 Example of a cervical cytology specimen

in the lithotomy position. With a speculum in the vagina and either using either a spatula and/or a brush, cells are scraped from the cervix and either spread across a glass slide and fixed with cytospray (or hairspray in some jurisdictions) (Fig. 6.2). Alternatively the cells are placed in a liquid-based media (such as Hologic's Thin Prep®, Bedford, MA), or BD SurePath™ (Franklin Lakes, NJ). This specimen is processed in a lab with various stains and read by a cytotechnologist and/or cytologist. The results are reported using the Bethesda 2001 classification system [20]. A few weeks after the test is obtained, the woman must return or call her physician's office for her results and disposition planning.

Efficacy

There has only been one randomized trial comparing a once-in-a-lifetime cervical cytology to no screening. Fifty-two villages in India, with a total of 131,746 healthy women aged 30–59 years, were randomly assigned to one of four groups [21]. These groups received screening by a single lifetime cervical cytology ($n=32{,}058$), HPV test ($n=34{,}126$), visual inspection by acetic acid ($n=34{,}074$), or standard care which involved giving women information on how to seek screening at local hospitals ($n=31{,}488$). The single lifetime cytology test had no significant impact on 8 years mortality (age-adjusted HR 0.89, 95 % CI 0.62–1.28, $p=0.53$). The single lifetime cytology test had no statistical impact on 8 years incidence of cervical cancer (age-adjusted HR 1.34, 95 % CI 0.99–1.81, $p=0.06$). The higher incidence of cervical cancer in the screened group is explained by the active detection of disease in the screened group and the fact that this was the first screen almost any woman had received. A single lifetime cytology test had no statistical impact on 8-year incidence of Stage 2 or higher cervical cancer (age-adjusted HR 0.75, 95 % CI 0.51–1.10, $p=0.14$).

Although there is no direct evidence from randomized trials for the efficacy of a single cervical cytology test in decreasing rates of cervical cancer, there is overwhelming epidemiologic data to infer the impact of cytology screening on reducing cervical cancer rates. These data come from two types of work. First, case–control studies have been reported from many jurisdictions around the world comparing the history of cervical cytology of women with cervical cancer and age-matched controls of those without cervical cancer (i.e. Canada, Columbia, Costa Rica, Finland, Japan, Italy, South Africa, Panama, Sweden, USA). These studies show consistently that the odds of developing cervical cancer are lower in those women who received at least one Pap test (in the order of OR 0.036) compared to those not screened [18, 22–34]. The second body of epidemiologic evidence is the correlation of incidence and mortality trends of cervical cancer in screened populations such as reported from Canada, the Nordic countries, and the UK [35–38].

The test parameters for conventional cervical cytology to define lesions of CIN 2 or worse are sensitivity 44–78 % and specificity 91–96 % [39, 40]. The low sensitivity means that, in those women with a normal test, it must be repeated frequently (i.e. at least every 3 years) to ensure that a lesion has not been missed or that a new lesion has not developed [15]. The high specificity means that those women without disease will have a normal test result.

Advantages

The advantages of cervical cytology are that the test is easy to learn to perform and the consumables (i.e. spatula) are low cost.

Limitations

Since cervical cytology has been available for at least 50 years, its limitations are well documented:

1. As discussed earlier, a single Pap test has low sensitivity, and this sensitivity can be improved with repeated cytological assessments over time. The low sensitivity can be related to process issues: for example, the physician may fail to sample the squamocolumnar junction (more common in perimenopausal or postmenopausal women). This high false-negative rate is a serious weakness [41].
2. A high rate of unsatisfactory smears can occur: for example, if the sample is not fixed appropriately, if cotton tips applicators are used to retrieve the specimen (as the cotton fibres create artefact on the slide), or if the woman has an infection. If the woman has an unsatisfactory smear, she should return for a repeat test. Liquid-based cytology has been developed to decrease the amount of time necessary to assess each specimen, to decrease the number of unsatisfactory cervical cytology reports, and to allow the residual fluid to be available for HPV assessment; it can be automated. However, a systematic review and meta-analysis of liquid-based cytology show that sensitivity and specificity are the same as for conventional cytology [40].
3. Another limitation is that evaluation of the cytology test is highly subjective. The cytologists and cytotechnologists must be trained to recognize various cellular patterns. Thus, at the laboratory level, there must be an ongoing system of quality assurance both in optimally staining the slides and pattern recognition.
4. The cost of infrastructure, including laboratory space, personnel, and information networks, can be daunting. Conventional cytology screening is resilient and the reagents are low in cost, compared to those jurisdictions that use liquid-based cytology, which requires expensive equipment, a reliable electrical source, and daily maintenance, which may not be available in all settings [42, 43].
5. The attitudes and beliefs of a woman influence her willingness to have a screening test. For example, a pelvic exam may not be acceptable to all women, and this may be related, in part, to the gender of the provider.
6. Access to the test may be a limitation. In some settings, the test is accessible only through reproductive health clinics. Thus, peri- and menopausal women, who are at the highest risk for dysplasia, may not attend and so be disadvantaged.
7. A cytology-based system requires that a woman return to see the physician repeatedly (for the test, for test results, and subsequent tests, resulting in reduced patient compliance as discussed later in this chapter). Out-of-pocket costs for health care and indirect costs of lost hours of productive work, child care expenses, or long distance travel can put a great burden on poor women. Thus, a cytology-based system may fail due to low compliance [42, 44–48].

Other Considerations from Experiences in Low-Resource Settings

In Central and South America, there was a high coverage in screening appropriate women, but the quality of cytology assessment was poor, and so rates of cervical cancer remain high [49]. Strategies to improve this problem included implementing telemedicine systems to help bring high-quality cytology assessment to remote settings. For example, the Italian NGO Associazione Patologi Oltre Frontiera (APOF) has worked since 2000 to help countries in Sub-Saharan Africa [50]. A pilot project in Chirundu, Southern Zambia, showed that it was feasible to train histology lab workers to screen Pap smears, take digital photographs of suspicious or positive cases, and then by digital scanner and satellite connection confirm a diagnosis within four days. Original slides are reviewed in Italy every 6 months for quality-control purposes.

Conclusion

Cervical cytology, especially if repeated periodically during a woman's lifetime, has resulted in a fall in cervical cancer rates; however, there are limitations not just with the test but the context in which it is applied. We will discuss these in more detail later in this chapter.

Visual Inspection (Otherwise Known as Direct Visual Inspection)

Visual inspection involves inspecting the cervix with the naked eye using a bright light source and is followed by the application of either a 3–5 % dilute acetic acid for one minute (known as visual inspection with acetic acid, VIA) or acetic acid test (AAT). If Lugol's iodine is used, this is called visual inspection with Lugol's iodine (VILI) or the Schiller's test.

Visual Inspection with Acetic Acid

With the application of acetic acid to the cervix, there is a reversible coagulation of intracellular proteins. If dysplasia is present, a pronounced white lesion is seen. A VIA test can be reported as "negative" if no lesion is seen, "positive" if there is detection of a well-defined aceto-white area close to the squamocolumnar junction (Fig. 6.3), and "suspicious for cancer" if an irregularly exophytic or ulcerative lesion is identified (Fig. 6.4) [51, 52]. VIA can only reliably be used in women where the squamocolumnar junction is visible on the ectocervix; thus, it should mainly be used in women 30–45 years old.

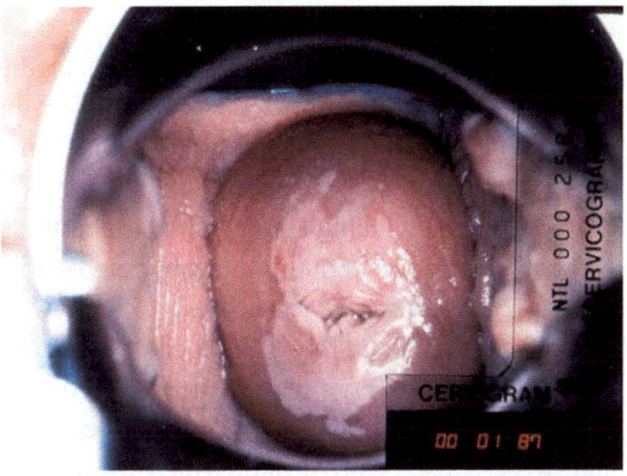

Fig. 6.3 Cervix after the application of 3-5 % vinegar showing a white lesion. This is an example of VIA positive

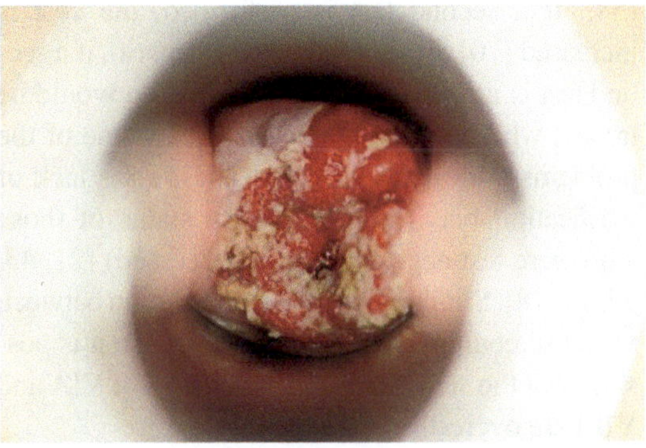

Fig. 6.4 Cervical cancer. This is an example of VIA suspicious for cancer

Efficacy

A cluster-randomized trial in the Dindigul district of India involved 49,311 women aged 30–59 years. They were randomized to health education or VIA. At 7 years, the VIA group had a lower incidence of cancer (HR 0.75 95 % CI 0.55–0.95) and lower mortality (HR 0.65, 95 % CI 0.47–0.89) [53].

A cluster-randomized trial in India involved 142,701 women aged 30–59 years. One group was given education alone. The three other groups involved a once-in-a-life time cervical cytology or VIA or oncogenic HPV test. Detection of CIN 2/3 was the same for all three screening tests at 0.7 % for VIA, 1 % for cytology, and 0.9 % for oncogenic HPV DNA [21].

The test parameters for VIA have been critically assessed, and the sensitivity ranges from 49–96 % and the specificity ranges from 49–98 % [54, 55].

Advantages

VIA has several advantages. It is inexpensive [9, 56, 57] . When used in already existing health centres, the instruments required for VIA are already present, and there are few disposables [9, 56–59]. VIA is easy to learn [57] and can be performed by a wide range of health-care workers (i.e. physician, nurse, midwife, local health-care worker) [52, 56, 57, 60–63]. The accuracy of VIA is the same as cervical cytology. Sensitivity is the same or higher than cervical cytology. VIA provides immediate results, which can be given to the woman during the same physician visit [9, 56–59, 63, 64]. VIA can be used in a screen-and-treat algorithm which decreases issues related to compliance (to be discussed later in this chapter). VIA does not require a lab infrastructure [59]. VIA can be associated with increasing screening coverage, which in part means laying down the framework to integrate novel, more sensitive technologies in the future [65].

Limitations

In VIA the acetic acid can cause a temporary stinging sensation for the woman.VIA is not suitable for older women because the squamocolumnar junction is not visible on the exocervix [57, 58]. VIA is a subjective test with high inter-rater variability, so substantial provider-training and ongoing quality assurance assessments are needed [55, 66–70]. Some fear that the quality assurance of VIA may be more difficult to control than the quality of cervical cytology [71]. VIA has a lower specificity and higher false-positive rate, which means that women need to be referred for a second test like colposcopy to determine if the disease is truly present. This might mean the colposcopy and pathology departments could be overwhelmed [58]. If a second test is performed, the cost is increased [70]. In a see-and-treat scenario, if a second test is not performed, many women would be treated who do not have disease [72]. One of the problems with many of the studies is the lack of verification bias (i.e. the disease status of those who were test negative was not assessed) [21, 43, 54, 73–78]. Similarly, there is a correlation between visual screening tests and colposcopy, so it is possible that the sensitivity and specificity of VIA and VILI are overestimated [55].

Some barriers to VIA uptake include the resistance of medical professionals to using a screening test other than cervical cytology. Some national policies restrict screening and treatment to physician providers, and they do not recognize or support use of VIA, especially when done by midwives or nurses.

Other Considerations

VIA lends itself to mobile telemedicine technology. In Gaborone, Botswana, four nurse midwives collected VIA images by mobile phone, and these were transferred to a website by MMS without need for an Internet connection. Unfortunately, in this study in a third of cases the images were insufficient [56, 79]. The concept of VIA image capture was assessed in El Salvador. Here, a digital camera gave the opportunity for a second assessment which resulted in a higher sensitivity than using the naked eye alone [80]. Capturing the images can be useful for getting further input from colleagues or physician staff, medical record storage, or quality assurance.

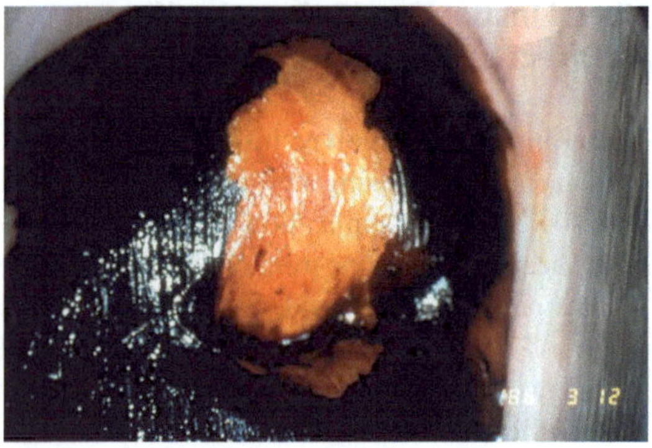

Fig. 6.5 Cervix after the application of Lugol's iodine. This is an example of VILLI positive

Visual Inspection with Lugol's Iodine

In visual inspection with Lugol's iodine (VILI), the cervix is washed with Lugol's iodine and the glycogenated cells of the vagina and cervix stain a deep mahogany brown. The non-glycogenated cells such as the glandular epithelium and areas of dysplasia do not stain. Findings are reported in terms of "VILI negative" (no lesion or abnormality), "VILI positive" (a lesion is identified) (Fig. 6.5), and "suspicious for cancer."

Efficacy

There are several studies assessing the use of VILI. A multi-centre study involving 49,000 women in India and Africa compared evaluations with VIA and VILI. The sensitivity of VILI was 92 % and the specificity was 85 % [64]. Another study involving 3,000 Latin-American women showed less optimistic findings, with sensitivity of 53 % and specificity of 78 % [81].

Advantages

VILI can be conducted by nurses or midwives after being trained. It requires minimal supplies (i.e. Lugol's iodine). Results are available at the time of test.

Limitations

Lugol's iodine is quite messy and can stain a person's clothes. Providers require training and ongoing quality reviews as the assessment is subjective. There are no studies on the efficacy of VILI in decreasing the incidence or mortality from cervical cancer.

VIA with Magnification

The AviScope™ is one example of VIA with Magnification. Here, the cervix is inspected with LED illumination with four-fold magnification of the cervix [82].There are no reports on efficacy. The advantage is better identification of lesions. The limitations in low-resource settings are the occurrences of power outages, power fluctuations, and difficulty in repairing equipment or getting parts [83].

Oncogenic HPV Test

A persistent oncogenic HPV infection is the known cause of cervical dysplasia and, ultimately, cancer. The genital tract can be swabbed for oncogenic HPV. There are a number of commercially available tests available for assessing for the presence or absence of oncogenic HPV types (i.e. HC2, HPV, DNA test produced by Qiagen (Hilden, Germany), also called the Digene® HPV test) or specific oncogenic HPV types (i.e. cobas® HPV test by Roche Molecular Diagnositics (Pleasanton, CA)). The number of HPV types varies slightly across tests.

The global estimates are that the overall age-adjusted prevalence of HPV is 10.5 %. Geographic variation of oncogenic HPV prevalence exists with the higher rates being noted in resource-poor regions (i.e. 35 % in Mongolia) [84]. Prevalence is known to decline as a woman ages. Using an HPV test in women over 30 years of age is more likely to pick up persistent HPV infection associated with dysplasia compared to the transient infection seen in younger women.

Efficacy

The efficacy of a once-in-a-lifetime oncogenic HPV test was evaluated in fifty-two clusters of villages in India, with a total of 131,746 healthy women between the ages of 30 and 59 years [21]. The villages were randomly assigned to four groups: one group underwent screening by a once-in-a-lifetime HPV test (34,126 women), and one group received the standard of care which involved giving women information on how to seek screening at local hospitals (31,488). The once-in-a-lifetime screen made an impact on mortality. Screening using a single lifetime HPV test made a significant impact on 8-year mortality when compared to no screening (age-adjusted HR 0.52, 95 %CI 0.33–0.83, $p=0.005$). There was no impact on overall incidence of cervical cancer (age-adjusted HR 1.05, 95 % CI 0.77–1.43, $p=0.76$). However, a randomized study from Finland using cancer registry data showed in 58,076 women that HPV testing with cytology triage was superior to cytology alone in identifying CIN 3 or worse (HR 1.77, 95 %CI 1.16–2.74) [85]. The study from India showed that only HPV testing had an impact on *the incidence of advanced cancer* (*Stage 2 or higher cancer*), by significantly decreased advanced cervical cancer (age-adjusted HR 0.47, 95 %CI 0.32–0.69, $p=0.0001$) [35].

There have been six randomized controlled trials in Europe and one in Canada evaluating HPV test, either alone or in combination with cytology. HPV DNA is more sensitive than cytology in women over 30 years (96 % compared to 53 %) but less specific (91 % compared to 96 %) [86–88]. The very high negative predictive value of HPV testing allows prolongation of the interval between tests (i.e. the test need only be repeated every 5 or more years) [22, 49, 88].

Twenty-five cross-sectional studies where women were concomitantly tested with Pap test and HC 2 HPV test also showed that the sensitivity for CIN 2/3 was 89.7 % (95 %CI 86.4–93.0) [22, 38]. Specificity was 85–90 % [22]. Unfortunately, the HC2 HPV test has consistently high sensitivity in Europe and North America [89, 90] but not in all low- and middle-resource countries. For example, sensitivity of HC2 HPV test in three cross-sectional studies in India were 50, 70, and 80 %; Peru was 77 %; Zimbabwe was 81 %; Brazil was 83 %; and South Africa was 88 % [15]. A cross-sectional comparison of screening performance of five screening methods (VIA, VILI, VIA with magnification (VIAM), cytology, and HPV) in 11 study sites in low-resource settings showed the following results for the detection of CIN 2 or worse: cytology (sensitivity was 57 %, specificity 93 %), VIA (sensitivity 79 % and specificity 85 %), and HPV (sensitivity 62 % and specificity 94 %) [40, 90].

Through funds from the Bill and Melinda Gates Foundation (Washington State), an HPV test (careHPV™, Qiagen, Hilden, Germany) was specifically developed with the issues unique to low-resource countries in mind. careHPV™ assesses for 14 oncogenic HPV types [16, 18, 31, 33, 35, 38, 44, 50, 51, 55, 57, 58, 65, 67]. It is affordable (<US$ 5 per test). The results are available in 3 h compared to 7 h for HC2. It requires very basic laboratory supplies—for example, no running water is required—making it simpler to perform. This test was evaluated in 2,400 women in Shanxi province, China. Sensitivity was 90 % and specificity was 84 % compared to cytology at 41 and 95 %, respectively [91].

Advantages

An oncogenic HPV test is objective, reproducible, and less demanding in terms of training, and it can be performed by a technician, and quality assurance is easier to demonstrate compared to cytology [11]. Because of the excellent negative predictive value of the test, it provides 5–10 years of reassurance against high-grade disease, thus allowing for an increase screening interval [92].

One of the unique attributes of the oncogenic HPV test is that it provides an opportunity for a woman to complete the test by herself without a pelvic exam. This self-sampling of the vagina, although less sensitive (74 %) and less specific (84 %) than a physician-acquired sampling test from the cervix, is a potential option for hard-to-reach populations (i.e. due to geographic isolation or populations where there is a cultural hesitancy to pelvic examinations). Self-sampling should increase population coverage among women who are uncomfortable with provider-conducted screening (i.e. fear of speculum exam, loss of privacy, resistance from spouse) [11, 93–102]. Self-sampling is cost-effective and reduces time to do screening [103]. It is highly accepted by women [103, 104].

Limitations

An oncogenic HPV test involves doing an endocervical swab and this should not be done in pregnancy [57]. Laboratory equipment and reagents are required even for the careHPV™ test [57]. Laboratory technicians do require some basic training [57]. There is a cost for the equipment to take and perform the test [57, 105]. Currently, the algorithms for using the test are not clearly defined. This is important as the lower specificity of the HPV test means that a "see-and-treat" policy would result in a high number of women with infection, but not dysplasia, being treated. Using a second test after a positive HPV test (prior to referral to colposcopy) could involve cytology or VIA triage, which increases the number of appointments, with the associated compliance problems, and increases cost [57].

In conclusion, screening does identify precancerous lesions and results in a stage shift to earlier stages of disease and therefore benefits women. This meets prerequisite four of the WHO guidelines for screening.

Diagnosis

In high-resource countries, women with an abnormal result on a screening test often go for further diagnostic assessment. This usually involves a colposcopic assessment with cervical biopsies. The colposcope was first introduced by Hans Hinselmann from Germany in 1925. It allows for magnification (5- to 15-fold) and illuminates the

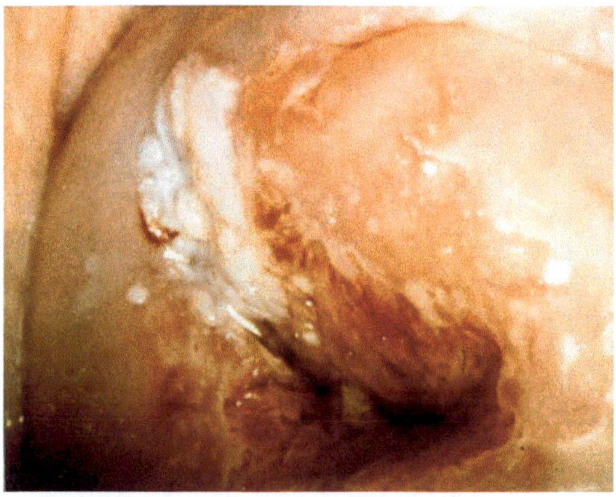

Fig. 6.6 Colpophotograph of a white lesion

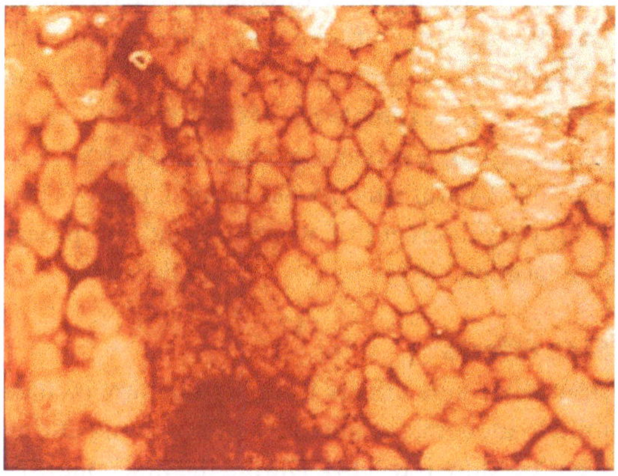

Fig. 6.7 Colpophotograph of mosaicism

cervix. The cervix is examined once the speculum is placed and then again after the application of acetic acid. Features indicative of high-grade dysplasia include a well-demarcated white lesion (Fig. 6.6) near the squamocolumnar junction, especially if there is an abnormal vessel pattern with punctuation or mosaicism (Fig. 6.7). The more severe the dysplasia, the more it is characterized by an opaque colour of the lesion, well-demarcated boarders, and a coarser vascular pattern. Visualizing the lesion with a green filter can often enhance the vascular pattern (Fig. 6.8). The adequacy of the colposcopic examination involves assessing whether the extent of the lesion can be seen, especially into the endocervical canal. Colposcopy is a subjective assessment and thus requires training and ongoing quality assurance. Many jurisdictions (i.e. British Columbia, Canada, and the UK) have an accreditation system for certifying and ongoing assessment of medical staff that perform colposcopy.

Efficacy

Although colposcopically directed biopsies have been the gold standard against which screening tests have been evaluated, when colposcopically directed biopsies are assessed against larger excisional biopsies or hysterectomy, the sensitivity of colposcopy is only 44–77 %, the specificity is 85–90 %, and the positive predictive value is low [106, 107]. More recently, the use of colposcopically directed biopsies was evaluated in China against routinely completing four quadrant biopsies and an endocervical sample. The latter procedure identified more disease ($p=0.03$ to $p<0.001$) [108–112].

Advantages

A colposcopic exam with biopsies means that only women with histologically proven high-grade dysplasia are offered treatment. Women with a cytology assessment that shows high-grade disease but a non-confirming biopsy are usually offered further assessment with a cone biopsy (to be discussed later in this chapter).

Limitations

A colposcopic examination requires at least two visits: one visit for assessment and one for the provision of results and counselling around next steps. Colposcopy is usually available only at specialized centres, and this increases the direct payment (for the assessment and the evaluation of the biopsies) and indirect costs (travel to attend the examination, childcare costs, lost time from work) that a woman assumes. For these reasons, women may not comply with this strategy. Colposcopy requires pattern recognition training for both colposcopists and pathologists.

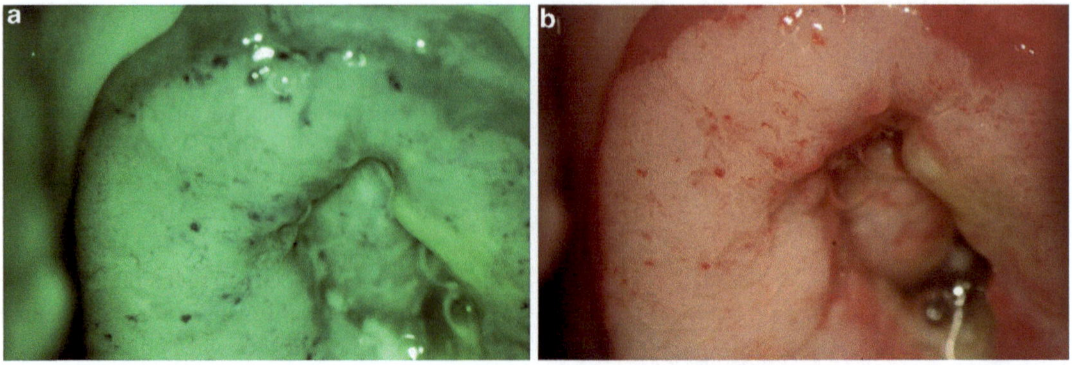

Fig. 6.8 Colpophotograph with the *green* filter (**a**) and without the *green* filter (**b**)

Colposcopy requires expensive colposcopy and pathology equipment that requires maintenance and replacement parts. Colposcopy requires a reliable electrical supply.

Treatment of Precancerous Lesions

Once high-grade disease is identified, there are several treatment options available for removing the lesion (i.e. cryotherapy, loop electrosurgical excisional procedure (LEEP), laser, cold-knife cone biopsy, and hysterectomy) for removing the lesion. Each option has its own attributes and limitations.

Cryotherapy

Cryotherapy has been in use for more than 40 years. Cryotherapy means the cells are exposed to temperatures of −20° C for more than one minute and so undergo cryonecrosis. Cryotherapy is mainly used to treat small lesions on the ectocervix. Cryotherapy leaves no histological sample for assessment. The procedure involves visualizing the cervix, the cryotherapy probe with its circular metal tip is applied to the ectocervix, and a refrigerant gas (either nitrous oxide or carbon dioxide) is allowed to flow through the instrument cooling the metal tip. With cervical tissue, the recommendation is to freeze for 3 min, allow a thaw for 5 min, and then refreeze for three minutes [113, 114].

Efficacy

With cryotherapy, 90 % of women with dysplasia are disease free at one year after treatment. Efficacy decreases as the severity of the disease increases; for example 83–100 % of CIN 1 cases are disease free at one year compared to 65–95 % of CIN 2 cases and 55–92 % of CIN 3 [115]. Eighty-five percent of women found the procedure acceptable [60].

Side Effects

Immediate side effects from cryotherapy include mild to moderate cramping and/or fainting during the procedure [60, 114]. During the first couple of weeks after the treatment, there is a profuse, watery, vaginal discharge [60, 114]. Cervicitis and/or PID can occur in 1 % of women [53, 57, 114], vaginal wall injury in 0.1–0.8 % [114], and hospitalization in 0.5–1 % [114]. Long-term complications can include cervical stenosis or infertility, but these are rare [114]. Following cryotherapy, it is difficult to assess the squamocolumnar junction in future colposcopic evaluations.

Advantages

Cryotherapy requires no anaesthesia or electricity. The equipment is portable, and the consumables are low in cost. With adequate training and supervision, primary health-care professionals (i.e. nurses) can provide cryotherapy [116].

Limitations

Cryotherapy is not recommended in the following situations: pregnancy; women who have large lesions involving more than three quadrants; a lesion which extends beyond the cryoprobe by 2 mm; endocervical lesions; a lesion that extends onto the vagina; situations where there are polyps, ulcers, a distorted or atrophic cervix; situations where cervicitis or PID is present; a bleeding diathesis; vaginal wall prolapsed causing inadequate visualization of the cervix; or any lesion suspicious for cancer. If a lesion has not resolved after two cryotherapy sessions, the patient should have a cone biopsy. The equipment must be properly decontaminated before reuse to prevent spread of infection (usually in 10 % bleach solution or 70 % ethyl alcohol). The costs of cryotherapy involve the cryotherapy unit ($400/unit), the carbon dioxide or nitrous oxygen gas, the tank, and the refrigerant. There has been an issue with clogging or blockage of the gas flow within the cryo unit, and various techniques exist to deal with these problems [117].

Loop Electrosurgical Excisional Procedure or Large Loop Excision of Transformation Zone

LEEP involves the use of a fine wire to excise a lesion from the cervix. The loops come in various sizes and shapes. The loops attach to a handheld apparatus that allows for cutting or coagulation settings. The handheld piece is attached to an electrosurgical power generator. A smoke evacuator is used to minimize the plume. When doing a LEEP, a specially coated speculum should be used. The cervix is usually washed with Lugol's iodine to ensure that the physician sees the extent of the lesion. Some physicians would use local anaesthetic to minimize the woman's discomfort during the procedure. Some physicians add epinephrine or vasopressin to minimize bleeding.

Efficacy

LEEP, laser, and cold-knife cone all have the same efficacy (reduction of invasive cancer by 95 % for at least 8 years) [106, 118–120].

Side Effects

Immediate side effects from a LEEP include cramping or pain. This pain is no different in severity or duration compared to cryotherapy [114]. During the first days after a treatment, all patients have some vaginal discharge [114] or bleeding. Significant bleeding can occur in 2 % of women and is usually related to the extent of the procedure and/or a superimposed infection [114]. Vaginal wall injuries occur in 0.4–4.4 % of women. Cervical stenosis is a long-term complication that occurs in 4–6 % of women [114]. Of all of the treatment options, LEEP is the maneuver that most likely allows preservation of the squamocolumnar junction for future assessments. Long-term complications can include premature rupture of membranes (OR 2.69, 95 % CI 1.62–4.46) [120, 121], preterm delivery (OR 1.81, 95 % 1.18–2.76), low-birth weight infants (<2,500 g) (OR 1.60, 95 % CI 1.01–2.52), and cervical stenosis [120, 122].

Advantages

LEEP can be used for small or large lesions of the cervix [123]. LEEP provides a histological specimen for confirmation of the extent and severity of disease. The LEEP specimen may involve one pass or multiple passes. Adequacy of excision is more difficult to assess when there have been multiple passes. Access to the coagulation setting on the handheld device allows an immediate resource to stop bleeding in the event that this is an issue.

Limitations

Compared to cryotherapy, LEEP requires more training and is usually only performed by physicians in specialized centres; these requirements have implications for patient access to care. It requires more equipment (i.e. electrocautery generator, one-time use loops, handheld disposable devise, smoke evacuator with tubing and filters, specialized speculums to minimize transduction of heat) and so the cost is higher. It requires a reliable electrical supply. Although LEEP provides a histological specimen, the cautery artefact at the edges of the sample may make it difficult to assess the adequacy of excision (i.e. margins) in some cases.

Laser

Laser involves using a very high energy light beam to either evaporate the cells of the high-grade lesions or excise them. The laser works by being attached to a colposcope. A smoke evacuator is necessary. Everyone in the room must wear eye protection and masks to filter evaporated particles/plume. Any flammable material (sheets, paper drapes) must either be moved away from the area of work or made wet to decrease the risk of fire.

Efficacy

As listed for LEEP.

Advantages

The advantages are the same as those listed for LEEP. The laser energy beam can be defocused to deal with immediate bleeding. The laser is very useful for dealing with lesions that extend onto the vagina/vulva.

Limitations

Laser requires very expensive equipment (i.e. laser power source, micromanipulator, colposcope, galvanized speculum, smoke evacuator with tubing and filter, eye protection for everyone in the room, CO_2 gas). It requires a reliable power supply. The laser requires access to replace parts. There is a need for both extensive training and experience for the physician operator, the nurse staffing the laser control panel, and a biomedical engineer for dealing with equipment issues. Although laser excision provides a histological specimen, due to cautery artefact, it may be difficult to assess the margins.

Cold-Knife Cone

A cold-knife cone is usually recommended for those lesions where (1) the endocervical extent of the disease is not visible; (2) the work-up suggests adenocarcinoma in situ or possible malignancy; or (3) there is a significant discrepancy between the cytology result with a negative colposcopically directed biopsy.

A cold-knife cone biopsy is performed in the operating room with the woman either under general anaesthesia or under epidural or spinal block. The physician washes the cervix with Lugol's iodine solution to outline the extent of the lesion. The cervix is infiltrated with Xylocaine® with epinephrine/vasopressin. Stay sutures are placed at 3 and 9 o'clock. A knife (i.e. "beaver blade") is used to remove the lesion, and the ultimate defect is in the shape of an inverted cone. Pathology can assess the severity of the lesion and if the lesion has been completely excised or if any of the margins (deep endocervical, lateral, or ectocervical) are involved. A post-cone endocervical curettage (ECC) helps define if disease is still present above the level of the excised specimen. Any bleeding from the defect in the cervix can be cauterized, sutured, covered in thickened ferrous sulphate, or packed with an agent like Surgicel R or Fibrillar TM (Ethicon, Somerville, NJ).

Side Effects

The immediate risks of a cold-knife cone biopsy are related to the anaesthesia risk from spinal, epidural, or general anaesthetic and bleeding. There is a 9 % post-cone bleeding risk, which usually occurs 7–10 days post-procedure and is usually related to a superimposed infection. Long-term sequelae include PTROM, preterm delivery (RR 2.19, 95 % CI 1.93–2.49), low-birth weight (2.53, 1.19–5.36), caesarean section (3.17, 1.07–9.40), and cervical stenosis [22, 124]. The future ability to assess the squamocolumnar junction is compromised by a cone biopsy.

Advantages

Cold-knife cone biopsy provides a histological specimen where margins can be easily assessed.

Limitations

Cold-knife cone biopsy requires access to an operating room, an anaesthetist, and surgeon. The cost is very high.

Hysterectomy

A hysterectomy may be recommended when screening and diagnostic tests show that disease persists after attempted conservative treatment.

Hysterectomy is the definitive way to remove cervical disease, especially in a woman who has completed her childbearing. A hysterectomy involves removing the cervix and uterus with or without the tube and ovaries. A hysterectomy can be completed by the vaginal route, by the abdominal route with a Pfannenstiel or vertical incision, or by laparoscopic approach.

Side Effects

The immediate risks are bleeding, infection, thromboembolic disease, and injury to surrounding structures (i.e. bladder, bowel, or ureters). Hysterectomy has the highest rate of complications. Recovery from surgery takes 4–6 weeks.

Advantages

Hysterectomy provides the best histological specimen for evaluation. It is definitive treatment for the cervical disease.

Limitations

Hysterectomy can only be performed in specialized centres. It is the most costly treatment strategy. It results in loss of fertility.

Assessment of Treatment Options

All five treatment options demonstrate that effective treatment is available for pre-invasive or early invasive disease, meeting the third WHO (i.e. prerequisite of effective treatment being available) [1]. Clearly, the first four treatment options for managing presymptomatic disease allow preservation of fertility with minimal side effects meeting the fourth WHO prerequisite (i.e. treatment of presymptomatic disease results in benefits beyond those obtained through treatment of symptomatic disease) [1].

Approaches to Screening, Diagnosis, and Treatment for Cervical Disease

There are several approaches to screening, diagnosis, and treatment of cervical disease. Three approaches are described here. The "traditional approach" is to screen using cervical cytology, diagnose disease using the colposcope, confirm disease with a biopsy, and then treat the disease using LEEP. An "intermediate approach" is to screen using an oncogenic HPV test, diagnose using either VIA or cervical cytology, and then treat with cryotherapy. The "screen-and-treat" approach is to screen with VIA and treat using cryotherapy at the same visit.

The "traditional approach" that has evolved in high-resource settings includes cervical cytology, colposcopic examination for those with an abnormal screen, biopsy confirmation, and LEEP. It involves multiple visits: a visit for the Pap test, a visit to get the results, a visit to another consultant for the colposcopy exam and biopsies, another visit for the results, a visit for the LEEP procedure, and one or more follow-up visits to ensure that the disease has been removed. To minimize loss to follow-up, various programmes have developed "call recall" systems to remind especially non-compliant women. This traditional approach is costly to the health-care system and to the woman (i.e. travel, childcare, lost time at work). This multiple visit approach has not been successful in low-resource settings for two reasons: low compliance and lack of access to treatment at the point of care. Thus, in low-resource settings, this strategy has resulted in poor outcomes.

The "screen-and-treat" approach, otherwise known as the "same visit treatment" or "see-and-treat" approach, is a single visit for screening and treatment. This approach minimizes the chance that an abnormal finding goes unmanaged. To be successful the screening test must provide results rapidly and accurately. The treatment must also be safe, appropriate to the training of the staff, and effective. For screen and treat to be successful, both components need to happen at the same visit. The infrastructure must be simple without the need for specialized care. The screening test could be a rapidly read cervical cytology, careHPV™ test, or VIA. Although attempted with cervical cytology, the problem is the time to complete the cytological assessment [51, 125]. The treatment can be cryotherapy or LEEP [59]; however, cryotherapy has many advantages in the low-resource setting.

Efficacy

As described previously, a "see-and-treat" approach was used in 80,000 women in India aged 30–59 years. There was a 25 % reduction in cervical cancer incidence and a 35 % reduction in cervical cancer deaths compared to a non-screened group [51, 73, 126].

A safety study of the "see-and-treat" approach in Thailand using VIA as the screening test and cryotherapy as the treatment showed that, among women who were VIA positive and were treated, 94.3 % were disease free at one year (i.e. VIA negative). These results have been replicated in other settings like Ghana [42]. However, such excellent results are not universal. For example, in Osmanabad, India, the success rate was only 50 % [21], and in Dindigul, in Southern India, there was no benefit [127].

A different "see-and-treat" approach was used in South Africa. Here 6,555 nonpregnant women aged 35–65 years received either HPV test (HC2), VIA, or no screening test. They were randomized to immediate or delayed treatment with cryotherapy. Treatment was given if the woman was HPV positive or if they were VIA positive. The rates of dysplasia were lower in both groups at 6 and 12 months. Safety and feasibility were confirmed [76]. In the subgroup of women followed to 36 months, those with a positive HPV test (HC2) and treatment had the greatest benefit [76].

A cost-effectiveness study assessed several screening strategies involving India, Kenya, Peru, South Africa, and Thailand. Screening women once in their lifetime at age 35 years with a one or two visit screening strategy involving VIA and cryotherapy at the same visit was the most cost-effective strategy [94, 128]. This strategy reduced lifetime risk of cancer by 25–36 % and cost less than $500 (international dollars) per year of life saved [93]. This strategy had a cost-effectiveness ratio less than the country's per capita GDP. According to the Commission on Macroeconomics and Health, this is considered very cost-effective [129]. To put this in the context of other well-known public health interventions, this strategy was as cost-effective as Hepatitis B vaccination in India, second treatment for TB in Peru, and malaria prevention with nets in Kenya.

Limitations

The limitations of this approach are the limitations listed for each of the components. In addition, some national decision makers will not accept the "see-and-treat" approach if cervical cytology and colposcopy are currently available within the country [130].

Cervical Cancer Prevention Programme

There are several of ways to implement a cervical screening programme. *Opportunistic cervical screening* means that the woman initiates the interaction to be screened, or a woman who sees a physician for another reason is offered the opportunity to be screened at that visit. In contrast, an *organized screening programme* involves a clear system of education, age-appropriate invitation to screening, access to screen and treatment, quality assurance, and programme evaluation.

According to the International Agency for Research on Cancer (IARC), there are eight essential features an organized screening programme:

1. A clearly defined target population
2. Eligible screening participants are identifiable (e.g. a list with names and addresses)
3. Processes are in place to maximize reach and encourage participation (e.g. personalized invitation letters)
4. Suitable field and lab facilities exist for collecting and analysing specimens
5. Systematic quality-control procedures are in place to assess how tests are performed and interpreted
6. Appropriate facilities exist for diagnosis, treatment, and follow-up of patients with confirmed abnormalities
7. An organized referral system is in place to manage any identified abnormalities and provide information about normal results
8. An organized performance measurement/monitoring system is in place to enable collection of relevant and timely epidemiological data [131]

Studies from the Nordic countries and the Netherlands have shown that when such programmes are in place there is a significant drop in cervical cancer incidence and mortality [132–135]. Next, we present examples from low-resource setting that highlight problems and successes in cervical cancer prevention.

Problems

Organization

It is important that an organized programme encompasses training of health-care providers involved in screening (family doctors, nurses, colposcopists, cytologist, cytotechnician). The literature focuses especially on training in cytology [136]. An example of why this is so important is that, in some countries such as Argentina, up until recently gynaecologists read the Pap test [137].

The programme needs to ensure equipment and supply chain, and high-quality lab services. Honduras is an example where 80 % of the population is screened, but there is an extremely high false-negative rate of Pap smears. In part, this is due to poor Pap smear quality as a result of lack of supplies such as fixatives, spatulas, and cytobrushes [90, 138].

An organized programme also needs to establish a referral pathway for assessment and treatment of women with abnormal results. Capacity needs to be developed to ensure treatment for pre-invasive (i.e. colposcopy, LEEP) and invasive disease (radical surgery and radiation therapy). In Central and South America, coverage is high but a woman's access to treatment is poor; thus, rates of cervical cancer remain high [49, 139, 140].

The population needs to be educated concerning cervical cancer and prevention opportunities. Studies show that participation in screening programmes is proportional to awareness and knowledge [141–143]. There are numerous studies from low-resource settings showing that women are unfamiliar with cervical cancer and HPV infection as the cause of cancer [142, 144–147].

Screening tests and the way they are implemented also need to be culturally relevant to ensure patient participation [148–150].

Extent of Use

It is clear that screening benefits older women (30 and above) and that overscreening harms women in their teens. Thus, the emphasis of screening should address participation rates in a target population. A review of cancer screening in 57 countries using data from 2002 found that only 18 % of 25- to 64-year-old women in developing countries had a pelvic exam and Pap test in the last 3 years [151]. Screening occurs at even lower rates of <1 % in Bangladesh, Ethiopia, and Myanmar; <10 % in Ethiopia, Bangladesh, and Malawi.

Data Registration

A centralized database for detailed information on the date and result of a screen and follow-up tests for abnormal results allows tracking for compliance with follow-up. When a review was conducted in Peru, it was identified that 56 % of women with high-grade Pap tests were lost to follow-up and 3 % died of cervical cancer [152].

Successes

Organization

Prior to undertaking a cervical screening programme, each country needs to define whether cervical cancer is a problem in their jurisdiction by assessing incidence and mortality from the disease. Next, they need to determine whether there is the political will to designate resources toward developing an effective plan, implementation, and monitoring [153]. A cervical cancer prevention programme involves more than just the screening test. A cervical screening programme encompasses all of the services, from provision of the test to diagnosis and treatment [81]. An organized programme involves national policies that define, among other things, the ages during which screening is to occur, the screening interval, and the method of screening. These guidelines are to be implemented on a population basis with effective recruitment strategies to achieve high coverage. This could involve access to a population-based cancer registry and a computerized call and recall system.

In Vietnam several agencies came together to launch a population-based Pap smear screening system in Ho Chi Minh City (150 women per day). They developed community outreach methods, quality control, and quality assurance programmes with a centralized cytology lab and access to curative treatment [129].

In Chile, prior to 1987, only 10 % of women were screened annually. In 1987, the Chilean Ministry of Health and WHO collaborated to train health professionals, establish a system of patient follow-up, improve cytology accuracy, and improve patient education. In 1990, screening coverage increased to 66 % for women aged 25–64 years. Mortality from cervical cancer fell by 39 % by 2001. This is a success story showing that reallocating resources and infrastructure led to a fall in cervical cancer rates [49, 90, 154].

Another aspect of organization involves incorporating screening into the existing health-care system. The system of HIV care in Africa has taught us that cervical cancer screening is feasible and acceptable within the setting of an HIV care and treatment clinic. An example of this is in Nyanza province on the shores of Lake Victoria in Kenya. Collaboration was built between the Family AIDS Care and Education Services Program (FACES) and the University of California, University of San Francisco, and Kenya Medical Research Institute, Nairobi, Kenya, to provide cervical cancer screening for HIV-positive women [155, 156].

A similar successful collaboration has been described in Zambia between the University Teaching Hospital in Lusaka and the University of Alabama at Birmingham, and the Center for Infectious Disease Research in Zambia and the Zambian Ministry of Health [105, 123, 157, 158].

A programme should encompass training of health-care providers like cytologists. The Argentine Society of Cytology [137] mandated certification of professionals by scientific organizations according to national and international standards to ensure professional standards. Certification of professionals was felt to be a prerequisite to lab certification.

A programme needs to identify mechanisms to ensure attendance for screening or follow-up. Transportation incentives increase adherence to follow-up [159, 160].

HIV care has taught health planners in Africa that if you want people to adhere to treatment you have to work with community health workers. They live in the villages with their neighbours. They are a source of education and reinforcement [161]. Personalized follow-up letters increase adherence to follow-up [159, 160]. Counselling and telephone calls increase adherence to treatment appointments and follow-up [159, 162].

Method of Quality Assurance

The Argentine Society of Cytology [137] currently mandates that first screen must be carried out by cytotechnicians under supervision of a pathologist who re-reads 100 % of abnormal smears and a percent of normals. Labs should read 10,000 smears annually [137].

Peru uses lab certification by the Peruvian Scientific Society of Cytology after they verify certain conditions, including that a certain number of Pap smears are read annually [137].

The United States implemented the Clinical Laboratory Improvement Amendment, which involves an evaluation of eight steps within the lab system as a means of evaluating and maintaining cytology quality [163].

Monitoring Systems are built for the purpose of evaluation through performance indicators and quality assurance (i.e. cytology assessment). Performance indicators can include documenting the coverage, interval from the test to reporting the results, proportion of unsatisfactory Pap tests, treatment compliance, timeliness of follow-up of abnormal results, sensitivity, specificity, and interval cancers. Use of these indicators has pointed to areas where improvement is needed.

When follow-up was assessed in three rural areas of Honduras that offered cytology screening, it was identified that when VIA was followed by immediate colposcopy, compliance was 83 %. When Pap test was followed up by an appointment to give results and then colposcopy, compliance was only 38 % [164].

The programme needs to have a designated management team responsible for planning, implementation, and evaluation [163, 165].

Conclusion

In this chapter, we identified four prerequisites necessary for defining whether a mass screening programme should be developed. We have shown that cervical cancer is one of the leading cancers in women, especially in low-resource settings, and it is a major cause of mortality. Cervical cancer is preceded by a long asymptomatic phase of disease. Several screening strategies can be used to identify precancer, and, if treated, the screening programme can decrease the occurrence of cancer or shift the presentation of cancer to earlier stage, which, when treated, results in low mortality. Organized screening programmes provide the best population prevention of disease with the lowest rate of harm. Various models of screening, diagnosis, and treatment exist and have been assessed within the low-, medium-, and high-resource settings. Given that the four WHO prerequisites have been met, each jurisdiction must decide on the model that meets the needs of that population. For low-resource settings with limited health infrastructure, a national "see-and-treat" programme with a once or twice in a lifetime assessment with VIA or HPV testing and cryotherapy for those with positive tests will lead to a quick reduction in cervical cancer rates at low cost with low technology. The emphasis should be on screening women aged 30–49. It is important that a screening programme address the populations' knowledge and awareness of cervical cancer and HPV, facilitate compliance with screening, followup on abnormal test result, and ensure quality control.

References

1. Wilson JMG, Jungner G. Principles and practice of screening for disease, Public health papers, vol. 34. Geneva: World Health Organization; 1968.
2. Cole P, Morrison AS. Basic issues in cancer screening. In: Miller AB, editor. Screening in Cancer. Geneva: UICC; 1978.
3. Jemal A, Bray F, Center MM, Ferlay J, Ward E, Forman D. Global Cancer Statistics. CA Cancer J Clin. 2011;61:69–90.
4. GLOBOCAN: country fact stat. 2008. http://globocan.iarc.fr/factsheets/populations/factsheet.asp?uno=900. Accessed 29 Dec 2011.
5. Maree JE, Wright SCD. Cervical cancer: does our message promote screening? A pilot study in a South African context. Eur J Oncol Nurs. 2011;15(2):118–23.
6. Shanta V, Krishnamurthi S, Gajalakshmi CK, Swaminathan R, Ravichandran K. Epidemiology of cancer of the cervix: global and national perspective. J Indian Med Assoc. 2000;98:49–52.
7. Ferlay J. Cancer incidence in five continents. Processing of data. IARC Sci Publ. 1992;120:39–44.
8. Ferlay J, Bray F, Pisani P, Parkin DM. GLOBOCAN 2002: cancer incidence, mortality and prevalence worldwide. Lyon: IARC; 2004.
9. Reeler A, Qiao Y, Dare L, Li J, Zhang AL, Saba J. Women's cancers in developing countries: from research to an integrated health systems approach. Asian Pac J Cancer Prev. 2009;10:519–26.
10. Kitchener HC, Castle PE, Cox JT. Achievements and limitations of cervical cytology screening. Vaccine. 2006;24:S63–70.
11. Arbyn M, Raifu AO, Bray F, Weiderpass E, Anttila A. Treads of cervical cancer mortality in the member states of the European Union. Eur J Cancer. 2009;45(15):2640–8.
12. Anorlu RI, Orakwue CO, Oyeneyin L, Abudu OO. Late presentation of patients with cervical cancer to a tertiary hospital in Lagos: what is responsible? Eur J Gynaecol Oncol. 2004;25:729–32.
13. McCredie MR, Sharples KJ, Paul C, Baranyai J, Medley F, Jones RW, et al. Natural history of cervical neoplasia and risk of invasive cancer in women with cervical intraepithelial neoplasia 3: a retrospective cohort study. Lancet Oncol. 2008;9:425–34.
14. McIndoe WA, McLean MR, Jones RW, Mullins PR. The invasive potential of carcinoma in situ of the cervix. Obstet Gynecol. 1984;64:451–8.
15. Cuzick J, Arbyn M, Sankaranarayanan R, Tsu V, Ronco G, Mayrand MH, et al. Overview of Human Papillomavirus-based and other novel options for cervical cancer screening in developed and developing countries. Vaccine. 2008;26S:K29–41.
16. Wikipedia the Free Encyclopaedia. Developing countries<>, last modified 30 Mar 2012. Available from: http://en.wikipedia.org/wiki/Developing_country.
17. The World Bank. How we classify countries. http://data.worldbank.org/about/country-classifications. 2011.
18. Andrae B, Kemetli L, Sparén P, Silfverdal L, Strander B, Ryd W, et al. Screening-preventable cervical cancer risks: evidence from a nationwide audit in Sweden. J Natl Cancer Inst. 2008;100(9):622–9.
19. DiCenso A, Guyatt G. Recommendations about screening. In: DiCenso A, Guyatt G, Ciliska D, editors. Evidence-based nursing. A guide to clinical practice. St. Louis, MO: Mosby; 2005. p. 526–41.

20. Solomon D, Davey D, Kuman R, Moriarty A, O'Connor D, Prey M. The 2001 Bethesda System: terminology for reporting results of cervical cytology. JAMA. 2002;287:2114–9.
21. Sankaranarayanan R, Nene BM, Shastri SS, Jayant K, Muwonge R, Budukh A. HPV screening for cervical cancer in rural India. N Engl J Med. 2009;360(14):1385–94.
22. IARC Working Group on evaluation of cervical cancer screening programmes. Screening for squamous cervical cancer: duration of low risk after negative results of cervical cytology and its implication for screening policies. Br Med J (Clin Res Ed). 1986;293(6548):659–64.
23. Sasieni PD, Cuzick J, Lynch-Farmery E. Estimating the efficacy of screening by auditing smear histories of women with and without cervical cancer. The National Co-ordinating Network for cervical screening Working Group. Br J Cancer. 1996;73(8):1001–5.
24. Nieminen P, Kallio M, Anttila A, Akama M. Organised versus spontaneous Pap smear screening for cervical cancer: a case–control study. Int J Cancer. 1999;83(1):55–8.
25. Decker K, Demers A, Chateau D, Musto G, Nugent Z, Lotocki R, et al. Papanicolaou test utilization and frequency of screening opportunities among women diagnosed with cervical cancer. Open Med. 2009;3(3):e140–7.
26. Hernandez-Avila M. Lacano[Ponce ED, de Ruiz PA, Romieu I. Evaluation of the cervical cancer screening programme in Mexico: a population-based case–control study. Int J Epidemiol. 1998;27:370–6.
27. Hoffman M, Cooper D, Carara H, Rosenberg I. Limited pap screening associated with reduced risk of Cervical Cancer in South Africa. Int J Epidemiol. 2003;32:573–7.
28. Jiménez PM, Thomas DB. Has the use of pap smears reduced the risk of invasive cervical cancer in Guadalajara, Mexico? Int J Cancer. 1999;82(6):804–9.
29. Makino H, Sato S, Yajima A, Komatsu S, Fukao A. Evaluation of the effectiveness of cervical cancer screening: a case–control study in Miyagi, Japan. Tohoku J Exp Med. 1995;175(3):171–8.
30. Talbott EO, Norman SA, Kuller LH, Ishii EK, Baffone KM, Dunn MS, et al. Refining preventive strategies for invasive cervical cancer: a population-based case–control study. J Womens Health (Larchmt). 1995;4(4):387–95.
31. Aristizabal N, Cuello C, Correa P, Collazos T, Haenszel W. The impact of vaginal cytology on cervical cancer risks in Cali, Colombia. Int J Cancer. 1984;34(1):5–9.
32. Berrino F, Gatta G, d'Alto M, Crosignani P, Riboli E. Efficacy of screening in preventing invasive cervical cancer: a case–control study in Milan, Italy. IARC Sci Publ 1986;(76):111–23.
33. Clarke EA, Anderson TW. Does screening by "Pap" smears help prevent cervical cancer? A case–control study. Lancet. 1979;2(8132):1–4.
34. Herrero R, Brinton LA, Reeves WC, Brenes MM, de Britton RC, Gaitan E, et al. Screening for cervical cancer in Latin America: a case–control study. Int J Epidemiol. 1992;21(6):1050–6.
35. Parkin DM. Screening for cervix cancer in developing countries. In: Miller AB, Chamberlain J, Day NE, Hakama M, Proroc PC, editors. Cancer screening. Cambridge: Cambridge University Press; 1991. p. 184–98.
36. Sasieni P, Adams J. Effect of screening on cervical cancer mortality in England and Wales: analysis of trends with an age period cohort model. BMJ. 1999;318(7193):1244–5.
37. Van der Aa MA, Pukkala E, Coebergh JW, Anttila A, Siesling S. Mass screening programmes and trends in cervical cancer in Finland and the Netherlands. Int J Cancer. 2008;122(8):1854–8.
38. Bulkmans NW, Rozendall L, Voorhoorhorst FJ, Snijders PJ, Meijer CJ. Long-term protective effect of high-risk human papillomavirus testing in population-based cervical screening. Br J Cancer. 2005;92(9):1800–2.
39. Fahey MT, Irwig L, Macaskill P. Meta-analysis of Pap test accuracy. Am J Epidemiol. 1995;141(7):680–9.
40. Arbyn M, Bergeron C, Klinkhamer P. Liquid compared with conventional cervical cytology. Obstet Gynecol. 2008;111(1):167–77.
41. Spence AR, Goggin P, Franco EL. Process of care failures in invasive cervical cancers: a systemic review and metaanalysis. Prev Med. 2007;45:93–106.
42. Blumenthal PD, Gaffikin L, Deganus S, Lewis R, Emerson M. Cervical cancer prevention: safety, acceptability, and feasibility of a single-visit approach in Accra, Ghana. Am J Obstet Gynecol. 2007;196(4):e1–407.e9.
43. Denny L, Quinn M, Sankaranarayanan R. Screening for cervical cancer in developing countries. Vaccine. 2006;24 Suppl 3:S71–7.
44. Huong DB, Phuong NK, Bales S. Rural health care in Vietnam and China: conflict between market reforms and social need. Int J Health Serv. 2007;37(3):555–72.
45. McIntyre D, Thiede M, Dahlgren G. What are the economic consequences for households of illness and of paying for health care in low- and middle-income country contexts? Soc Sci Med. 2006;62(4):858–65.
46. Houts PS, Lipton A, Harvey HA. Nonmedical costs to patients and their families associated with outpatient chemotherapy. Cancer. 1984;53(11):2388–92.
47. Stommel M, Given CW, Given BA. The cost of cancer home care to families. Cancer. 1993;71(5):1867–74.
48. Ohaeri JU, Campbell OB, Ilesanmi AO. The psychosocial burden of caring for some Nigerian women with breast cancer and cervical cancer. Soc Sci Med. 1999;49(11):1541–9.
49. Sepulveda C, Prado R. Effective cervical cytology screening programmes in middle-income countries:

the Chilean experience. Cancer Detect Prev. 2005; 29(5):405–11.
50. Micheli A, Sanz N, Mwangi-Powell F, Coleman MP, Neal C, Ullrich A, et al. International collaborations in cancer control and the Third International Cancer Control Congress. Tumori. 2009;95:579–96.
51. Megevand E, Van Wyk W, Knight B, Bloch B. Can cervical cancer be prevented by a see, screen, and treat program? A pilot study. Am J Obstet Gynecol. 1996;174(3):923–8.
52. University of Zimbabwe/JHPIEGO Cervical Cancer Project. Visual inspection with acetic acid for cervical-cancer screening: test qualities in a primary-care setting. Lancet. 1999;353(9156):869–73.
53. Sankaranarayanan R, Esmy PO, Rajkumar R, Muwonge R, Swaminathan R, Shanthakumari S. Effect of visual screening on cervical cancer incidence and mortality in Tamil Nadu, India: a cluster randomised trial. Lancet. 2007;370(9585):398–406.
54. Sangwa-Lugoma G, Mahmud S, Nasr SH, Liaras J, Kayembe PK, Tozin RR, et al. Visual inspection as a cervical cancer screening method in a primary health care setting in Africa. Int J Cancer. 2006;119(6): 1389–95.
55. Arbyn M, Sankaranarayanan R, Muwonge R. Pooled analysis of the accuracy of 5 cervical cancer screening tests assessed in eleven studies in Africa and India. Int J Cancer. 2008;123:153–60.
56. Quinley KE, Gormley RH, Ratcliffe SJ, Shih T, Szep Z, Steiner A, et al. Use of mobile telemedicine for cervical cancer screening. J Telemed Telecare. 2011;17(4):203–9.
57. Ngan HYS, Garland SM, Bhatla N, Pagliusi SR, Chan KKL, Cheung ANY, et al. Asia Oceania Guidelines for the implementation of programs for cervical cancer prevention and control. J Cancer Epidemiol. 2011;2011:794861. doi:10.1155/2011/794861.
58. Safaeian M, Solomon D. Cervical cancer prevention—cervical screening: science in evolution. Obstet Gynecol Clin North Am. 2007;34(4):739–60, ix.
59. Gaffikin L, Blumenthal PD, Emerson M, Limpaphayom K. Safety, acceptability and feasibility of a single-visit approach to cervical-cancer prevention in rural Thailand: a demonstration project. Lancet. 2003;361(9360):814–20.
60. FIGO Global Guidance for Cervical Cancer Prevention and Control. http://www.figo.org/files/figo-corp/English_version.pdf. 2009.
61. Mergevand E, Denny L, Dehaeck K, Soeters R, Bloch B. Acetic acid visualization of the cervix: an alternative to cytologic screening. Obstet Gynecol. 1996;88(3):383–6.
62. Sankaranarayanan R, Black RJ, Swaminathan R, Parkin DM. An overview of cancer survival in developing countires. IARC Sci Publ. 1998;(145):135–73.
63. Denny L. The prevention of cervical cancer in developing countries. Br J Obstet Gynaecol. 2005;112: 1204–12.
64. Sankanranarayanan R, Basu P, Wesley RS, Mahe C, Keita N, Mbalawa CC. Accuracy of visual screening for cervical neoplasia: results from an IARC multicentre study in India and Africa. Int J Cancer. 2004;110(6):907–13.
65. WHO. New options for cervical cancer screening and treatment in low-resource settings. Geneva: World Health Organization; 2010.
66. Jeronim J, Sciffman M. Colposcopy at a crossroads. Am J Obstet Gynecol. 2006;195:349–53.
67. WHO Department of Reproductive Health and Research and Department of Chronic Diseases and Health Promotion. Comprehensive cervical cancer control. Geneva: WHO; 2006.
68. Almonte M, Ferreccio C, Winkler JL. Cervical screening by visual inspection, HPV testing, liquid based and conventional cytology in Amazonian Peru. Int J Cancer. 2007;121:796–802.
69. Sellors J, Jeronimo J, Sanakaranarayanan R. Assessment of the cervix after acetic acid wash: interrater agreement using photographs. Obstet Gynecol. 2002;99:635–40.
70. Sherigar B, Dalal A, Durdi G. Cervical cancer screening by visual inspection with acetic acid-interobserver variability between nurse and physician. Asian Pac J Cancer Prev. 2010;11:619–22.
71. Wright TC, Denny L, Kuhn L, Pollack A, Lorincz A. HPV DNA testing of self-collected vaginal samples compared with cytologic screening to detect cervical cancer. JAMA. 2000;283:81–6.
72. Park IU, Diaz ML, Bowey C, Magaril R, Ferris DG, on behalf of the INCCA Foundation. Cervical cancer prevention in the developing world. JLGTD. 2007;11(4):273.
73. Sankaranarayanan R, Gaffikin L, Jacob M, Sellors J, Robles S. A critical assessment of screening methods for cervical neoplasia. Int J Gynecol Obstet. 2005;89(Supp 2):S2–14.
74. Mittra I, Mishra GA, Singh S, Aranke S, Notani P, Badwe R, et al. A cluster randomized controlled trial of breast and cervix cancer screening in Mumbai India: methodology and interim results after three rounds of screening. Int J Cancer. 2010;126(4): 976–84.
75. Velázquez-Hernández N, Sánchez-Anguiano LF, Lares-Bayona EF, Cisneros-Pérez V, Milla-Villeda RH, Arreola-Herrera Fde A, et al. Comparison of the diagnostic utility for visual inspection with acetic acid and cervical cytology. Ginecol Obstet Mex. 2010;78(5):261–7.
76. Denny L, Kuhn L, Hu CC, Tsa WY, Wright TC. Human papillomavirus-based cervical cancer prevention: long-term results of a randomized screening trial. J Natl Cancer Inst. 2010;102(20):1557–67.
77. Dinshaw K, Mishra G, Shastri S, Badwe R, Kerkar R, Ramani S, et al. Determinants of compliance in a cluster randomised controlled trial on screening of breast and cervix cancer in Mumbai, India. 1. Compliance to screening. Oncology. 2007;73(3–4): 143–53.
78. Doh AS, Nkele NN, Achu P, Essimbi F, Essame O, Nkegoum B. Visual inspection with acetic acid and

cytology as screening methods for cervical lesions in Cameroon. Int J Gynaecol Obstet. 2005;89(2): 167–73.
79. Jamshida R, Blumenthal P. Digital assessment of the reproductive tract (DART). J Acquir Immune Defic Syndr. 2004;37:S171–3.
80. Cremer M, Jamshidi RM, Muderspach L, Tsao-Wei D, Felix JC, Blumenthal PD. Digital camera assessment for detection of cervical intraepithelial neoplasia in rural El Salvador. Int J Gynecol Obstet. 2005;91(1):42–6.
81. Sarian LO, Derchain SF, Naud P. Roteli-MartensC, Longatto-Filho A, Tatti S. Evaluation of visual inspection with acetic acid (VIA), Lugol's iodine (VILI), cervical cytology and HPV testing as cervical screening tools in Latin America. This report refers to partial results from the LAMS (Latin American Screening study. J Med Screen. 2005;12(3):142–9.
82. Sellors JW, Winkler JL, Kreysar DF. Illumination optics and clinical performance of a hand-held magnified visual inspection device (Avi Scope) a comparison with colposcopy. J Acquir Immune Defic Syndr. 2004;37 Suppl 3:S160–6.
83. Robyler D, Park SY, Adewole I, Follen M. Objective screening for cervical cancer in developing nations: lessons from Nigeria. Gynecol Oncol. 2007;107(1 Suppl 1):S94–7.
84. Dondog B, Clifford GM, Vaccarella S, Waterboer T, Unurjargal D, Avirmed D. Human papillomavirus infection in Ulaanbaatar, Mongolia: a population-based study. Cancer Epidemiol Biomarkers Prev. 2008;17(7):1731–8.
85. Anttila A, Kotaniemi-Talonen L, Leinonen M, Hakama M, Laurila P, Tarkkanen J, et al. Rate of cervical cancer, severe intraepithelial neoplasia, and adenocarcinoma in situ in primary HPV DNA screening with cytology triage: randomized study within organized screening programme. BMJ. 2010;340:c1804.
86. Cuzick J, Clavel C, Petry KU. Overview of the European and North American Studies on HPV testing in primary cervical cancer screening. Int J Cancer. 2006;119(5):1095–101.
87. Grce M. Primary and secondary prevention of cervical cancer. Expert Rev Mol Diagn. 2009;9(8): 851–64.
88. Bulkmans NW, Berkhof J, Rozendaal L. Human papillomavirus DNA testing for the detection of cervical intraepithelial neoplasia grade 3 and cancer. 5 year follow-up of a randomised controlled implementation trial. Lancet. 2007;370(9601):1764–72.
89. Longatto-Filho A, Erzen M, Branca M, et al. Human Papillomavirus testing as an optional screening tool in low-resource settings of Latin America: experience from the Latin America Screening Study. Int J Gynecol Cancer. 2006;16:955–62.
90. Ditzian LR, David-West G, Maza M, Hartmann B, Shirazian T, Cremer M. Cervical cancer screening in low- and middle-income countries. Mt Sinai J Med. 2011;78:319–26.
91. Qiao YL, Sellors JW, Eder PS. A new HPV-DNA test for cervical-cancer screening in developing regions: a cross sectional study of clinical accuracy in rural China. Lancet Oncol. 2008;9(10):929–36.
92. Sherman ME, Lorincz AT. Scott Dr. Baseline cytology, human papillomavirus testing and risk for cervical neoplasia: a 10-year cohort analysis. J Natl Cancer Inst. 2003;95:46–52.
93. Olgilvie GS, Patrick DM, Schulzer M, Sellors JW, Petric M, Chambers K, et al. Diagnostic accuracy of self collected vaginal specimens for human papillomavirus compared to clinician collected human papillomavirus specimens: a meta-analysis. Sex Transm Infect. 2005;81(3):207–12.
94. Goldie SJ, Gaffikin L, Goldhaber-Fiebert JD, Gordillo-Tobar A, Levin C, Mahe C. Cost effectiveness of cervical-cancer screening in five developing countries. N Engl J Med. 2005;353(2):2158–68.
95. Arbyn M, Sasieni P, Meijer CJ, Clavel C, Koliopoulos G, Dillner J. Chapter 9: Clinical applications of HPV testing: a summary of meta-analyses. Vaccine. 2006;24 Suppl 3:S78–89.
96. Salmeron J, Lazcano-Ponce E, Lorincz A, Hernandez M, Hernandez P, Leyya A, et al. Comparison of HPV-based assays with papanicolaou smears for cervical cancer screening in Morelos State, Mexico. Cancer Causes Control. 2003;14:505–12.
97. Sellors JW, Lorincz AT, Mahony JB, Mielzunska I, Lutwun A, Roth P. Comparison of self-collected vaginal, vulvar and urine samples with physician-collected cervical samples for human papilloma virus testing to detect high grade squamous intraepithelial lesions. Can Med Assoc J. 2000;163:513–8.
98. Nobbenhui MA, Helmerhorst TJ, van den Bruie AJ, Rozendaal L, Jaspaars LH, Voorhorst FJ. Primary screening for high risk HPV by home obtained cervicovaginal lavage is an alternative screening tool for unscreened women. J Clin Pathol. 2002;55:435–9.
99. Longatto-Filho A, Toletli-Martins C, Hammes L, Etlinger D, Pereira SM, Erzen M. Self sampling for human papillomavirus (HPV) testing as cervical cancer screening option. Experience from the LAMS study. Eur J Gynaecol Oncol. 2008;29(4):327–32.
100. Petignat P, Faltin DL, Bruchim I. Are self-collected samples comparable to physician-collected cervical specimens for human papillomavirus DNA testing? A systematic review and meta-analysis. Gynecol Oncol. 2007;105:530–5.
101. Pengsaa P, Sriamporn S, Kripetcharat O. A comparison of cytology with Pap smears taken by a gynaecologist with a self-sampling device. Asian Pac J Cancer Prev. 2003;4:99–102.
102. Barbee L, Kobetz E, Menard J. Assessing the acceptability of self-sampling for HPV among Haitian immigrant women: CBPR in action. Cancer Causes Control. 2010;21:421–31.
103. Balasubramanian A, Kulasingam SL, Baer A. Accuracy and cost-effectiveness of cervical cancer screening by high-risk human papillomavirus DNA testing of self-collected vaginal samples. J Low Genit Tract Dis. 2010;14:185–95.

104. Howe SI, Vargas DE, Granada D, Smith JK. Cervical cancer prevention in remote rural Nicaragua: a program evaluation. Gynecol Oncol. 2005;99 Suppl 3:232–5.
105. Mwanahamuntu MH, Sahasrabuddhe VV, Kapambwe S, Praendler KS, Chibwesha C, Mkumba G, et al. Advancing cervical cancer prevention initiatives in resource-constrained settings: insights from the cervical cancer prevention program in Zambia. PLoS Med. 2011;8(5):e1001032.
106. Mitchell MF, Tortolero-Luna G, Cook E, Whittaker L, Rhodes-Morris H, Silva E. A randomized clinical trial of cryotherapy, loop electrosurgical excision for treatment of squamous intraepithelial lesions of the cervix. Obstet Gynaecol. 1998;92:737–44.
107. Howe DT, Vincenti AC. Is large loop excision of the transformation zone (LLETZ) more accurate than colposcopially directed punch biopsy in the diagnosis of cervical intraepithelial neoplasia? Br J Obstet Gynaecol. 1991;98(6):588–91.
108. Pretorius RG, Belinson JL, Burchette RJ, Hu S, Zhang X, Qiao YL. Regardless of skill, performing more biopsies increases the sensitivity of colposcopy. J Low Genit Tract Dis. 2011;15(3):180–8.
109. Pretorius RG, Bao YP, Belinson JL, Burchette RJ, Smith JS, Qiao YL. Inappropriate gold standard bias in cervical screening studies. Int J Cancer. 2007;121(10):2218–24.
110. Cagle AJ, Hu SY, Sellors JW, Bao YP, Lim JM, Li SM, et al. Use of an expanded gold standard to estimate the accuracy of colposcopy and visual inspection with acetic acid. Int J Cancer. 2010;126(1): 156–61.
111. Pretorius RG, Kim RJ, Belinson JL, Elson P, Qiao YL. Inflation of sensitivity of cervical cancer screening tests secondary to correlated error in colposcopy. J Low Genit Tract Dis. 2006;10(1):5–9.
112. Pretorius RG, Zhang WH, Belinson JL, Huang MN, Wu LY, Zhang X. Colposcopically directed biopsy, random cervical biopsy, and endocervical curettage in the diagnosis of cervical intraepithelial neoplasia II or worse. Am J Obstet Gynecol. 2004;191(2): 430–4.
113. Sellors JW, Sankaranarayanan R. Colposcopy and treatment of cervical intraepithelial neoplasia: a beginner's manual. Lyon, France: IARC;2003/2004.
114. Chamot E, Kristense S, Stringer JSA, Mwanahamuntu MH. Are treatments for cervical precancerous lesions in less-developed countries safe enough to promote scaling up of cervical screening programs? A systematic review. BMC Womens Health. 2010;10:1–11.
115. Castro W, Gage J, Gaffikin L, Ferreccio C, Sellors J, Sherris J. Effectiveness, safety and acceptability of cryotherapy: a systematic literature review. Cervical cancer prevention: issues in depth, No. 1. Alliance for Cervical Cancer Prevention; 2003.
116. Blumenthal PD, Lauterbach M, Sellors JW, Sankaranarayanan R. Training for cervical cancer prevention programs in low-resource settings: focus on visual inspection with acetic acid and cryotherapy. Int J Gynecol Obstet. 2005;89(Supp 2):S30–7.
117. Seamans Y, Loesel C, Jeronimo J, Sellors J, Castle PE. Effect of cough technique and cryogen gas on temperatures achieved during simulated cryotherapy. BMC Womens Health. 2007;7:16.
118. Soutter WP, De Barros Lopes A, Fletcher A, et al. Invasive cervical cancer after conservative treatment for cervical intraepithelial neoplasia. Lancet. 1997;349:978–80.
119. Alvarez RD, Helm CW, Edwards RP, et al. Prospective randomized trial of LLETZ versus laser ablation in patients with cervical intraepithelial neoplasia. Gynecol Oncol. 1994;52:175–9.
120. Kyrgiou M, Koliopoulos G, Martin-Hirsch P, Arbyn M, Prendiville W, Paraskevaidis E. Obstetric outcomes after conservative treatment for intraepithelial or early invasive cervical lesions: systematic review and meta-analysis. Lancet. 2006;367(9509):489–98.
121. Arbyn M, Kyrfiou M, Raifu AO, Koliopoulos G, Martin-Hirsch P, Prendiville W. Perinatal mortality and other severe adverse pregnancy outcomes associated with treatment of cervical intraepithelial neoplasia; metaanalysis. BMJ. 2008;337:a1284.
122. Crane JMG. Pregnancy outcome after loop electrosurgical excision procedure: a systematic review. Obstet Gynecol. 2003;102:1058–62.
123. Pfaendler KW, Mwanahamuntu MH, Sahasrabuddhe VV, Mudenda V, Stringer JS, Parham GP. Management of cryotherapy-ineligible women in a "screen-and-treat" cervical cancer prevention program targeting HIV-infected women in Zambia: lessons from the field. Gynecol Oncol. 2008;110(3): 402–7.
124. Bruinsma FJ, Quinn MA. The risk of preterm birth following treatment for precancerous changes in the cervix: a systematic review and meta-analysis. BJOG. 2011;118(9):1031–41.
125. Denny L, Kuhn L, De Souza M, Pollack AE, Dupree W, Wright Jr TC. Screen-and-treat approaches for cervical cancer prevention in low-resource settings: a randomized controlled trial. JAMA. 2005;294(17):2173–81.
126. Sankaranarayanan R, Rajkumar R, Esmy PO. Effectiveness, safety and acceptability of 'see and treat' with cryotherapy by nurses in a cervical screening study in India. Br J Cancer. 2007;96(5): 738–43.
127. Alliance for Cervical Cancer Prevention (ACCP). New evidence on the impact of cervical cancer screening and treatment using HPV DNA tests, visual inspection, or cytology. http://www.rho.org/files/ACCP_screening_factsheet_July09.pdf. [cited 2009 July].
128. Goldie SJ, Kuhn L, Denny L, Pollack A, Wright TC. Policy analysis of cervical cancer screening strategies in low-resource settings: clinical benefits and cost-effectiveness. JAMA. 2001;285(24):3107–15.

129. Goldhaber-Fiebert JD, Goldie SJ. Estimating the cost of cervical cancer screening in 5 developing countries. Cost Eff Resour Alloc. 2006;4:13.
130. Suba EJ, Murphy SK, Donnelly AD, Furia LM, Huynh ML, Raab SS. Systems analysis of real-world obstacles to successful cervical cancer prevention in developing countries. Am J Public Health. 2006; 96(3):480–7.
131. Organization WH. Cancer prevention (Chap. 16). In: Dos Santos Silva I, editor. Cancer epidemiology. Lyon: IARC Nonserial Publication; 1999. p. 355–83.
132. Arbyn M, Rebolj M, de Kok IM, Fender M, Becker N, O'Reilly M, et al. The challenges of organising cervical screening programmes in the 15 old member states of the European Union. Eur J Cancer. 2009;45(15):2671–8.
133. Anttila A, Nieminen P. Cervical cancer screening programme in Finland with an example on implementing alternative screening methods. Coll Antropol. 2007;31 Suppl 2:17–22.
134. Lynge E, Clausen LB, Guignard R, Poll P. What happens when organization of cervical cancer screening is delayed or stopped? J Med Screen. 2006;13(1): 41–6.
135. de Kok IM, van der Aa MA, van Ballegooijen M, Siesling S, Karim-Kos HE, van Kemenade FJ, et al. Working Group Output of the Netherlands Cancer Registry. Trends in cervical cancer in the Netherlands until 2007: has the bottom been reached? Int J Cancer. 2011;128(9):2174–81.
136. Franco EI, Duarte-Franco E, Frenzy A. Early detection of cervical cancer with visual inspection methods. Salud Publica Mex. 2003;45(Supp 3):S5367–75.
137. Arrossi S, Paolino M, Sankaranarayanan R. Challenges faced by cervical cancer prevention programs in developing countries: a situational analysis of program organization in Argentina. Rev Panam Salud Publica. 2010;28(4):249–57.
138. Perkins RB, Langrish SM, Stern LJ, Burgess JF, Simon CJ. Impact of patient adherence and test performance on the cost-effectiveness of cervical cancer screening in developing countries: the case of Honduras. Womens Health Issues. 2010;20(1): 35–42.
139. Yabroff KR, Washington KS, Leader A, Neilson E, Mandelblatt J. Is the promise of cancer-screening programs being compromised? Quality of follow-up care after abnormal screening results. Med Care Res Rev. 2003;60(3):294–331.
140. Yabroff KR, Kerner JF, Mandelblatt JS. Effectiveness of interventions to improve follow-up after abnormal cervical cancer screening. Prev Med. 2000;31(4): 429–39.
141. Kelly AW, Fores CM, Wollan PC. A program to increase breast and cervical cancer screening for Cambodian women in a Midwestern community. Mayo Clin Proc. 1996;71:437–44.
142. Pearlman DN, Clark MA, Rakowski W, Ehrich B. Screening for breast and cervical cancers: the importance of knowledge and perceived cancer survivability. Health. 1999;28:93–112.
143. Gupta A, Kumar A, Stewart DE. Cervical cancer screening among South Asian women in Canada: the role of education and acculturation. Health Care Women Int. 2002;23:123–34.
144. Francis SA, Nelson J, Liverpool J, Soogun S, Mofammere N, Thorpe RJ. Examining attitudes and knowledge about HPV and cervical cancer risk among female clinic attendees in Johannesburg, South Africa. Vaccine. 2010;28(50):8023–42.
145. Idestrom M, Milsom I, Ellstrom AA. Knowledge and attitudes about the pap smear screening program. A population-based study of women aged 20–59. Acta Obstet Gynecol Scand. 2002;81: 962–7.
146. Waller J, Mccaffery K, Wardle J. Beliefs about the risk factors for cervical cancer in a British population sample. Prev Med. 2004;38:745–53.
147. Yucel U, Ceber E, Ozenturk G. Efficacy of a training course given by midwives concerning cervical cancer risk factors and prevention. Asian Pac J Cancer Prev. 2009;10:437–42.
148. Waller J, McCaffery K, Forrest S, Szarewski A, Cadman L, Wardle J. Awareness of human papillomavirus among women attending a well women clinic. Sex Transm Infect. 2003;79(4):320–2.
149. Lambert EC. College student's knowledge of human papillomavirus and effectiveness of a brief educational intervention. J Am Board Fam Pract. 2001; 14(3):178–83.
150. Ramirez JE, Ramos DM, Clayton L, Kanowitz S, Moscicki AB. Genital human papillomavirus infection: knowledge, perception of risk, and actual risk in a nonclinic population of young women. J Womens Health. 1997;6(1):113–21.
151. Gakidou E, Nordhagen S, Obermeyer Z. Coverage of cervical cancer screening in 57 countries: low average levels and large inequalities. PLoS Med. 2008;5(6):e132.
152. Gage JC, Ferreccio C, Gonzales M, et al. Followup care of women with an abnormal cytology in a low-resource setting. Cancer Detect Prev. 2003;27: 466–71.
153. Herdman C, Sherris J. Planning appropriate cervical cancer prevention programs. Seattle, WA: PATH. http://www.path.org/publications/files/cxca-planning-appro-prog-guide.pdf. 2000.
154. Murillo R, Almonte M, Pereira A, Ferrer E, Gamboa OA, Jeronimo J, et al. Cervical cancer screening programs in Latin America and the Caribbean. Vaccine. 2008;26 Suppl 11:L37–48.
155. Huchko MJ, Bukusi EA, Cohen CR. Building capacity for cervical cancer screening in outpatient HIV clinics in the Nyanza province of western Kenya. Int J Gynaecol Obstet. 2011;114:106–10.
156. Chirenje ZM, Rusakaniko S, Akino V, Millingo M. A randomised clinical trial of loop electrosurgical excision procedure (LEEP) versus cryotherapy in the treatment of cervical intraepithelial neoplasia. J Obstet Gynaecol. 2001;21(6):617–21.
157. Mwanahamuntu MH, Sahasrabuddhe VV, Praendler KS, Mudenda V, Hicks ML, Vermund SH, et al.

Implementation of 'see and treat' cervical cancer prevention services linked to HIV care in Zambia. AIDS. 2009;23(6):N1–5.
158. Parham GP, Mwanahamuntu MH, Pfaendler KS, Sahasrabuddhe VV, Myung D, Mkumba G, et al. eC3—A modern telecommunications matrix for cervical cancer prevention in Zambia. J Low Genit Tract Dis. 2010;14(3):167–73.
159. Choconta-Piraquive LA, Alvis-Guzman N, Hoz-Restrepo FDL. How protective is cervical cancer screening against cervical cancer mortality in developing countries? The Colombian case. BMC Health Serv Res. 2011;10(270):1–6.
160. Marcus AC, Crane LA, Kaplan CP, Reading AE, Savage E, Funning J, et al. Improving adherence to screening follow-up among women with abnormal Pap smears: results from a large clinic-based trial of three intervention strategies. Med Care. 1992;30(3):216–30.
161. Carmichael M. Not just an illness of the rich. Scientific America. March 2011. p. 66–70.
162. Engelstad LP, Stewart S, Otero-Sabogal R, Leung MS, Davis PI, Pasick RJ. The effectiveness of a community outreach intervention to improve follow-up among underserved women at highest risk for cervical cancer. Prev Med. 2005;41(3–4):741–8.
163. IARC. Handbook of cancer prevention, Cervix cancer screening, vol. 10. Lyon: IARC; 2005.
164. Park DM, Bray F, Ferlay J, Pissani P. Global cancer statistics, 2002. CA Cancer J Clin. 2005;55:74–108.
165. ACCP. Planning and implementing cervical cancer prevention and control programs. A manual for managers. http://whqlibdoc.who.int/paho/2004/a92126.pdf. 2004.

Ovarian Cancer Screening and Early Detection in Low- and Middle-Income Countries

7

Trevor Tejada-Bergés, Edward L. Trimble, and Mahesh K. Shetty

Abstract

The burden of ovarian cancer worldwide and the rationale for and against screening are discussed. Sonography is very useful in identifying and triaging patients with adnexal masses who require surgical intervention. A detailed description of sonography in the characterization of adnexal masses is presented.

Introduction

The burden of cancer is increasing dramatically in economically disadvantaged countries. In 2008, about 12.7 million cancer cases and 7.6 million cancer deaths were estimated worldwide, and 56 % of the cases and 64 % of the deaths occurred in the economically developing world [1]. In females, breast cancer remains the most frequently diagnosed cancer followed by cervical cancer. Despite an overall lower incidence of ovarian cancer in low- or middle-income countries (LMICs), management of ovarian cancer is a significant problem. The incidence of ovarian cancer worldwide is estimated at 225,500 cases with 140,200 deaths. Of these, 125,500 of the incident cases and 75,700 of the deaths occur in developing countries [1]. Furthermore, as more effective preventative, screening, and treatment strategies are established for cancers of the cervix and breast, it seems reasonable to expect that the problem of ovarian cancer will increase.

Yet, there is a paucity of data aimed at understanding ovarian cancer and its treatment in LMICs. Most of the available data stems from work in high-income countries (HIC), and there is a growing recognition that much of this work may not be applicable to the realities in LMICs [2]. To complicate matters further, grouping countries under a vague category like LMICs can be misleading and carries the danger of suggesting that their values and belief systems are always comparable. This grouping represents a large and heterogeneous group of countries both in terms

T. Tejada-Bergés (✉)
Department of Obstetrics and Gynecology, Women and Infants' Hospital, Providence, RI 02905, USA
e-mail: TTejadaBerges@wihri.org

E.L. Trimble
Department of Health and Human Services, Center for Global Health, National Cancer Institute, National Institutes of Health, Rockville, MD 20852, USA
e-mail: trimblet@ctep.nci.nih.gov

M.K. Shetty
Woman's Center for Breast Care and MRI, Woman's Hospital of Texas, Houston, TX 77054, USA
e-mail: mshetty@womens-radiology.com

M.K. Shetty (ed.), *Breast and Gynecological Cancers: An Integrated Approach for Screening and Early Diagnosis in Developing Countries*, DOI 10.1007/978-1-4614-1876-4_7,

of financial resources and cultural and religious values. Even within LMICs, there will undoubtedly be pockets of women with greater resources who are able to avail themselves of the most advanced medical technology. All of this needs to be kept in mind when considering treatment strategies for countries with limited resources.

While studies comparing survival in HIC and LMICs are limited, the available evidence indicates what one might intuitively suspect. There is a significant survival discrepancy between women diagnosed with ovarian cancer in HIC as compared to LMICs. In a study from Mumbai, India, the authors reported a 5-year relative survival of 25.4 % for women diagnosed with ovarian cancer [3]. For their part, Redaniel and colleagues [4] compared the survival among Philippine residents and Filipino-Americans and Caucasians living in the US and found that the 5-year absolute survival was lower in Philippine residents (44 %) as compared to Filipino-Americans (53.1 %), despite a more favorable distribution of age and cancer morphology and a similar stage distribution. Not surprisingly, they attributed this to differences in access to health care.

Despite improvements in surgery, postoperative care, and chemotherapy options, the overall survival from ovarian cancer has improved only slightly in the past decades. Ovarian cancer still carries the highest case-fatality rate of all gynecologic malignancies. Early detection by screening or early clinical diagnosis is an important goal of ovarian cancer control, as survival is closely linked to stage at presentation. While studies have demonstrated that it is possible to detect-screen some cases of ovarian cancer at an early stage, the benefit in terms of overall mortality reduction has not been proven. As of 2012, in the USA there is no large organization that recommends screening women at average risk for ovarian cancer, including the American College of Obstetrics and Gynecology (ACOG), the US Preventive Services Task Force (USPSTF), or the Society of Gynecologic Oncology (SGO). None of the available studies have focused on the realities of LMICs or have evaluated these screening methods in countries with limited resources. Out of necessity, therefore, for the purposes of this chapter, we must look to studies done in HIC. The goal of this chapter is to review the current data on ovarian cancer screening and to emphasize areas of particular interest to countries with limited resources. It highlights the lack of published data from countries with limited resource and should serve as impetus to improve the body of data available.

Rationale for Screening and Challenges to Screening Test Implementation

There is a clinical rationale for ovarian cancer screening. Survival from ovarian cancer is closely related to the stage of disease at presentation. The 5-year survival among women with stage I disease ranges between 80 and 90 %, but this falls to approximately 40–45 % among women with metastatic stage III disease. The poor prognosis is largely due to the fact that more than 75 % of women are diagnosed with ovarian cancer when the disease has progressed to stage III or IV. Some experts estimate that if 75 % of ovarian cancers could be detected in stages I or II, the number of women dying of the disease could be reduced by 50 % [5].

The World Health Organization (WHO) established a set of principles to guide the development of an effective screening strategy [6]. In order to be successful, most of these criteria should be met. Evaluating potential screening tests for ovarian cancer has been extremely challenging on a number of fronts, and, while some of the criteria outlined by the WHO for an effective screening test are met, others remain an obstacle. This is particularly true when considering the economic, political, social, and religious realities in LMICs. There is no denying that ovarian cancer is an important health problem, but the relative rarity of the disease carries important health care policy implications. Should countries with limited resources focus on screening for this or any rare disease for that matter? Would this limit funding for more common diseases, such as cervical cancer, which may be more amenable to mass screening? As outlined by the WHO, in order to justify this approach, the cost of screening needs to be counterbalanced by the benefits to society at large, taking into account the money available as a whole. How one measures this "cost effectiveness" in countries with LMICs is not fully agreed upon.

When considering screening tests for any disease, it is important not only to consider the inherent efficiency of the test but also how it performs in the "real world." The predictive value of a test and, specifically, the positive predictive value (PPV) refer to the likelihood that the disease is present if the test is "positive" and is greatly influenced by the overall prevalence of disease. The predictive ability of a screening test for ovarian cancer is particularly important since an accurate diagnosis typically requires a major surgical intervention. A high PPV is required in order to minimize the morbidity of screening procedures. Given that the prevalence of ovarian cancer is so low (estimated at 1 in 2,500 in postmenopausal women), an effective screening test for ovarian cancer would require extremely high sensitivity and specificity in order to yield the maximum PPV. In many developed countries, epidemiologists consider a 10 % PPV to be the minimum value in order to be considered cost effective. By definition, even a "high" PPV like 10 % would result in ten surgeries for every case of cancer detected. Whether this approach would be acceptable to LMICs is not clear. From a purely financial perspective, this seems unlikely given that the average expenditure per capita in LMICs is just a fraction of what is spent in HIC.

A major challenge to the development of a screening test for ovarian cancer is that there is no established histologic precursor in ovarian cancer or defined molecular events that precede malignant transformation. According to the WHO guidelines, case finding in a screening program is typically a continuous process. This is an extension of the concept that cancers have an identifiable natural history, with preinvasive changes leading, over time, to an invasive cancer. This latent period allows for periodic testing to diagnose cancers either in their preinvasive stage or at the earliest possible invasive stage, such that curative treatments are available. There are recent data that suggest that, in a proportion of patients who are carriers of a BRCA 1 or 2 mutation, the initial precursor lesion occurs in the fallopian tube [7, 8]. Whether this will apply to the majority of women with a clinical diagnosis of ovarian cancer is undetermined at this time.

Another issue that is not fully explored in the current screening regimens being evaluated, but which is of particular importance in LMICs, is the potential loss to follow-up of patients with abnormal testing. Most effective cancer screening algorithms capitalize on the ability to pursue repeated testing at specific intervals of time. Given that in LMICs most medical resources are centered around large urban areas and transportation to and from these areas is often limited, other strategies have been devised in order to minimize the consequences of loss to follow-up, such as "screen-and-treat" for cervical cancer control. As part of a solution to this problem, the WHO suggested the concept of "task-shifting" to allow trained nonmedical personnel to go out into communities and implement screening practices [9]. Since the definitive diagnosis and treatment of ovarian cancer require a major surgical procedure, this concept is not easily translatable to screening for ovarian cancer. Nonetheless, it does highlight the importance of evaluating different strategies that would take into account the limitations "on the ground."

Finally, the impact on ovarian cancer mortality can only be confirmed in a prospective, randomized, controlled trial, but the low prevalence in the general population means that very large cohorts studied over a long time period are needed to evaluate the ability of a specific test. Prior to embarking on and recommending such a costly venture as mass screening for ovarian cancer, it seems prudent to await the results of these trials to determine whether they have a significant impact on mortality reduction.

Approaches to Screening for Epithelial Ovarian Cancer

The most commonly studied screening modalities for screening and early detection of ovarian cancer include clinical pelvic examination, ultrasound examinations, serum biomarkers, or a combined modality approach.

Pelvic Examinations

In the past, many organizations routinely recommended pelvic examinations with the goal of trying to detect asymptomatic ovarian masses and in the hope of detecting early stage ovarian cancers. In countries with limited economic resources, this strategy is especially appealing. Despite this, there are no published data available that support this practice in terms of a mortality reduction from ovarian cancer. The majority of ovarian cancers detected on a pelvic examination are advanced in stage, and there is no evidence that cancer detected on the basis of a routine pelvic examination alters morbidity or mortality. Despite the lack of evidence for a survival advantage, recent data demonstrate that practitioners continue to believe this is an effective screening strategy. One study in the US reported that 68 % of obstetrician/gynecologists routinely perform pelvic examinations for the purpose of ovarian cancer screening and believe that this procedure is useful to screen for gynecologic cancers (OR 3.8, CI 2.6–55) [10]. While there are certainly other arguments to be made for annual gynecologic examinations as a component of well-woman care, the benefit of pelvic exams as a screening test for ovarian cancer seems minimal at best.

Ovarian Cancer Symptom Index

One of the challenges often cited in detecting ovarian cancer is the relative absence of symptoms among women with early ovarian cancer. Remarkably, even advanced cases of ovarian cancer often present with nonspecific signs or symptoms. This has led ovarian cancer to be called a "silent killer." But numerous studies that evaluated symptoms among women with ovarian cancer confirmed that, at least retrospectively, symptoms may be present for several months, although they are often vague in nature [11, 12]. A large survey of 1725 women with ovarian cancer in the US and Canada confirmed that 95 % of women with ovarian cancer recall developing symptoms an average of 3–6 months before their diagnosis [13]. The most common symptoms were abdominal (77 %), gastrointestinal (70 %), pain (58 %), constitutional (50 %), urinary (34 %), and pelvic (26 %). Remarkably, gynecologic symptoms were the least common. In their follow-up study, Goff and colleagues [14] reported on the frequency and duration of symptoms among women with ovarian cancer. Cancer patients reported symptoms which occurred 20–30 times per month, as compared with 2–3 times per month among control patients. In addition, symptoms among women with ovarian cancer were significantly shorter in duration, usually less than 3–6 months as compared to controls. Large population-based studies have substantiated these findings [15, 16].

This information was recently used to develop an ovarian symptom index (SI) that might be helpful for the purposes of screening [17]. The index is considered to be positive in women who report 1 of 6 symptoms (bloating, increased abdominal size, difficulty eating, early satiety, and abdominal or pelvic pain) more than 12 times/month and in whom the symptoms are present for less than 1 year. The overall sensitivity and specificity for detecting ovarian cancer were 70 % and 86 %, respectively, and it was lowest among women with early stage disease (57 %). Other investigators reported limited utility to the use of SI when evaluated retrospectively. Rossing and coworkers [18] surveyed women about their symptoms before diagnosis and compared this with age-matched controls and found the sensitivity of the SI was low for early stage disease (62.3 %) with a PPV of 1 %.

Although current data do not indicate that focusing on symptom index results in an increased detection rate of early stage ovarian cancer, current trials are evaluating whether the combined use of symptom index with other modalities, including US or biomarkers would improve early detection [19–21]. Given the limited availability of other more costly options, this would seem to be of interest for LMICs. At a minimum, these data emphasize that ovarian cancer is not truly a "silent killer." Whether these symptoms can be capitalized upon for the early detection of ovarian cancer remains unclear.

Ultrasound Screening for Ovarian Cancer

An alternative to the use of pelvic examinations and symptoms for screening of ovarian cancer involves the use of ultrasonography. Imaging of the ovary permits an assessment of variations in ovarian size and morphology, which may precede the development of metastatic disease. The increased availability of ultrasound over the past few decades has prompted its use in multiple large-scale screening studies. Furthermore, relatively low cost and portable US units have become increasingly available in countries with limited resources, and this makes it appealing as a means of screening and early detection. A detailed description of assessment of the ovary by ultrasound appears in the next section.

Transvaginal ultrasound (TVUS) offers benefits over transabdominal ultrasound (TAUS), including an enhanced ability to detect subtle morphologic changes in the ovaries and has been proposed as a more specific alternative as a screening test for ovarian cancer [22, 23]. Studies of TVUS for the detection of early stage ovarian cancer have yielded mixed results. In one of the largest studies, Van Nagell and colleagues [24] reported their findings on more than 25,000 women screened with TVUS at a single institution. Eligible women included all women ≥50 years and women ≥25 years with a documented family history of ovarian cancer. Initial abnormality criteria included (1) ovarian volume of more than 10 cm^3 in a postmenopausal woman, (2) ovarian volume of more than 20 cm^3 in a premenopausal woman, or (3) any cystic ovarian lesion with a papillary projection. Three hundred and sixty-four women (1.4 %) with a persisting ovarian tumor on TVUS underwent surgery. Of these, 29 women were found to have invasive ovarian cancer, among whom 14 (48 %) had stage I disease. Nine patients had a false negative screen and received a diagnosis of ovarian cancer within 12 months (interval cancers). The sensitivity of TVUS screening was calculated to be 85 %, and the specificity was 98.7 %. The PPV of an abnormal screen was 14 %. The 5-year survival rate among screen-detected patients of 77 % compared favorably with historic controls.

Over time, the protocol for reporting abnormal findings has changed. Since 2006, unilocular ovarian cysts <10 cm in women with a normal serum CA125 were considered normal and, since 2009, multilocular cysts with a normal CA125 were considered normal. In a more recent follow-up publication, Van Nagell and coworkers [25] reported on the long-term survival of women with ultrasound screen-detected ovarian cancer. Specificity and PPV for primary invasive epithelial ovarian cancer were 98.5 % and 8.9 %, respectively. Eleven operations were performed per primary cancer detected, and 70 % of the 47 screen-detected cancers were either stage I or II. Twelve women developed ovarian cancer within 12 months of a negative screen. In addition to an apparent "stage-shift" to earlier stage disease, the reported 5-year survival of women with ovarian cancer in the screening arm, which includes both screen-detected invasive ovarian cancer and interval cancers, was 74.8 % compared to 53.7 % in an unscreened cohort from the same institution ($p<0.01$). While promising, these results are not the results of a randomized trial. Furthermore, they reflect the experience of a single institution with years of experiences. Reports demonstrate considerable variation among observers in interpreting ultrasonographic images, and the sensitivity of imaging has been low in external validation studies [26]. These results may be difficult to reproduce in the general community, and this is of particular relevance to countries with limited resources. An additional criticism to this trial revolves around the inclusion criteria. Given that many patients were considered to be at greater than average risk due to their family history, the PPV may be higher than the value that would be expected in the general population.

The data from the ultrasound arm of the UK Collaborative Trial of Ovarian Cancer Screening (UKCTOCS) highlight the importance of obtaining results from a multicentered randomized controlled trial prior to making assertions about the generalizability of the results of ultrasound-based screening to the population at large. The UKCTOCS is currently the largest ongoing randomized controlled screening trial of ovarian cancer. In one arm of this trial, 48,230 women were randomly assigned to screening with annual TVUS as one arm of a randomized trial comparing multimodality screening, TVUS, and no screening [27]. The study involves 13 participating regional centers in the UK. Recognizing the importance of maintaining high quality ultrasonography, the study required all ultrasonographers to undergo an initial program of accreditation with a reaccreditation process every 2 years to ensure that scanning standards and uniformity were maintained [28]. The initial prevalence screen found 45 primary ovarian and fallopian tube cancers. Of these, 25 were invasive cancers and, of these, 12 were stage I or II. The reported sensitivity, specificity, and PPV for primary ovarian and tubal cancers were 84.9 %, 98.2 %, and 5.3 %, respectively. Additional testing was required in 12 % of participants ($n=5779$), and surgery was performed in 1.8 % of women ($n=845$). Specificity was lower for TVUS alone compared to multimodal screening, and nine times as many surgeries were performed for an abnormal TVUS compared to multimodal screening. This has implications in the setting of LMICs, where the financial burden of the screening tests, in addition to the costs of evaluating false positives, could easily outstrip any overall benefit.

Both the financial costs of the actual screening tests and the diagnostic surgeries that ensue, as well as the potential morbidity of any unnecessary surgeries as a result of a false-positive screen, cannot be underestimated, particularly in countries with limited resources. While it certainly appears that ultrasound evaluation as a component of early diagnosis of ovarian cancer is encouraging and needs to be further assessed, there is currently no role for mass screening at this time in LMICs. This is especially true in light of a recent review that evaluated training opportunities for ultrasound in LMICs [29]. Generalist and obstetric physicians and even nonmedical personnel perform the majority of ultrasound scans in LMICs, with little to no formal training in ultrasonography. In the authors' estimation, training in LMICs often does not meet the minimum criteria outlined by the WHO, such as the number of scans performed under direct supervision and the length of training programs that is recommended.

While the current data do not support mass population ultrasound-based screening for ovarian cancer, the use of ultrasound may provide other potential benefits in LMICs. One opinion piece even suggested that this modality should be considered for breast cancer screening, and it would be compatible with the concept of "task-shifting" as suggested by the WHO [30]. One limitation to screening in LMICs is the distance and general inaccessibility of screening programs. Transportation to centers where these technologies are available is a challenge. The use of portable ultrasound machines by nonmedical ultrasonographers may help circumvent several of these problems. In HIC, training of nonmedical sonographers has proven to be an acceptable manner to "extend" the ability of physicians to care for a larger number of patients. With proper training and support, it stands to reason that this approach may be feasible in LMICs. In addition, sonographers may be more accepting of deployment out of a capital city, for example. The results of ultrasound are also immediately available and do not require a return visit to obtain results. If an abnormality is identified, protocols can be developed to ensure that follow-up tests are pursued and, if indicated, surgery scheduled in an appropriate manner. Whether such a regimen is logistically feasible and culturally acceptable to women in LMICs and whether governments would choose to implement these policy changes is unclear. The national commitment to develop cancer control services is the single most important factor for cancer control in all countries, including LMICs.

Serum Biomarkers: Cancer Antigen 125

Serum biomarkers have been intensely studied for the early detection of ovarian cancer. This strategy is attractive since measurement of tumor markers is widely available, affordable, and minimally invasive and can be repeated at predetermined, appropriate intervals. Furthermore, as opposed to ultrasound-based screening, the results are not operator dependent. One of the most widely evaluated is the cancer antigen 125 (CA125), which is a high molecular weight glycoprotein expressed by a large proportion of epithelial ovarian cancers. Since its discovery, CA125 has become established as a tumor marker for epithelial ovarian cancer. The initial report of CA125 found that the tumor marker was elevated in the serum of approximately 80 % of women with advanced-stage ovarian cancer and in only 1–2 % of the normal population [31]. Enthusiasm was high initially that this might be a good means of screening for ovarian cancers. However, further studies have demonstrated that both the sensitivity and specificity of CA125 is inadequate for its use as a stand-alone screening test. First of all, it lacks sensitivity. It is raised only in approximately 50 % of stage I epithelial ovarian cancers [32]. Likewise, the specificity of the test is poor overall, and, while it is elevated in 75–90 % of patients with advanced disease, false-positive results have been noted in many medical disorders, both benign and malignant, including endometriosis, uterine fibroids, liver cirrhosis, PID, peritonitis, pancreatitis, and renal failure [33–35].

In one study from Sweden, serum CA125 levels were measured annually among 5,550 women over the age of 40 years [36]. An elevated CA125 prompted increased surveillance with sequential CA125 every 3 months, pelvic exams, and TAUS every 6 months. If the CA125 doubled or was >95 U/mL, or if an adnexal mass was identified on ultrasound, patients were offered an exploratory laparotomy. Among participants, 175 women were found to have an elevated CA125, and 6 ovarian cancers were identified (2 stage IA, 2 stage IIB, and 2 stage II), but three women with normal CA125 levels also developed ovarian cancer. The group reported a specificity of 97 % among women <50 years of age compared to 99 % among women >50 years of age. Similar studies were reported by others and demonstrated that, despite high rates of specificity ranging from 98.6 to 99.4 %, the PPV was too low to serve as a stand-alone screening modality [37, 38].

The NCI-sponsored Prostate, Lung, Colorectal, and Ovarian (PLCO) Cancer Screening Trial provided evidence that annual screening with CA125 is not an effective screening regimen for detection of early ovarian cancer [39]. In the ovarian portion of the PLCO trial, 78,237 asymptomatic women between 55 and 74 years of age were randomly assigned to screening, including baseline measurements of CA125 and TVUS followed by annual CA125 for 6 years and TVUS for 3 years. Controls consisted of women who received routine gynecologic care alone. The subjects were followed for approximately 13 years (median 12.4 years). At baseline, the initial prevalence screen of 28,816 women found the CA125 was abnormal in 436 women (1.5 %) and the TVUS was abnormal in 4.7 % of women. Nearly one in three women who had a positive screening test underwent surgery ($n=570$). Among these, 29 neoplasms were identified (26 ovarian, 2 fallopian, and 1 primary peritoneal), resulting in a PPV for invasive cancer of 3.7 % [40]. Nine of these were LMPs. Only two of the invasive cancers were stage I. The estimated PPV of an abnormal ultrasound was 1 %. If both tests were abnormal, the PPV increased to 23.5 %; however, if only those subjects where both tests were abnormal had been evaluated, the majority (12 of 20) of invasive cancers would have been missed. The final results of the PLCO trial demonstrate no benefit in terms of reduction in mortality to screening with annual TVUS and CA125. In addition, there was no difference in the stage of ovarian cancer identified. The majority presented with advanced disease, stage III, or IV (77 %). Mortality rates were not significantly different among the two groups (RR 1.21, CI 0.91–1.54). False positives were identified in 3,285 women, and approximately one-third of those women underwent a diagnostic surgery ($n=1080$). Of significant concern, among those women who underwent surgery for a false-positive finding, approximately 15 % had a serious complication ($n=166$).

Development of Risk of Malignancy Algorithm

One important observation is that, among women with an elevated CA125 who develop ovarian cancer compared to women with an elevated

CA125 who do not, there is a progressive elevation of the CA125 over time. Retrospective analysis of serial CA125 levels seems to indicate that, for most women without ovarian cancer, the CA125 profile will remain relatively flat, but, for women who develop ovarian cancer, the CA125 profile shows a progressive increase [41]. This may occur even within a reportedly "normal" level of CA125 and has led some researchers to suggest that there is a time frame within which a rising, albeit "normal" CA125 can help identify patients at greatest risk of developing ovarian cancer. Capitalizing on this finding would help to increase the sensitivity of the screening test while maintaining a high level of specificity. This risk of ovarian cancer algorithm (ROCA) calculates the risk of ovarian cancer for an individual, comparing each individual serial CA125 level to the pattern in known cases of ovarian cancer and control. Skates and colleagues [42] demonstrated that a higher sensitivity was obtained for CA125 if the rate of change in CA125 serum levels is used as predictor rather than a single, fixed cut-off value and increased the sensitivity for detection of ovarian cancer from 70 to 86 %, while maintaining a high level of specificity (98 %). The ROCA is currently being evaluated in a number of trials, including both average risk and high risk women. The largest of these is the UKCTOCS.

Multimodal Screening

The most promising approach to screening for ovarian cancer seems to involve a multimodality approach, capitalizing on the combination of serum markers and ultrasonography. Three large randomized trials have evaluated the combination of screening with serum CA125 and ultrasound either sequentially or concurrently. As noted previously, the PLCO demonstrated no benefit to screening with annual CA125 and TVUS. More encouraging results were reported in a randomized controlled trial of 83,000 postmenopausal women in Japan [43]. In this study, 42,000 women were invited to participate in annual screening with pelvic ultrasound and CA125. The control group received standard care at the discretion of the provider. At a follow-up of 9.2 years, there was no significant difference in the detection of ovarian cancer among those patients undergoing screening (27 cases) vs. controls (32 cases). However, there was a nonsignificant trend toward earlier disease in the screened group. Thirty-three surgeries were performed to detect each case of ovarian cancer. Overall mortality data have not yet been reported for this trial.

A subsequent study by Jacobs and colleagues [44] evaluated sequential screening with CA125 and ultrasound in volunteers without a family history of ovarian cancer. If the serum CA125 was abnormally elevated, the women underwent TAUS. If the imaging was abnormal, they were offered a diagnostic laparotomy. A total of 41 women underwent surgery, and 11 had ovarian cancer (two stage IA, one stage IB, one stage IIA, and seven stage III or IV). Eight women had a false-negative screen and developed ovarian cancer in the subsequent 12 months. The authors reported a PPV of 26.8 % for ovarian cancer. Based on these prevalence data, the authors performed a pilot randomized trial of screening among 22,000 postmenopausal women aged >45 years [45]. Women randomized to screening underwent three annual screening evaluations that involved measurements of serum CA125, TVUS if the CA125 was elevated, and referral to a gynecologist if the ultrasound was abnormal. Among the screened women, there were 468 with abnormally elevated CA125. Cancer was detected in six of these women. The PPV was estimated at 21 %. During the follow-up period, an additional ten women were diagnosed with ovarian cancer among the screened women and 20 in the control group. The median survival for women with ovarian cancer among the screened group was 72.9 months and in the control group was 41.8 months ($p = 0.0112$).

The UKCTOCS distinguishes itself from the PLCO trial in that it defines an abnormal CA125 according to the ROCA score. The UKCTOCS randomized 202,638 women in a 1:1:2 ratio into (1) a multimodality screening arm, where CA125 was the primary screening test using the ROCA, and ultrasound was used as a secondary screen if the CA125 was deemed abnormal; (2) a ultrasound-based screening arm; and (3) a control arm. The study was designed to have a 90 % power to detect a 30 % reduction in mortality due to screening. The initial prevalence results of UKCTCOS trial seem promising. The prevalence screen found 42 primary ovarian and tubal tumors in the multimodality arm. Eight of these were borderline tumors, but 16 of the other 34 (47 %) were stage I or II invasive cancers. The sensitivity, specificity, and PPV in the initial screen were 89.5 %, 99.8 %, and 35.1 %, respectively, when borderline tumors are excluded. Approximately 2 operations (2.3:1) were performed for every screen-detected cancer in the multimodality group. This was significantly higher in the ultrasound group (18.8:1). The UKCTOCS completed 10 years of screening in December 2011, and follow-up results are expected in 2014/2015.

As a "proof of principle," screening using CA125 levels and ultrasound has demonstrated that ovarian cancer can be identified at an early stage in asymptomatic women; however, these screening tests are associated with a significant false-positive rate and require large number of diagnostic surgeries in order to detect one case of ovarian cancer. Additionally, there is no proven benefit in terms of mortality reduction. Realistically, even if these trials demonstrate a survival advantage, it is unclear if these data will be generalizable to the situation in LMICs. Putting aside the crippling financial burden this would place on LMICs for a moment, the overall lower prevalence of this disease in economically developing countries means that the PPV of any of these screening modalities is likely to be lower than what has been reported. One foreseeable impact would be to increase the number of women requiring diagnostic surgeries, resulting in an increase in the overall cost to society and potentially an increase in the morbidity to the individual woman, as was demonstrated in the PLCO trial.

Prevention of Ovarian Cancer

It is appropriate to discuss other options that could potentially be helpful in decreasing or preventing the disease in the first place. Is it possible to prevent ovarian cancer? While this approach is relevant to all women facing the possibility of this diagnosis, this is of particular importance in countries where resources are limited. Exploring these options requires an understanding of the etiology and risk factors for this disease. Up to this point, the etiology of this disease, or group of diseases, remains elusive; however, certain risk factors have been identified, and some may be amenable to exploring as a means of reducing the overall incidence of the disease.

Lifestyle and environmental factors such as exercise and diet have not demonstrated conclusively to have a link to ovarian cancer; however, reproductive and endocrine factors do seem to play a significant role in modifying the risk of ovarian cancer. Increased parity has a demonstrated protective effect on the development of ovarian cancer. An analysis of 12 US case–control studies found a decreasing risk of ovarian cancer with increasing parity [46]. Each additional pregnancy conferred a risk reduction of approximately 14 %. They found no association with the age of first pregnancy. Similar findings were reported in a subsequent report [47]. However, this latter study did find an effect of age at childbirth with subsequent risk of ovarian cancer. In their study, a delay in pregnancy appeared to confer an additional protective effect when compared to women who gave birth before 20 years of age. Breastfeeding has also been reported to provide a protective effect on ovarian cancer risk, reducing the risk by approximately 40 % in the collaborative US analysis [46].

Data demonstrate that beyond the potential benefits to society from family planning, this approach may also help reduce a woman's risk of developing ovarian cancer. As such, research in this area deserves special attention. Nandakumar and coworkers [48] reported on a case–control study of ovarian cancer in Bangalore, India, using data from a population-based registry. They examined the effect of tobacco, alcohol, dietary practices, and reproductive factors in the development of ovarian cancer. Ninety-seven patients with a diagnosis of ovarian cancer were matched with 194 controls. Only a history of practising family planning was associated with a decreased risk of ovarian cancer. More specifically, tubal surgery reduced the risk of developing ovarian cancer ($OR = 0.25$; $p = 0.02$). Other reproductive factors did not appear to influence the risk of ovarian cancer. Similar reductions in ovarian cancer were reported in the collaborative analysis of US case–control studies (OR 0.59, CI 0.38–0.53) 46 and other studies [49–51].

Finally, the protective effects of the combined oral contraceptive pill against ovarian cancer are also well documented and should be further explored in LMICs. The cancer and steroid hormone study (CASH) demonstrated that oral contraceptive use reduces the risk of ovarian cancer by up to 40 % [52]. The protective effect appears to be proportional to the duration of use; however, even short periods of use conferred a benefit and persist beyond the time of use. Numerous other studies have confirmed these results [46].

Sonographic Evaluation of the Ovaries

Sonography has been well validated as a modality of choice for the characterization of adnexal masses. While large masses are best evaluated through a transabdominal as well as an endovaginal approach, smaller masses are optimally examined by endovaginal sonogram including color and spectral Doppler assessment. Characterization of adnexal masses is important in the management of a patient with an adnexal mass to minimize unnecessary surgical interventions, since only a small percentage of surgically removed adnexal masses are proven malignant. Of the 5–10 % of women with adnexal masses who undergo surgery, the malignancy rate is only 13–21 %. When CA 125 is used, 10–20 surgeries have to be performed to find one cancer [53]. There is a need to gain a better understanding of the morphologic features and ovarian masses so as to reliably distinguish non-neoplastic abnormalities from tumors and benign from malignant tumors. Such knowledge will help improve management and outcomes in patients with an adnexal mass.

Adnexal masses discovered clinically or identified during the course of a pelvic ultrasound performed for a pelvic symptom may be non-neoplastic (Fig. 7.1a–d), benign neoplastic (Fig. 7.2a–d), or a malignant ovarian neoplasm (Figs. 7.3a–d and 7.4a–d). The role of ultrasound is to accurately characterize these masses to allow for optimal management. Pattern recognition involves initial exclusion of non-neoplastic entities. Non-neoplastic masses including functional cysts, hemorrhagic cysts, inflammatory tubo-ovarian masses, and endometriomas are in most instances managed conservatively (Fig. 7.1a–d). Once non-neoplastic causes have been excluded, a more detailed analysis is carried out to distinguish a benign from a malignant mass. Characterization of an ovarian mass has significant surgical approach management implications. Benign cysts are generally excised via a laparoscopic approach; probably, benign neoplasms may require laparotomy and those that are suspicious for malignancy require extensive surgical debridement.

There have been different approaches studied for characterization of adnexal masses. The most commonly used is a subjective assessment using a pattern recognition approach; other methods include a simple descriptive scoring systems, mathematically developed scoring systems, and logistic regression models.

Subjective Assessment of Adnexal Masses

Subjective assessment of adnexal masses based on gray scale and Doppler ultrasound findings is the most widely used and an accepted method for discriminating benign from malignant masses. The accuracy of pattern recognition is, however, dependent on the operator's skill and experience. A prospective preoperative study involving 300 women with pelvic masses reported 92 % accuracy with an experienced investigator who was provided with hard copy images of a pelvic ultrasound examination and a brief clinical history which included age of the patient, menstrual status, family history of ovarian cancers, history of surgery, and presenting symptoms [54]. Less experienced operators were found to have a lower accuracy and interobserver

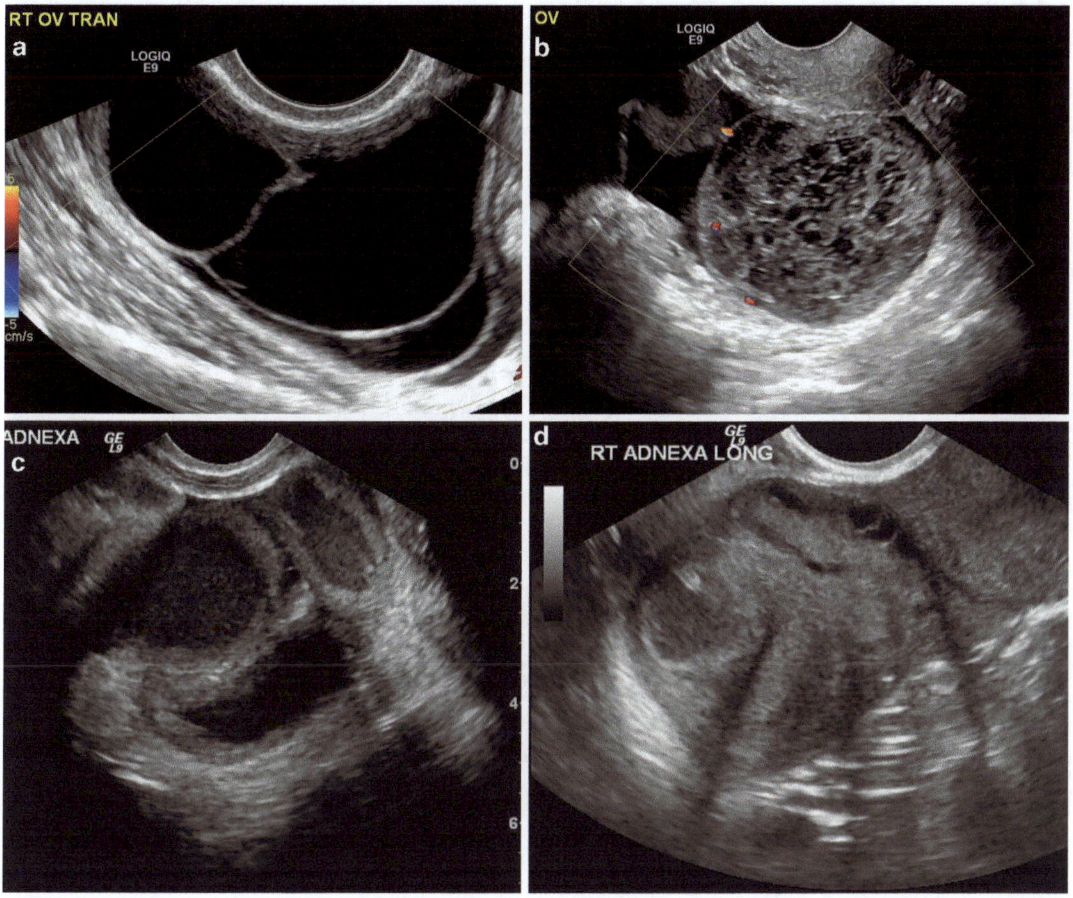

Fig. 7.1 Benign non-neoplastic abnormalities of the ovary. (**a**) A multiseptate cyst that was proved to be a functional cyst at laparoscopy. (**b**) Hemorrhagic cyst: unilocular cyst with a lacy internal pattern characteristic of a hemorrhagic cyst. (**c**) Endometrioma: multiloculated thick-walled cyst with low level internal echoes in a histologically proven endometrioma. (**d**) A complex mass in the left adnexa with a cystic component inseparable from the left ovary was proven to be a chronic tubo-ovarian abscess

agreement, with accuracy rates ranging from 82 to 87 %. A combination of real-time and Doppler parameters were utilized to provide a benign or a malignant preoperative diagnosis in 300 women. Doppler parameters included pulsatility index (PI), resistive index (RI), peak systolic velocity (PSV), and time averaged peak velocity (TAPV). Ascites was noted if >5 mm in the Pouch of Douglas. Subjective assessment included assessment of the size, locularity, echogenicity, papillary surface, and internal surface of the tumor. There were a large number of malignancies with 31 % stage I cancers, which are harder to diagnose compared to advanced stage invasive cancers. Ten percent were borderline tumors. Cystadenofibromas and tubo-ovarian abscesses were the most challenging and correctly identified in only 25 % of the cases by all six operators [54].

There have been attempts to improve accuracy and bring standardization to characterization of adnexal tumors The international ovarian tumor analysis (IOTA) group was such an initiative to standardize terms used in the characterization of adnexal masses by sonography and Doppler evaluation. The variability of diagnostic accuracy in the characterization of adnexal masses has been attributed to a lack of uniformity in the descriptors of adnexal pathology. The outcome of the consensus presented by the IOTA

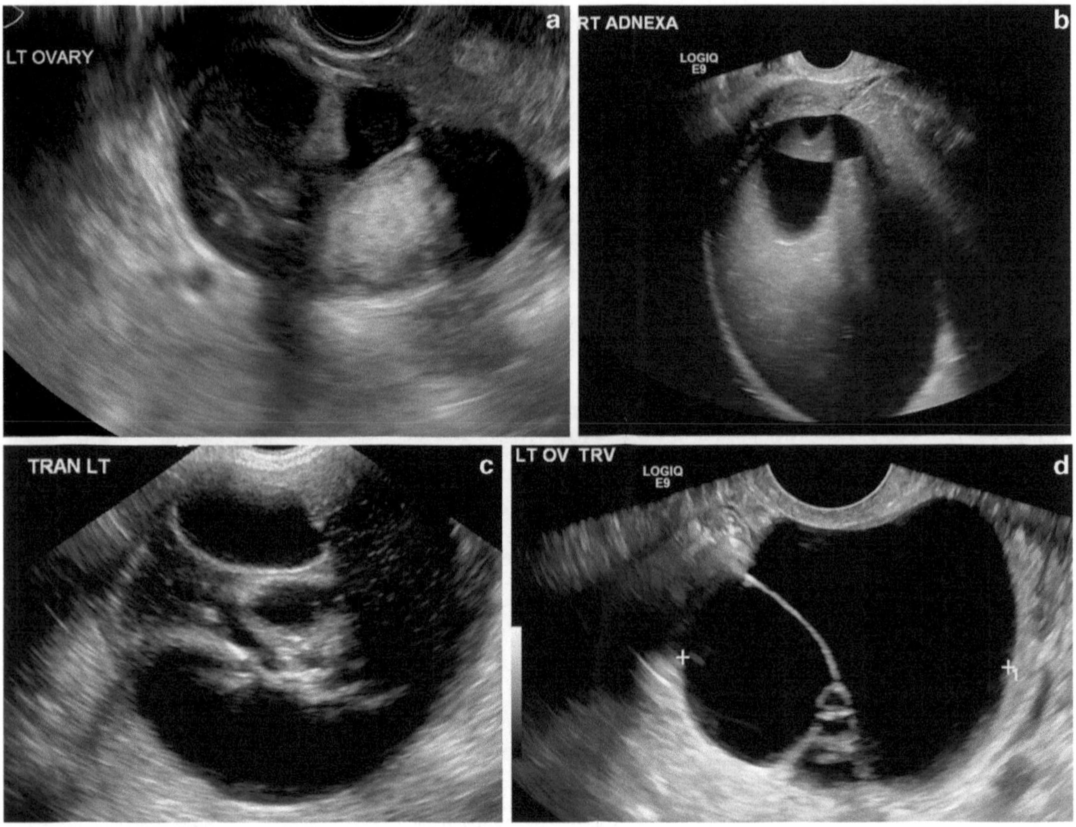

Fig. 7.2 Benign tumors of the ovary. (**a**) A complex cystic mass with a characteristic regional high echogenicity in a mature cystic teratoma. (**b**) A large complex cystic mass with multiple loculations and low level internal echoes representing mucin in a mucinous cystadenoma. (**c**) A complex cystic mass with multiple thick internal septations and few low-level internal echoes in a mucinous cystadenoma. (**d**) A large cystic mass with multiple internal septations in a serous cystadenoma

group involved definition of the morphological features, qualitative classification of masses into six categories, quantitative assessment of morphology, and a description of the vascular features of the adnexal masses [55].

Morphological Features of Ovarian Masses

An adnexal mass is described as a solid mass or a cystic mass. In a solid mass, the appearance of the external wall and presence of acoustic shadowing if present is documented. In a cystic tumor, internal septations, papillary projections, internal wall, and contents of a cyst are described. Presence of free pelvic fluid is noted when present. These particular features are described in detail next.

A septum is defined as a thin strand of tissue running across the cyst cavity from one internal surface to the contralateral side. An incomplete septum is one that is not complete in some scanning planes. A solid mass is one that demonstrates high echogenicity. A blood clot is distinguished from a solid tumor by the presence of internal movement when gentle pressure is applied with the transducer; presence of vascularity is suggestive of a solid tumor. When these are unhelpful in distinguishing blood clots from solid tumors, the lesion is classified as solid. A solid papillary projection is defined as a solid projection into a cyst that is greater or equal to 3 mm. Hyperreflective

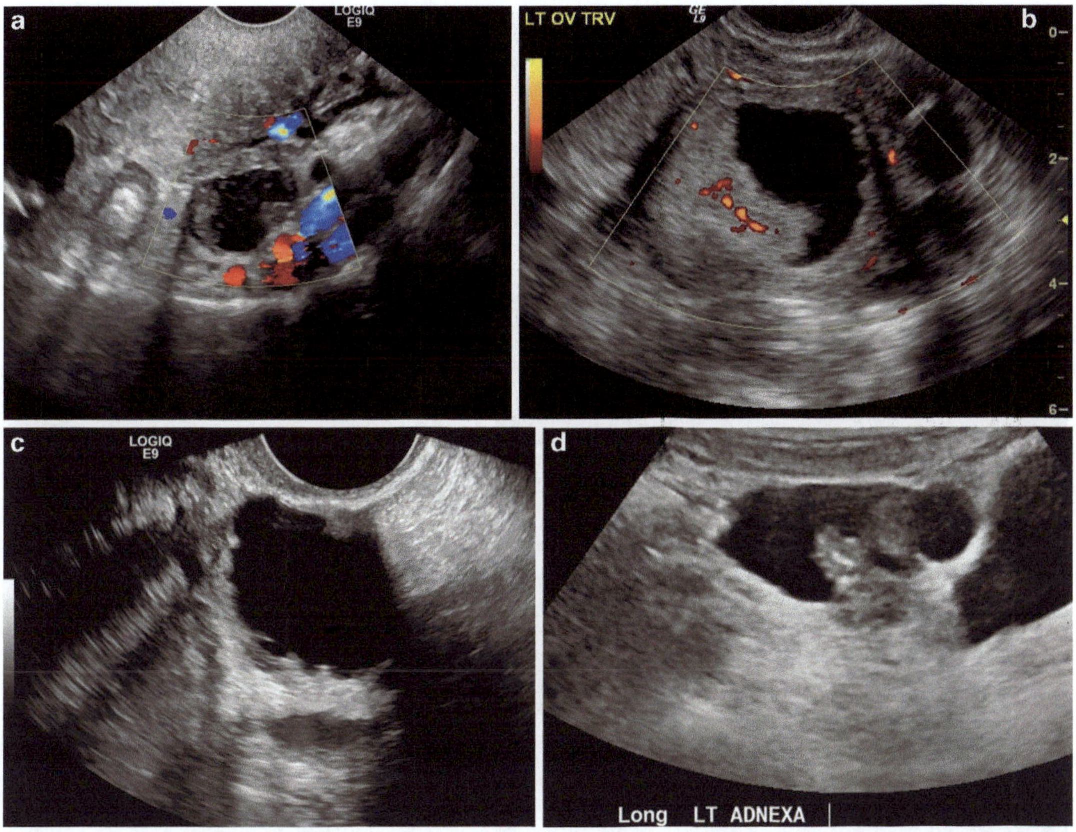

Fig. 7.3 Malignant epithelial ovarian tumors. (**a**) A small complex cystic mass with irregular mural nodules histologically proven to be an endometrioid carcinoma of the ovary. (**b**) A complex cystic mass with a large mural soft tissue mass that at surgery showed a serous cyst adenocarcinoma of the ovary. (**c**) Unilocular cyst with thick and irregular internal and external wall in a serous cystadenocarcinoma of the ovary. (**d**) A unilocular cyst with a papillary projection in a mucinous cystadenocarcinoma of the ovary

and avascular area in a dermoid is not a papillary projection. Sludge seen in the internal wall of an endometrioma is also not classified as a papillary projection. Solid papillary projections may be smooth or irregular. The internal wall of a cystic lesion is described as being smooth or irregular. In case of a solid mass, the external wall may be described as being smooth or irregular. The cystic contents may be described as anechoic as in simple cysts, low level echoes as seen in mucinous tumors, ground glass as in endometriotic cysts, and a lacy pattern with internal threadlike structures as in a hemorrhagic cyst. Acoustic shadows refer to loss of acoustic echoes posterior to the lesions. Fluid outside of the pouch of Douglas is considered ascites; this finding is noted if present [55].

Qualitative Classification of Lesions

The masses are classified under one of six groups. A unilocular cyst is a cyst without a septum, solid components, or papillary projections. A unilocular, solid cyst is a unilocular cyst without a measurable solid component or a papillary projection. A multilocular cyst is cyst with at least one complete septum but no measurable solid component or a papillary projection. Multilocular solid cyst contains a measurable solid component or a papillary projection. A solid tumor is a tumor where the solid components comprise 80 % or more of the tumor in a two-dimensional plane. An unclassifiable lesion is one that is so because of poor visualization [55].

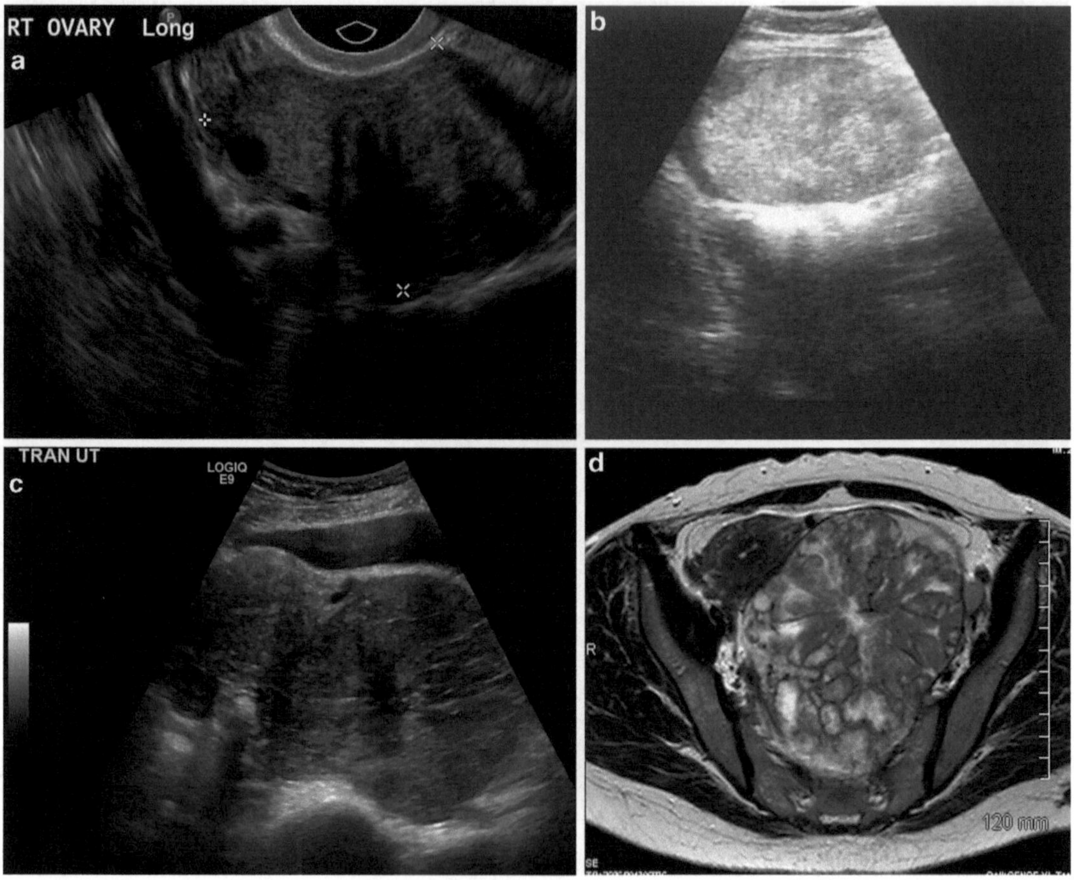

Fig. 7.4 Solid tumors of the ovary. (**a**) A round hypoechoic solid mass in the right ovary with posterior acoustic shadowing histologically proven to be an ovarian fibroma. (**b**) A large heterogeneous solid mass in the left adnexa proven to be a Sertoli-Leydig cell sex cord stromal tumor of the left ovary. (**c**) MRI: axial T2-weighted image in the same patient demonstrates a mixed signal intensity solid mass separate from the uterus. (**d**) An enlarged ovary with a heterogeneously predominantly hyperechoic solid mass that proven to be an endodermal sinus tumor of the ovary

Quantitative Assessment of Lesions

Quantitative assessment was described to define ways to measure morphologic features of an adnexal mass. The size of the lesion as well as the ovary is measured as the largest three dimensions in three planes. The thickness of the thickest septum is measured. The largest papillary projection is measured in two perpendicular planes; when more than one, the number and presence of vascularity is recorded. The number of locules is counted. In cystic solid tumors, the largest solid component is measured in three planes. The amount of fluid in the Pouch of Douglas is measured as the largest anteroposterior diameter in the sagittal plane in mm [55].

Vascular Features of Adnexal Masses

The entire tumor is assessed by color Doppler. A subjective assessment of the flow is made based on color Doppler imaging using a scoring system. Score of 1 is given when there is no blood flow. A score of 2 when only minimal flow is detected, score of 3 indicates moderate flow, score of 4 is assigned to an adnexal tumor that is highly vascular. Spectral sampling of areas of vascularity is then performed. The set of results where the highest time averaged maximum velocity and the corresponding values for the pulsatility index (PI), resistance index (RI), and peak systolic velocity (PSV) are selected. [55]

These descriptors for use in the assessment of adnexal lesions were primarily developed to be used in protocols for research studies with specific objectives as a way of standardizing results, allowing for meaningful comparisons of study results. In routine clinical practice, recording all of these end points may neither be essential nor practical. Terminology as pointed out by the authors of the IOTA group is supposed to undergo continuous reassessment and modifications as new research studies are conducted and presented. These descriptions are a very useful set of standardized terminology that can be useful guidelines in gynecological imaging. The validity of the IOTA consensus has been studied in prospective multicenter trials [56].

Based on the sonographic features described by the IOTA group and a series of clinical features, a logistic regression model has also been developed and tested in a multicenter trial involving 1066 patients. The investigators reported a total of 12 independent prognostic variables: (1) personal history of ovarian cancer, (2) hormonal therapy, (3) age, (4) maximum diameter of lesion, (5) pain, (6) ascites, (7) blood flow within a solid papillary projection, (8) presence of an entirely solid tumor, (9) maximal diameter of solid component, (10) irregular internal cyst walls, (11) acoustic shadows, and (12) a color score of intratumoral blood flow. They showed that the model containing all 12 variables gave an area under the receiver operating characteristic curve of 0.95 for the development data set (=754 patients). The corresponding value for the test data set (=312 patients) was 0.94, and a probability cutoff value of 0.10 gave a sensitivity of 93 % and a specificity of 76 %. Fourteen malignant masses, including ten borderline tumors, were incorrectly classified as benign, and 23 % of the benign masses were classified as malignant. The current practice of subjective assessment of adnexal masses does well with experienced imagers. This model may therefore suit the less experienced operators more and help them to improve the accuracy [56].

Pattern recognition by an experienced operator is still the better method for evaluating adnexal tumors and has been shown in studies comparing it with IOTA models [56, 57]. A study attempting to prospectively evaluate mathematical models to predict malignancy found that all IOTA models performed well and similarly with sensitivity and specificity ranging from 92 to 96 % to 74 to 84 %, respectively, compared to a sensitivity of 90.2 % and specificity of 92.9 % for the pattern recognition approach [57].

Unclassifiable Adnexal Masses

The pattern recognition approach for classifying adnexal masses has been in wide use; however, a small but significant number of adnexal masses cannot be classified at sonographic evaluation. About 7–10 % of adnexal masses that are considered appropriate for surgical removal may not be classified as benign or malignant by experienced ultrasound operators. This can lead to unavoidable extensive surgical procedure being carried out in women with benign ovarian neoplasms. Occasionally, this may also lead to an initial undertreatment of women who needed more extensive surgery.

In one study, 7 % of adnexal masses (244/3511) considered appropriate for surgical removal could not be classified by an experienced ultrasound examiner as benign or malignant using subjective assessment of gray-scale and Doppler ultrasound findings [58]. Multilocular cysts with more than ten locules and masses with small solid components seem to be more difficult to classify than other types of tumors. The histological diagnoses that presented the greatest diagnostic difficulties were borderline tumors, cystadeno fibromas, and fibromas. A group of investigators attempted to use logistic regression models to estimate the risk of malignancy in women with ovarian masses that were unclassifiable based on subjective assessment and Doppler ultrasound findings and to compare it with use of serum CA 125 and risk of malignancy index (RMI). Logistic regression models to estimate the risk of malignancy, CA 125 measurements, and the RMI were found to be not helpful in unclassifiable masses. These findings are disappointing because, if a mass cannot be reliably classified as benign, it is likely to be treated as potentially malignant [58].

Gynecological Imaging Report and Data System

A methodology for standardizing final interpretation of an adnexal mass based on sonographic features has been proposed. This proposes structured reporting system based on ultrasound features is the Gynecologic Imaging-Report and Data System (GI-RADS), similar to the widely used BI-RADS (American College of Radiology. Illustrated breast imaging reporting and data system, third edition. Reston, VA: American College of Radiology, 1998). GIRADS was initially suggested in 2009 [59]. The concept was to provide a summarized standardized report of ultrasound findings that would provide an estimated risk of malignancy for an adnexal mass and categorize them as grade 1 (= definitely benign), grade 2 (= very probably benign), grade 3 (= probably benign), grade 4 (= probably malignant), and grade 5 (= very probably malignant) (Table 7.1). A prospective multicenter study was conducted by the same group that had proposed use of GIRADS to test its efficacy and value. This study involved 432 adnexal masses in 372 women over a 3-year period. Transvaginal ultrasound was used and examination performed by one of three experts in gynecological ultrasound [60]. The established pattern recognition approach was used to categorize masses into one of four groups (2–5). Normal ovaries received a grade 1. Reporting was provided to referral clinicians with recommendation based on the degree of suspicion. Recommendations were as follows: grade 2 for a follow-up scan, grade 3 laparoscopic surgery, and grade 4 or 5 referral to gynecological oncologist. There were 112 malignant and 320 benign lesions. Sensitivity was 99.1 %, specificity was 85.9 %, and PPV and NPV was 71.1 % and 99.6 %, respectively. GI-RADS reporting system performed well in identifying adnexal masses at high risk for malignancy and seemed like a useful tool to guide clinical management of adnexal masses characterized by ultrasonography [59, 60].

Gray Scale and Doppler Imaging Features of Adnexal Masses

Morphologic features that are suggestive of malignancy include thick irregular wall and septa, papillary projections, and solid hyperechoic loculi. Color Doppler ultrasound may help in differentiating solid tumors from nonvascularized structures such as blood clots; it also identifies vessels for Spectral Doppler interrogation [61, 62]. Benign lesions generally are less vascular and tend to have vessels that are more peripheral in location; malignant tumors tend to neovascularize centrally. Malignant neovascularity tends to lack smooth muscle and hence demonstrate low resistance, high diastolic flow, and low systolic diastolic variation, and arteriovenous shunting. Both the pulsatility and resistive index increase with increasing distal resistance, and hence these are low in malignant tumors compared to benign tumors. RI less than 0.4–0.8 and PI less than 1.0 are the norm [62] (Fig. 7.5a). Limitations of Doppler US include operator dependence, absence of standard criteria, and technical difficulty in eliciting signals from tumors; moreover, in premenopausal women, there is lower specificity due to lowered blood vessel resistance caused by physiological changes (Fig. 7.5b) and conditions such as endometriosis and tubal inflammation leading to an overlap with findings associated with malignant lesions [62]. Premenopausal women sensitivity and specificity of color Doppler ultrasound was 80 and 67 % only compared to 93 and 83 %, respectively, in postmenopausal women [63]. Gray scale assessment of morphologic features yields a sensitivity of 94 % and a specificity of 87 % and a PPV of 60 %, which improves to a 94, 99, and 94 % with addition of spectral waveform analysis [64]. In addition to the morphologic features that are mentioned here as being characteristic of malignancy, large size of an ovarian mass is an important factor in predicting malignancy in an ovarian mass. Tumors exceeding 10 cm have been reported to be significantly more likely associated with ovarian malignancy [62]

Table 7.1 Gynecologic imaging report and data system (GI-RADS) classification system for adnexal masses

GI-RADS grade	Diagnosis	Estimated probability malignancy (%)	Detail
1	Definitive benign	0	Normal ovaries identified and no adnexal mass seen
2	Very probably benign	<1	Adnexal lesions thought to be of functional origin, e.g., follicles, corpora lutea, hemorrhagic cysts
3	Probably benign	1–4	Neoplastic adnexal lesions thought to be benign, such as endometrioma, teratoma, simple cyst, hydrosalpinx, paraovarian cyst, peritoneal pseudocyst, pedunculated myoma, or findings suggestive of pelvic inflammatory disease
4	Probably malignant	5–20	Any adnexal lesion not included in GI-RADS 1–3 and with one or two findings suggestive of malignancy*
5	Very probably malignant	>20	Adnexal masses with three or more findings suggestive of malignancy*

*Thick papillary projections, thick septations, solid areas and/or ascites, defined according to IOTA criteria [12], and vascularization within solid areas, papillary projections or central area of a solid tumor on color or power Doppler assessment [5]

Source: Reprinted with permission of John Wiley & Sons Inc. from Amor F, Alcazar Al, Vaccaro H, Leon M, Iturra A. GI-RADS reporting system for ultrasound evaluation of adnexal masses in clinical practice: a prospective multicenter study. Ultrasound Obstet Gynecol 2011; 38: 450–455.

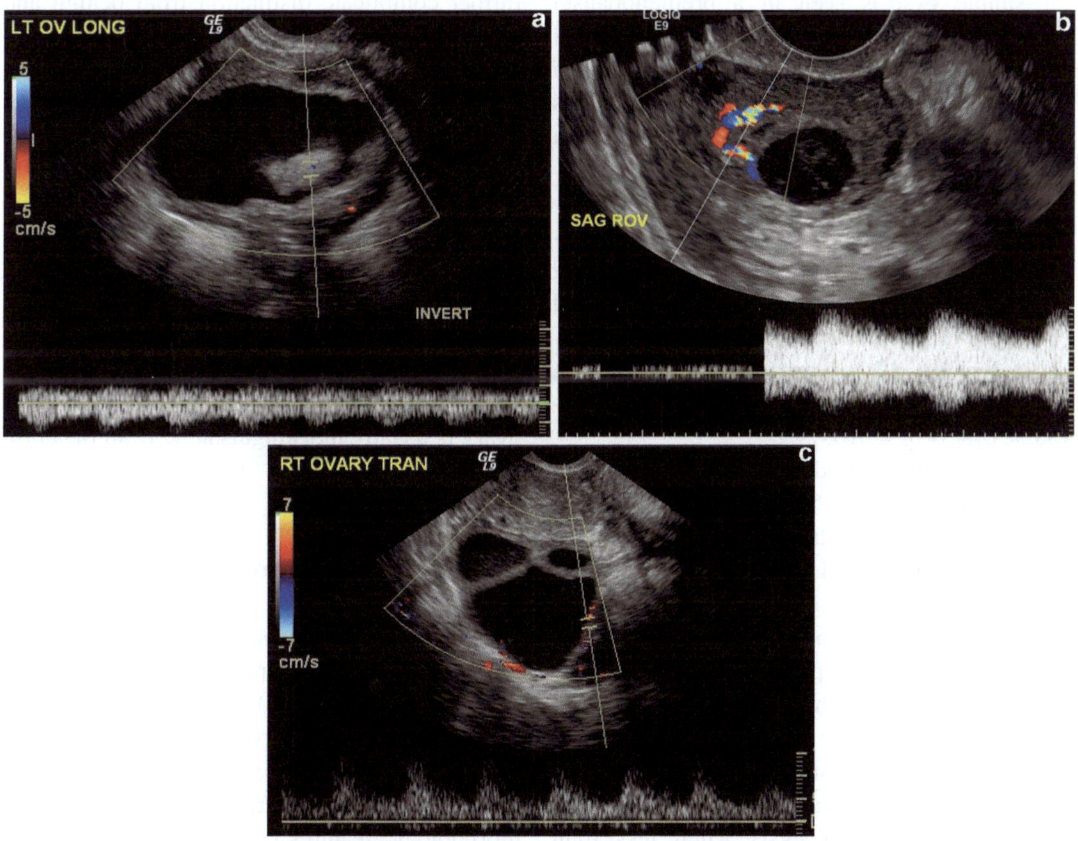

Fig. 7.5 Spectral Doppler pattern of adnexal masses. (**a**) Low resistance arterial flow pattern in a malignant ovarian tumor. (**b**) Low resistance arterial flow pattern in a physiologic corpus luteum. (**c**) High resistance arterial flow pattern in an endometrioma

Differential Diagnosis and Pitfalls in Sonographic Assessment of Adnexal Masses

Functional Cysts

These are follicular cysts resulting from a failure of follicle to rupture or corpus luteal cysts resulting from hemorrhage into the corpus luteum. Functional cysts are anechoic with thin smooth walls and posterior acoustic enhancement. Functional cysts are usually unilocular and occasionally multilocular (Fig. 7.1a). Although cystadenomas can appear similar and unilocular, papillary projections and nodular septa are more often seen in ovarian neoplasms. Doppler US is generally not helpful in distinguishing functional cysts from ovarian neoplasms. When a unilocular simple cyst is seen in a premenopausal woman, the standard practice is to recommend follow up in 6–8 weeks based on the assumption that most functional cysts will resolve. It has been suggested that a 6–12-month follow up is a more useful practice, unless the patient is symptomatic, in distinguishing the more commonly encountered functional cysts from the less common cystadenoma, which can have an imaging appearance of a simple cyst [65]. Functional cysts may be complicated by presence of hemorrhage which will then appear as a cyst with a lacy internal pattern characteristic of a hemorrhagic cyst (Fig. 7.1b).

The Society of Radiologists in Ultrasound (SRU) consensus conference in 2009 recommended that sonographic follow up not be pursued on asymptomatic simple ovarian cysts that are smaller than or equal to 5 cm in premenopausal or perimenopausal women because they are likely to be physiologic. Small neoplastic cysts are encountered in postmenopausal women and seen in up to 20 % of cases, most commonly in the first decade of postmenopause. SRU guidelines suggest no follow up for simple unilocular cysts when less than 1 cm, and, when less than 3 cm, the opinion was that there may not be a need for a follow-up examination [66].

Endometrioma

Endometrioma is lined by endometrial glands, and the wall may get progressively thick, fibrotic, and irregular. These appear as a cystic mass with diffuse low level echoes and a spectrum of appearances ranging from cystic to complex cystic and solid. Hyperechoic foci in the wall when seen result from cholesterol clefts. When the appearance is of a complex cystic mass, an endometrioma can be confused with ovarian malignancies [62] (Fig. 7.1c). Of the benign non-neoplastic causes, endometriomas can pose some of the most difficult challenges in differential diagnosis due to the wide spectrum of appearance ranging from simple unilocular cysts to complex cystic masses; chronic hematomas in endometriomas can simulate solid ovarian neoplasms, and vascularity of such endometriotic nodules may further complicate distinction from benign and malignant ovarian tumors. In developed countries, MRI is a useful modality to diagnose endometriomas due to the unique imaging characteristics of blood products in an endometrioma. While acute pelvic inflammatory diseases with tubo-ovarian abscess are easily distinguished from a neoplastic process, differential diagnostic dilemma may occasionally arise in women with a chronic tubo-ovarian complexes in those improperly or inadequately treated for PID. These may appear as adnexal masses with solid and cystic components, some peripheral vascularity; the ovary is usually indistinguishable from the complex mass (Fig. 7.1d).

Mature Cystic Teratomas

Mature cystic teratomas are the most common ovarian tumors and are often asymptomatic, being incidentally identified during a routine pelvic examination or a pelvic ultrasound. Since ectodermal elements predominate, these tumors are more often called dermoid tumor. The classic morphologic features described are regional or diffuse high echogenicity, shadowing echogenicity, hyperechoic lines, and dots and fat-fluid levels. In most instances, sonography accurately diagnoses mature cystic teratomas, although, in rare instances, distinction from endometriomas and ovarian malignancy may be challenging. Immature teratoma is a malignant tumor that also demonstrates fat; this tumor is typically large and may show large solid components and coarse calcifications [62] (Fig. 7.2a).

Epithelial Neoplasms of the Ovary

These comprise 60 % of benign and 85 % of malignant tumors. The most frequent types are serous and mucinous types; rarer types include endometroid, clear cell, and Brenner tumor. Epithelial tumors are benign (Fig. 7.2b–d) or borderline or malignant (Fig. 7.3a–d) based on the histology and clinical behavior. Ultrasound features of a benign neoplasm are a unilocular cyst, thin walls, few thin septations, absent mural nodularity, or papillary projections (Fig. 7.2b–d). Unlike malignant tumors, benign tumors do not show stromal invasion or evidence of metastasis. Malignant epithelial tumors are often large at diagnosis and complex cystic with thick irregular septations and or papillary projections or mural nodules. Apart from morphologic features of the primary tumor, pelvic organ invasion, ascites, peritoneal or omental deposits, and adenopathy are signs of malignancy. Serous epithelial tumors are the most common of the epithelial tumors, and mucinous tumors are less common, larger, more likely to be multiloculated, and tend to have low level internal echoes [62] (Fig. 7.2b, c).

Solid Tumors of the Ovary

Solid tumors of the ovary are comprised mainly of sex cord/stromal and Brenner tumor, the latter being an epithelial tumor. Sex cord/stromal tumors arise from stromal cells such as fibromas (Fig. 7.4a), theca cells or Leydig cells (Fig. 7.4b, c) or from primitive sex cords. Granulosa cell tumors are functional sex cord tumors of low malignant potential (Fig. 7.4d). They present early because of the hormonal effects such as excessive bleeding or precocious puberty. Small percentages of cases metastasize to distal sites.

In one series of 500 ovarian tumors, there were 117 solid ovarian tumors; 16.2 % of these solid tumors were benign, 83.8 % malignant. Epithelial tumors were the most common (28.2 %), followed by germ cell tumors (22.2 %), sex cord stromal tumors (21.4 %), and metastatic tumors (19.7 %) [67]. Stromal tumors arise from gonadal stroma and include fibromas (Fig. 7.3a), thecomas, and fibrothecomas. The thecal component cause estrogenic effects. Ascites is seen in association in about 40 % of cases. These are rare tumors most often seen in middle-aged women; they are solid tumors with posterior acoustic shadowing. Unusual appearance includes hyperechogenicity and increased sound transmission [62]. Brenner's is another group of solid ovarian tumors. In one series of 29 Brenner's tumor, five were borderline or malignant and 24 were benign [68]. The benign tumors were solid and had very little blood flow on Doppler interrogation. The malignant tumors were less solid and more vascularized than the benign tumors. Calcifications were not a discriminatory feature. Brenner's tumors are rare, and the majority of Brenner's tumors are benign and unilateral [68]. In one series of 63 patients with solid ovarian masses, there were no malignancies; all tumors demonstrated minimal vascularity, posterior acoustic shadowing, and minimal cystic components [68]. Ultrasound can accurately predict benignity of solid ovarian neoplasms. In another recently reported series of 43 solid tumors, 29 were managed conservatively with no malignancy diagnosed at follow up. These masses were all characterized by well-circumscribed borders, homogenous echotexture, posterior acoustic shadowing, and minimal or no vascularity or a cystic component [69]. Sex cord and stromal tumors of the ovary, therefore, present as solid masses, are seen in all age groups, are hormonally active and have a better prognosis than epithelial tumors. About 70 % of these tumors are stage I at diagnosis and hence amenable to surgical removal with a consequent good prognosis [70].

Borderline Tumors of the Ovary

Borderline ovarian tumors (BOT) are entity separate from benign and invasive ovarian tumors. These tumors are more prevalent in younger women of child bearing age and carry a prognosis better than invasive cancers. They are often seen in asymptomatic women during routine physical and or sonographic examination of the pelvis. Fertility sparing surgery is an option in younger women who have a borderline tumor. There are two histological groups: a serous (typical serous and micropapillary) type and a mucinous (gastrointestinal and endocervical) type. Typically associated morphologic features include unilocular cyst with a positive ovarian crescent sign and extensive papillarities arising from the inner wall. An ovarian crescent sign refers to presence of normal ovarian tissue, often with small follicles adjacent to the tumor, often encircling the tumor. A multilocular nodule in a unilocular cyst is also a recognized appearance of BOTs. One group reported a high specificity but a sensitivity of only 68.6 %. The lower sensitivity using the pattern recognition approach was due to high proportion of unilocular cysts that did not exhibit the typical features described in association with these tumors [71].

Pitfalls in the Diagnosis of Adnexal Masses

Recognized pitfalls in the differential diagnosis include non-ovarian lateral pelvic masses such as cystic pedunculated fibroids (Fig. 7.6a, b), complex hydrosalpinges (Fig. 7.6d, e), or paratubal cysts and peritoneal inclusion cysts. The latter develop in patients who have had surgery, trauma, infection, or endometriosis, and result from fluid trapped in between adhesions surrounding an ovary; a compressed, deformed ovary may then appear like a solid component of a complex cystic adnexal mass and be mistaken for ovarian malignancy (Fig. 7.6f, g). Torsed ovary when enlarged may take on an abnormal appearance, and, in a patient with subacute pelvic pain, this may be mistaken for an ovarian neoplasm [65] (Fig. 7.6c).

Real time gray scale and Doppler sonography remains the best available imaging modality to characterize adnexal masses, and its value has been extensively studied and validated in both symptomatic as well as a screening modality in women with normal or elevated risk for ovarian cancer.

Conclusions

In the absence of a low-cost, simple, and effective screening strategy for the early detection of ovarian cancer, the treatment of this disease will continue to challenge care-givers in LMICs. Even if the large randomized trials that are currently in place demonstrate a reduction in mortality, it seems unlikely that countries with limited resources will adopt these approaches in the near future. Most of the treatment will continue to be aimed at women with advanced disease. Extrapolation of "gold-standard" treatment in developed countries to countries with limited resources is problematic. It is important that we not hold patients "hostage" to a recommended treatment regimen based on articles or textbooks that are geared primarily to countries with high resources. As an example, in countries with few resources, where realistically the only diagnostic test available is an ultrasound, this may be sufficient to warrant exploratory surgery, particularly, when the burden of paying for tests falls largely on the patient herself.

A standardized approach for the treatment of ovarian cancer in LMICs based on the available resources is currently lacking. Outlining such an approach is outside the scope of this chapter; however, the need for global research and educa-

Fig. 7.6 (continued) (**c**) A torsed ovary in a patient with polycystic ovarian disease preoperatively diagnosed as a suspicious for ovarian malignancy. (**d**, **e**) A tubular anechoic structure with incomplete septum representing a hydrosalpinx. (**f**, **g**) Peritoneal inclusion cysts: A normal sized ovary with small follicles suspended in a complex cystic area representing fluid trapped in adhesions around the ovary in a patient with prior pelvic surgery

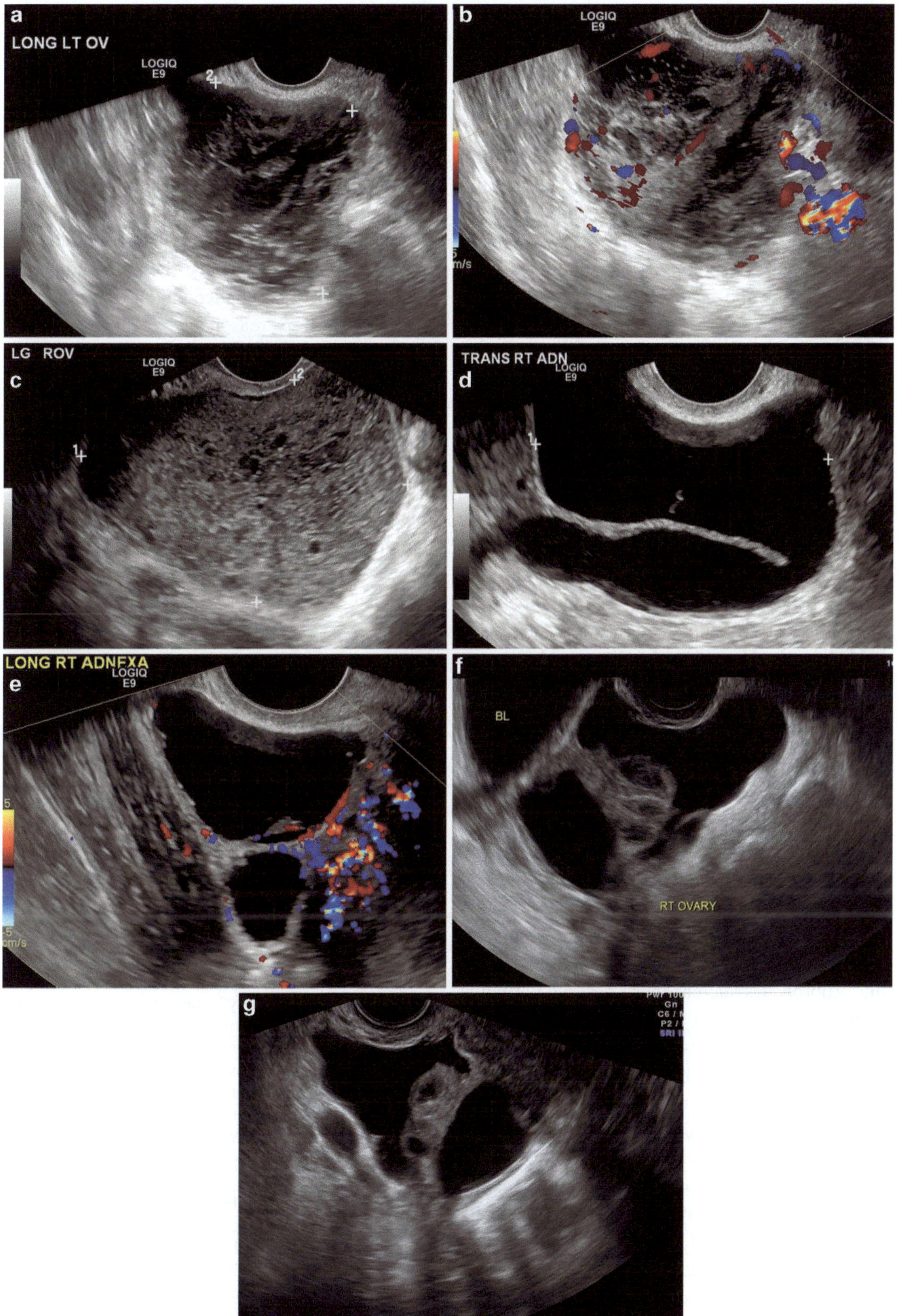

Fig. 7.6 Pitfalls in the differential diagnosis of ovarian tumors. (**a**, **b**) A pedunculated fibroid with cystic degeneration diagnosed preoperatively as a complex cystic adnexal mass suggestive of a benign ovarian neoplasm.

tional and clinical care partnerships in cancer care must be recognized if we hope to reduce disparity between LMICs and high resource countries [2]. An approach akin to that taken by the breast health global initiative (BHGI) may be helpful. Using an evidence-based approach, the BHGI attempts to stratify goals of care based on available resources. A similar set of guidelines might help countries and health ministries with LMIC budgets for the care of women with ovarian cancer. Clearly, every country needs to make decisions "on the ground" as to what they can recommend or mandate. Research into LMICs needs to focus on those realities and explore preventative strategies and treatment options that are feasible under their particular circumstances. As an example, for many years, the standard of care in HIC has involved primary cytoreductive or "debulking" surgery followed by adjuvant chemotherapy. By and large, this remains the standard in most developed countries. The recent publication by Vergote and colleagues [72] compared a neoadjuvant chemotherapeutic approach to the standard approach of up-front surgery. They found that neoadjuvant chemotherapy followed by interval debulking surgery was not inferior to primary debulking surgery. In addition, potential benefits were reported. The largest residual tumor was ≤ 1 cm in the majority of patients after interval debulking (80.6 %) as compared to 41.6 % of patients after primary debulking, and postoperative rates of adverse effects and mortality tended to be lower after interval debulking. Approaches such as these deserve particular attention in the setting of LMICs. A primary surgical approach requires very specialized surgical training as well as high-level postoperative care. This type of specialty training and postoperative care is not always available in LMICs, and it is certainly is not available in most countries outside of larger urban centers. The use of neoadjuvant chemotherapy may circumvent the need for this highly specialized training or, at least, minimize its need in LMICs.

In addition, standard chemotherapy regimens for ovarian cancer, which include platinum- and taxane-based combination chemotherapies in HIC, are often not available in LMICs. Yet, research exploring the efficacy of other regimens that are not "state of the art" is limited and needs to be encouraged. Understandably, most journals focus on "state-of-the-art" regimens for chemotherapy. The article by Sterling and colleagues [73] demonstrates how limited the available data are for comparative trials of ovarian cancer chemotherapy in LMICs. Identifying the best chemotherapy options in LMICs is challenging; however, there is a need to develop "reasonable" regimens and then explore their applicability, acceptability, and efficacy in these settings. In our quest to evaluate novel and more effective treatment options for ovarian cancers in HIC, we need to make sure that we continue to evaluate the effectiveness of available options in LMICs, lest, we inadvertently promote an even greater disparity in survival outcomes than those that already exist.

References

1. Jemal A, Bray F, Center MM, et al. Global Cancer Statististics. CA Cancer J Clin. 2011;61:69–90.
2. Lyerly HK, Abernethy AP, Stockler MR, et al. Need for Global Partnership in Cancer Care: Perceptions of Cancer Care Researchers Attending the 2010 Australia and Asia Pacific Clinical Oncology Research Development Workshop. J Clin Oncol. 2011;7(5):324–9.
3. Yeole BB, Kumar AV, Kurkure A, Sunny L. Population-based survival from cancers of breast, cervix and ovary in women in Mumbai, India. Asian Pac J Cancer Prev. 2004;5(3):308–15.
4. Redaniel MTM, Laudico A, Mirasol-Lumague MR, Gondos A, GL U, Toral JA, Benavides, Brenner H. Ovarian cancer survival population differences: a "high-resolution study" comparing Philippine residents, and Filipino-Americans and Caucasians living in the US. BMC Cancer. 2009;9:340.
5. Van Nagell JR, Pavlik Jr EJ. Ovarian Cancer Screening. Clin Obstet Gynecol. 2012;55(1):43–51.
6. Wilson JMG, Jungner G. Principles and practice of screening for disease. WHO Chronicle. Geneva: World Health Organization; 1968;22(11):473. Public health Papers #34.
7. Kurman RT, Shih I. The origin and pathogenesis of epithelial ovarian cancer: a proposed unifying theory. Am J Surg Pathol. 2010;34:433–43.
8. Crum CP, McKeon FD, Xian W. BRCA, the Oviduct, and the Space and Time Continuum of Pelvic Serous Carcinogenesis. Int J Gynecol Cancer. 2012;22:S29–34.
9. WHO Report. Task-shifting to tackle health worker shortages, March 2007 (http://www.who.int/healthsystems/task_shifting_booklet.pdf).

10. Stormo AR, Cooper CP, Hawkins NA, Saraiya M. Physician characteristics and beliefs associated with use of pelvic examinations in asymptomatic women. Prev Med. 2012;54(6):415–21.
11. Smith EM, Anderson B. The effects of symptoms and delay in seeking diagnosis among women with cancers of the ovary. Cancer. 1985;56:2727–32.
12. Flam F, Einhorn N, Sjovall K. Symptomatology of ovarian cancer. Eur J Obstet Gynecol Reprod Biol. 1988;27:53–7.
13. Goff BA, Mandel L, Muntz HG, et al. Ovarian carcinoma diagnosis Cancer. 2000;89:2068–75.
14. Goff BA, Mandel LS, Melancon CH, et al. Frequency of symptoms of ovarian cancer in women presenting to primary care clinics. JAMA. 2004;291:2705–12.
15. Smith LH, Morris CR, Yasmeen S, et al. Ovarian cancer: can we make the clinical diagnosis earlier? Cancer. 2005;104:1398–407.
16. Laurie G, Thompson PJ, McDuffie KE, et al. Prediagnostic symptoms of ovarian carcinoma: a case–control study. Gynecol Oncol. 2009;114:231–6.
17. Goff BA, Mandel LS, Drescher CW, et al. Development of an ovarian cancer symptom index: possibilities for earlier detection. Cancer. 2007;109(2):221–7.
18. Rossing MA, Wicklund KG, Cushing-Haugen KL, et al. Predictive value of symptoms for early detection of ovarian cancer. J Natl Cancer Inst. 2010;102:222–9.
19. Goff BA, Lowe KA, Kane JC, et al. Symptom triggered screening for ovarian cancer: a pilot study of feasibility and acceptability. Gynecol Oncol. 2012;124:230–5.
20. Andersen MR, Goff BA, Lowe KA, et al. Combining a symptom index with CA125 to improve detection of ovarian cancer. Cancer. 2008;113:484–9.
21. Andersen MR, Goff BA, Lowe KA, et al. Use of a Symptom Index, CA125, and HE4 to predict ovarian cancer. Gynecol Oncol. 2010;116:378–83.
22. Sassone AM, Timor-Tristsch IE, Artner A, Westhoff C, Warren WB. Transvaginal sonographic characterization of ovarian disease: evaluation of a new scoring system to predict ovarian malignancy. Obstet Gynecol. 1991;78:70–6.
23. Van Nagell JR, DePriest Jr PD, Reedy MB, et al. The efficacy of transvaginal sonographic screening in asymptomatic women at risk for ovarian cancer. Gynecol Oncol. 2000;77:350–6.
24. Van Nagell JR, DePriest Jr PD, Ueland FR, et al. Ovarian cancer screening with annual transvaginal sonography: findings of 25,000 women screened. Cancer. 2007;109:1887–96.
25. Van Nagell JR, Jr MRW, DeSimone CP, et al. Long-term survival of women with epithelial ovarian cancer detected by ultrasonographic screening. Obstet Gynecol. 2011;118:1212–21.
26. Mol BV, Boll D, De Kanter M, et al. Distinguishing the benign and malignant adnexal mass: an external validation of prognostic models. Gynecol Oncol. 2001;80:162–7.
27. Menon U, Gentry-Maharaj A, Hallett R, et al. Sensitivity and specificity of multimodal and ultrasound screening for ovarian cancer, and stage distribution of detected cancers: results of the prevalence screen of the UK Collaborative Trial of Ovarian Cancer Screening (UKCTOCS). Lancet Oncol. 2009;10:327–40.
28. Menon U. The UKCTOCS Experience – Reasons for Hope? Int J Gynecol Cancer. 2012;22:S18–20.
29. Lagrone LN, Sadasivam V, Kushner AL, Groen RS. A review of training opportunities for ultrasonography in low and middle income countries. Trop Med Int Health. 2012;17:808–19.
30. Galukande M, Kiguli-Malwadde E. Rethinking breast cancer screening strategies in resource-limited settings. Afr Health Sci. 2010;10(1):89–92.
31. Bast Jr RC, Klug TL, St John E, et al. A radioimmunoassay using a monoclonal antibody to monitor the course of epithelial ovarian cancer. N Engl J Med. 1983;309:883–7.
32. Jacobs I, Bast Jr RC. The CA125 tumour-associated antigen: a review of the literature. Hum Reprod. 1989;4:1–12.
33. Mol BW, Bayram N, Lijmer JG, et al. The performance of CA-125 measurement in the detection of endometriosis: a meta-analysis. Fertil Steril. 1998;70:1101–8.
34. Zuckerman E, Lanir A, Sabo E, et al. Cancer antigen 125: a sensitive marker of ascites in patients with liver cirrhosis. Am J Gastroenterol. 1999;94:1613–8.
35. Sjövall K, Nilsson B, Einhorn N. The significance of serum CA125 elevation in malignant and nonmalignant diseases. Gynecol Oncol. 2002;85:175–8.
36. Einhorn N, Sjövall K, Knapp RC, et al. Prospective evaluation of serum CA125 levels for early detection of ovarian cancer. Obstet Gynecol. 1992;80:14–8.
37. Zurawski Jr VR, Orjaseter H, Andersen A, Jellum E. Elevated serum CA125 levels prior to diagnosis of ovarian neoplasia: relevance for early detection of ovarian cancer. Int J Cancer. 1988;42:677–80.
38. Jacobs I, Davies AP. BridgesJ et al. Prevalence screening for ovarian cancer in postmenopausal women by CA 125 measurement and ultrasonography. BMJ. 1993;306:1030–4.
39. Buys SS, Partridge E, Black A, et al. Effect of screening on ovarian cancer mortality. The Prostate, Lung, Colorectal and Ovarian (PLCO) Cancer Screening Randoized Controlled Trial. JAMA. 2011;305:2295–303.
40. Buys SS, Partridge E, Greene MH, et al. Ovarian cancer screening in the Prostate, Lung, Colorectal and Ovarian (PLCO) Cancer Screening Trial: findings from the initial screen of a randomized trial. Am J Obstet Gynecol. 2005;193:1630–9.
41. Skates SJ. Ovarian cancer screening: development of the Risk of Ovarian Cancer Algorithm (ROCA) and ROCA Screening Trials. Int J Gynecol Cancer. 2012;22:S24–6.
42. Skates SJ, Xu FJ, Yu YH, et al. Toward an optimal algorithm for ovarian cancer screening with longitudinal tumor markers. Cancer. 1995;76:2004–10.
43. Kobayashi H, Yamada Y, Sado T, et al. A randomized study of screening for ovarian cancer: a multicenter study in Japan. Int J Gynecol Cancer. 2008;18:414–20.

44. Jacobs I, Davies AP, Bridges J, et al. Prevalence screening for ovarian cancer in postmenopausal women by CA125 measurement and ultrasonography. BMJ. 1993;306:1030–4.
45. Jacobs IJ, Skates SJ, MacDonald N, et al. Screening for ovarian cancer: a pilot randomized controlled trial. Lancet. 1999;353:1207–10.
46. Whittemore AS, Harris R, Itnyre J. Characteristics relating to ovarian cancer risk: Collaborative analysis of 12 US case–control studies. Am J Epidemiol. 1992;136:1184–203.
47. Adami HO, Hsie CC, Lambe M, et al. Parity, age at first childbirth, and risk of ovarian cancer. Lancet. 1994;344:1250–4.
48. Nandakumar A, Anantha N, Dhar M, et al. A case–control investigation on cancer of the ovary in Bangalore, India. Int J Cancer. 1995;63(3):361–5.
49. Hankinson SE, Hunter DJ, Colditz GA, et al. Tubal ligation, hysterectomy, and risk of ovarian cancer: A prospective study. JAMA. 1993;270:2813–8.
50. Irwin KL, Weiss NS, Lee NC, Peterson HB. Tubal sterilization, hysterectomy, and the subsequent occurrence of epithelial ovarian cancer. Am J Epidemiol. 1991;134:362–9.
51. Rosenblatt KA, Thomas DB. Reduced risk of ovarian cancer in women with a tubal ligation or hysterectomy. The World Health Organization Collaborative Study of Neoplasia and Steroid Contraceptives. Cancer Epidemiol Biomarkers Prev. 1996;5:933–5.
52. The Cancer and Steroid Hormone Study of the Centers for Disease Control and the National Institute of Child Health and Human Development. The reduction in risk of ovarian cancer associated with oral-contraceptive use. N Engl J Med. 1987;316:650–5.
53. Consensus NIH. Conference. Ovarian cancer: screening, treatment, and follow-up—NIH Consensus Development Panel on Ovarian Cancer. JAMA. 1995;273:491–7.
54. Timmerman D, Schwartzberg P, Collins WP, et al. Subjective assessment of adnexal masses with the use of ultrasonography: an analysis of interobserver variability and experience. Ultrasound Obstet Gynecol. 1999;13:11–6.
55. Timmerman D, Valentin L, Bourne TH, Collins WP, Verrelest H, Vergote I. Terms definitions and measurements to describe the sonographic features of adnexal tumors. A consensus opinion from the International Ovarian Tumor Analysis [IOTA] Group. Ultrasound Obstet Gynecol. 2000;16:500–5.
56. Timmerman D, Testa AC, Bourne TH. Logistic regression model to distinguish between the benign and malignant adnexal mass before surgery: a multicenter study by the International Ovarian Tumor Analysis Group. J Clin Oncol. 2005;23:8794–801.
57. Holsbeke CV, Calster BV, Testa AC. Prospective internal validation of mathematical models to predict malignancy in adnexal masses: results from the international ovarian tumor analysis study. Clin Cancer Res. 2009;15(2):684–91.
58. Valentin L, Ameye L, Savelli L, Fruscio R, Leone FPG, Czekierdowski A, et al. Adnexal masses difficult to classify as benign or malignant using subjective assessment of gray-scale and Doppler ultrasound findings: logistic regression models do not help. Ultrasound Obstet Gynecol. 2011;38:456–65.
59. Amor F, Vaccaro H, Alcazar JL, Leon M, Craig JM, Martinez J. Gynecologic imaging reporting and data system: a new proposal for classifying adnexal masses on the basis of sonographic findings. J Ultrasound Med. 2009;28:285–91.
60. Amor F, Alcázar JL, Vaccaro H, León M, Iturra A. GI-RADS reporting system for ultrasound evaluation of adnexal masses in clinical practice: a prospective multicenter study. Ultrasound Obstet Gynecol. 2011;38:450–5.
61. Twickler DM, Moschos E. Ultrasound and assessment of ovarian cancer risk. AJR Am J Roentgenol. 2010;194:322–9.
62. Jeong YY, Outwater EK, Kang HK. Imaging Evaluation of Ovarian Masses. Radiographics. 2000;20:1445–70.
63. Reles A, Wein U, Lichtenegger W. Transvaginal color Doppler sonography and conventional sonography in the preoperative assessment of adnexal masses. J Clin Ultrasound. 1997;25:217–25.
64. Timor-Tritsch LE, Lerner JP, Monteagudo A, Santos R. Transvaginal ultrasonographic characterization of ovarian masses by means of color flow-directed Doppler measurements and a morphologic scoring system. Am J Obstet Gynecol. 1993;168:909–13.
65. Patel MD. Pitfalls in the sonographic evaluation of adnexal masses. Ultrasound Q. 2012;28(1):29–40.
66. Levine D, Brown DL, Andreotti RF, et al. Management of asymptomatic ovarian and other adnexal cysts imaged at US: Society of Radiologists in Ultrasound Consensus Conference Statement. Radiology. 2010;256:943–54.
67. Tyagi SP, Maheswari V, Tyagi N, et al. Solid tumors of the ovary. J Ind Med Assoc. 1993;91(9):227–30.
68. Dierickx I, Valentin L, Holsbeke C, et al. Imaging in Gynecological disease (7): clinical and ultrasound features of Brenner tumors of the ovary. Ultrasound Obstet Gynecol. 2012;40(6):706–13. doi:10.1002/uog.11149 [Epub ahead of print].
69. Wang S, Johnson S. Prediction of benignity of solid adnexal masses. Arch Gynecol Obstet. 2012;285(3):721–6.
70. Jung SE, Rha SE, Lee JM, et al. CT and MRI Findings of Sex Cord–Stromal Tumor of the Ovary. AJR. 2005;185:207–15.
71. Yazbek J, Raju KS, Ben-Nagi J, et al. Accuracy of ultrasound subjective 'pattern recognition' for the diagnosis of borderline ovarian tumors. Ultrasound Obstet Gynecol. 2007;29:489–95.
72. Vergote I, Tropé CG, Amant FN, et al. Neoadjuvant chemotherapy or primary surgery in stage IIIC or IV ovarian cancer. N Engl J Med. 2010;363(10):943–53.
73. Sterling L, van Lonkhuijzen L, Nyangena J, Orango E, Strother M, Busakhala N, Rosen B. Protocol development for ovarian cancer treatment in Kenya: a brief report. Int J Gynecol Cancer. 2011;21(2):424–7.

Endometrial Cancer: Risk Factors and Early Diagnosis in Low-Resource Countries

8

Siriwan Tangjitgamol, John Kavanagh, and Mahesh K. Shetty

Abstract

Many risk factors are recognized for the development of endometrial cancer (EMC). A strong risk factor for hereditary nonpolyposis colonic cancer is an indication for EMC screening. Any women at risk must be counseled and evaluated in detail about their risk for many cancers, especially colonic and EMC. This is usually done in higher levels of health service rather than in a low resource setting. Also, the data concerning risk have been derived in these higher resource settings and are not necessarily transferable to other populations. For EMC, the screening methods comprise an annual transvaginal ultrasound beginning at 30–35 years of age and periodic endometrial sampling. EMC screening is not recommended in any woman with low or moderate risk or those without familial predisposition. Nevertheless, patients should be educated for the signs or symptoms suggesting an endometrial lesion, such as postmenopausal bleeding. An endometrial biopsy with a small cannula is considered an initial diagnostic step. This procedure can be performed in an out-patient setting while uterine curettage is reserved for a woman with inadequate, inconclusive, or hyperplasic tissue from endometrial biopsy. Transvaginal ultrasonography may be useful as an adjunct in selected cases depending on the availability, physician training, or resource setting. Hysteroscopy, as a diagnostic and therapeutic maneuver, requires specialized operative skill and may not be available in limited health care environments.

S. Tangjitgamol
Department of Obstetrics and Gynecology,
Vajira Hospital, Bangkok 10300, Thailand
e-mail: siriwanonco@yahoo.com

J. Kavanagh
Department of Obstetrics and Gynecology,
Chulalongkorn University, Bangkok 10330, Thailand
e-mail: jjkavanaghmd@gmail.com

M.K. Shetty (✉)
Woman's Center for Breast Care and MRI,
Woman's Hospital of Texas,
Houston, TX 77054, USA
e-mail: mshetty@womens-radiology.com

M.K. Shetty (ed.), *Breast and Gynecological Cancers: An Integrated Approach for Screening and Early Diagnosis in Developing Countries*, DOI 10.1007/978-1-4614-1876-4_8,

Introduction

Endometrial cancer (EMC) is the third most-common gynecologic cancer after breast and cervical cancers worldwide. EMC appears more important in terms of number of new cases than in terms of mortality [1, 2].

A trend of increasing incidence of EMC was seen in the global statistic report 2008 compared to 2002. This increase was in both developed and developing countries [1, 2]. A total number of 145,000 new cases in 2008 were reported in developing countries and 142,300 in developed countries [1]. The corresponding figures of mortality had also increased to a total of 41,000 and 32,000 deaths, respectively. These resulted in a higher "mortality to new case ratio" in developing than in developed countries: 0.28 compared to 0.23.

Early diagnosis is a key factor for success in cancer treatment. This is particularly true for EMC. Early detection of the cancer as well as timely treatment usually results in a good outcome. Aside from stage of disease and an appropriate intervention, intrinsic risks of cancer development and characteristic features of each cancer type are also important prognostic factors. EMC has been classified according to different pathophysiologic pathways. Type I involves exposure to high levels of estrogen while type II is independent of hormone exposure [3]. Type I is represented by endometrioid histology while type II is composed of high grade histologies with more aggressive behavior, i.e., serous or clear cell carcinomas. In later years, EMC associated with Lynch syndrome has been added as type III [4].

With the burden of cancer in low and middle income countries leading to increases in cancer-related morbidity, mortality, and economic cost, it is prudent to evolve cancer control strategies aimed at improving outcome while minimizing toxicity and cost. Towards that goal, guidelines should encompass the entire management spectrum from primary prevention, screening, and diagnosis at one end to palliative treatment of advanced EMC at the other end.

We have published an article involving management of EMC in Asia in 2009 [5]. The specific recommendations involving screening, diagnosis, and treatment were made according to the evidence-based consensus panel process to create resource-sensitive guidelines. The model was the breast cancer management framework formulated by the Breast Health Global Initiative (BHGI) [6]. This Initiative has developed and applied to a four-tier system as follows: basic level, limited level, enhanced level, and maximal level resources. This chapter will focus on the risk factors and screening together with early diagnosis of EMC in low resource settings or at the basic and limited levels.

Risk Factors

As mentioned earlier, EMC can arise through three different pathophysiologic pathways based on the relationship with the levels of estrogen and familial risk. Some characteristic features of three types of EMC are shown in Table 8.1. Any conditions that are associated with the high status of estrogen are risk factors, particularly for type I EMC. The risk relationship to each factor is variable. Some recognized risk factors are exemplified in the following sections.

High Estrogen Level

The source of estrogen may be endogenous or exogenous. Estrogen as a single entity increases relative risk between 3.1 and 15 [7, 8]. This depends on the amount and duration of exposure [8, 9]. The recommendation for hormonal replacement therapy in a perimenopausal woman with an intact uterus is a combined use of estrogen and progesterone [10]. Herbal or traditional medicines may contain estrogen constituents, either natural or manmade. Long-term users of these estrogen-containing substances may have a risk of EMC.

Another source of estrogen is endogenous, i.e., hormone-producing tumors [11], polycystic ovary syndrome, or chronic anovulation [12].

Table 8.1 Characteristic features in each type of endometrial cancer

	Type I (low grade)	Type II (high grade)	Type III (familial)
Age at diagnosis	Perimenopause	Late postmenopause	Approximately 10 years younger than common age incidence in type I
Risk factors	Estrogen related	Not estrogen related	Familial risk (Lynch syndrome)
Endometrial background	Hyperplastic	Atrophic	–
Diabetes mellitus, obesity	Often associated	No association	No association
Grading and pathology	Low grade, endometrioid, mucinous, villoglandular	High grade, non-endometrioid CA: clear cell or serous CA	More commonly non-endometrioid CA
Stage	Low stage	advanced stage	–
Myometrial invasion	Minimal	Deep	–
Clinical course and prognosis	Slow progressive, favorable prognosis	Aggressive behavior, unfavorable prognosis	–

Modified with permission from Sorosky JI. Endometrial cancer. Obstet Gynecol 2012;120:383–97

These conditions can cause high circulating estrogen levels without or inadequate counteracting progesterone. A prolonged high estrogen will subsequently result in endometrial hyperplasia and eventually carcinoma.

Endometrial Hyperplasia

The risk of progression of endometrial hyperplasia to EMC can be as high as 47 % [13]. Although histochemical stains, analysis of ploidy or molecular studies may help in distinguishing endometrial hyperplasia from EMC [14–16], these tests require special laboratory techniques and may not be available in basic or limited resource settings. Standard histologic evaluation remains the most important tool for a diagnosis [17]. One must also be aware that EMC may readily coexist with endometrial hyperplasia in up to 43 % cases [18].

Tamoxifen Use

Tamoxifen, an antiestrogen, is used in the adjuvant treatment for hormone receptor positive breast cancer. However, the compound exerts a weak estrogenic activity on the endometrium and can stimulate endometrial proliferation, hyperplasia, and cancer. The risk of developing EMC seems to depend on the duration and dose of tamoxifen [19]. The relative risk ranged from 1.9 to 7.5 [20–23], with an absolute annual risk of about 2 per 1,000 patients [24, 25]. Many factors contribute to this wide range of risk, including the failure of some studies to control for confounding risk factors such as concurrent use of hormone replacement therapy or obesity [20, 21]. Furthermore, the conclusions of many studies are limited by the retrospective nature of those studies.

Proven benefits in preventing or controlling recurrences of breast cancer and occurrence of cancer in the contra lateral breast must be weighed against its risk. Findings from the ATAC (Arimidex, Tamoxifen, Alone or in Combination) trial suggested that an aromatase inhibitor, i.e., anastrozole, was superior to tamoxifen as adjuvant therapy for breast cancer. It is hoped that tamoxifen-induced EMC will become a diminishing problem [26]. However, the relatively higher cost of an aromatase inhibitor makes the continued usage of tamoxifen more likely in developing countries. This risk factor for EMC will probably persist for several years.

Obesity

The incidence of EMC is relatively higher in obese woman. Any woman with a 5 kg/m^2 increase of body mass index (BMI) will have 1.59-fold relative risk of EMC [27].

Diabetes Mellitus and Hypertension

A woman with diabetes mellitus and hypertension, with or without obesity, will have higher risk of EMC. This relationship is related to an insulin-resistance with associated higher levels of insulin-like growth factors and hyper-insulinemia [27–29].

Familial Genetic Factor

Although there has been no specific or highly predictive genes directly related to familial EMC, there is an increased chance that EMC will occur in a first-degree relative of a patient with the diagnosis. The better recognized familial cancer related to EMC is hereditary nonpolyposis colorectal cancer or Lynch syndrome. Any woman affected with this syndrome will have a lifetime risk of 27–71 % for EMC, much higher than the 3 % risk in the general population. The age at diagnosis in these women is approximately 46–54 years old or generally younger than that of a sporadic case of EMC [30, 31].

Women with Lynch syndrome who are diagnosed with colorectal cancer will have a sixfold increased risk of developing EMC compared to the general population. Indeed, approximately one fourth of them will have EMC within the following 10 years [32].

Breast Cancer

Women with a history of breast cancer certainly have a higher risk of developing EMC due to common risk factors such as obesity and nulliparity. A woman with breast cancer who carries the BRCA1 gene mutation has a relative risk of approximately 2.6, especially when she is also a tamoxifen user [33].

Nulliparity

The risk of EMC is inversely related to the number of pregnancies. This is somewhat related to the anovulatory condition which is frequently found in woman with fertility problems [34].

Nutrition

There have been no definitive data regarding the modification of caloric or food intake to reduce the risk of EMC [35]. Long-term consumption of phytoestrogen from soy bean products [36] or alcohol intake [37] may be a risk factor for endometrial hyperplasia and cancer. On the other hand, coffee or green tea beverages have been reported as protective factors [38, 39].

Screening

There is no proven role for screening in asymptomatic women who are at average or medium-risks for the development of EMC. These risk groups include women with nulliparity, late menopause, or even receiving tamoxifen therapy [19]. Screening should only be considered for high-risk women who may be genetic mutation carriers of Lynch syndrome or those with suspected autosomal predisposition to colon cancer [40]. An annual transvaginal ultrasonography and endometrial aspiration biopsy for endometrial assessment should be started at 30–35 years of age [41]. Some researchers have proposed beginning at a younger age of 25 years [42]. One systematic review made the recommendation that individuals with an inherited predisposition to Lynch syndrome begin genetic counseling and basic medical surveillance at age 21 [43]. Colonoscopy should start at ages 20–25 years (or 10 years less than the youngest age of diagnosis

Table 8.2 Summary for screening and diagnosis

	Consensus based on level of resource			
Areas of discussion	Basic	Limited	Enhanced	Maximal
Screening				
Normal women[a]	No	No	No	No
High-risk women[b]	No	No	Yes	Yes
Diagnosis[c]	Yes	Yes	Yes	Yes

Reprint with permission of Elsevier from Tangjitgamol S, Anderson BO, See HT, Lertbutsayanukul C, Sirisabya N, Manchana T et al. Asian Oncology Summit. Management of endometrial cancer in Asia: consensus statement from the Asian Oncology Summit 2009. Lancet Oncol 2009;10:1119–27

[a]Screening for endometrial cancer in average or medium risks women is not recommended except for history taking and physical examination including pelvic examination which could be done in all levels

[b]Screening in high-risk women requires detailed familial history and genetic evaluation, endometrial biopsy, and ultrasound of the pelvis in addition to complete physical and pelvic examination. These are generally not available in basic and limited settings

[c]Diagnostic tools include endometrial sampling biopsy or uterine curettage with or without transvaginal ultrasound evaluation depending on the availability of the instrument and the operative setting

in the family) for every 1–2 years, and endometrial sampling and transvaginal ultrasound of the uterus (and ovaries) should begin at ages 30–35 years [43]. These recommendations should be individualized after appropriate discussion with the patient and probably be best conducted by an expert with genetic counseling support. In basic or limited resource medical levels, this may be difficult. The management of such families in populations where the genetics are either ill undefined or unavailable remains a major clinical challenge.

Some authors have proposed genetic testing for first-degree relatives of woman aged <50 years with double primary cancers of colorectum and endometrium. In addition, the patients should have measurements of the serum cancer antigen (CA) 125 and endometrial biopsy with optional hysteroscopy [44]. DNA replication errors, which represent microsatellite-marker analyses of tumor DNA [45], and associated germ line mutations in MLH1, MSH2, and MSH6 [44] are reported in women with Lynch syndrome. These tests require special laboratory techniques which may not be available or are too expensive in the basic or limited resource settings.

The summary of EMC screening based on the four tiers of resource settings is shown in Table 8.2 [5].

Early Diagnosis

Although women with average- or medium-risks for EMC are not recommended for a routine screening, all women should be educated for abnormal symptoms or signs associated with endometrial lesions.

Indications

Cervical cytology is not an acceptable method used to screen for or used to make a diagnosis of endometrial pathology because of its low sensitivity. Nevertheless, the presence of endometrial cells on a pap smear in a postmenopausal woman or atypical glandular cell in a woman aged ≥35 years old are indications for endometrial tissue assessment [46].

Abnormal uterine bleeding is the most common sign and symptom of EMC found in 90 % of the patients [47]. Five to twenty percent of postmenopausal women with uterine bleeding have EMC. The presence of such bleeding is certainly an indication for an evaluation of endometrial tissue pathology. Other indications are pyometria in a postmenopausal woman, abnormal bleeding in a woman ≥40 years old, or a younger age woman with risk factors for endometrial lesions [47].

Ultrasonography

A detailed discussion on endometrial sonography appears next. Transvaginal ultrasonography, which is a noninvasive procedure, can suggest a possible cause of endometrial lesion. This is especially true when caused by an atrophic endometrium. The latter is the most common cause of postmenopausal uterine bleeding. A postmenopausal woman with an endometrial thickness of less than 4–5 mm has minimal risk for significant endometrial pathology [48, 49]. The risk of EMC in women with postmenopausal bleeding but whose endometrial thickness on transvaginal ultrasound is less than 5 mm is only 1 in 917 [48]. Nevertheless, this negative predictive value of the endometrial thickness has been validated only in postmenopausal women. Aside from this caveat, additional limitations of ultrasound exist, i.e., the presence of fibroids, previous surgery, marked obesity, and an axial uterus [49]. Figures 8.1, 8.2, 8.3, 8.4, 8.5, 8.6, and 8.7 show various physiologic and pathologic changes of endometrium seen on transvaginal ultrasonography.

Obtaining Endometrial Tissue for Histopathology

The operative procedure to obtain endometrial tissue for pathology can be achieved by endometrial sampling which is considered a gold standard. An endometrial aspiration biopsy can be performed through a plastic cannula (e.g., Pipelle®, Cooper Surgical, Trumbull, CT) instrument which is widely available at present. The procedure can be done in an out-patient setting. The cost is nominal compared to conventional uterine curettage under anesthesia. The pathology obtained by endometrial biopsy correlates well with that obtained by uterine curettage, with 85–98 % accuracy compared to the standard dilatation and curettage [50, 51]. One systemic review and meta-analysis compared the results from endometrial sampling to those from hysteroscopic biopsy or hysterectomy in over 7,000 women [50]. Less than 5 % had inadequate tissue for diagnosis. The sensitivity of endometrial biopsy to determine EMC and endometrial hyperplasia was 99.6 % in postmenopausal women and 91 % in premenopause. The specificity ranged from 98 to 100 %.

Nevertheless, histologic tumor grading from a small piece of tissue obtained by endometrial biopsy may not be highly accurate. Tumor grade from a hysterectomy specimen is upgraded from the earlier biopsy sample in approximately 30 % [52, 53]. This issue should be particularly concerning when hysterectomy for EMC is intended in the basic or limited settings wherein complete surgical staging including lymph node surgicopathological evaluation may not possible.

Another limitation of endometrial biopsy, aside from the accurate grading, is when the endometrial pathology is focal or involving an area less than 50 % of the uterus. Such conditions may result in inadequate diagnostic tissue as often as 15 % of cases (Fig. 8.8a) [54]. A formal uterine curettage is then required to rule out the presence of malignancy. Also, hyperplasic endometrial tissue in the endometrial biopsy is an indication for uterine curettage because of the possibility of coexisting EMC. This has even greater importance if complete surgical staging for EMC is not possible or a standard practice in that particular setting. Figure 8.8a–f shows the histopathology of inadequate tissue for diagnosis (Fig. 8.8a), simple and complex hyperplasia (Fig. 8.8b, c), and various types of endometrial carcinoma (Fig. 8.8d–f).

Uterine curettage is necessary when the index of suspicion for EMC is high, when the biopsy is inconclusive or inadequate, or when unexplained recurrent uterine bleeding without a clear etiology [54]. In these events, hysteroscopy to directly evaluate gross endometrial lesion and to assist in selecting area for tissue biopsy is another useful procedure. Although this hysteroscopy may cause dissemination of EMC cells into the peritoneum, the impact on survival has not been evidenced [55]. Nevertheless, hysteroscopy requires special expertise and additional expense. Hysteroscopy use in basic and limited resources may not be practical.

Figure 8.9 shows an algorithm of procedures used for EMC diagnosis.

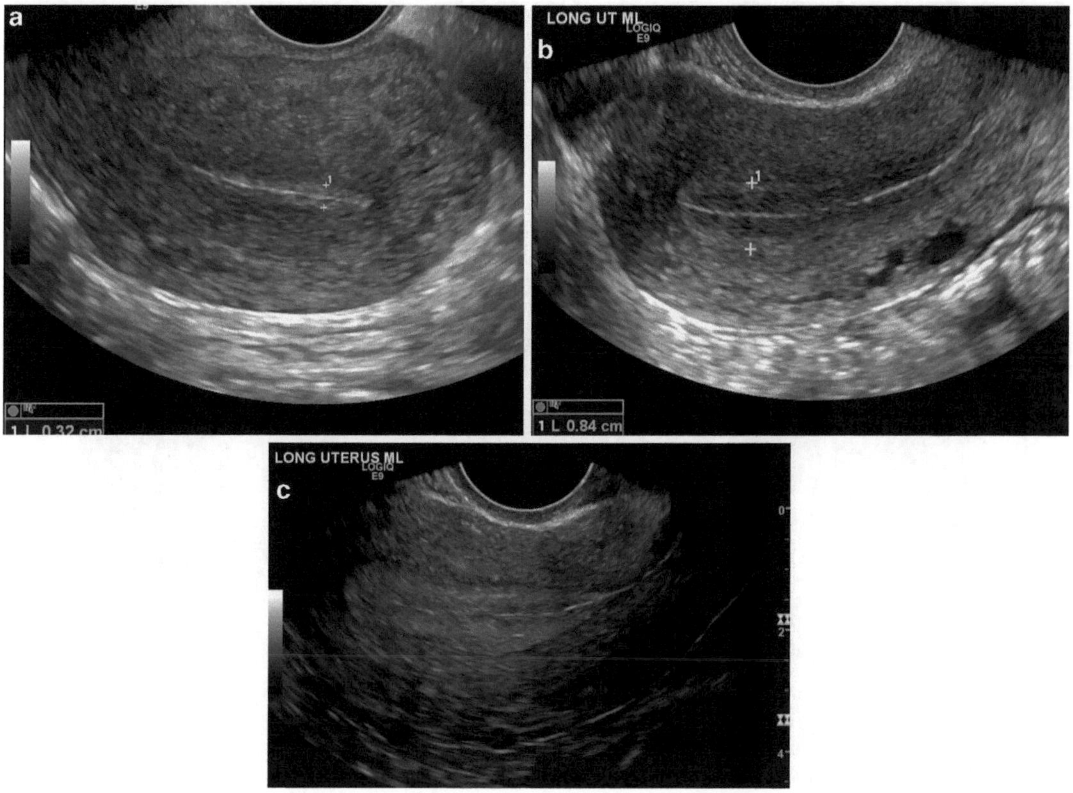

Fig. 8.1 Transvaginal sonographic images of the premenopausal endometrium. (**a**) Menstrual phase. (**b**) Proliferative phase. (**c**) Secretory phase

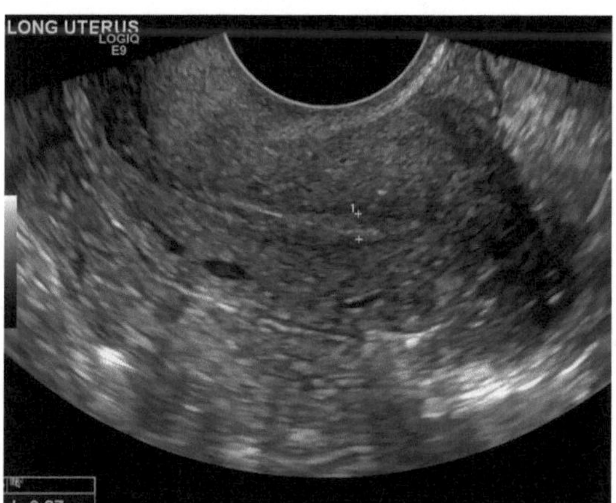

Fig. 8.2 Sixty-five-year-old postmenopausal woman with abnormal bleeding. Sagittal endovaginal sonogram demonstrated a thin 3 mm endometrium suggestive of endometrial atrophy

Endometrial Sonography

The endometrial lining of the uterus is optimally evaluated by sonography. The endometrial stripe is well visualized on transabdominal ultrasound with a full bladder; however, the most detailed analysis of the endometrium is best performed by endovaginal sonography (EVS). Higher resolution of the transducer combined with a shorter distance to the area of interest results in superior visualization of the endometrium and allows optimal measurement of the endometrial thickness and assessment of endometrial abnormalities. EVS in the symptomatic postmenopausal woman with endometrial sampling in those with an abnormal endometrium is of proven benefit in the early detection of EMC.

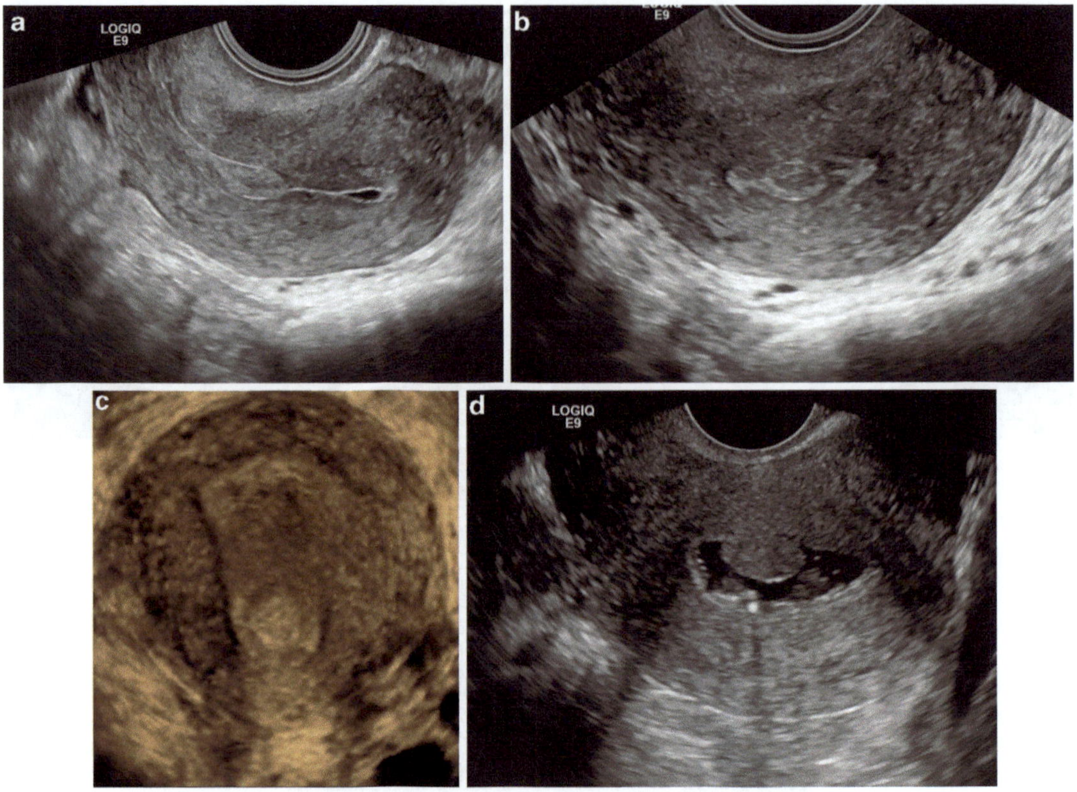

Fig. 8.3 Sonographic images demonstrating an endometrial polyp in the uterus. (**a**) An image in the sagittal plane demonstrating an intracavitary hyperechoic mass suggestive of a polyp. (**b**) An image in the transverse plane showing the polyp in the endometrial cavity. (**c**) 3D Image of the uterus shows an intracavitary mass. (**d**) Sonohysterogram demonstrates a broad based polyp outlined by saline distended endometrial cavity

Normal Appearance of the Endometrium

Ultrasound is the primary imaging modality for assessment of the endometrium. The spectrum of normal appearance of the endometrium varies depending on the menstrual status of the patient and the phase of the menstrual cycle.

Premenopausal Endometrium

In a premenopausal woman, the appearance of endometrium varies depending on the phase of the menstrual cycle. During the menstrual phase, the endometrium is the thinnest and appears as an echogenic line measuring 4 mm or less (Fig. 8.1a). The thickness is measured during an endovaginal scan in the sagittal plane of the uterus with cursors placed at the echogenic border with the myometrium. During the proliferative phase of the menstrual cycle (days 6–14), the endometrium becomes thicker and progressively echogenic relative to the myometrium [56]. In the preovulatory phase, the endometrium assumes a multilayered appearance with a hyperechoic basal layer, a hypoechoic inner layer, and a thin central echogenic layer; the endometrial thickness can measure up to 11 mm (Fig. 8.1b). Such a multilayered appearance disappears after ovulation. There is progressive thickening and increased echogenicity of the endometrium in the secretory phase during which a thickness of 16 mm may be reached (Fig. 8.1c). During the secretory phase, there may also be increased echogenicity and posterior acoustic enhancement of the endometrium; such an appearance has been attributed to the presence of stromal edema and distended glands [56]. An understanding of the physiologic cyclic changes in the appearance of the endometrium is important in order to distinguish normal from endometrial hyperplasia.

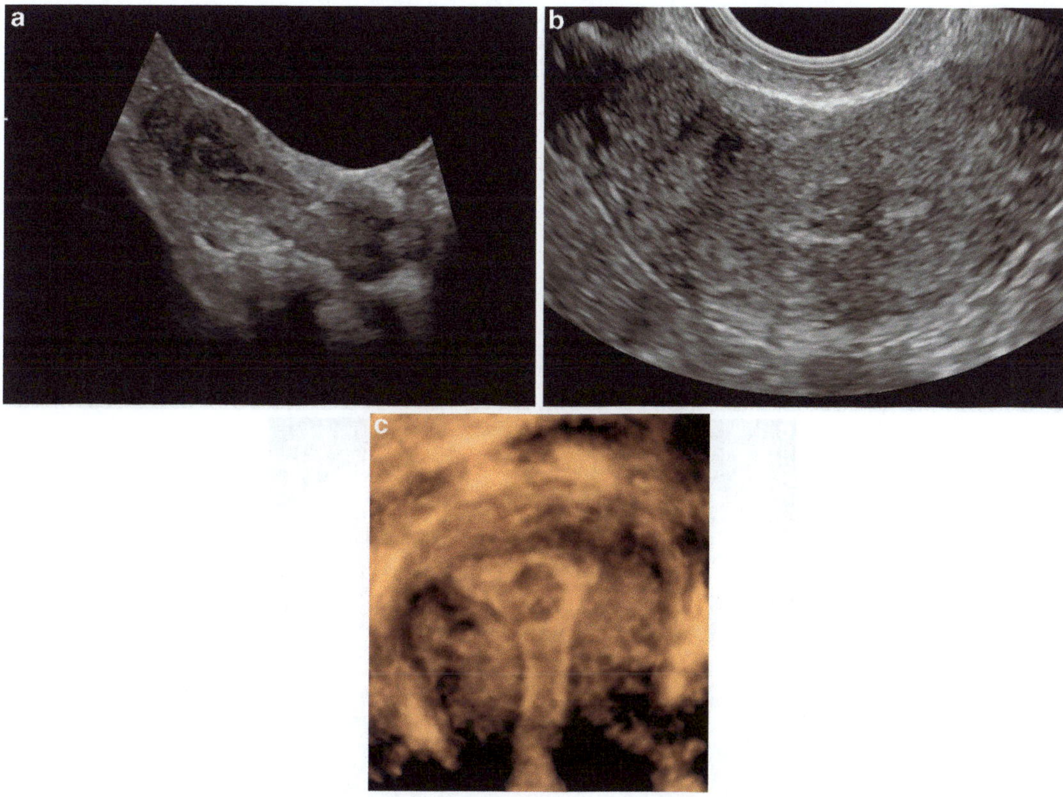

Fig. 8.4 Sonographic images demonstrating an intracavitary fibroid. (**a**) Sagittal image of the uterus on a transabdominal scan demonstrates a hypoechoic intracavitary mass proven to be an intracavitary fibroid. (**b**) An image in the transverse plane on endovaginal scan showing the intracavitary mass. (**c**) A 3D Image demonstrating the intracavitary fibroid

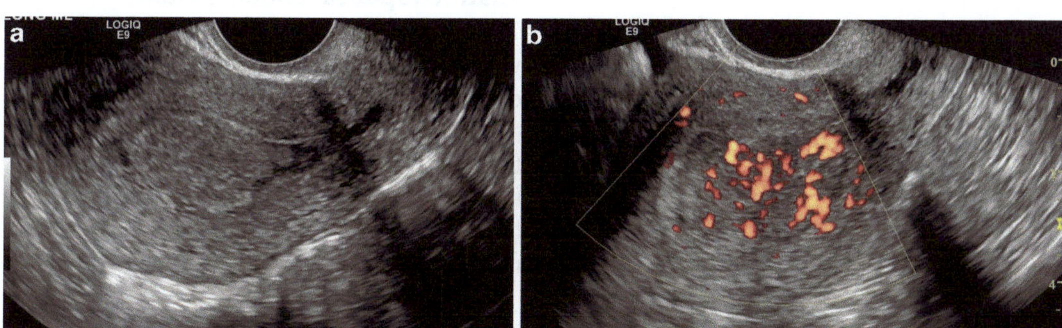

Fig. 8.5 A 31-year-old woman with abnormal uterine bleeding and history of polycystic ovarian disease. Endovaginal sonographic images show abnormally thickened endometrium with increased blood flow seen on color Doppler imaging. Histology showed complex endometrial hyperplasia. (**a**) Sagittal image of the uterus. (**b**) Color Doppler image of the endometrium demonstrating increased vascularity within the thickened endometrium

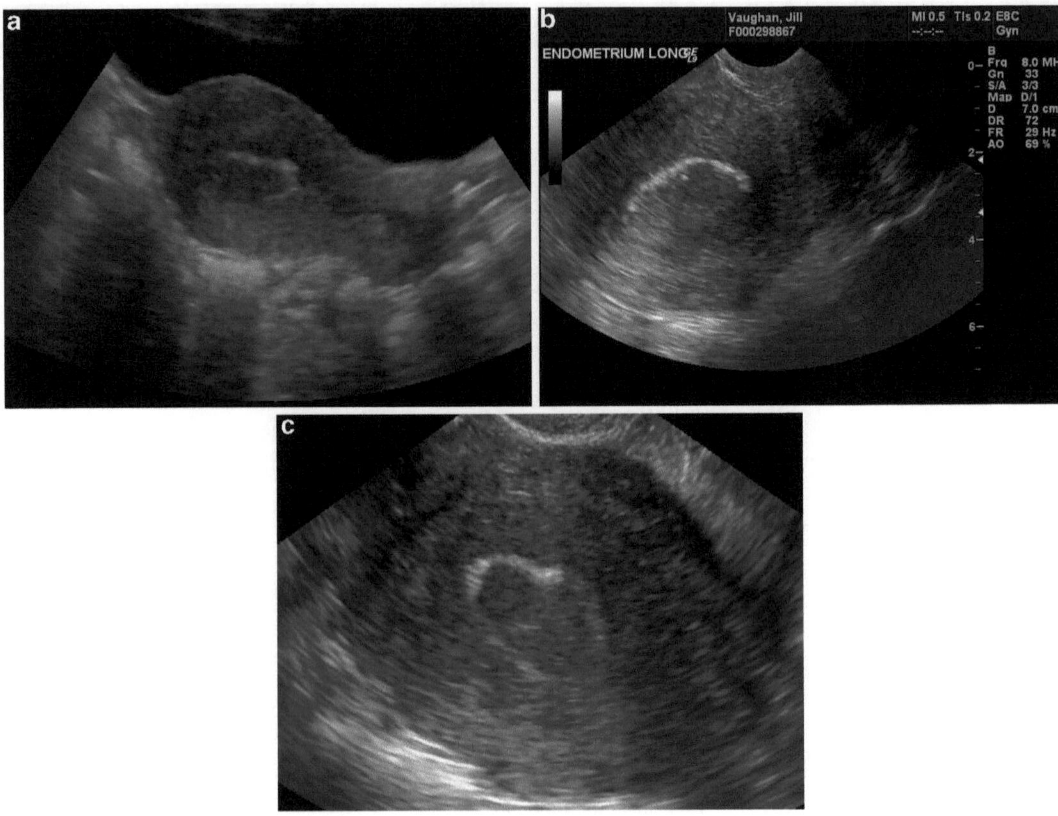

Fig. 8.6 Fifty-six-year-old postmenopausal woman with abnormal uterine bleeding. Sonographic images demonstrate a hypoechoic endometrial mass. Histology showed endometrial cancer. (**a**) Sagittal image of the uterus on a transabdominal scan. (**b**) Sagittal image of the uterus on an endovaginal scan. (**c**) Transverse image of the uterus on an endovaginal scan

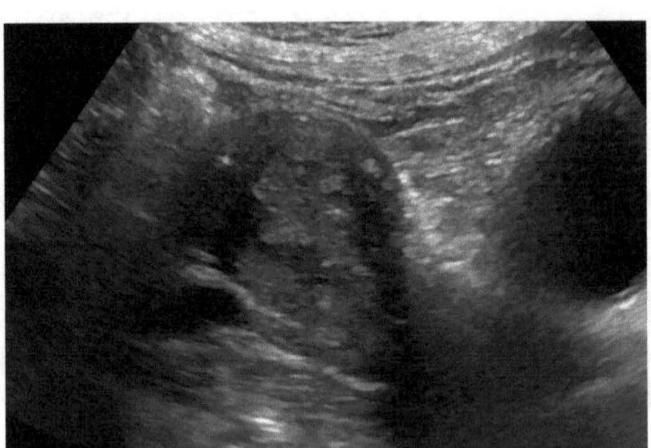

Fig. 8.7 Sixty-year-old postmenopausal woman with abnormal uterine bleeding. Transabdominal sonogram of the uterus in a sagittal plane demonstrates an irregularly thickened endometrium. Histology showed endometrial cancer

Postmenopausal Endometrium

The normal endometrium in a postmenopausal woman is thin, homogenous, and echogenic and does not significantly change during menopause [57]. A thickness of less than 5 mm without focal thickening is considered a normal appearance for the endometrium in a postmenopausal woman (Fig. 8.2). In those on hormone replacement, a thickness of up to 8 mm is considered normal [56].

Endometrial Abnormalities

Benign endometrial abnormalities account for nearly 90 % of postmenopausal bleeding. The most common cause accounting for 75 % of the cases is endometrial atrophy. Other causes include

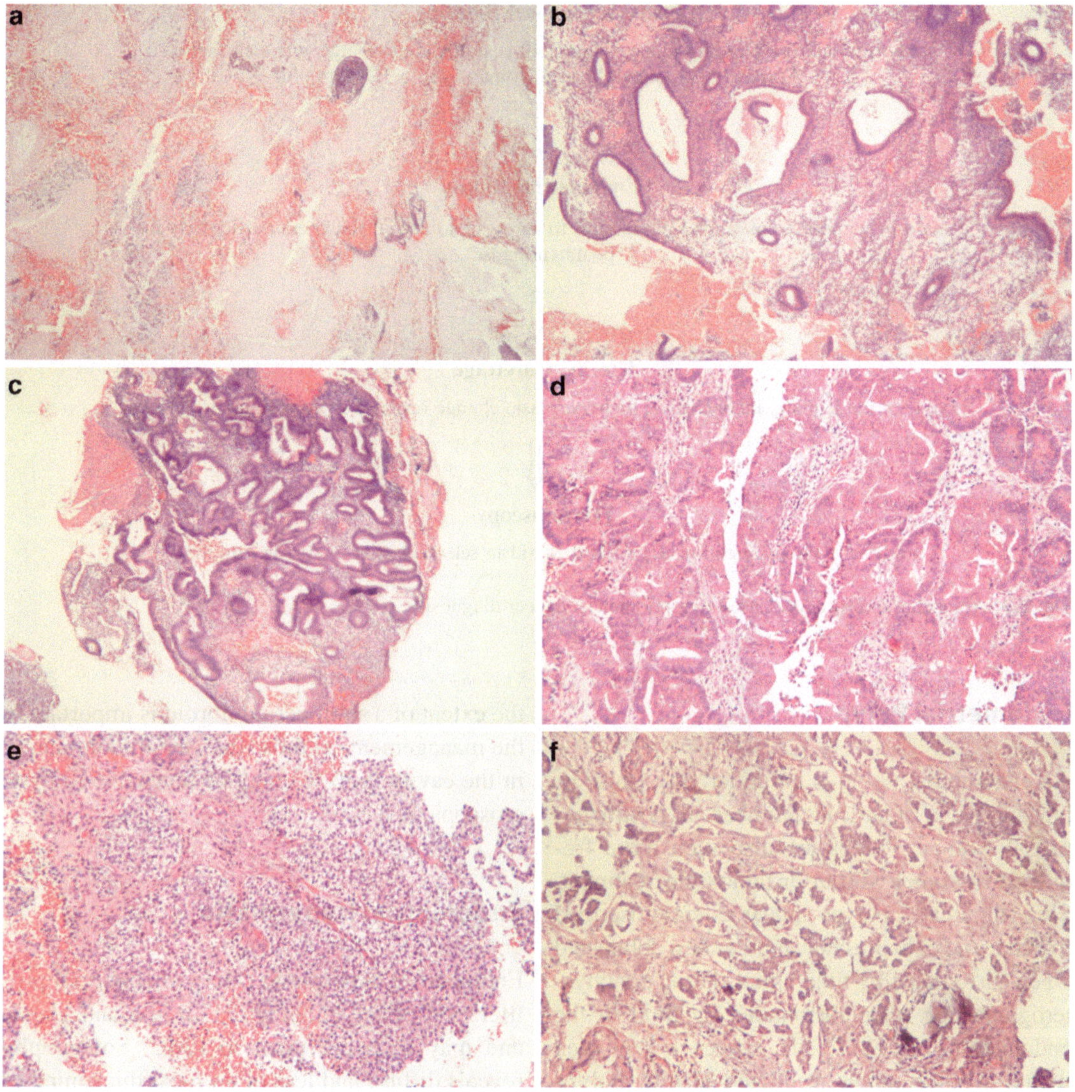

Fig. 8.8 (**a**–**f**) Spectrum of histopathological abnormalities of the endometrium. (**a**) shows inadequate specimen with only few tiny pieces of endometrial tissue floating in mucinous material. (**b**) shows fragments of endometrial tissues with slightly glandular proliferation and some cystic dilated glands. (**c**) demonstrates features of complex hyperplasia with endometrial glandular proliferation in tubular pattern in excess of stromal tissue. (**d**) shows endometrioid carcinoma evidenced from aspiration biopsy. (**e**) shows a small piece of tissue from endometrial biopsy that exhibits characteristic feature of clear cell carcinoma with papillary structure lined by epithelial cells with clear cytoplasm. (**f**) shows serous carcinoma characterized by papillary structures of malignant glands and foci of psammoma bodies

endometrial polyps, submucosal fibroids, endometrial hyperplasia, and estrogen withdrawal. About 10 % of cases of postmenopausal bleeding are caused by endometrial carcinoma [58]. Imaging assessment of the endometrium is best performed after the bleeding has stopped, if feasible. Some of the common benign endometrial abnormalities are described next.

Post-Menopausal Bleeding

Abnormal uterine bleeding in a woman ≥ 40 years or younger age with risk factors
Atypical glandular cells in a woman aged ≥ 35 years old

⇩

Endometrial Biopsy

with or without transvaginal ultrasound to assess endometrial thickness particularly in postmenopause

⇩

Uterine Curettage

in case of inadequate, inconclusive, or hyperplasic change revealed from endometrial biopsy

⇩

Hysteroscopy

to directly visualize endometrium and to aid in selecting area for tissue sampling

Fig. 8.9 Algorithm of procedures used for endometrial cancer diagnosis

Endometrial Polyp

An endometrial polyp is an underlying cause of bleeding in a significant number of postmenopausal women. Polyps are also seen more frequently in women who are on tamoxifen treatment. Sonographically, polyps appear as circumscribed hyperechoic or hypoechoic masses best delineated when surrounded by fluid either during sonohysterography or when surrounded by fluid in the endometrial cavity. Cystic spaces when seen within a polyp represent dilated glands. Polyps may be pedunculated or broad-based and sessile; often, a vascular stalk is demonstrated on color Doppler imaging (Fig. 8.3a–d).

Fibroids

Uterine leiomyomas may cause abnormal bleeding when they are submucosal or intracavitary. They appear as hypoechoic masses protruding into the endometrial cavity or lying predominantly in the endometrial cavity when intracavitary (Fig. 8.4a–c). Fibroids have a heterogeneous appearance and often demonstrate posterior acoustic shadowing. Sonographic assessment of the extent of a submucosal fibroid is important in the management, as those that are predominantly in the cavity (>50 %) may be amenable to hysteroscopic resection.

Endometrial Hyperplasia

Endometrial hyperplasia refers to abnormal proliferation of the endometrial stroma and glands and may be a precursor to EMC. Sonography reveals diffuse and less often focal thickening of the endometrium; endometrial thickness often exceeds 10 mm (Fig. 8.5a, b). The sonographic appearance of endometrial hyperplasia can overlap with that of EMC and distinction then can only be made by endometrial biopsy [56].

Endometrial Adenocarcinoma (EMC)

In endometrial carcinoma, the endometrium is thickened and has a heterogeneous and irregular appearance. There may be an overlap in the appearance with benign endometrial abnormalities such a polyps and endometrial hyperplasia. A specific sign of EMC is focal thickening and irregularity as well as irregularity of the endometrium-myometrium border, a finding that is also indicative of an invasive disease [56] (Figs. 8.6a–c and 8.7). Sonography can be used to assess the depth of myometrial invasion, a finding that has a bearing on the likelihood of lymph node involvement and, consequently, on the staging and surgical management of a patient with EMC. Myometrial invasion greater than 33 % has a negative impact on prognosis. In one study, ultrasound was shown to accurately identify deep myometrial invasion in all cases where there was one [59]. Ultrasound may, however, be limited in identifying myometrial invasion in women with adenomyosis and/or fibroids, where it can overdiagnose myometrial invasion [59]. Ultrasound accuracy in predicting myometrial invasion has been compared to intraoperative frozen section sampling. In a series of 155 patients with endometrial malignancy, sensitivity, specificity, positive, and negative predictive values and accuracy of ultrasound was 75, 89, 86, 79, and 81 %. Intraoperative frozen section performed better than sonography at 92, 92, 89, 94, and 92 %. The authors of this study concluded that, although ultrasound did well in identifying myometrial invasion, for optimal surgical management in patients with EMC, intraoperative frozen section to determine myometrial extent is still recommended [60]. In another series comparing 64 women with EMC, TVS and TVS with CDI performed as well as intraoperative frozen section and the more expensive MRI in determining the depth of deep myometrial invasion [61].

Triaging of Women with Postmenopausal Bleeding

Abnormal vaginal bleeding is a frequent symptom encountered in a gynecological practice. In most instances, 98 % of women in one series, particularly in young premenopausal patients, the underlying cause are benign endometrial abnormalities such as a polyp, fibroid, or hyperplasia [62]. In postmenopausal women, one should add endometrial atrophy to the list of benign causes for bleeding. These benign causes account for 90 % of cases; in the remaining 10 % of women, EMC is the underlying abnormality. Sonography, therefore, is of value since benign endometrial diseases are readily diagnosed and is also a cost-effective alternative to blind endometrial biopsy [63]. Advantages of endovaginal ultrasound over endometrial biopsy include a less invasive procedure, no complication or pain, and equal or better sensitivity particularly in benign endometrial diseases [64]. A study reported a 0.6 % prevalence of EMC in women with PMB with sonographic measured endometrial thickness of 4 mm or less and 19 % when 5 mm or thicker. It has been suggested that, based on these findings, endometrial biopsy may not be required when thickness is less than 4 mm [64]. The false negative rates with EVS are better than the reported false negative rate of 5–15 % for office-based endometrial sampling. Ultrasound is also able to visualize the entire extent of the endometrium compared to the blind office-based biopsy [65–68]. Office-based endometrial sampling has several recognized limitations. Some of these include insufficient sampling, especially when abnormalities are small and focal, difficulty in gaining access to endometrial cavity due to cervical stenosis, and difficulty in diagnosing some of the benign causes of PMB. Ultrasound has the advantage of being able to see the entire endometrial lining and to accurately identify benign causes of endometrial bleeding such as polyps, fibroids, and atrophy. In one study of women with known EMC, 17 % the samples were found to be negative for malignancy [63].

Performing EVS to triage patients for sampling is therefore the most sensible approach. It has been shown that use of sonography to triage patients has a cost savings of 16 % in women with normal or average risk [68]. A study group of 339 postmenopausal women with bleeding reported that 13 % (44/339) had EMC or AEH (1.5 %). There were no cancers in women with an endometrial thickness of <4 mm. The reliability of endometrial thickness (cutoff value 4 mm) as a diagnostic test for EMC was: sensitivity, 100 %; specificity, 60 %; positive predictive value, 25 %; and negative predictive value, 100 %. Transvaginal sonographic scanning is an excellent tool for the determination of whether further investigation with curettage or some form of endometrial biopsy is necessary [69]. The consensus group of the Society of Radiologists in Ultrasound recommends that a cutoff of 5 mm be used. The group concluded that either the US or office-based endometrial biopsy can be used in the initial evaluation of a postmenopausal woman with vaginal bleeding [70].

The triage of patients with postmenopausal bleeding proposed by Goldstein is most appropriate: (1) no anatomic pathology best treated expectantly; (2) a global endometrial process, in which case random blind endometrial sampling is appropriate; or (3) a focal endometrial abnormality in which case endometrial sampling should be done with the visualization offered by hysteroscopy [71]. The issue of postmenopausal women having a thickened endometrium that is found incidentally with no associated bleeding needs to be addressed, as this may occur not infrequently; reported in 10–17 %, such a finding in the absence of bleeding is not an indication for endometrial biopsy [71]. It is also important to understand that, in a symptomatic woman, when the entire endometrium is not seen or is obscured by a fibroid, sonographic evaluation must be considered incomplete. Such a scenario should prompt endometrial sampling to exclude EMC. In a study of 4,454 women with PMB, in whom 5.9 % were diagnosed with EMC, in 174 of 4,454 women (4 %), the endometrium was not visualized on sonography. In this subgroup where the endometrium was not well seen, there were 26 EMCs, proving the need to perform additional testing such as hysteroscopy and/or endometrial sampling [72].

Screening for Endometrial Cancer with Ultrasound

Screening for EMC in the asymptomatic patient is not justified and has not been shown to be of proven benefit. A study of 1,926 women from the general population found just one case of cancer and four cases of atypical endometrial hyperplasia [73]. However, there may be benefit in EMC screening postmenopausal women who are at an elevated risk for EMC [74] as has been discussed earlier in this chapter. A nested case–control study of postmenopausal women who underwent TVS in the United Kingdom Collaborative Trial of Ovarian Cancer Screening (UKCTOCS) was performed to evaluate the role of sonography in screening for EMC. UKCTOCS is a prospective trial of ovarian cancer screening; endometrial thickness was measured as part of this study, providing an opportunity to determine the value of this measurement as a possible screening tool for EMC. The cohort of 37,038 women included 136 women who developed EC or AEH. One hundred and thirty-three had endometrial thickness measured, and three had endometrial abnormalities. One hundred and twelve women were asymptomatic during the last EVS, and 24 were symptomatic. The control group had 36,888 women, and in this group there were 23 cases of EMCs. The endometrium had a thickness of >5 mm in 81 % of women diagnosed with EC; 33 of these were symptomatic and 74 asymptomatic. The positive predictive value and the negative predictive value for a cutoff of endometrial thickness of 5 mm in the symptomatic group was 30.8 and 93.1 % compared to only 1.4 and 99.9 % in the asymptomatic group [74]. These investigators concluded that TVS has a high sensitivity for diagnosing EMC and may be of benefit to screen women at risk for developing EMC, but they did not advocate its use to screen asymptomatic women.

Diagnosis of Endometrial Cancer with Ultrasound

The value of endometrial sonographic assessment in the diagnosis of EMCs in the symptomatic population has been extensively studied. A meta-analysis of 35 studies including a cohort of 5,892 women reported that 96 % of women with EMC had an abnormal finding on EVS; 92 % of women with endometrial disease malignant and nonmalignant such as polyp and atypical hyperplasia had abnormal findings using a cutoff value of 5 mm. Ultrasound did equally well in identifying endometrial disease irrespective of whether women were on HRT [75]. However, hormone replacement did affect the findings in women without endometrial disease; in those who were not on HRT, ultrasound performed better, being abnormal only in 8 % with a normal histology compared to 23 % in women who were on HRT. For a postmenopausal woman with vaginal bleeding, the probability of EMC dropped from a pre-test value of 10 % to a postnormal test value of only 1 %. Overall, ultrasound has a very high sensitivity for EMC in the range of 96 %, but specificity is low especially in those on HRT as discussed above [75].

Postmenopausal Bleeding in Women Under 50 Years of Age

The significance of postmenopausal bleeding in women under the age of 50 has also been reported. In a study group of 4,454 women with postmenopausal bleeding, 260 women (5.8 %) were younger than 50 years, 130 women had an endometrium of thickness less than 5 mm and hence did not undergo biopsy but were followed for 1–5 years, and in the remaining group biopsy was performed. There were no cancers in women under the age of 50 years. These findings may suggest that the need to investigate women under the age of 50 years is probably less urgent [76].

Role of 3D Power Doppler Ultrasound in Diagnosis of Endometrial Cancer

3D power Doppler angiography has been evaluated as adjunctive tool to 2D real-time ultrasound in the diagnosis and staging of EMC [77, 78]. In a series of 99 women with PMB and an endometrium of thickness >5 mm, 3D-PDA was used prior to endometrial biopsy. There were 44 EMCs in this group of patients. Endometrial volume, vascularity index, and vascularity flow index were all shown to be significantly higher in malignant versus benign conditions; of these, the vascularity index was reported to be the best predictor of malignancy [77]. In another series, 99 women with known EMC were interrogated with endovaginal 3D ultrasound and power Doppler angiography. Endometrial volume and 3D-PDA indices such as vascularization index, flow index, and vascularization flow index were calculated using a virtual organ computer-assisted method. Only endometrial volume and vascularity index were associated with myometrial invasion, of which only endometrial volume correlated with depth of myometrial invasion, and vascularity index was associated with the tumor grade. This is easy to understand since tumor size determines the depth of myometrial invasion, and there is greater degree of angiogenesis and consequently flow in high grade tumors [78].

Contrast Enhanced Ultrasound Evaluation of the Endometrium [79–81]

The value of using contrast enhancement during sonographic assessment of the endometrium has been studied in small group of patients. The examination involves administration of intravenous SonoVue® (Bracco, Milan, Italy). A slow bolus injection of 2.5 mL SonoVue is followed by a flush with 5 mL saline that is administered through an intravenous catheter placed in an arm vein. This technique may hold promise as an adjunct to transvaginal sonography such as in identifying malignancy in women with a thin otherwise normal appearing endometrium, in determining the presence of deep myometrial invasion, and in distinguishing benign from malignant abnormalities [79–81]. One study of 35 patients with EMCs reported an accuracy of 85.3 % for determining myometrial infiltration depth when using arcuate vascular plexus involvement as a marker for deep myometrial invasion. The added value of increased tumor-to-tissue contrast made it useful in women with an otherwise normal appearing thin endometrium. The utility of distinguishing benign from malignant abnormalities was studied in a small series of 17 women with EC and 17 with benign abnormalities. Doppler indices were measured before and after contrast enhancement: the pulsatility index and the resistive index were measured before and following administration of intravenous ultrasound contrast.

These indices were considerably lower in vessels of malignant tumors than in benign endometrial polyps after enhancement by intravenous contrast. There was no difference between benign and malignant lesions in PI, RI velocity index, flow index, or velocity flow index before contrast enhancement or in VI, FI, or VFI after contrast enhancement [79–81].

In summary, sonographic assessment of the symptomatic postmenopausal patient proceeds by triaging patients into three groups—one without an abnormality who can be treated expectantly, one with a global endometrial abnormality who can undergo blind endometrial biopsy, and one with a focal abnormality who needs to undergo biopsy under hysteroscopic visualization. A significant number of postmenopausal women without symptoms may have a thickened endometrium (10–17 %) [71], and invasive endometrial sampling may not be appropriate in these women unless there are coexisting risk factors such as obesity, diabetes, and history of polycystic ovarian disease. Similarly, polyps in asymptomatic women with endometrial polyps may not need endometrial sampling since less than 0.1 % may have EMC in the polyp [82]. Endometrial assessment by sonography is indicated to exclude cancer in any woman older than 35 years having anovulatory uterine bleeding [71]. Finally, a note from the American College of Obstetricians and Gynecologists: the gynecological committee is of the opinion that when a thin distinct endometrial echo of 4 mm or less is seen on transvaginal sonography, risk of malignancy is less than 1 in 917 and therefore endometrial biopsy is not required [71].

Conclusion

Risk factors of EMC should be recognized. Although there have been no clear data regarding the different risks in developing or developed countries, each factor should be related to the characteristics of the women in each population area. Screening is recommended only in high-risk women with genetic predisposition. This requires genetic counseling services and specialized laboratory evaluations. Also, the familial risk data and reported genetic abnormalities may not be applicable to all population subsets. The appropriate methods of genetic management remain a significant clinical challenge in developing countries. Therefore, there are no recommendations for screening with basic and limited resource availability. Instead, early diagnosis and timely treatment are the fundamental principles of endometrial management in low resource countries. This can be achieved by proper patient education and prompt investigation for any abnormal signs or symptoms suggesting endometrial lesions. Histopathology is mandatory for a diagnosis and can be obtained with a biopsy in the outpatient setting, which is cost-efficient and well tolerated by patients. Ultrasonography is a cost-effective modality to triage patients so as to offer endometrial aspiration biopsy only to those who have an endometrial abnormality. In those few instances where abnormality is determined to be focal by sonography and aspiration biopsy is inconclusive, a dilation and curettage procedure can be performed.

References

1. Ferlay J, Shin HR, Bray F, Forman D, Mathers C, Parkin DM. Estimates of worldwide burden of cancer in 2008: GLOBOCAN 2008. Int J Cancer. 2010;127:2893–917.
2. Parkin DM, Bray F, Ferlay J, Pisani P. Global cancer statistics, 2002. CA Cancer J Clin. 2005;55:74–108.
3. Sherman ME. Theories of endometrial carcinogenesis: a multidisciplinary approach. Mod Pathol. 2000;13:295–308.
4. Sorosky JI. Endometrial cancer. Obstet Gynecol. 2008;111:436–47.
5. Tangjitgamol S, Anderson BO, See HT, Lertbutsayanukul C, Sirisabya N, Manchana T, et al. Asian Oncology Summit. Management of endometrial cancer in Asia: consensus statement from the Asian Oncology Summit 2009. Lancet Oncol. 2009;10:1119–27.
6. Anderson BO, Yip CH, Smith RA, Shyyan R, Sener SF, Eniu A, et al. Guideline implementation for breast healthcare in low-income and middle-income countries: overview of the Breast Health Global Initiative Global Summit 2007. Cancer. 2008;113:2221–43.
7. Henderson BE. The cancer question: an overview of recent epidemiologic and retrospective data. Am J Obstet Gynecol. 1989;161:1859–64.

8. Persson I, Adami HO, Bergkvist L, Lindgren A, Pettersson B, Hoover R, et al. Risk of endometrial cancer after treatment with oestrogens alone or in conjunction with progestogens: results of a prospective study. BMJ. 1989;298:147–51.
9. Persson I, Weiderpass E, Bergkvist L, Bergstrom R, Schairer C. Risks of breast and endometrial cancer after estrogen and estrogen-progestin replacement. Cancer Causes Control. 1999;10:253–60.
10. Rossouw JE, Anderson GL, Prentice RL, LaCroix AZ, Kooperberg C, Stefanick ML, et al. Risks and benefits of estrogen plus progestin in healthy postmenopausal women: principal results from the Women's Health Initiative randomized controlled trial. JAMA. 2002;288:321–33.
11. Aiman J, Forney JP, Parker Jr CR. Secretion of androgens and estrogens by normal and neoplastic ovaries in postmenopausal women. Obstet Gynecol. 1986;68: 1–5.
12. Coulam CB, Annegers JF, Kranz JS. Chronic anovulation syndrome and associated neoplasia. Obstet Gynecol. 1983;61:403–7.
13. Silverberg SG. Hyperplasia and carcinoma of the endometrium. Semin Diagn Pathol. 1988;5:135–53.
14. Fenoglio CM, Crum CP, Ferenczy A. Endometrial hyperplasia and carcinoma. Are ultrastructural, bio chemical and immunocytochemical studies useful in distinguishing between them? Pathol Res Pract. 1982;174:257–84.
15. Sherman ME, Silverberg SG. Advances in endometrial pathology. Clin Lab Med. 1995;15:517–43.
16. Silverberg SG. Problems in the differential diagnosis of endometrial hyperplasia and carcinoma. Mod Pathol. 2000;13:309–27.
17. Kendall BS, Ronnnett BM, Isacson C, et al. Reproducibility of the diagnosis of endometrial hyperplasia, atypical hyperplasia, and well differentiated carcinoma. Am J Surg Pathol. 1998;22:1012–9.
18. Trimble C, Kauderer J, Zaino R, Silverberg S, Lim PC, Burke JJ, et al. Concurrent endometrial carcinoma in women with biopsy diagnosis of atypical endometrial hyperplasia: a Gynecologic Oncology Group study. Cancer. 2006;106:812–9.
19. Committee on Gynecologic Practice, The American College of Obstetricians and Gynecologists. ACOG committee opinion. Tamoxifen and endometrial cancer. Int J Gynecol Obstet. 2006;107:1475–8.
20. Formander T, Rutqvist LE, Cedermark B, Glas U, Mattsson A, Silfverswärd C, et al. Adjuvant tamoxifen in early breast cancer: occurrence of new primary cancers. Lancet. 1989;2:117–20.
21. Andersson M, Storm HH, Mouridse HT. Carcinogenic effects of adjuvant tamoxifen treatment and radiotherapy for early breast cancer. Acta Oncol. 1992;31: 259–63.
22. Fisher B, Costantino JP, Redmond CK, et al. Endometrial cancer in tamoxifen-treated breast cancer patients: findings from the National Surgical Adjuvant Breast and Bowel Project (NSABP) B-14. J Natl Cancer Inst. 1994;86:527–37.
23. Curtis RE, Boice Jr JD, Shriner DA, et al. Second cancer after adjuvant tamoxifen therapy for breast cancer. J Natl Cancer Inst. 1996;88:8332–4.
24. Cohen I. Endometrial pathologies associated with postmenopausal tamoxifen treatment. Gynecol Oncol. 2004;94:256–66.
25. Magriples U, Naftolin F, Schwartz PE, Carcangiu ML. High grade endometrial carcinoma in tamoxifen-treated breast cancer patients. J Clin Oncol. 1993;11:485–90.
26. Cuzick J, Sestak I, Baum M, Buzdar A, Howell A, Dowsett M, et al. Effect of anastrozole and tamoxifen as adjuvant treatment for early-stage breast cancer: 10-year analysis of the ATAC trial. Lancet Oncol. 2010;11:1135–41.
27. Renehan AG, Tyson M, Egger M, Heller RF, Zwahlen M. Body-mass index and incidence of cancer: a systematic review and meta-analysis of prospective observational studies. Lancet. 2008;371:569–78.
28. Soliman PT, Wu D, Tortolero-Luna G, Schmeler KM, Slomovitz BM, Bray MS, et al. Association between adiponectin, insulin resistance, and endometrial cancer. Cancer. 2006;106:2376–81.
29. Zhang Y, Liu Z, Yu X, Zhang X, Lü S, Chen X, et al. The association between metabolic abnormality and endometrial cancer: a large case-control study in China. Gynecol Oncol. 2010;117:41–6.
30. Meyer LA, Broaddus RR, Lu KH. Endometrial cancer and Lynch syndrome: clinical and pathologic considerations. Cancer Control. 2009;16:14–22.
31. Ollikainen M, Abdel-Rahman WM, Moisio AL, Lindroos A, Kariola R, Järvelä I, et al. Molecular analysis of familial endometrial carcinoma: a manifestation of hereditary nonpolyposis colorectal cancer or a separate syndrome? J Clin Oncol. 2005;23: 4609–16.
32. Obermair A, Youlden DR, Young JP, Lindor NM, Baron JA, Newcomb P, et al. Risk of endometrial cancer for women diagnosed with HNPCC-related colorectal carcinoma. Int J Cancer. 2010;127:2678–84.
33. Beiner ME, Finch A, Rosen B, Lubinski J, Moller P, Ghadirian P, et al. The risk of endometrial cancer in women with BRCA1 and BRCA2 mutations. A prospective study. Gynecol Oncol. 2007;104:7–10.
34. Parazzini F, Negri E, La Vecchia C, Benzi G, Chiaffarino F, Polatti A, et al. Role of reproductive factors on the risk of endometrial cancer. Int J Cancer. 1998;76:784–6.
35. Prentice RL, Thomson CA, Caan B, Hubbell FA, Anderson GL, Beresford SA, et al. Low-fat dietary pattern and cancer incidence in the Women's Health Initiative Dietary Modification Randomized Controlled Trial. J Natl Cancer Inst. 2007;99:1534–43.
36. Unfer V, Casini ML, Costabile L, Mignosa M, Gerli S, Di Renzo GC. Endometrial effects of long-term treatment with phytoestrogens: a randomized, double-blind, placebo-controlled study. Fertil Steril. 2004;82: 145–8. quiz 265.
37. Setiawan VW, Monroe KR, Goodman MT, Kolonel LN, Pike MC, Henderson BE. Alcohol consumption

and endometrial cancer risk: the multiethnic cohort. Int J Cancer. 2008;122:634–8.
38. Bravi F, Scotti L, Bosetti C, Gallus S, Negri E, La Vecchia C, et al. Coffee drinking and endometrial cancer risk: a metaanalysis of observational studies. Am J Obstet Gynecol. 2009;200:130–5.
39. Tang NP, Li H, Qiu YL, Zhou GM, Ma J. Tea consumption and risk of endometrial cancer: a metaanalysis. Am J Obstet Gynecol. 2009;201:605.e1–8.
40. Smith RA, Cokkinides V, Brawley OW. Cancer screening in the United States, 2009: a review of current American Cancer Society guidelines and issues in cancer screening. CA Cancer J Clin. 2009;59:27–41.
41. Lynch HT, de la Chapelle A. Hereditary colorectal cancer. N Engl J Med. 2003;348:919–32.
42. Brown GJ, St John DJ, Macrae FA, Aittomäki K. Cancer risk in young women at risk of hereditary nonpolyposis colorectal cancer: implications for gynecologic surveillance. Gynecol Oncol. 2001;80:346–9.
43. Lindor NM, Petersen GM, Hadley DW, Kinney AY, Miesfeldt S, Lu KH, et al. Recommendations for the care of individuals with an inherited predisposition to Lynch syndrome: a systematic review. JAMA. 2006;296:1507–17.
44. Aaltonen LA, Salovaara R, Kristo P, Canzian F, Hemminki A, Peltomaki P, et al. Incidence of hereditary nonpolyposis colorectal cancer and the feasibility of molecular screening for the disease. N Engl J Med. 1998;338:1481–7.
45. Lu KH, Schorge JO, Rodabaugh KJ, Daniels MS, Sun CC, Soliman PT, et al. Prospective determination of prevalence of lynch syndrome in young women with endometrial cancer. J Clin Oncol. 2007;25:5158–64.
46. Wright TC, Massad S, Dunton C, Spitzer M, Wilkinson EJ, Solomon D, for the 2006 American Society for Colposcopy and Cervical Pathology—sponsored Consensus Conference ASCCP. 2006 consensus guidelines for the management of women with abnormal cervical cancer screening tests. Am J Obstet Gynecol. 2007;197:346–55.
47. Sorosky JI. Endometrial Cancer. Obstet Gynecol. 2012;120:383–97.
48. Karlsson B, Granberg S, Wikland M, Ylöstalo P, Torvid K, Marsal K, et al. Transvaginal ultrasonography of the endometrium in women with postmenopausal bleeding—a Nordic multicenter study. Am J Obstet Gynecol. 1995;172:1488–94.
49. Goldstein S. The role of transvaginal ultrasound or endometrial biopsy in the evaluation of the menopausal endometrium. Am J Obs Gyn. 2009;201:5–11.
50. Dijkhuizen FP, Mol BW, Brolmann HA, Heintz AP. The accuracy of endometrial sampling in the diagnosis of patients with endometrial carcinoma and hyperplasia: a meta-analysis. Cancer. 2000;89:1765–72.
51. Lipscomb GH, Lopatine SM, Stovall TG, Ling FW. A randomized comparison of the Pipelle, Accurette, and Explora endometrial sampling devices. Am J Obstet Gynecol. 1994;170:591–4.
52. Larson DM, Johnson KK, Broste SK, Krawisz BR, Kresl JJ. Comparison of D&C and office endometrial biopsy in predicting final histopathologic grade in endometrial cancer. Obstet Gynecol. 1995;86:38–42.
53. Frumovitz M, Singh DK, Meyer L, Smith DH, Wertheim I, Resnik E, et al. Predictors of final histology in patients with endometrial cancer. Gynecol Oncol. 2004;95:463–8.
54. Clark TJ, Mann CH, Shah N, Khan KS, Song F, Gupta JK. Accuracy of outpatient endometrial biopsy in the diagnosis of endometrial hyperplasia. Acta Obstet Gynecol Scand. 2001;80:784–93.
55. Obermair A, Geramou M, Gucer F, Denison U, Graf AH, Kapshammer E, et al. Impact of hysteroscopy on disease-free survival in clinically stage I endometrial cancer patients. Int J Gynecol Cancer. 2000;10: 275–9.
56. Nalaboff KM, Pellerito JS, Ben-Levi E. Imaging the endometrium: disease and normal variants. Radiographics. 2001;21:1409–24.
57. Zalud I, Conway C, Schulman H, et al. Endometrial and myometrial thickness and uterine blood low in postmenopausal women: the influence of hormonal replacement therapy and age. J Ultrasound Med. 1993;12:737–41.
58. Fleischer AC. Sonographic assessment of endometrial disorders. Semin Ultrasound CT MR. 1999;20: 259–66.
59. Sahakain V, Syrop C, Turner D. Endometrial carcinoma: transvaginal ultrasonography prediction of depth of myometrial invasion. Gynecol Oncol. 1991; 43:217–9.
60. Savelli L, Testa AC, Mabrouk M, Zannoni L, Ludovisi M, Seracchioli R, et al. A prospective blinded comparison of the accuracy of transvaginal sonography and frozen section in the assessment of myometrial invasion in endometrial cancer. Gynecol Oncol. 2012;124(3):549–52.
61. Ozdemir S, Celik C, Emlik D, Kiresi D, Esen H. Assessment of myometrial invasion in endometrial cancer by transvaginal sonography, Doppler ultrasonography, magnetic resonance imaging and frozen section. Int J Gynecol Cancer. 2009;19(6):1085–90.
62. Dubinsky TJ. Value of sonography in the diagnosis of abnormal vaginal bleeding. J Clin Ultrasound. 2004;32:348–53.
63. Gull B, Carlsson SA, Karlsson B, et al. Transvaginal ultrasound in the endometrium in women with postmenopausal bleeding: is it always necessary to perform an endometrial biopsy? Am J Obstet Gynecol. 2000;182:509.
64. Einerth Y. Vacuum curettage by the Vabrar method: a simple procedure for endometrial diagnosis. Acta Obstet Gynecol Scand. 1982;61:373–6.
65. Lidor A, Ismajovich B, Confino E, David MP. Histopathological findings in 226 women with postmenopausal uterine bleeding. Acta Obstet Gynecol Scand. 1986;65:41–3.
66. Ferenczy A, Shore M, Guralnick M, Gelfand MM. The Kevorkian curette: an appraisal of its effectiveness in endometrial evaluation. Obstet Gynecol. 1979;54:262–7.

67. Stovall TG, Photopulos GJ, Poston WM, Ling FW, Sandles LG. Pipelle endometrial sampling in patients with known endometrial carcinoma. Obstet Gynecol. 1991;77:954–6.
68. Medverd JR, Dubinsky TJ. Cost analysis model: US versus endometrial biopsy in evaluation of peri- and postmenopausal abnormal vaginal bleeding. Radiology. 2002;222:619–27.
69. Gull B, Karlsson B, Milsom I, Granberg S. Can ultrasound replace dilation and curettage? A longitudinal evaluation of postmenopausal bleeding and transvaginal sonographic measurement of the endometrium as predictors of endometrial cancer. Am J Obstet Gynecol. 2003;188:401–8.
70. Goldstein RB, Bree RL, Benson CB, Benacerraf BR, Bloss JD, Carlos R, et al. Evaluation of the woman with postmenopausal bleeding: Society of Radiologists in Ultrasound—sponsored consensus conference statement. J Ultrasound Med. 2001;20:1025–36.
71. Goldstein SR. Modern evaluation of the endometrium. Obstet Gynecol. 2010;116(1):168–76.
72. Burbos N, Musonda P, Crocker SG, Morris EP, Nieto JJ, Duncan TJ. Management of postmenopausal women with vaginal bleeding when the endometrium cannot be visualized. Acta Obstet Gynecol Scand. 2012;91(6):686–91.
73. Fleischer AC, Wheeler JE, Lindsay I, et al. An assessment of the value of ultrasonographic screening for endometrial disease in postmenopausal women without symptoms. Am J Obstet Gynecol. 2001;184:70–5.
74. Jacobs I, Gentry-Maharaj A, Burnell M, et al. Sensitivity of transvaginal ultrasound screening for endometrial cancer in postmenopausal women: a case-control study within the UKCTOCS cohort. Lancet Oncol. 2011;12:38–48.
75. Smith-Bindman R, Kerlikowske K, Feldstein VA. Endovaginal ultrasound to exclude endometrial cancer and other endometrial abnormalities. JAMA. 1998;280(17):1510–7.
76. Burbos N, Musonda P, Crocker SG, Morris EP, Nieto JJ, Duncan TJ. Outcome of investigations for postmenopausal vaginal bleeding in women under the age of 50 years. Gynecol Oncol. 2012;125(1):120–3.
77. Alcazar JL, Galvan R. Three-dimensional power Doppler ultrasound scanning for the prediction of endometrial cancer in women with postmenopausal bleeding and thickened endometrium. Am J Obstet Gynecol. 2009;200:44.e1–6.
78. Galvan R, Merce L, Jurado M, et al. Three-dimensional power Doppler angiography in endometrial cancer: correlation with tumor characteristics. Ultrasound Obstet Gynecol. 2010;35:723–9.
79. Liu ZZ, Jiang YX, Dai Q, Yang M, Zhu QL, Zhao DC, et al. Imaging of endometrial carcinoma using contrast-enhanced sonography. J Ultrasound Med. 2011;30(11):1519–27.
80. Lieng M, Qvigstad E, Dahl GF, Istre O. Flow differences between endometrial polyps and cancer: a prospective study using intravenous contrast-enhanced transvaginal color flow Doppler and three-dimensional power Doppler ultrasound. Ultrasound Obstet Gynecol. 2008;32(7):935–40.
81. Song Y, Yang J, Liu Z, Shen K. Preoperative evaluation of endometrial carcinoma by contrast-enhanced ultrasonography. BJOG. 2009;116(2):294–8; discussion 298–9.
82. Ferrazzi E, Zupi E, Leone FP, Savelli L, Omodei U, Moscarini M, et al. How often are endometrial polyps malignant in asymptomatic postmenopausal women? A multicenter study. Am J Obstet Gynecol. 2009;200:235.e1–6.

Breast and Gynecologic Cancer Prevention in Low-Resource Countries

9

William Kofi Bosu, Terri L. Cornelison, and Brandy M. Heckman-Stoddard

Abstract

This chapter focuses on the prevention of breast, ovarian, endometrial, and cervical cancers through a discussion of risk factors and active interventions for prevention. The priority options available to most low resource countries (LRCs) are to improve health lifestyles and to promote early diagnosis of symptomatic cancer. Avoiding alcohol misuse, smoking, adult weight gain, obesity, physical inactivity, shortened or absent duration of breastfeeding are amenable to individual or group actions. Enacting and enforcing national legislation to reduce lifetime exposure to risk factors and to introduce and expand HPV vaccination programs are needed. The benefits of chemoprevention studies may only be felt in LRCs when low cost options are proven effective in locally relevant resource-limited settings.

Abbreviations

AHA	American Heart Association
AIs	Aromatase inhibitors
BCPT	Breast Cancer Prevention Trial
BHGI	Breast Global Health Initiative
BPM	Bilateral prophylactic mastectomy
BSE	Breast self-examination
BSO	Bilateral salpingo-oophorectomy
CBE	Clinical breast examination
CDC	Centers for Disease Control and Prevention
CPM	Contralateral prophylactic mastectomy
DDT	Dichlorodiphenyltrichloroethane
DMPA	Depot medroxyprogesterone acetate
ELF-EMF	Extremely low frequency-electromagnetic fields
EPIC	European Prospective Investigation into Cancer and Nutrition
ER	Estrogen receptor
HBOC	Hereditary breast and ovarian cancer

W.K. Bosu (✉)
Disease Control and Prevention Department,
Ghana Health Service, Accra, Ghana
e-mail: Billy.Bosu@ghsmail.org; Wbosu@wahooas.org

T.L. Cornelison • B.M. Heckman-Stoddard
Division of Cancer Prevention,
National Cancer Institute, 6130 Executive Blvd,
EPN 2128/2129, Rockville, MD 20892, USA
e-mail: cornelit@mail.nih.gov;
heckmanbm@mail.nih.gov

M.K. Shetty (ed.), *Breast and Gynecological Cancers: An Integrated Approach for Screening and Early Diagnosis in Developing Countries*, DOI 10.1007/978-1-4614-1876-4_9,

FDA	Food and Drug Administration
HNPCC	Hereditary nonpolyposis colorectal cancer
HPV	Human papilloma virus
HRT	Hormonal replacement therapy
IARC	International Agency for Research on Cancer
IBIS	International Breast Cancer Intervention Study
IOM	Institute of Medicine
LRCs	Low resource countries
MORE	Multiple Outcomes of Raloxifene Evaluation
NCD	Non-communicable disease
NSABP	National Surgical Adjuvant Breast and Bowel Project
OCs	Oral contraceptives
PARP	Poly adenosine diphosphate ribose polymerase
PLCO	Prostate, lung, colorectal, and ovarian
RCTs	Randomized controlled trials
SERMs	Selective estrogen receptor modulators
STAR	Study of Tamoxifen and Raloxifene
US	United States
USPSTF	US Preventive Services Task Force
VTE	Venous thromboembolic events
WCRF	World Cancer Research Fund
WHI	Women's Health initiative

Introduction

Prevention is not only an important strategy, but it is also the most cost-effective strategy to control breast and gynecologic cancers. Two general prevention strategies are [1] the avoidance or removal of known carcinogenic exposures, and [2] use of active interventions such as drugs, vaccines, nutrients, and behavioral modifications (dietary alterations, physical activity) to reduce cancer risk. This chapter focuses on the prevention of breast, ovarian, endometrial, and cervical cancers through a discussion of risk factors and active interventions to reduce risk as they relate to low resource countries (LRCs).

Risk factors

Breast Cancer

Worldwide, breast cancer is the most common cancer in women. The risk factors associated with breast cancer are complex and include demographic, genetic, biologic, reproductive, hormonal, and environmental factors. Age, gender, and family history are among the strongest risk factors for breast cancer, although it is well known that serum levels of endogenous sex hormones are also strongly associated with an increased risk of breast cancer [1].

Positive family history is a known risk factor for breast cancer. In the Nurses' Health Study, women whose mothers were diagnosed before age 50 had a 69% increased risk and those whose mothers were diagnosed at 50 or older had a 37% increased risk of developing breast cancer compared to women with no family history [2]. Women with either mother or sister diagnosed before age 50 had a 70% increased risk, while those diagnosed at age 50 or older had a 30% increased risk. In Nigeria, positive family history of breast cancer in first- and second-degree relatives was the strongest risk factor associated with breast cancer after adjusting for sociodemographic, reproductive, lifestyle, and anthropometric factors [3].

The non-modifiable risk factors for breast cancer are increasing age (>50 years), gender, ethnicity, early menarche (<12 years), late menopause (>55 years), family history (≥1 first-degree relative diagnosed with breast cancer, particularly if diagnosed at <50 years of age), and breast density. Women with dense tissue in more than 60–75% of their breast are at a four to sixfold increased risk of breast cancer than those with no densities [4]. The contribution of these non-modifiable risk factors to breast cancer is not insignificant. In Germany, they account for 37–48% of invasive breast tumors, depending on the subtype [5].

However, there are modifiable risk factors that also contribute significantly to breast cancer risk.

Danaei and colleagues estimate that heavy alcohol use (5%), overweight and obesity (9%), and physical inactivity (10%) together account for about 21% of breast cancer deaths globally [6]. The population attributable risk fraction due to these risk factors is 27% for high-income countries and 18% for low- and middle-income countries, the difference coming from the higher fractions for alcohol use and overweight and obesity in high-income countries. The contribution of physical inactivity to the risk of breast cancer is independent of obesity [7].

Other modifiable risk factors include postmenopausal hormonal replacement therapy (HRT), use of oral contraceptives, and breastfeeding. HRT, specifically estrogen plus progesterone, has been linked to an increase in breast cancer [8]. After an increased risk was reported in 2002 in the United States (US), there was a precipitous decline in breast cancer incidence by 6.7% in 2003, especially in ER-positive tumors [9], that has been attributed to the widespread discontinuation of HRT. However, fewer breast cancers were reported in the estrogen-alone arm than in the placebo group among women with a prior hysterectomy, although not statistically significant [10]. In vitro estrogen has been shown to induce apoptosis of previously estrogen-deprived cells, supporting this finding [11]. Exogenous hormone use earlier in life has also been linked to breast cancer risk. The Collaborative Group on Hormonal Factors in Breast Cancer found that women who were current or recent users of birth control pills had a slightly higher risk of developing breast cancer than women who had never used the pill, and this observation was confirmed in the Nurses' Health Study [12, 13]. Some studies have shown that breastfeeding for more than 1 year slightly lowers breast cancer risk or both ER-positive and ER-negative breast cancer [14, 15]. This is hypothesized to work through lowering the number of menstrual cycles in a women's lifetime.

In the prostate, lung, colorectal, and ovarian (PLCO) cancer screening trial [16], earlier age at menarche (<12 years) and early menopause (<45 years) were less strongly associated with breast cancer than was expected. Only severe obesity (body mass index (BMI; kg/m^2) of 35 or more) was statistically significantly associated with breast cancer [16]. While the study confirmed increasing age, nulliparity, positive family history of breast cancer, and use of menopausal hormone therapy as increasing the risk of breast cancer, findings also suggested that the associations between breast cancer and age at menarche, age at menopause, and obesity in the United States (US) might be changing.

A recent review by the Institute of Medicine (IOM) concluded that the use of combination hormone therapy products, current use of oral contraceptives (OCs), exposure to ionizing radiation, overweight, and obesity among postmenopausal women, and alcohol consumption were clearly associated with increased breast cancer risk, while greater physical activity was associated with a reduced risk [17]. It identified the following actions as potentially reducing the risk for breast cancer, even if some are not easily implementable:

- Eliminating exposure to unnecessary medical radiation throughout life
- Avoiding use of combination estrogen–progestin menopausal hormone therapy, unless it is medically necessary
- Avoiding active and passive smoking
- Limiting alcohol consumption
- Increasing physical activity
- Minimizing overweight and weight gain
- Chemoprevention using tamoxifen or raloxifene for some high-risk women

Additionally, there are environmental hazards that may contribute to breast cancer risk. Based on limited epidemiological evidence and evidence from animal studies, the International Agency for Research on Cancer (IARC) classifies exposure to ethylene oxide as a carcinogen associated with lymphoid tumors and breast cancer [18]. The IOM review concluded that there was also clear evidence benzene and 1,3-butadiene were associated with increased risk of breast cancer [17]. Besides industry, it identified transport-related air pollution, and industrial and tobacco smoke as settings through which the public could be exposed.

In 2007, IARC classified night-shift work as a Group 2A human carcinogen, probably carcinogenic to humans [19]. Denmark has started compensation payouts to women with breast cancer who have no known risk factors other than working a night shift at least once weekly over the past 20 years [20]. The IOM review of environmental causes of breast cancer concluded that the role of dichlorodiphenyltrichloroethane (DDT), a widely used pesticide in LRCs, was inconclusive but early-life exposures may be etiologic [17].

Risk for breast cancer is increased by early life exposure to ionizing radiation, with the risk persisting through life and increasing in a dose–response fashion. X-rays and gamma rays are classified as breast carcinogens in premenopausal women [21]. Studies have found no significant association between nonionizing radiation (microwaves appliance, mobile telephony, infrared or radio waves) and breast cancer [17]. IARC classifies extremely low frequency-electromagnetic fields (ELF-EMF) as possibly carcinogenic.

The role of occupational exposure and radiation in most LRCs is inadequately assessed but is probably low. Reducing occupational risk of breast cancer requires occupational safety measures such as environmental monitoring, health screening, education, and legislation to reduce harmful exposures. Many LRCs require international assistance to regulate their atomic energy industry. Unfortunately, occupational safety measures are not well established in many LRCs.

Epithelial Ovarian Cancer

Need to emphasize the focus on Low Resource Countries and reduce the reference to the epidemiology in US. Ovarian cancer shares many risk factors with breast cancer including age, family history, genetic risk, obesity, menstrual history, and hormone replacement therapy use. Ovarian cancer risk increases with age, with 63 as the median age of diagnosis, and fewer than 5% of ovarian cancers diagnosed before the age of 40 [22].

A family history of breast, ovarian, or colorectal cancer increases the risk of ovarian cancer due to genetic predisposition. Hereditary breast and ovarian cancer (HBOC) syndrome and hereditary nonpolyposis colorectal cancer (HNPCC) syndrome account for 10% of all ovarian cancer. The lifetime risk of ovarian cancer in these populations ranges from 9% in HNPCC to 28–60% in BRCA-1 carriers [23–25]. The higher risk estimates come from studies, which followed high-risk clinic populations.

Obesity is a risk factor for ovarian cancer, with over 85% of reports showing a positive association between obesity and ovarian cancer. In addition, obesity is a poor prognostic factor. A recent meta-analysis showed that women who are obese prior to an advanced ovarian cancer diagnosis have a 45% increase in risk of cancer mortality [26, 27].

The ovary is hormonally responsive, and hormone replacement therapy has been shown to be associated with an increase in ovarian cancer risk, with a stronger association for estrogen alone than estrogen plus progesterone [28]. In the Women's Health Initiative (WHI), randomized trial of 17,000 postmenopausal women randomized to 0.625 mg unconjugated estrogen plus 2.5 mg medroxyprogestrone acetate or placebo, the hazard ratio for estrogen plus progestin versus placebo for invasive ovarian cancer was 1.58 (95% CI 0.77–3.24), suggestive of an increased risk although not statistically significant [29]. The NCI Study of Hormone Therapy and Ovarian Cancer supported the increase [30].

Additionally, nonhormonal factors have been linked to an increase in the risk of ovarian cancer. Talcum powder applied to genital region has been associated with an increase risk in ovarian cancer [31]. Smoking has been associated with an increase in mucinous ovarian cancer but not serous [32].

The majority of studies have consistently reported that tubal ligation is associated with a 50% decrease in ovarian cancer risk, with an overall summary relative risk of 0.63, (95% CI 0.44–0.91) [33]. However, the WHO Collaborative Study of Neoplasia and Steroid Contraceptives found a nonsignificant reduction for tubal ligation (odds ratio (OR), 0.72; 95% confidence interval (CI), 0.48–1.08) and hysterectomy (OR, 0.58; 95% CI, 0.26–1.27) [34]. These differences in risk estimates could be explained by adjustment factors, with the most adjusted estimates showing the strongest association. Additionally, Rosenblatt and colleagues suggest that different types of ovarian cancer may be affected differentially by tubal ligation.

In contradistinction with breast cancer, oral contraceptives significantly lower the risk of ovarian cancer by up to 50%. A case–control study in Thailand showed that depot medroxyprogesterone acetate (DMPA) was associated with a 39% decrease in ovarian cancer, with an 83% decrease in risk in women who used DMPA for more than 3 years [35].

Parity is associated with a decreased risk of ovarian cancer. Women who were ever pregnant have a 30–60% less risk of ovarian cancer than nulliparous women, and multiple pregnancies exert an increasingly protective effect [36, 37]. In addition, breastfeeding decreases the risk of ovarian cancer. It is presumed that the protective effect of parity and breastfeeding are due to decreased endogenous estrogen exposure over a lifetime. Ovulation-inducing drugs (clomiphene) have been previously shown to be associated with an increase in ovarian cancer risk, but recent studies with the ability to control for significant confounders including nulliparity found no increase in risk [38].

Endometrial Cancer

The risk factors for endometrial cancer are age, family history, genetic risk, unopposed estrogen, a higher number of total menstrual cycles, obesity, diabetes, and polycystic ovarian syndrome; these represent a complex etiology involving both endogenous and exogenous hormonal factors.

However, the greatest risk factors for endometrial cancer are obesity and unopposed estrogen. Women who are more than 30 pounds or 13.6 kg above ideal body weight have a threefold increased risk of endometrial cancer [39, 40]. Women with more than 50 pounds or 22.7 kg above ideal body weight have a tenfold increased risk of endometrial cancer. This high risk is comparable only to the 9.5-fold increased risk of endometrial cancer due to unopposed estrogen [25].

Family history of colorectal or endometrial cancer also poses a significant risk. The lifetime risk of endometrial cancer in women with HNPCC ranges from 20 to 60% [24, 41–44]. Due to this increased risk, international guidelines promote gynecologic surveillance beginning between age 25 and 35 with transvaginal ultrasound or endometrial aspiration [45, 46]. BRCA1 and BRCA2 mutation have not been associated with an increase in endometrial cancer [46].

Tamoxifen has been associated with increased risk of endometrial cancer. The National Surgical Adjuvant Breast and Bowel Project (NSABP) Prevention (P)-1: Breast Cancer Prevention Trial (BCPT) [47, 48], the Royal Marsden Hospital tamoxifen randomized chemoprevention trial [49, 50], the Italian Tamoxifen Prevention Study [51, 52], and the International Breast Cancer Intervention Study (IBIS)-1 [53, 54] all showed an increase in the relative risk (RR) of endometrial cancer in the tamoxifen-treated group.

Oral contraceptives, hormone-induced intrauterine devices, and pregnancy are associated with a decrease in endometrial cancer risk [55]. The protective effect of parity may be restricted to the first pregnancy [25, 56].

Cervical Cancer

Cervical cancer is the most common gynecologic cancer worldwide. Annually, nearly 500,000 women are diagnosed with cervical cancer, and more than 250,000 die from this disease. The single most important risk factor for cervical cancer is human papilloma virus (HPV). HPV is associated with over 99% of cervical cancers and is considered the primary etiological factor.

Immunosuppression, by human immunodeficiency virus or an autoimmune disease, increases the risk of cervical cancer. HPV infections are more prevalent in HIV-infected women and tend to be more persistent [57]. While immunosuppression does not increase the risk of exposure to HPV, it does compromise host ability to clear HPV infection. *Chlamydia trachomatis* and herpes simplex virus, both sexually transmitted infections, are considered cofactors in HPV-associated neoplasia, possibly through induction of cervical inflammation [58].

Additional risk factors that have been described for cervical cancer, such as multiple pregnancies, early first coitus, multiple sexual partners, and poverty, are actually linked to an increased risk of HPV exposure and infection. When HPV presence is accounted for, these risk factors associated with sexual behavior are no longer considered independent factors of risk. Smoking remains an independent risk factor for cervical cancer.

Hormonal contraceptive use has been associated with an increase in the risk of cervical cancer, with the greatest effect in women who have used hormonal contraceptives for longer than 10 years. However, there are some data that this risk decreases when use ceases [59].

Active Interventions

Active interventions can be offered to mitigate an increased risk of cancer. These interventions include behavioral modification such as physical activity, pharmaceutical agents such as tamoxifen for breast cancer reduction, or a prophylactic HPV vaccine for cervical cancer prevention, or even prophylactic surgical removal of the tissue at risk.

Behavior Modification

Compliance with the World Cancer Research Fund (WCRF) 2008 recommendations to increase weight management, physical activity, healthy food intake, breastfeeding, and decrease alcohol consumption have been associated with decreased risk of developing breast cancer and several other cancers in the European Prospective Investigation into Cancer and Nutrition (EPIC) study [60]. A one-point increment in a composite score of the WCRF recommendations was associated with a 5% (95% CI 3–7%) lower risk of developing breast cancer after a median follow-up period of 11.0 years. Within the context of noncommunicable disease (NCD) control, healthier lifestyles that should be promoted include avoiding exposure to tobacco, avoiding harmful use of alcohol, engaging in moderate- to vigorous-intensity physical activity, and achieving weight reduction for overweight or obese women. Campaign efforts to promote healthier lifestyles can be undertaken for a combination of health benefits beyond just cancer prevention.

Until recently, the association between tobacco consumption and breast cancer was tenuous or inconclusive. IARC and IOM reached different conclusions about the role of tobacco in breast cancer [17, 61]. In prospective studies, the risk of breast cancer is higher in premenopausal women who start smoking at an early age, postmenopausal women who smoke, and premenopausal women exposed to secondhand smoke [62]. A recent meta-analysis found that women who smoked before their first pregnancy (regardless of whether or not they continued to smoke after the pregnancy) had a 10% greater risk of breast cancer than women who had never smoked [63]. However, in LRCs, where tobacco consumption, particularly among women, is much lower than in high-income countries, tobacco cessation campaigns may have a smaller effect on breast cancer prevention specifically, even though there is an expected overall health benefit for the general population [64].

The WHO's Framework Convention for Tobacco Control of 2003 has provided a catalyst for many LRCs which have ratified it to strengthen their tobacco control measures [65]. In 2008, WHO launched a package of six proven tobacco control measures, labeled by the acronym MPOWER based on the first letters of each of the measures. The policy package calls for:

M: monitoring tobacco use and prevention polices
P: protecting people from tobacco smoke
O: offering help to people to quit tobacco use
W: warning about the dangers of tobacco
E: enforcing bans on tobacco advertising, promotion, and sponsorship
R: raising taxes on tobacco

Some LRCs (e.g., Niger, Kenya, Uganda, Tanzania) have banned smoking in public places by law. In LRCs which have not legislated a ban in public smoking, there is wide public support for such a smoking policy [66]. A major obstacle is the political will to pass and actively enforce legislation in countries where tobacco is a key revenue and employment source. Many women in LRCs are engaged in tobacco farming as their main livelihood source. Crop substitution farming with subsidies and alternative livelihoods are less economically viable in LRCs and has been generally unsuccessful [67].

It is estimated that about 4% of the breast cancers in developed countries are attributable to alcohol [68]. For developing countries, alcohol has a negligible contribution to the incidence of breast cancer due to the low consumption of 0.4 g per day. Studies suggest that a 10% increase in the proportion of persons consuming 10 g ethanol per day corresponds to a 0.8% increase in the incidence of breast cancer in women [69]. It is recommended that, if alcoholic beverages are consumed, they should be limited to two standard beverages daily for men and one standard beverage daily for women [70, 71]. Many LRCs lack policies or legislation to regulate the alcohol industry. The alcoholic beverage industry exploits this gap, advertises aggressively in the mass media, and markets their products through event sponsorship. Some brewery companies have been known to sponsor tame national policies to regulate the industry [72]. As with tobacco, policies and legislation should aim to regulate production, distribution, marketing, and advertising and to prevent and manage the adverse health effects of alcohol.

The systematic review of WCRF 2008 found that the association between body fatness and breast cancer varies according to the menopausal status of women, with an increase risk of breast cancer for postmenopausal women who are overweight and obese, while premenopausal women have a decreased risk of cancer [73]. However, the WCRF panel judged that the level of physical activity probably reduces the risk of breast cancer in premenopausal and postmenopausal women [73]. In a systematic review of published studies, IARC found that physical activity reduced the risk of breast cancer by 20–40% when compared to sedentary activity [7]. A study in Tunisia confirmed the beneficial effect of lifetime physical activity for breast cancer in postmenopausal women but not in premenopausal women [74]. Various organizations such as WRCF, WHO, and the Centers for Disease Control and Prevention (CDC) recommend that adults engage in a combination of moderate- and vigorous-intensity physical activities for at least 30 min each day on most days of the week. Every adult should also perform activities that maintain or increase muscular strength and endurance at least 2 days in a week. Studies show that even minimal physical activity is more beneficial than little or no physical activity [75].

Operationalizing physical activity recommendations can be challenging in LRCs where gym membership programs or keep-fit-clubs are costly options. Persons should therefore be encouraged to do everyday manual tasks (washing, walking, dancing, sweeping) with more effort for fitness. Persons engaged in sedentary occupations—market women or men, sedentary traders, typists, etc. who are more difficult to target individually—could be reached through labor groups. At the organizational or strategic level, physical activity should be encouraged in schools, workplaces, and in communities.

The role of physical activity for ovarian cancer prevention remains uncertain, as findings of benefit have been inconsistent. Half the studies suggest that physical activity modestly decreases risk, and half the studies suggest no association. A recent meta-analysis of studies examining recreational physical activity and ovarian cancer risk estimated a 20% reduced risk for the most active versus least active women [27]. For endometrial cancer, the epidemiologic evidence to date suggests that physical activity is probably protective, with a risk reduction of about 20–30% for those with the highest levels of physical activity compared to those with the lowest levels [76]. A recent case–control study showed that women who reported light to moderate physical activity had a 34% lower risk of endometrial cancer [77].

The WCRF, American Heart Association (AHA), and other professional organizations propose a number of recommendations to limit weight gain and to avoid obesity [71, 78, 79]. Weight reduction measures require a combination of healthy eating and physical activity. LRCs should develop guidelines on healthy eating based on locally available foods and beverages.

Recommended nutrient values should be translated into measures that are easy to understand and implement. Notwithstanding the observation that many dietary factors are not associated specifically with breast cancer [73], it is recommended that persons limit consumption of energy-dense foods, avoid sugary beverages, eat adequate amounts of a variety of fruits and vegetables, consume a high fiber diet, and limit consumption of fast foods. Western countries are introducing taxes on unhealthy foods and beverages (fat taxes) with a view to encouraging consumption of healthy foods [80]. It is not clear what impact such a measure will have in LRCs.

Many LRCs celebrate international events such as the World Heart Day, World Diabetes Day, World No Tobacco Day, and World Cancer Day to highlight the importance of health promoting behavior. Political blocks are getting increasingly involved, particularly where the event has a United Nations backing, such as the World Diabetes Day. Since 2009, the African Union has declared the last Friday in February is to be celebrated by Member States as the Africa Healthy Lifestyles Day.

It is crucial to enact and enforce legislation that regulates tobacco and alcohol, ensures healthy foods, and reduces exposure to harmful radiation. And understanding that the legislative processes in LRCs can be very slow as competing priorities limit government funds to control chronic noncommunicable diseases (NCDs), there is scope to mobilize funds from the private sector. WHO recommends that taxes from alcohol and tobacco as well as the levies from drunk driving as cost-effective ways to impact the burden of NCD, and there are examples of countries that have successfully allocated revenue from raising taxes to funding health promotion or expanding health insurance services at the primary health-care level [81].

Pharmaceutical Agents and Vaccines

Results from clinical trials have shown that two selective estrogen receptor modulators (SERMs)—tamoxifen and raloxifene—are effective in preventing breast cancer among high-risk persons. The FDA approved the two drugs in October 1998 and September 2007, respectively. SERMs act by blocking the action of estrogen in breast tissue and are effective in preventing estrogen receptor (ER) positive cancers but not ER negative cancers. In an overview of seven randomized controlled trials (RCTs), tamoxifen achieved an overall reduction of invasive cancers by 38% after 10 years of follow up and a 50% reduction in the incidence of ER-positive cancers [82, 83]. Raloxifene has similar effects to tamoxifen but has the advantage of a better safety profile. In the Multiple Outcomes of Raloxifene Evaluation (MORE) trial, a 3-year treatment with raloxifene reduced the risk of invasive breast cancer among postmenopausal women with osteoporosis by 76% and of ER-positive breast cancer by 90%, but it did not reduce ER-negative breast cancer [84]. Breast experts recommend tamoxifen as the drug of choice because of the long history of use, and it can be used in premenopausal and postmenopausal women. Raloxifene is only approved as a breast cancer prevention treatment for postmenopausal women. A recent analysis of the National Surgical Adjuvant Breast and Bowel Project Study of Tamoxifen and Raloxifene (STAR) data at a median follow-up of 81 months revealed a significant difference in invasive breast cancer between the two treatment groups, with a 24% higher rate with raloxifene compared to tamoxifen (RR, 1.24; 95% CI, 1.05–1.47) [85]. However, raloxifene continued to be associated with fewer cancers than expected in the absence of a preventive intervention, such that raloxifene would reduce the risk of invasive breast cancer by approximately 38% when compared to placebo.

The main adverse effects of tamoxifen are invasive endometrial cancer and venous thromboembolic events (VTE) such as stroke, pulmonary embolism, or deep venous thrombosis. Women <50 years are at low risk of these effects [86]. In the MORE trial, raloxifene increased the risk of VTE but not of endometrial cancer [84].

The choice for each patient who might benefit from tamoxifen chemoprevention must be based on a careful assessment of risk, benefit, patient preference, and complication management capability. The risk of breast cancer can be assessed using online assessment tools (based on older age, number of first-degree relatives with breast cancer, age at first menstrual period, age at first live birth, medical history of any breast cancer, a history of atypical hyperplasia on a breast biopsy, and the woman's race) or the Gail index [87]. The US Preventive Services Task Force (USPSTF) recommends tamoxifen for women at high risk of breast cancer in their 40s or in their 50s without a uterus who also have a low risk for thromboembolic events. The American Society of Clinical Oncology recommends tamoxifen for women with a 5-year projected risk for breast cancer greater than or equal to 1.66%.

Despite the FDA approval and public interest, there has been low uptake of tamoxifen by patients [48, 88]. In 2005, only 0.08% of US women aged 40–79 years without a personal history of breast cancer took tamoxifen for chemoprevention [89]. Multifactorial reasons relating to both providers and patients have been proposed including the physicians' assessment of risk-benefit ratio, exaggeration of harms associated with tamoxifen, and underestimation of risk of breast cancer. A systematic review found that perceived vulnerability to breast cancer was associated with increased uptake while concern with adverse effects was associated with decreased uptake [88].

Another pharmaceutical category, aromatase inhibitors (AIs), acts against estrogen synthesis through the inhibition of the cytochrome P450 enzyme aromatase. In adjuvant trials to prevent contralateral tumors, AIs reduced the risk of breast cancer nearly 50% better than tamoxifen, suggesting an overall reduction of about 75% in ER-positive tumors [83, 90]. AIs are better tolerated and do not have the VTE and gynecologic adverse effects associated with tamoxifen, although they carry a higher risk of bone mineral loss. Exemestane reduced the occurrence of invasive breast cancer by 65% and ER-positive or PR-positive breast cancer by 73% in high-risk postmenopausal women after a median follow-up period of 35 months [91]. No serious adverse effects were attributable to exemestane. Exemestane is not FDA approved at the time of this writing. A summary of the key features and findings for various RCTs of SERMs and AIs have been described in a recent review [92].

Owing to the limitations of SERMs and AIs, there are planned or ongoing prevention trials to evaluate other drug categories. Bisphosphonates are one promising group of drugs, as two large observational studies (WHI and The Breast Cancer in Northern Israel Study) observed a reduction of 28–32% among postmenopausal users [93, 94]. In the Northern Israel study, there was a greater reduction for ER-negative tumors in bisphosphonate users than nonusers.

Other drugs of interest for breast cancer prevention are retinoids, statins, and COX-2 inhibitors. Poly adenosine diphosphate ribose polymerase (PARP) inhibitors are of interest for breast and ovarian cancer prevention in BRCA-1 and BRCA-2 carriers. Metformin is an interesting potential cancer prevention agent that may have broad impact, specifically in obesity-related cancers such as postmenopausal breast cancer or endometrial cancer. Aspirin is another agent that currently is being debated, with the definitive trials difficult to do because of the widespread use of the agent and the over-the-counter availability. Aspirin has been linked to a decrease in cancer incidence and mortality [95, 96].

A comprehensive review found that OCs were associated with a 19% (95% CI 9, 29%) increased risk of breast cancer in premenopausal women [97]. Overall, OCs slightly increase the risk of cervical, breast, and liver cancers while decreasing the risk of endometrial and ovarian cancers. IARC argues that the net effect could be beneficial [98], even though IARC classifies OCs as a human carcinogen. Based on risk–benefit analysis, the WHO has determined that, for most healthy women, OCs are more beneficial than potentially harmful [99]. Studies are needed to determine how OCs decrease ovarian and endometrial cancer risk so the protective effect can be maintained in future formulations. Progesterone has been used to treat atypical endometrial hyper Studies are needed to determine optimal progesterone formulation and dose for effective endometrial tissue response.

What is the relevance of these chemoprevention findings for low resource and other settings? The relative risks associated with tamoxifen and breast cancer and the adverse events from the NSABP P-1 trial were applied to local data in

Korea, where breast cancer prevalence is much lower than in the US [100]. Sensitivity analysis showed that women younger than 40 years of age were most likely to benefit from tamoxifen. Older women taking tamoxifen were estimated to have a higher risk of stroke than women in the US. However, the simulation study in Korea did not consider the hormone receptor status, a factor known to strongly predict the effectiveness of tamoxifen [101]. In Africa, the relatively higher proportion of ER-negative or triple-negative tumors suggests that chemoprevention with SERMs and AIs may not be as beneficial as in the West. Newer approaches such as the use of kinase inhibitors are needed for hormone receptor-negative tumors [102]. Also, metformin may have some action against hormone receptor-negative tumors and is already used in LRCs to treat diabetes. There is limited experience with the use of risk assessment for cardiovascular disease in many LRCs despite availability of user-friendly colored charts for many years. Nevertheless, lessons learned in Western countries regarding difficulties experienced with the risk/benefit assessment of tamoxifen by providers and reasons for the reduced uptake may be translatable to LRCs.

Compliance is another potential challenge given the unfavorable experience with response to follow-up care in LRCs with respect to screening. For instance, in Egypt, more than half of women recalled after a screening mammogram were lost to follow up. In Eastern Nigeria [103], 29% of women refused a diagnostic biopsy for breast cancer [104]. In Western countries, a meta-analysis found that 23–28% of patients discontinued their tamoxifen or AIs prematurely during at least 4 years of follow-up [105]. Asian researchers suggest that targeting women with premalignant breast lesions might be a more feasible option and may improve compliance than targeting healthy women at high risk of breast cancer [106]. However, this does not seem to be the case based on a retrospective analysis of 2,942 women with atypical lesions treated in Boston area hospitals, only 18.9% of whom took chemoprevention whether tamoxifen, raloxifene (Evista), and/or exemestane (for any duration) [107].

Reproductive health decisions will need to be informed by issues other than, but in conjunction with, breast cancer risk. For instance, LRCs must also consider benefits and effect of changes in the age at first full-term birth, parity, and duration of breast feeding. At the population level, increasing education, technology, and socioeconomic development means that women in LRCs will increasingly have earlier menarche, later age at first full-term birth, fewer children, and shorter duration of breastfeeding—all factors that will contribute to increased risk of breast cancer. It has been estimated that these changes engendered by modernization could increase the risk of breast cancer by 25% or higher [69].

The main message for LRCs with respect to reproductive health-related prevention is to educate women to avoid prolonged exposure to exogenous hormones, to breastfeed each infant for as long as possible, and to avoid hormone-replacement therapy unless absolutely necessary [12, 14, 73, 108]. HRT in LRCs is rarely prescribed even to those patients who can afford it. In Ghana, for example, the majority of women use a combination of nonhormonal medications and alternative medicine, including dietary modifications, exercise, hydrotherapy, use of herbs, and other lifestyle changes to self-manage their menopausal symptoms [109]. Whereas in the US, Caucasian women will opt for a variety of medication as their first-line intervention, ethnic minorities will prefer medication as a final choice only when alternative methods have failed [110].

Due to the use of vaccines to protect against childhood disease and the infrastructure to distribute these vaccines, LRCs may benefit from the development of vaccine preventive interventions. Despite the FDA approval of two HPV vaccines for primary prevention and the successful completion of HPV vaccine delivery and monitoring projects in four developing countries, most LRCs have not yet implemented HPV vaccination as part of their cervical cancer prevention programs [111, 112]. The main reason is due to the high cost of the three doses of the HPV vaccine. But there are also sociocultural and religious barriers, low population awareness, limited infrastructure capacity, and heightened concerns about vaccine safety. Ideally, all developed vaccines should use technology to maintain vaccine stability when refrigeration is not available, induce immunity with a single dose, and be available at a low cost for implementation in LRCs. Second and third generation HPV vaccines are being developed to meet these goals to reduce cervical cancer in LRCs. At present, the available HPV vaccines are prophylactic vaccines, which mean that they can only prevent HPV infection in people who have not yet been exposed to the virus. Therefore, therapeutic vaccines are also needed to eliminate HPV in the overwhelmingly high number of people who already have persistent HPV infection. Breast cancer vaccines are also under development but are currently only under investigation in patients with metastatic disease to reduce tumor load and in patients with early stage disease to reduce the risk of recurrence. Unlike cervical cancer, an infectious agent has not been identified in the etiology of breast cancer, and so a prophylactic vaccine is not feasible.

Surgical Interventions

Fifty-one variants of 40 genes have been found to be significantly associated with breast cancer [113]. Of these, 14 variants of nine genes show moderate to strong evidence of an association [114]. The breast cancer susceptibility genes include four rare high-penetrance genes (BRCA1, BRCA2, TP53, and PTEN). Mutations in the BRCA-1 and BRCA-2 genes are rare, with a frequency of less than 0.5%. They are estimated to cause 2–5% of all breast cancer cases. Overall, hereditary breast cancer susceptibility genes, including BRCA-1 and BRCA-2, account for 5–10% of all breast cancers. BRCA mutation carriers have a 40–65% lifetime risk of breast cancer, have an 11–40% lifetime risk of ovarian cancer, and tend to have a younger age of onset than noncarriers [115, 116].

A cochrane review of eight trials found that that cancer genetic risk-assessment services for familial breast cancer help to reduce anxiety, improve the accuracy of the perceived risk of breast cancer, and increase knowledge about breast cancer and genetics [116]. Options available to genetically high-risk women are nonsurgical interventions including chemoprevention and surgery. Surgical interventions include (bilateral (BPM) or contralateral) prophylactic mastectomy (CPM), bilateral salpingo-oophorectomy (BSO), or a combination of these. The improved assessment of genetic risk has been associated with increased uptake of surgery to prevent breast cancer, to prevent its recurrence, and to improve survival. Selection bias, small sample sizes, insufficient follow-up periods, and various confounders have affected the studies. In the absence of a positive family history of breast cancer, the incidence of contralateral breast cancer is rare, occurring in about 2.7% of patients after 4.8 years of follow-up [117].

A cochrane review involving 20 studies found that BPM reduced the incidence and mortality of breast cancer, particularly in women with BRCA1/2 mutations [118]. A risk reduction of 85–100% was reported after a median follow-up period of 13.4 years in BRCA1/2 carriers who underwent BPM. The review also found that CPM prevents cancer in the contralateral breast, although its impact on survival is less clear. The gain in preventing cancer in the contralateral breast must be balanced against morbidity and mortality from the primary tumor. CPM has been shown to improve disease-free and overall survival, after adjusting for various prognostic factors, and has been more beneficial for patients with hormone receptor-negative disease [119].

Accumulating data support the efficacy of BSO in significantly reducing the risk of both gynecologic cancers (ovary, fallopian tube, peritoneal) and breast cancer in women who carry BRCA-1 or BRCA-2 mutations. In the Prevention and Observation of Surgical Endpoints Study, the relative risk of ovarian/fallopian tube/peritoneal cancer after BSO was 0.04 (95% CI 0.01–0.16) [120].

A hysterectomy may also be performed in women with HNPCC, in women planning to take tamoxifen, or in women who wish to take unopposed estrogen due to the increased risk of endometrial cancer. It may also be an option for women with unresolved atypical endometrial hyperplasia.

Surgery is always controversial, and often screening is recommended in place of surgery in high-income countries. In women with a known high-risk condition in LRCs, surgery may be a better option.

Early Detection

Early detection is the major focus of breast cancer prevention programs in LRCs. It targets two categories of persons. One group is those with symptomatic breast cancer who, for various reasons, delay seeking care or are not diagnosed or treated early in health facilities. The other group is the asymptomatic group who are at risk of developing breast cancer.

Early Reporting and Diagnosis

For persons with symptoms of breast cancer, some of whom wait up to 5 years before seeking professional care, the objective is to get them to report to health facilities early enough to improve their clinical outcomes [121]. This should increase the proportion of cases that are diagnosed at earlier stages (downstaging). The strategy requires qualitative studies to gain a better understanding of underlying reasons for delay, intensive education to improve breast awareness, and education on symptoms, early warning signs, and curability of breast cancer. Education should not only target women themselves but also the alternative care providers and the spiritualists who take up their care and unduly detain them before referral. It is also important to engage community leaders, religious leaders, husbands, and all those who may influence the decision to seek formal health care. Governments, national partners, and international partners should support civil society and nongovernmental organizations involving breast cancer survivors in this education drive to demystify the perceived fatalism associated with breast cancer.

LRCs should prioritize early diagnosis of persons with symptomatic disease over those without symptoms [122–124]. It is more cost effective to do so as the number of symptomatic cases is so much less than that for asymptomatic women and would obviate the need for expensive mammographic screening [125]. As the objective of clinical downstaging is achieved and the proportion of advanced stage and early detection become similar, the benefit to breast cancer outcome becomes less evident and more attention could be focused on detection among asymptomatic patients.

Capacity should be built to diagnose and treat the cases which reach the hospital. Reporting to the health facility may be hindered by geographical, sociocultural, and financial barriers [126]. It is often convenient to blame patients for delays in getting a diagnosis, but there are health service factors that are implicated. In a study of the cause of delays in diagnosis of breast cancer in Tunisia, the investigators found that factors related to the patient accounted for 92.5% of the delays and those related to the medical personnel accounted for 24% of cases [127]. Referrals systems can be complicated, and patients may visit several facilities at several levels of care before receiving appropriate care. Delays in receiving a diagnosis occur when there are only few histopathologists in the country, and often they are located in the teaching hospitals where biopsy specimens have to be sent (at the patients' expense), and the heavy workload may result in several months' wait before results are obtained. Patient navigation systems should be urgently introduced or improved to ensure patients receive care early once they make contact with the formal health care system [128, 129].

Even after patients are diagnosed in the hospital, other obstacles have to be overcome in order to improve clinical outcomes. Patients may refuse diagnostic procedures and treatment or abscond from follow-up care [130]. Refusals or default from care may be due to financial or geographical barriers. In Nigeria, patients had to be referred to the nearest radiotherapy facility, which was about 600 km on a poorly navigable road from the Breast Clinic, this being one of only four functional radiotherapy facilities in the country [103].

General Breast Health Awareness

There is low awareness of breast and gynecologic health in many LRCs, fuelled by cultural barriers, low literacy levels, absence of active and sustained educational programs, lack of local champions (e.g., breast cancer survivors, celebrities, opinion leaders), low interest from governments and their development partners, and consequent limited funding. There is sometimes confusion in the terms (e.g., breast awareness versus breast self-examination) that are used in educational efforts for breast cancer [131]. Low breast awareness is not limited to the lay public. Female health professionals including doctors have knowledge gaps in risk factors, and there are unsatisfactory breast self-examination, unsatisfactory clinical breast examination practices, and inaccurate beliefs about treatment [132, 133]. Among health professionals in a tertiary hospital in Lagos, Nigeria, only a quarter believed that prayer cannot cause a breast cancer lesion to disappear, and 64% believed that alternative or herbal medicines were not effective treatment to cure breast cancer [133]. In Iran, 40% of adult females were not sure if they could get breast cancer by touching a person with the disease [134]. In Ghana, 20% of women believed that keeping coins under the breasts was a risk factor for breast cancer [135]. There is often pessimism and fatalism associated with breast cancer [136, 137].

In general, the absence of pain in a breast lesion, ignorance about signs and symptoms, belief in divine protection, belief in spiritual healing, preference for herbal medications, fear of mastectomy, strong cultural values, and financial constraints are major barriers for women to seeking early breast care. Some women believe that a woman is not complete without her breasts and so will prefer to die than to live without the breasts [135]. The common misconception that breast cancer is contagious leads to stigma, breakdown of marriages, and discrimination [138]. It is thus not entirely surprising that 60–91% of patients in some countries report with advanced disease, some 10–12 months after their first symptoms [121, 139, 140]. A vicious cycle is created in which late reporting results in poor outcomes, which in turn reinforce the belief that hospitals cannot effectively manage breast cancer.

Current approaches to sensitizing the public to breast cancer in some LRCs include the celebration of breast awareness month (Pink October), World Cancer Day on February 4, and, more recently, the Susan G. Komen Race for the Cure. These events tend to be large celebrations designed to draw public attention to the problem of breast cancer, its signs, its risk factors, its complications, and the availability of treatment. They provide opportunity to engage politicians and policy makers on how best to approach the breast cancer problem.

A structured and systematic approach to improving health behavior and practices is urgently needed. "Business-as-usual" and noninteractive approaches involving unstructured talks on radio, on TV, and at health facilities are not likely to succeed. Educational programs should be evidence led and designed to respond to prevailing knowledge, beliefs, and behaviors, using persuasive culturally sensitive communication strategies. International organizations, civil society organizations, sociologists, psychologists, health promotion specialists, journalists, survivors, and community leaders are an important resource that should be consulted to develop appropriate toolkits, multimedia materials, educational materials, etc., to help raise awareness on breast cancer. Where educational materials are lacking, health officials in LRCs do not need to start from scratch. They could adapt materials available from other LRCs or several that are freely available online from international organizations such as the NCI, CDC, British Cancer Society, and Imperial Cancer Research Fund. Several principles regarding the development, delivery, content, and target group for strategic health communication across the continuum of breast cancer care in LRCs have been published [141].

In western countries, breast cancer awareness campaigns have been successful in raising greater public awareness and uptake of screening services, raising funds, and creating more effective treatments. There is now concern that public awareness may be exploited for commercial gain (e.g., getting women to test for BRCA1 and BRCA2 status) and for courting political and electoral favors [142]. While the concerns of public health officials in LRCs are clearly different, it is important to take lessons from the issues raised.

Screening

As discussed in Chap. 4, implementing screening programs for apparently healthy women to detect premalignant breast cancer is quite challenging. There are strong opinions in the literature on the value of breast self-examination (BSE) and clinical breast examination (CBE) in both LRCs and high-income countries. What is generally agreed upon is that that mammographic screening should not be the priority of most LRCs [122, 123, 125]. BSE has been widely discredited as having no value in early detection and may even be harmful [143–147]. However, the Breast Global Health Initiative (BHGI) has cautioned against completely rejecting BSE. As it argues, the aim of BSE in LRCs is not simply to get women to regularly examine their breasts but also to become more aware of breast symptoms [125]. Several studies show that, at least in the short term, BSE improves knowledge and practices relating to breast health [148–150]. There is more support for the role of clinical breast examination (CBE) in early detection [151–153].

The lack of efficacy of SBE has been discussed at length with many researchers dismissing it as a worthwhile practice. However, in LRCs, SBE could be a useful entry point to promote and reinforce breast awareness. The consequent increase in benign tumors that may overwhelm the clinics may be a reasonable price to pay if SBE results in downstaging and better clinical outcomes for breast cancer. There is more confidence in the efficacy of CBE, though indisputable evidence is lacking. This practice is endorsed by several experts, including the BHGI for LRCs, and may be effective in detecting breast cancer [154]. The priority of early detection should be to mobilize women with symptomatic disease to report early to health facilities [122, 155]. Mammography is more useful for diagnosis than for mass screening in LRCs. However, it remains an attractive high technology device that advocacy groups and politicians in LRCs use as a measure of commitment to women's health. Mammographic screening should not be the priority in breast cancer control in most LRCs. Early detection of gynecological cancers is discussed in Chaps. 6, 7, and 8; the challenges with early detection are covered further in Chap. 12.

Tools for National Control Programs in LRCs

Many LRCs do not have an integrated policy or strategic plan on NCDs, individual NCDs, or risk factors (tobacco, alcohol, physical inactivity, unhealthy diet). In a survey conducted among 130 countries, WHO found that the proportion of countries with national policies or plans for NCD control ranged from 14% in the African region to 58% in the European region [156]. Even among 22 high-NCD burden low- and middle-income countries, only 59% had an operational integrated NCD policy and 85% had a cancer policy [157]. Countries with plans often do not include specified targets. Some progress has been made with several countries now having plans and programs, partly due to increasing prioritization of NCDs and improved capacity to develop plans and programs [158]. Cancer control plans should be updated preferably every 5 years.

The national health policy should articulate NCDs as a clear priority anchored to overall health system strengthening and improved primary health care. Some countries incorporate cancer plans into their integrated NCD policy and plans. Others have a stand-alone cancer policy or plan. Countries with more developed cancer programs may develop separate plans for common cancers such as cancers of the cervix, breast, prostate, and liver. It is not efficient to have several NCD component parallel programs as this makes coordination difficult and involves duplication of efforts.

WHO and other international organizations have developed tools to guide countries (particularly low- and middle-income countries) to advocate, plan, and implement effective cancer control programs [154, 159, 160]. WHO advocates that countries should establish comprehensive national cancer control programs that include primary prevention, screening, early diagnosis, and palliative care, and these programs should be integrated into national NCD programs. Plans on prevention and control of breast and gynecologic cancer should include advocacy, health promotion, resource mobilization, financing, capacity building, screening, early detection, with built-in methods to monitor and evaluate progress. Legislative backing of a national cancer program (as in Kenya) would help secure governmental funding for cancer-related interventions.

Conclusion

The differences in breast and gynecologic cancer mortality and access to preventive care between LRCs and the rich economies represent some of the worst global disparities. Preventing cancers implies reducing risk of the disease and detecting potential or premalignant lesions early. The priority options available to most LRCs are to improve health lifestyles and to promote early diagnosis of symptomatic cancer. Avoiding alcohol misuse, smoking, adult weight gain, obesity, physical inactivity, and shortened or absent duration of breastfeeding is amenable to individual or group actions. Enacting and enforcing national legislation to reduce lifetime exposure to risk factors and to introduce and expand HPV vaccination programs are needed.

Unlike in Western countries, awareness of breast and gynecologic health is very low among women in resource-constrained settings. There is not just the absence of accurate information but also the presence of harmful, fatalistic, and stigmatizing attributions that contribute to delays in seeking care. There is considerable scope for improving public education to improve knowledge and behavior as several studies have shown. Most women with breast cancer first notice lumps in their breast, but they do not take the appropriate action until the symptoms progress [161].

Owing to the variety of resource levels in LRCs, often a combination of interventions should be implemented to prevent breast cancer. Establishing centers of excellence is capital intensive, but it is important to provide diagnosis and quality care for breast cancer cases that are identified. Strengthening of health systems, capacity building, infrastructure, and research and health information management is all very important, since this is a prerequisite to effective breast cancer control in LRCs. In particular, political will is needed to support the implementation of national policies, plans, and programs that are developed. A major constraint to progress is the financial investment required to implement interventions. One approach to saving costs is gaining efficiency through the integration of services. The Mumbai trial and other studies demonstrate the feasibility of integrating breast cancer control together with cervical cancer control and other health services [15, 162, 163]. Other financing options are taxation of unhealthy products, resource mobilization from development partners, and the private sector and health insurance.

Monitoring and evaluation are crucial to assess progress and outcome of interventions. Most of the evidence available for breast cancer prevention is based on studies conducted in Western countries. Locally relevant studies, especially those relating to a better understanding of the biology and etiology of the disease in resource-limited settings, and behavioral research to understand care-seeking patterns are essential. The benefits of chemoprevention studies are not likely to be felt in LRCs in the near future unless low-cost options are available. International and regional cooperation is vital to ensure successful programs.

References

1. Key T, Appleby P, Barnes I, Reeves G. Endogenous sex hormones and breast cancer in postmenopausal women: reanalysis of nine prospective studies. J Natl Cancer Inst. 2002;94:606–16.
2. Colditz GA, Kaphingst KA, Hankinson SE, Rosner B. Family history and risk of breast cancer: nurses' health study. Breast Cancer Res Treat. 2012;133:1097–104.
3. Okobia M et al. Case–control study of risk factors for breast cancer in Nigerian women. Int J Cancer. 2006;119:2179–85.
4. Boyd NF, Lockwood GA, Byng JW, Tritchler DL, Yaffe MJ. Mammographic densities and breast cancer risk. Cancer Epidemiol Biomarkers Prev. 1998;7:1133–44.
5. Barnes BB, Steindorf K, Hein R, Flesch-Janys D, Chang-Claude J. Population attributable risk of invasive postmenopausal breast cancer and breast cancer subtypes for modifiable and non-modifiable risk factors. Cancer Epidemiol. 2011;35:345–52.
6. Danaei G, Vander Hoorn S, Lopez AD, Murray CJ, Ezzati M, Comparative Risk Assessment collaborating group (Cancers). Causes of cancer in the world: comparative risk assessment of nine behavioural and

environmental risk factors. Lancet. 2005;366: 1784–93.
7. International Agency for Research on Cancer. IARC handbooks of cancer prevention, Weight control and physical activity, vol. 6. Lyon: IARC; 2002.
8. Rossouw JE et al. Risks and benefits of estrogen plus progestin in healthy postmenopausal women: principal results From the Women's Health Initiative randomized controlled trial. JAMA. 2002;288:321–33.
9. Ravdin PM et al. The decrease in breast-cancer incidence in 2003 in the United States. N Engl J Med. 2007;356:1670–4.
10. Chlebowski RT et al. Estrogen alone in postmenopausal women and breast cancer detection by means of mammography and breast biopsy. J Clin Oncol. 2010;28:2690–7.
11. Jordan VC, Ford LG. Paradoxical clinical effect of estrogen on breast cancer risk: a "new" biology of estrogen-induced apoptosis. Cancer Prev Res (Phila). 2011;4:633–7.
12. Collaborative Group on Hormonal Factors in Breast Cancer. Breast cancer and hormonal contraceptives: collaborative reanalysis of individual data on 53 297 women with breast cancer and 100 239 women without breast cancer from 54 epidemiological studies. Lancet. 1996;347:1713–27.
13. Hunter DJ et al. Oral contraceptive use and breast cancer: a prospective study of young women. Cancer Epidemiol Biomarkers Prev. 2010;19:2496–502.
14. Collaborative Group on Hormonal Factors in Breast Cancer. Breast cancer and breastfeeding: collaborative reanalysis of individual data from 47 epidemiological studies in 30 countries, including 50302 women with breast cancer and 96973 women without the disease. Lancet. 2002;360:187–95.
15. Ma H, Bernstein L, Pike MC, Ursin G. Reproductive factors and breast cancer risk according to joint estrogen and progesterone receptor status: a meta-analysis of epidemiological studies. Breast Cancer Res. 2006;8:R43.
16. Lacey Jr JV et al. Breast cancer epidemiology according to recognized breast cancer risk factors in the Prostate, Lung, Colorectal and Ovarian (PLCO) Cancer Screening Trial Cohort. BMC Cancer. 2009;9:84.
17. IOM (Institute of Medicine). Breast cancer and the environment: a life course approach. Washington, DC: The National Academies Press; 2012.
18. Baan R et al. A review of human carcinogens–Part F: chemical agents and related occupations. Lancet Oncol. 2009;10:1143–4.
19. Straif K et al. Carcinogenicity of shift-work, painting, and fire-fighting. Lancet Oncol. 2007;8:1065–6.
20. The Lancet. Breast cancer on the night shift. Lancet. 2009;373:1054.
21. International Agency for Research on Cancer. Ionizing radiation, Part 1: X- and gamma (γ)-radiation, and neutrons, IARC monographs on the evaluation of carcinogenic risks to humans, vol. 75. Lyon: IARC; 2000.
22. American Cancer Society. Cancer facts and figures 2012. In: American Cancer Society, editor. Atlanta, GA; 2012.
23. Boyd J. Molecular genetics of hereditary ovarian cancer. Oncology. 1998;12:399–406; discussion 409–10, 413.
24. Aarnio M et al. Cancer risk in mutation carriers of DNA-mismatch-repair genes. Int J Cancer. 1999; 81:214–8.
25. Ziel HK. Estrogen's role in endometrial cancer. Obstet Gynecol. 1982;60:509–15.
26. Yang HS, Yoon C, Myung SK, Park SM. Effect of obesity on survival of women with epithelial ovarian cancer: a systematic review and meta-analysis of observational studies. Int J Gynecol Cancer. 2011;21: 1525–32.
27. Olsen CM et al. Obesity and the risk of epithelial ovarian cancer: a systematic review and meta-analysis. Eur J Cancer. 2007;43:690–709.
28. Zhou B, Sun Q, Cong R, Gu H, Tang N, Yang L, et al. Hormone replacement therapy and ovarian cancer risk: a meta-analysis. Gynecol Oncol. 2008; 108(3):641–51.
29. Anderson GL, Judd HL, Kaunitz AM, Barad DH, Beresford SA, Pettinger M, et al. Effects of estrogen plus progestin on gynecologic cancers and associated diagnostic procedures: the Women's Health Initiative randomized trial. JAMA. 2003;290(13):1739–48.
30. Lacey Jr JV, Brinton LA, Leitzmann MF, Mouw T, Hollenbeck A, Schatzkin A, et al. Menopausal hormone therapy and ovarian cancer risk in the National Institutes of Health-AARP Diet and Health Study Cohort. J Natl Cancer Inst. 2006;98:1397–405.
31. Gertig DM et al. Prospective study of talc use and ovarian cancer. J Natl Cancer Inst. 2000;92:249–52.
32. Collaborative Group on Epidemiological Studies of Ovarian Cancer, Beral V, Gaitskell K, Hermon C, Moser K, Reeves G, et al. Ovarian cancer and smoking: individual participant meta-analysis including 28 114 women with ovarian cancer from 51 epidemiological studies. Lancet Oncol. 2012;13:946–56.
33. Hankinson SE et al. Tubal ligation, hysterectomy, and risk of ovarian cancer. A prospective study. JAMA. 1993;270:2813–8.
34. Rosenblatt KA, Thomas DB. Reduced risk of ovarian cancer in women with a tubal ligation or hysterectomy. The World Health Organization Collaborative Study of Neoplasia and Steroid Contraceptives. Cancer Epidemiol Biomarkers Prev. 1996;5:933–5.
35. Wilailak S et al. Depot medroxyprogesterone acetate and epithelial ovarian cancer: a multicentre case–control study. BJOG. 2012;119:672–7.
36. Daly M, Obrams GI. Epidemiology and risk assessment for ovarian cancer. Semin Oncol. 1998;25: 255–64.
37. Greene MH, Clark JW, Blayney DW. The epidemiology of ovarian cancer. Semin Oncol. 1984;11:209–26.
38. Kurta ML et al. Use of fertility drugs and risk of ovarian cancer: results from a U.S.-based case-control

study. Cancer Epidemiol Biomarkers Prev. 2012;21: 1282–92.
39. Trope CG, Sabbatini PJ, Zaino RJ. Corpus: epithelial tumors. In: Hoskins WJ et al., editors. Principles and practice of gynecologic oncology. 4th ed. Philadelphia: Lippincott Williams & Wilkins; 2005.
40. Tretli S, Magnus K. Height and weight in relation to uterine corpus cancer morbidity and mortality. A follow-up study of 570,000 women in Norway. Int J Cancer. 1990;46:165–72.
41. Vasen HF et al. Cancer risk in families with hereditary nonpolyposis colorectal cancer diagnosed by mutation analysis. Gastroenterology. 1996;110:1020–7.
42. Watson P, Vasen HF, Mecklin JP, Jarvinen H, Lynch HT. The risk of endometrial cancer in hereditary nonpolyposis colorectal cancer. Am J Med. 1994;96:516–20.
43. Dunlop MG et al. Cancer risk associated with germline DNA mismatch repair gene mutations. Hum Mol Genet. 1997;6:105–10.
44. Lancaster JM et al. Society of Gynecologic Oncologists Education Committee statement on risk assessment for inherited gynecologic cancer predispositions. Gynecol Oncol. 2007;107:159–62.
45. Burke W et al. Recommendations for follow-up care of individuals with an inherited predisposition to cancer: I. hereditary nonpolyposis colon cancer. JAMA. 1997;277:915–9.
46. Mehasseb MK, Latimer JA. Controversies in the management of endometrial carcinoma: an update. Obstet Gynecol Int. 2012;2012:676032. doi:10.1155/2012/676032.
47. Fisher B et al. Tamoxifen for prevention of breast cancer: report of the National Surgical Adjuvant Breast and Bowel Project P-1 Study. J Natl Cancer Inst. 1998;90:1371–88.
48. Fisher B et al. Tamoxifen for the prevention of breast cancer: current status of the National Surgical Adjuvant Breast and Bowel Project P-1 study. J Natl Cancer Inst. 2005;97:1652–62.
49. Powles TJ, Ashley S, Tidy A, Smith IE, Dowsett M. Twenty-year follow-up of the Royal Marsden randomized, double-blinded tamoxifen breast cancer prevention trial. J Natl Cancer Inst. 2007;99: 283–90.
50. Powles T et al. Interim analysis of the incidence of breast cancer in the Royal Marsden Hospital tamoxifen randomised chemoprevention trial. Lancet. 1998;352:98–101.
51. Veronesi U et al. Prevention of breast cancer with tamoxifen: preliminary findings from the Italian randomised trial among hysterectomised women. Italian Tamoxifen Prevention Study. Lancet. 1998;352:93–7.
52. Veronesi U et al. Tamoxifen for the prevention of breast cancer: late results of the Italian Randomized Tamoxifen Prevention Trial among women with hysterectomy. J Natl Cancer Inst. 2007;99:727–37.
53. Cuzick J. Continuation of the International Breast Cancer Intervention Study (IBIS). Eur J Cancer. 1998;34:1647–8.
54. Cuzick J et al. First results from the International Breast Cancer Intervention Study (IBIS-I): a randomised prevention trial. Lancet. 2002;360:817–24.
55. Merritt MA, Cramer DW. Molecular pathogenesis of endometrial and ovarian cancer. Cancer Biomark. 2011;9:287–305.
56. Parazzini F, La Vecchia C, Negri E, Fedele L, Balotta F. Reproductive factors and risk of endometrial cancer. Am J Obstet Gynecol. 1991;164:522–7.
57. Sun XW et al. Human papillomavirus infection in women infected with the human immunodeficiency virus. N Engl J Med. 1997;337:1343–9.
58. Castle PE, Giuliano AR. Chapter 4: Genital tract infections, cervical inflammation, and antioxidant nutrients—assessing their roles as human papillomavirus cofactors. J Natl Cancer Inst Monogr. 2003; 31:29–34.
59. Smit JS et al. Cervical cancer and use of hormonal contraceptives: a systematic review. Lancet. 2003;361:1159–67.
60. Romaguera D et al. Is concordance with World Cancer Research Fund/American Institute for Cancer Research guidelines for cancer prevention related to subsequent risk of cancer? Results from the EPIC study. Am J Clin Nutr. 2012;96:150–63.
61. Secretan B et al. A review of human carcinogens? Part E: tobacco, areca nut, alcohol, coal smoke, and salted fish. Lancet Oncol. 2009;10:1033–4.
62. Luo J et al. Association of active and passive smoking with risk of breast cancer among postmenopausal women: a prospective cohort study. BMJ. 2011; 342:d1016.
63. DeRoo LA, Cummings P, Mueller BA. Smoking before the first pregnancy and the risk of breast cancer: a meta-analysis. Am J Epidemiol. 2011;174: 390–402.
64. World Health Organization. WHO report on the global tobacco epidemic, 2008: the MPOWER package. Geneva: WHO; 2008.
65. World Health Organization. WHO framework convention on tobacco control. Geneva: WHO; 2003.
66. Owusu-Dabo E, Lewis S, McNeill A, Gilmore A, Britton J. Support for smoke-free policy, and awareness of tobacco health effects and use of smoking cessation therapy in a developing country. BMC Public Health. 2011;11:572.
67. World Health Organization. Study group on economically sustainable alternatives to tobacco growing (in relation to Articles 17 and 18 of the Convention). FCTC/COP/3/11. Conference of the Parties to the WHO framework convention on tobacco control third session, Durban, 17–22 Nov 2008.
68. Collaborative Group on Hormonal Factors in Breast Cancer. Alcohol, tobacco and breast cancer—collaborative reanalysis of individual data from 53 epidemiological studies, including 58515 women with breast cancer and 95067 women without the disease. Br J Cancer. 2002;87:1234–45.
69. McCormack VA, Boffetta P. Today's lifestyles, tomorrow's cancers: trends in lifestyle risk factors

for cancer in low- and middle-income countries. Ann Oncol. 2011;22:2349–57.
70. British Medical Association. Alcohol misuse: tackling the UK epidemic. Feb 2008.
71. World Cancer Research Fund and American Institute for Cancer Research. Food, nutrition, physical activity, and the prevention of cancer: a global perspective. London: AICR; 2007.
72. Bakke Ø, Endal D. Alcohol policies out of context: drinks industry supplanting government role in alcohol policies in Sub-Saharan Africa. Addiction. 2010;105:22–8.
73. World Cancer Research Fund/American Institute of Cancer Research. The associations between food, nutrition and physical activity and the risk of breast cancer. Washington, DC: AICR; 2008.
74. Awatef M et al. Physical activity reduces breast cancer risk: a case–control study in Tunisia. Cancer Epidemiol. 2011;35:540–4.
75. Church TS, Earnest CP, Skinner JS, Blair SN. Effects of different doses of physical activity on cardiorespiratory fitness among sedentary, overweight or obese postmenopausal women with elevated blood pressure: a randomized controlled trial. JAMA. 2007;297: 2081–91.
76. Kaaks R, Lukanova A, Kurzer MS. Obesity, endogenous hormones, and endometrial cancer risk: a synthetic review. Cancer Epidemiol Biomarkers Prev. 2002;11:1531–43.
77. Arem H et al. Physical activity and endometrial cancer in a population-based case–control study. Cancer Causes Control. 2011;22:219–26.
78. World Health Organization & Food and Agricultural Organization. Diet, nutrition and the prevention of chronic diseases: report of a joint WHO/FAO expert consultation. Geneva: WHO; 2003.
79. American Heart Association Nutrition Committee et al. Diet and lifestyle recommendations revision 2006: a scientific statement from the American Heart Association Nutrition Committee. Circulation. 2006;114:82–96.
80. Mytton OT, Clarke D, Rayner M. Taxing unhealthy food and drinks to improve health. BMJ. 2012; 344:e2931.
81. World Health Organization. Global status report on noncommunicable diseases 2010. Geneva: WHO; 2011.
82. Cuzick J. Use of selective estrogen receptor modulators in the prevention of breast cancer: an overview of the randomized trials. Cancer Res 2009;69; Abstract no. 905.
83. Cuzick J et al. Preventive therapy for breast cancer: a consensus statement. Lancet Oncol. 2011;12: 496–503.
84. Cummings SR et al. The effect of raloxifene on risk of breast cancer in postmenopausal women: results from the MORE randomized trial. Multiple outcomes of raloxifene evaluation. JAMA. 1999;281:2189–97; Erratum in: JAMA 1999;2282(2122):2124.
85. Vogel VG et al. Update of the National Surgical Adjuvant Breast and Bowel Project Study of Tamoxifen and Raloxifene (STAR) P-2 Trial: preventing breast cancer. Cancer Prev Res (Phila). 2010;3:696–706.
86. Iqbal J et al. Endometrial cancer and venous thromboembolism in women under age 50 who take tamoxifen for prevention of breast cancer: a systematic review. Cancer Treat Rev. 2012;38:318–28.
87. Gail MH et al. Weighing the risks and benefits of tamoxifen treatment for preventing breast cancer. J Natl Cancer Inst. 1999;91:1829–46.
88. Ropka ME, Keim J, Philbrick JT. Patient decisions about breast cancer chemoprevention: a systematic review and meta-analysis. J Clin Oncol. 2010;28:3090–5.
89. Waters EA, Cronin KA, Graubard BI, Han PK, Freedman AN. Prevalence of tamoxifen use for breast cancer chemoprevention among U.S. women. Cancer Epidemiol Biomarkers Prev. 2010;19:443–6.
90. Cuzick J. Aromatase inhibitors for breast cancer prevention. J Clin Oncol. 2005;23:1636–43.
91. Goss PE et al. Exemestane for breast-cancer prevention in postmenopausal women. N Engl J Med. 2011;364:2381–91.
92. Bozovic-Spasojevic I, Azambuja E, McCaskill-Stevens W, Dinh P, Cardoso F. Chemoprevention for breast cancer. Cancer Treat Rev. 2012;38:329–39.
93. Chlebowski RT et al. Oral bisphosphonate use and breast cancer incidence in postmenopausal women. J Clin Oncol. 2010;28:3582–90.
94. Rennert G, Pinchev M, Rennert HS. Use of bisphosphonates and risk of postmenopausal breast cancer. J Clin Oncol. 2010;28:3577–81.
95. Rothwell PM et al. Short-term effects of daily aspirin on cancer incidence, mortality, and non-vascular death: analysis of the time course of risks and benefits in 51 randomised controlled trials. Lancet. 2012;379:1602–12.
96. Rothwell PM et al. Effect of daily aspirin on risk of cancer metastasis: a study of incident cancers during randomised controlled trials. Lancet. 2012;379: 1591–601.
97. Kahlenborn C, Modugno F, Potter DM, Severs WB. Oral contraceptive use as a risk factor for premenopausal breast cancer: a meta-analysis. Mayo Clin Proc. 2006;81:1290–302.
98. Cogliano V et al. Carcinogenicity of combined oestrogen-progestagen contraceptives and menopausal treatment. Lancet Oncol. 2005;6:552–3.
99. World Health Organization. Carcinogenicity of combined hormonal contraceptives and combined menopausal treatment. WHO, HRP, Sept 2005.
100. Kim DU, Min JW, Kim YM, Chang MC. Estimating the risks and benefits of tamoxifen for prophylactic breast cancer chemoprevention in Korea. J Breast Cancer. 2012;15:51–6.
101. Early Breast Cancer Trialists' Collaborative Group. Relevance of breast cancer hormone receptors and other factors to the efficacy of adjuvant tamoxifen: patient-level meta-analysis of randomised trials. Lancet. 2011;378:771–84.

102. Uray IP, Brown PH. Chemoprevention of hormone receptor-negative breast cancer: new approaches needed. Recent Results Cancer Res. 2011;188: 147–62.
103. Anyanwu SNC, Egwuonwu OA, Ihekwoaba EC. Acceptance and adherence to treatment among breast cancer patients in Eastern Nigeria. Breast. 2011;20:S51–5.
104. Salem DS, Kamal RM, Helal MH, Hamed ST, Abdelrazek NA, Said NH, et al. Women Health Outreach Program; a New Experience for all Egyptian Women. J Egypt Natl Canc Inst. 2008;20: 313–22.
105. Chlebowski RT, Geller ML. Adherence to endocrine therapy for breast cancer. Oncology. 2006;71:1–9.
106. Sasano H, Suzuki T. Chemoprevention of breast cancer among Asian women—its perspective and problems. Biomed Pharmacother. 2006;60:266–8.
107. Coopey SB, Mazzola E, Buckley JM et al. Clarifying the risk of breast cancer in women with atypical breast lesions. San Antonio Breast Cancer Symposium. 2011; Abstract S4–4.
108. Collaborative Group on Hormonal Factors in Breast Cancer. Breast cancer and hormone replacement therapy: collaborative reanalysis of data from 51 epidemiological studies of 52,705 women with breast cancer and 108,411 women without breast cancer. Lancet. 1997;350:1047–59.
109. Odiari EA, Chambers AN. Perceptions, attitudes, and self-management of natural menopausal symptoms in Ghanaian women. Health Care Women Int. 2012;33:560–74.
110. Im EO, Ko Y, Hwang H, Chee W. "Symptom-specific or holistic": menopausal symptom management. Health Care Women Int. 2012;33:575–92.
111. LaMontagne DS et al. Human papillomavirus vaccine delivery strategies that achieved high coverage in low- and middle-income countries. Bull World Health Organ. 2011;89:821–30B.
112. Bello FA, Enabor OO, Adewole IF. Human papilloma virus vaccination for control of cervical cancer: a challenge for developing countries. Afr J Reprod Health. 2011;15:25–30.
113. Zhang B, Beeghly-Fadiel A, Long J, Zheng W. Genetic variants associated with breast-cancer risk: comprehensive research synopsis, meta-analysis, and epidemiological evidence. Lancet Oncol. 2011;12:477–88.
114. Ghoussaini M et al. Genome-wide association analysis identifies three new breast cancer susceptibility loci. Nat Genet. 2012;44:312–8.
115. Balmaña J, Díez O, Rubio IT, Cardoso F, ESMO Guidelines Working Group. BRCA in breast cancer: ESMO clinical practice guidelines. Ann Oncol. 2011;22:31–4.
116. Hilgart JS, Coles B, Iredale R. Cancer genetic risk assessment for individuals at risk of familial breast cancer. Cochrane Database Syst Rev;2012: CD003721.
117. Herrinton LJ et al. Efficacy of prophylactic mastectomy in women with unilateral breast cancer: a cancer research network project. J Clin Oncol. 2005;23:4275–86.
118. Lostumbo L, Carbine NE, Wallace J. Prophylactic mastectomy for the prevention of breast cancer. Cochrane Database Syst Rev 2010;CD002748.
119. Brewster AM et al. Association between contralateral prophylactic mastectomy and breast cancer outcomes by hormone receptor status. Cancer. 2012;118:5637–43.
120. Rebbeck TR et al. Prophylactic oophorectomy in carriers of BRCA1 or BRCA2 mutations. N Engl J Med. 2002;346:1616–22.
121. Clegg-Lamptey JNA, Hodasi WM. A study of breast cancer in Korle Bu Teaching Hospital: assessing the impact of health education. Ghana Med J. 2007;41:72–7.
122. Corbex M, Burton R, Sancho-Garnier H. Breast cancer early detection methods for low and middle income countries, a review of the evidence. Breast. 2012;21:428–34.
123. Harford JB. Breast-cancer early detection in low-income and middle-income countries: do what you can versus one size fits all. Lancet Oncol. 2011;12:306–12.
124. World Health Organization. Cancer control: knowledge into action. WHO guide for effective programmes, module 3. Early detection. Geneva: WHO; 2007.
125. Smith RA et al. Breast cancer in limited resource countries: early detection and access to care. Breast J. 2006;12:S16–26.
126. Anderson BO. Understanding social obstacles to early breast cancer detection is critical to improving breast cancer outcome in low- and middle-resource countries. Cancer. 2010;116:4436–9.
127. Landolsi A et al. Reasons of diagnostic delay of breast cancer in Tunisian women (160 patients in the central region of Tunisia). Tunis Med. 2010;88:894–7.
128. Dye TD et al. Complex care systems in developing countries: breast cancer patient navigation in Ethiopia. Cancer. 2010;116:577–85.
129. Mousa SM, Seifeldin IA, Hablas A, Elbana ES, Soliman AS. Patterns of seeking medical care among Egyptian breast cancer patients: relationship to late-stage presentation. Breast. 2011;20:555–61.
130. Clegg-Lamptey J, Dakubo J, Attobra YN. Why do breast cancer patients report late or abscond during treatment in Ghana? A pilot study. Ghana Med J. 2009;43:127–31.
131. Thornton H, Pillarisetti RR. 'Breast awareness' and 'breast self-examination' are not the same. What do these terms mean? Why are they confused? What can we do? Eur J Cancer. 2008;44:2118–21.
132. Ghanem S et al. Knowledge of risk factors, beliefs and practices of female healthcare professionals towards breast cancer, Morocco. Pan Afr Med J. 2011;10:21.
133. Ibrahim NA, Odusanya OO. Knowledge of risk factors, beliefs and practices of female healthcare professionals

towards breast cancer in a tertiary institution in Lagos, Nigeria. BMC Cancer. 2009;9:76.
134. Nafissi N, Saghafinia M, Motamedi MH, Akbari ME. A survey of breast cancer knowledge and attitude in Iranian women. J Cancer Res Ther. 2012;8:46–9.
135. Opoku SY, Benwell M, Yarney J. Knowledge, attitudes, beliefs, behaviour and breast cancer screening practices in Ghana, West Africa. Pan Afr Med J. 2012;11:28.
136. Mayo R, Hunter A. Fatalism toward breast cancer among the women of Ghana. Health Care Women Int. 2003;24:608–16.
137. De Ver Dye T et al. A mixed-method assessment of beliefs and practice around breast cancer in Ethiopia: implications for public health programming and cancer control. Glob Public Health. 2011;6:719–31.
138. Hamad HMA. Cancer initiatives in Sudan. Ann Oncol. 2006;17:viii32–6.
139. Ibrahim NA, Oludara MA. Socio-demographic factors and reasons associated with delay in breast cancer presentation: a study in Nigerian women. Breast Cancer Res. 2012;21:416–8.
140. Burson AM et al. Clinical and epidemiologic profile of breast cancer in Tanzania. Breast Dis. 2010;31: 33–41.
141. Kreps GL, Sivaram R. Strategic health communication across the continuum of breast cancer care in limited-resource countries. Cancer. 2008;113:2331–7.
142. The Lancet Oncology. Breast-cancer awareness: too much of a good thing? Lancet Oncol. 2007;8:1041.
143. Hackshaw AK, Paul EA. Breast self-examination and death from breast cancer: a meta-analysis. Br J Cancer. 2003;88:1047–53.
144. Thomas DB et al. Randomised trial of breast self-examination in Shanghai: final results. J Natl Cancer Inst. 2002;94:1445–57.
145. Kösters JP, Gøtzsche PC. Regular self-examination or clinical examination for early detection of breast cancer. Cochrane Database Syst Rev 2003; CD14003373.
146. Nelson HD et al. Screening for breast cancer: an update for the U.S. Preventive Services Task Force. Ann Intern Med. 2009;151:W237–742.
147. Semiglazov VF et al. Results of a prospective randomized investigation [Russia (St.Petersburg)/ WHO] to evaluate the significance of self-examination for the early detection of breast cancer. Vopr Onkol. 2003;49:434–41 [In Russian].
148. Shalini, Varghese D, Nayak M. Awareness and impact of education on breast self examination among college going girls. Indian J Palliat Care 2011;17:150–4.
149. Moodi M, Mood MB, Sharifirad GR, Shahnazi H, Sharifzadeh G. Evaluation of breast self-examination program using Health Belief Model in female students. J Res Med Sci. 2011;16:316–22.
150. Shepherd JH, McInerney PA. Knowledge of breast self-examination in Sierra Leone. Curationis. 2007;30:38–44.
151. Duffy SW, Tabar L, Vitak B, Warwick J. Tumor size and breast cancer detection: what might be the effect of a less sensitive screening tool than mammography? Breast J. 2006;12:S91–5.
152. Miller AB, To T, Baines CJ, Wall C, for the Canadian National Breast Screening. Canadian National Breast Screening Study-2: 13-year results of a randomized trial in women aged 50–59 years. J Natl Cancer Inst 2000;92:1490–9.
153. Sankaranarayanan R et al. Clinical trials of cancer screening in the developing world and their impact on cancer healthcare. Ann Oncol. 2011;22:vii20–8.
154. El Saghir NS et al. Breast cancer management in low resource countries (LRCs): consensus statement from the Breast Health Global Initiative. Breast Cancer Res. 2011;20:S3–11.
155. Harford JB et al. Problem solving for breast health care delivery in low and middle resource countries (LMCs): consensus statement from the Breast Health Global Initiative. Breast. 2011;20:S20–9.
156. Alwan A. Assessment of national capacity for NCD prevention and control. Geneva: WHO; 2001.
157. Alwan A et al. Monitoring and surveillance of chronic non-communicable diseases: progress and capacity in high-burden countries. Lancet. 2010;376: 1861–8.
158. Leowski J, Krishnan A. Capacity to control noncommunicable diseases in the countries of South-East Asia. Health Policy. 2009;92:43–8.
159. World Health Organization. Cancer control: knowledge into action. WHO guide for effective programmes; module 1. Planning. Geneva: WHO; 2006.
160. Sloan FA, Gelband H. Institute of Medicine Committee on Cancer Control in Low- and Middle-Income Countries. Cancer control opportunities in low- and middle-income countries: The National Academies Press; 2007.
161. Dye TD, Bogale S, Hobden C, Tilahun Y, Deressa T, Reeler A. Experience of initial symptoms of breast cancer and triggers for action in Ethiopia. Int J Breast Cancer. 2012;2012:908547.
162. Kim JJ, Salomon JA, Weinstein MC, Goldie SJ. Packaging health services when resources are limited: the example of a cervical cancer screening visit. PLoS Med. 2006;3:e434.
163. Mittra I et al. A cluster randomized, controlled trial of breast and cervix cancer screening in Mumbai, India: methodology and interim results after three rounds of screening. Int J Cancer. 2010;126:976–84.

Combined Screening for Breast and Gynecological Cancers Using Mobile Clinics: The Barretos Experience (Brazil)

10

Adhemar Longatto Filho, Thiago Buosi Silva, Silvana Rodrigues, and Raphael Luiz Haikel Jr.

Abstract

A mobile clinic is an effective method for providing cancer screening services for women and is particularly suited for women residing in remote locations with limited access to health care. The Barretos experience of providing such services to screen for breast and gynecological cancers is presented in this chapter.

Introduction

The Department of Cancer Prevention of Barretos Cancer Hospital (Brazil) started its activities in 1994 with one of the most popular preventive tests: the Papanicolaou smear for uterine/cervical cancer diagnosis. In the beginning, the Department of Cancer Prevention was composed of two enthusiasts of prevention: Dr. Paulo Prata and Dr. Edmundo Mauad, who saw, before anyone else in the institution, the needs of cancer prevention and that this prevention should be done following the most stringent academic criteria. The herculean task began with the construction of a portable table used to perform Pap tests in the private homes of women, a table that was patented years later.

The first screening program for cervical cancer took place in a poor suburb of the city of Barretos, Brazil. It consisted of two physician-creators of the project and a technical nurse equipped with a bicycle and a portable table upon which to perform Pap tests. The nurse would bike through the poor areas of the city and offer the Pap test to women, who performed the exams in their own homes (Fig. 10.1).

This scenario experienced an important change when this activity began to draw the attention of governments and the press. In 1998, Mrs. Creuza Saure, a technical nurse, received the Woman of the Year award from UNESCO; using her bike, she had performed over 1,700 Pap tests and uncovered seven confirmed cases of cervical carcinoma.

From this exposure and with the certainty that this was the correct path to follow, the hospital, in 1998, purchased a vehicle, a VW Kombi

A.L. Filho (✉)
Department of Pathology, São Paulo State University, Dr. Arnaldo Avenue, 455, São Paulo 01246-903, Brazil
e-mail: longatto16@hotmail.com

T.B. Silva • S. Rodrigues • R.L. Haikel Jr.
Department of Cancer Prevention, Barretos Cancer Hospital, Antenor Duarte Vilela Street, 3113, Barretos 14784-400, Brazil
e-mail: tbuosi@gmail.com; silvana.rodrigues@gmail.com; raphaelhjr@gmail.com

M.K. Shetty (ed.), *Breast and Gynecological Cancers: An Integrated Approach for Screening and Early Diagnosis in Developing Countries*, DOI 10.1007/978-1-4614-1876-4_10,

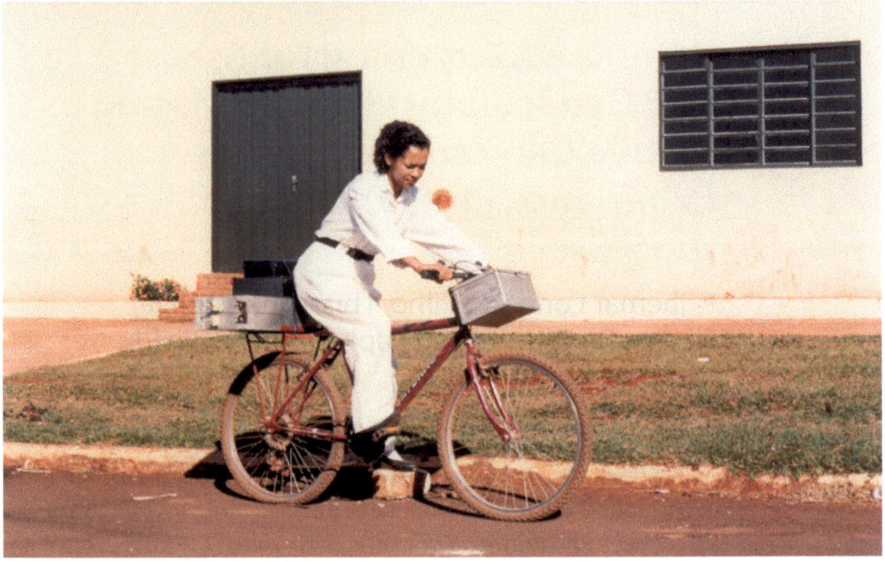

Fig. 10.1 Mrs. Creuza Saure riding her bike along the Barretos peripheral streets in early 1994. The gynecological table is located behind the bike, and the material used to collect Pap smears is located in the front

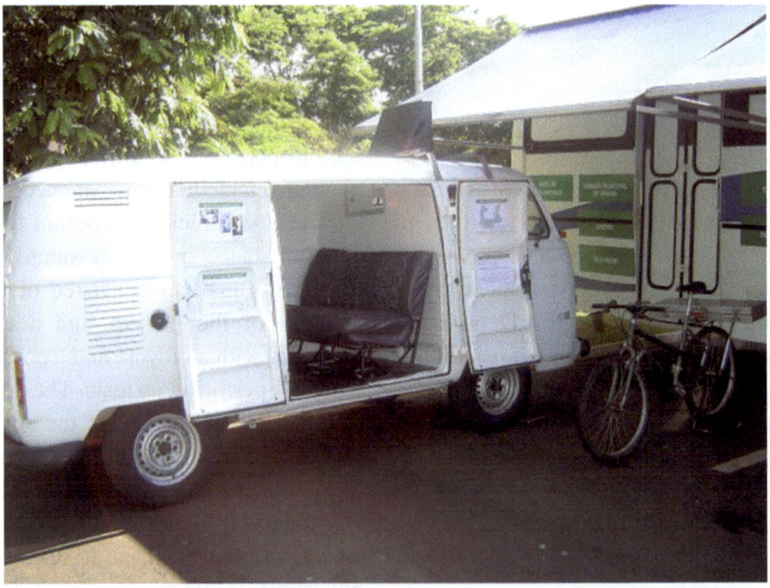

Fig. 10.2 The Kombi car was adapted to include a gynecological table used to collect pap smears

(Fig. 10.2), which was adapted, to allow for the collection of Pap smears in its interior, and which was used to initiate activities in the rural community near the city of Barretos. Concomitantly with this "innovation," the first sociocultural problems emerged because the husbands in the rural communities would not let their wives participate in the examination, as they feared exposure. The solution to this problem was to seek the help of the Barretos Military Police, who instructed police officers to help the security team. Furthermore, educational initiatives were critically important in order to optimize the explanation of the preventative cancer examina-

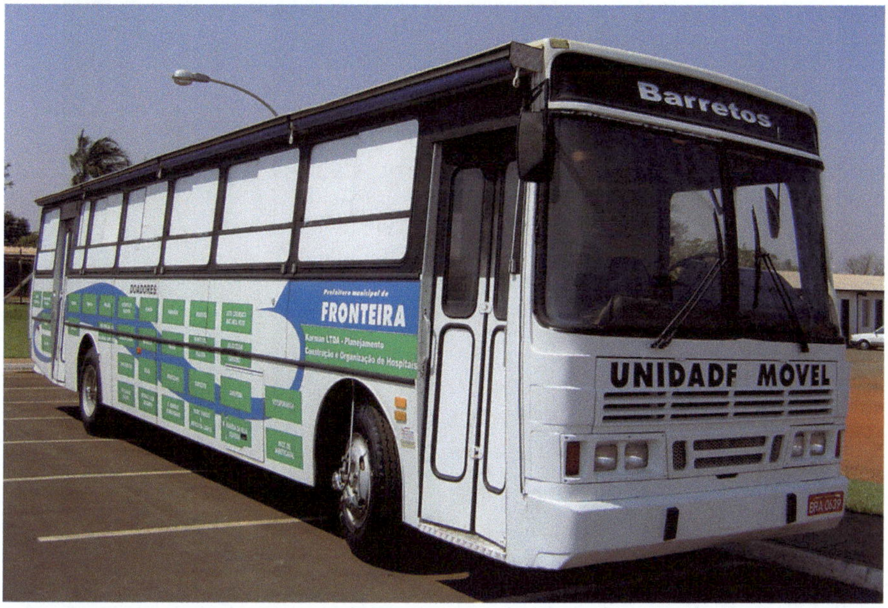

Fig. 10.3 This vehicle was our first complete ambulatory prepared for the road. It collected cervicovaginal samples, blood samples for PSA analysis, and allowed for treatment of small suspicious skin lesions

tion to the members of community, especially to the men of the town, as both these groups represented important barriers to the success of the program.

As the positive impact of this campaign increased, this "mobile idea" of implementing prevention became well-accepted by the female population and by the county's political authorities. In 2002, after the publication of the results obtained in the rural areas, Barretos Cancer Hospital acquired, through donations, its first large Mobile Unit 1 (MU1) [1]. This MU1 (Fig. 10.3) was a modified bus, carefully equipped to care for patients with regard to cervical cancer and prostate cancer prevention using the conventional Pap test, a digital rectal examination, and PSA analysis; additionally, the bus was equipped to handle detection of suspicious skin lesions and had the appropriate infrastructure to engage in minor surgical treatment within the mobile unit. The combination of different technological options and highly skilled professionals is essential to improving breast cancer detection [2, 3].

MU1 worked from 2001 to 2004, providing service in four states in Brazil (Sao Paulo, Minas Gerais, Goiás, and Mato Grosso do Sul). During these years, the team from MU1 did 57,395 cytopathological tests, 6,583 exams for prostate prevention, and 6,560 exams for skin care. All cases of cancer were referred to and treated at Barretos Cancer Hospital. Table 10.1 presents the number of tests performed in 10 years and the number of cases detected. Figure 10.4 shows the gynecological table that was part of MU1.

Table 10.1 The number of mammograms and Pap test performed during 2002–2012 (August) (The results of 2012 are partial)

Year	Mammography examinations (*n*)	Pap tests (*n*)
2002	0	423
2003	5,925	8,400
2004	6,919	11,447
2005	5,242	18,568
2006	6,932	22,136
2007	7,878	17,098
2008	31,054	20,111
2009	41,496	14,020
2010	37,267	19,921
2011	58,874	26,818
2012	38,480	15,663
Total	240,067 (100.0)	174,605

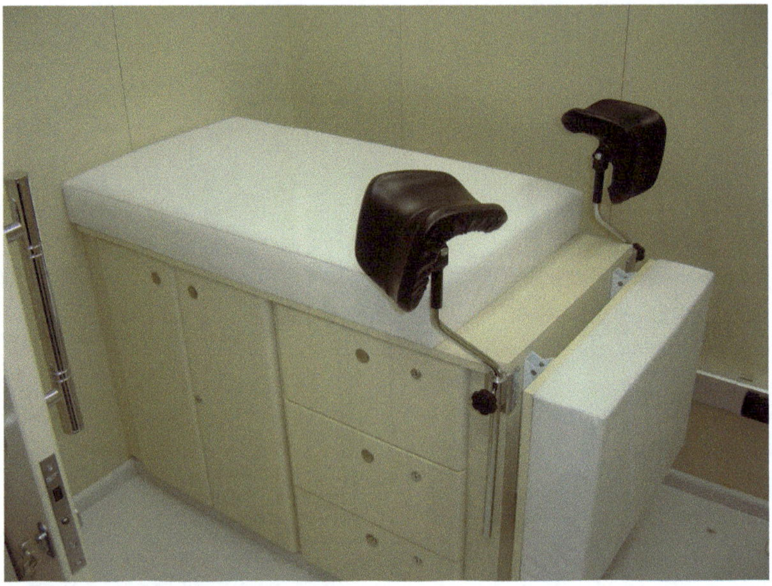

Fig. 10.4 This is an example of a gynecological table we used to put in the gynecological ambulatories of mobile units

The Years of Growing Expansion

The commitment to development, so characteristic of Barretos Cancer Hospital, was a catalyst for the exponential growth in cancer prevention activities and recruitment of professionals in the Department of Cancer Prevention starting in 2003. At this time, the Department of Cancer Prevention, which had experienced a rather timid start, had only approximately 16 professionals, taking into account all the medical doctors, nurses, technical professionals in radiology, and administrative professionals.

One of the most important initiatives was the introduction of the first mammographic screening programs that received recognition in Brazil, using the structure of the Barretos Cancer Hospital and the first mobile mammography unit, the Mobile Unit 2 (MU2) (Figs. 10.5 and 10.6). This unit was built on the platform of a bus, and it had a room with a mammography unit, a dark room, and rooms used to collect Pap smears. Figure 10.7 shows the statistics for Pap smears examined during 10 years in different Brazilian States.

This unit is still in operation and travels through 18 cities in the Regional Health Directorate of Barretos City (Diretório Regional de Saúde—DRS-V). It is responsible for screening an area with a total of more than 500,000 inhabitants and with a target audience (namely women aged 40–69 years old) that comprises more than 55,000 women. Furthermore, to the best of our knowledge, MU2 represented the first organized program of mammographic screening for breast cancer in this region and, probably, in Brazil. Figure 10.8 shows the statistics for mammograms examined in São Paulo and Bahia Juazeiro.

The Introduction of Trailers

In 2004, the bus-based MU1 was replaced by our first trailer (MU3), and, from this moment on, any boundaries to this cancer prevention program have been laid low. The MU3 truck (Fig. 10.9) that was designed for cervical cancer, prostate cancer, and skin cancer prevention was launched on September 8, 2004, in the Amazonian state of Rondonia, over

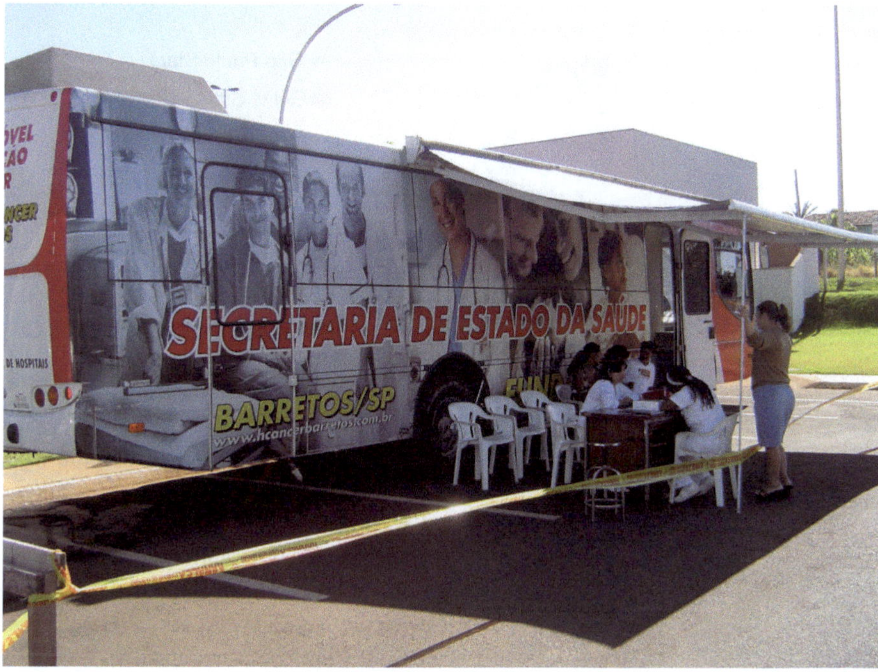

Fig. 10.5 Mobile Unit 2

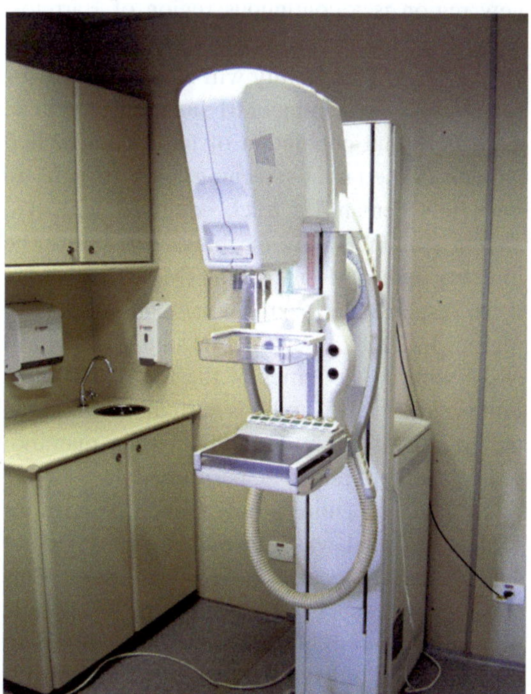

Fig. 10.6 Analog mammogram equipment in Mobile Unit 2. This was the first MU equipped with such equipment

2,000 km from the town of Barretos. At the end of 2011, the number of medical visits made by this mobile unit totaled approximately 125,000: 39,084 for cervical cancer prevention, 44,779 for prostate exams, and 40,394 for skin examinations; over 5,200 surgeries were also performed on MU3. These are amazing facts, considering the difficulties facing the vehicle when trying to negotiate inhospitable and remote areas (Fig. 10.10) or compete with the slow pace of the herds or animals on roads (Fig. 10.11).

2007 was a milestone year for the Department of Cancer Prevention and also perhaps for this new paradigm of hospital because the first combined fixed/mobile unit for cancer prevention was launched in the Brazilian northwest. This unit was designed to be located in Juazeiro County in the state of Bahia, a city with limited medical resources and with most of its population living in very poor conditions. Therefore, since 2007, this mobile unit that serves ten cities in the interior of Bahia (and that is an arm of the mammographic screening program of Barretos Cancer Hospital) helped increase early detection of breast cancer even in areas devoid of roads.

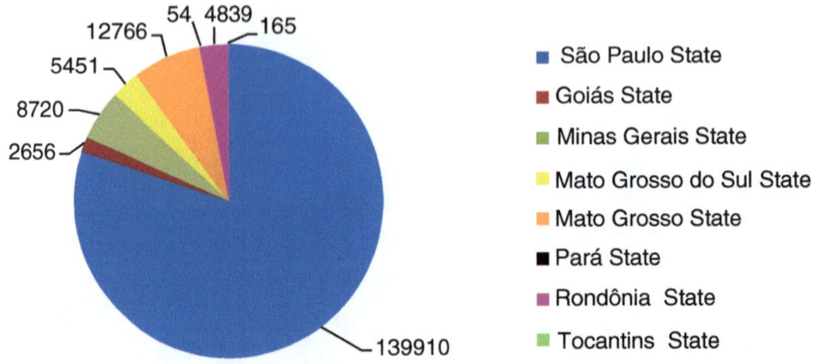

Fig. 10.7 The total number of Pap tests are depicted per State in Brazil for 2002–2011

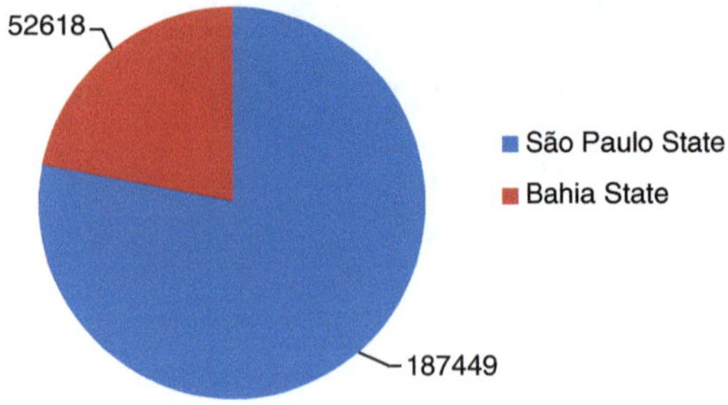

Fig. 10.8 The total number of mammograms examined in São Paulo and Bahia (Juazeiro) States for 2002–2011

Since 2007, more than 50,000 mammograms were performed in the region of Juazeiro and more than 200 cases of invasive breast cancer were diagnosed. The time elapsed since the introduction of this breast cancer program is not yet sufficient to modify the mortality curves and overall survival rates, but the 5-year period decisively improved the detection of breast cancer in its initial stages, thereby reaching levels comparable to the richest Brazilian states.

After this first, historical, qualitative leap in the prevention of breast cancer by Barretos Cancer Hospital, a remarkable new partnership in 2008 with the Avon Foundation for Women profoundly supported breast cancer prevention in Barretos by allowing for the construction of large, new headquarters for the Department of Cancer Prevention, filled with the most modern equipment and staffed by well-trained professionals (Figs. 10.12 and 10.13). Currently, all mammograms are performed by medical doctors rigorously trained in mammogram interpretation; meticulous systems to ensure the high quality, both internally and externally, for diagnoses have been implemented. We started a program for continued education and quality assurance, and a control system has been developed in association with the National Expert and Training Centre for Breast Cancer Screening (LRCB) in Holland.

With the growth of the Department and with the construction of a new building, another area was introduced into the screening program. This new region is a contiguous region of Barretos, and the screening headquarters are located at the city of Jales. This facility will be responsible for breast cancer screening in 61 small cities with an estimated total population of more than 60,000 women in the target screening ages. In order to meet this demand, a truck equipped with two analog mammography machines was built. The unit was named Mobile Unit 4 (MU4), and today it is responsible for the examination of that region. In 2008, a new mobile unit was built to assist with the activities of the MU2. This new unit is called MU5, and it is currently working in the region of Barretos, allowing for mammograms and Pap tests to be performed.

In 2010, an entirely new branch of Barretos Cancer Hospital was constructed in the city of Jales, remotely located in São Paulo State. This was long overdue. Following this, the first mobile unit with two digital mammogram machines (Mobile Unit 6, MU6) (Figs. 10.14 and 10.15) was launched with a very patient-friendly design that included a comfortable waiting room (Fig. 10.16).

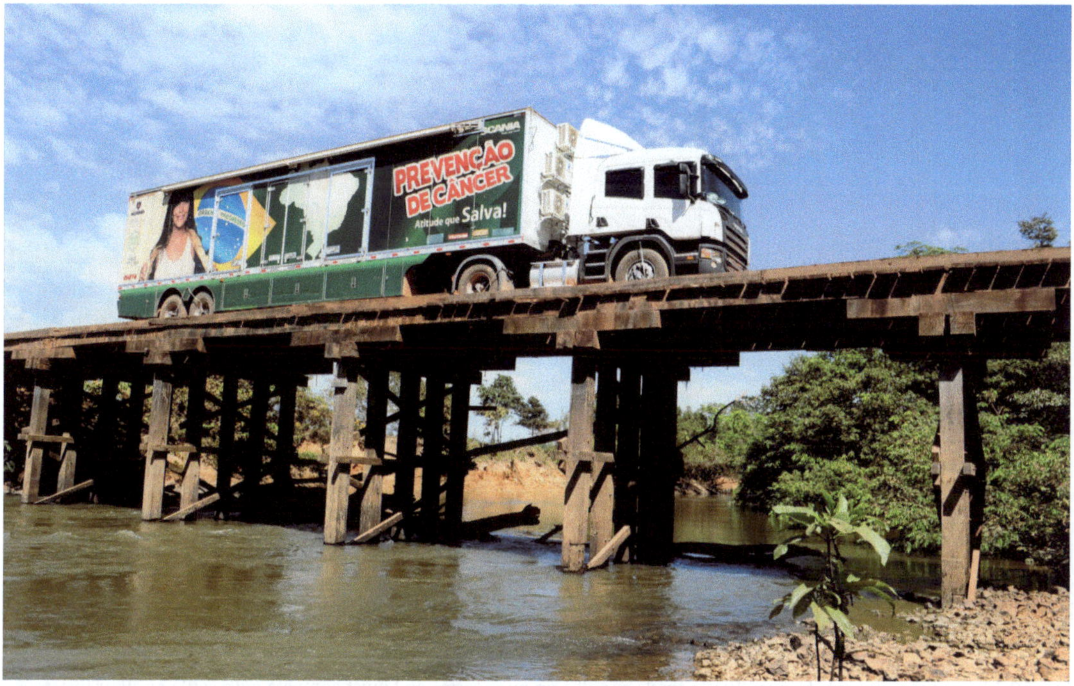

Fig. 10.9 Mobile Unit 3 crossing a wooden bridge in a rural area of Brazil

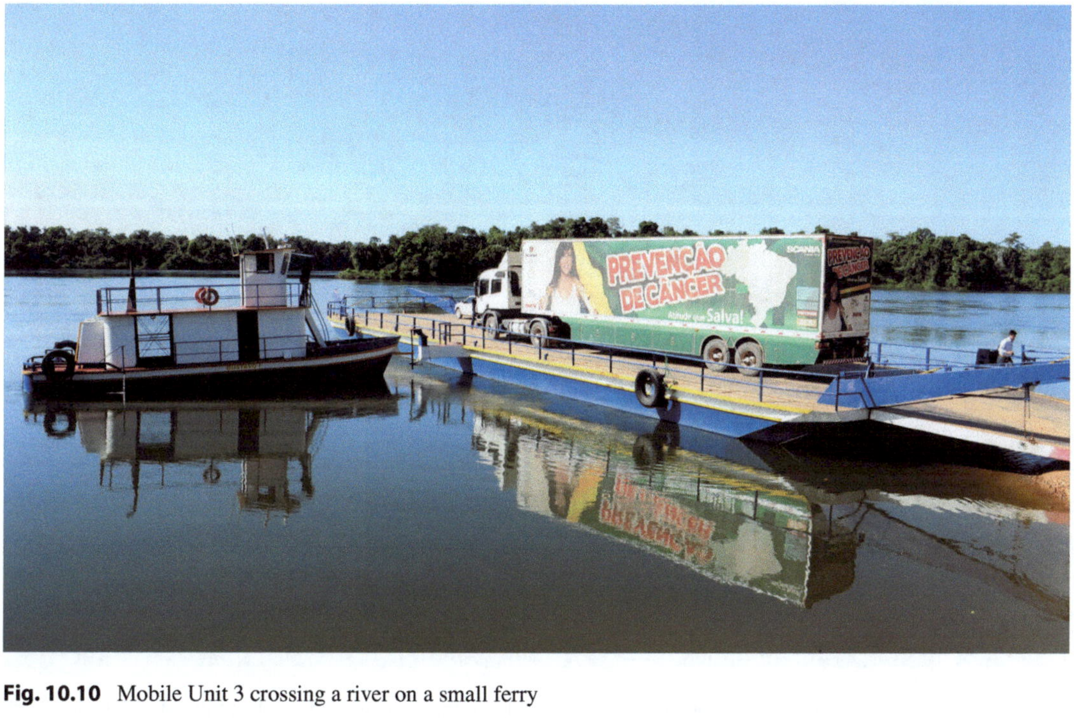

Fig. 10.10 Mobile Unit 3 crossing a river on a small ferry

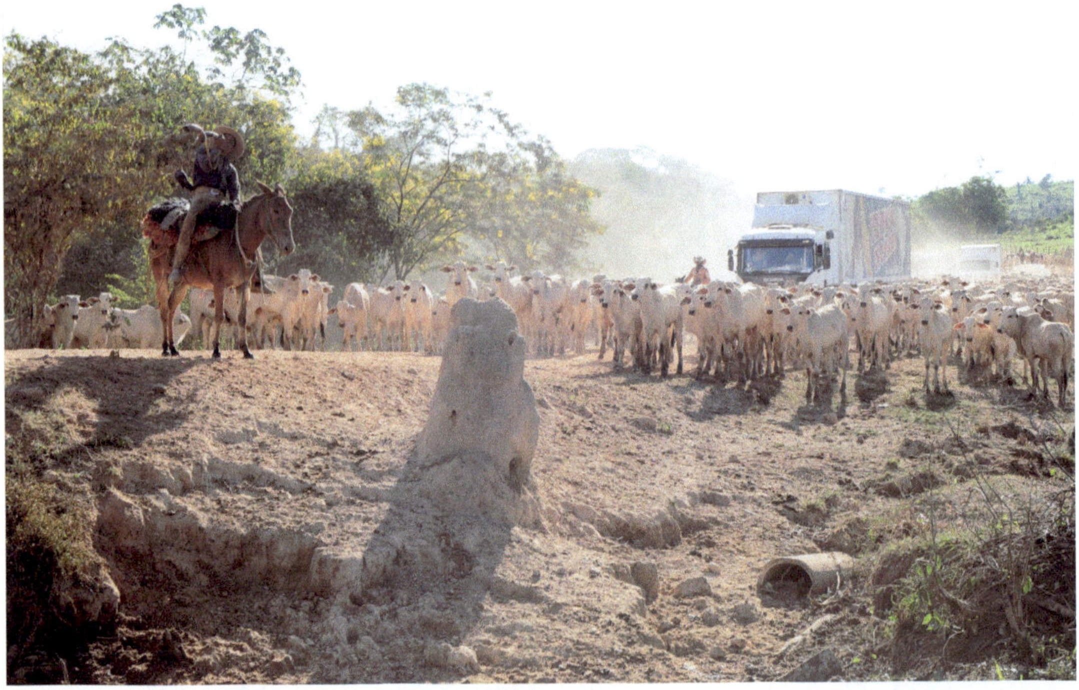

Fig. 10.11 The mobile units frequently use roads or paths on huge farms and must compete with cattle or other livestock

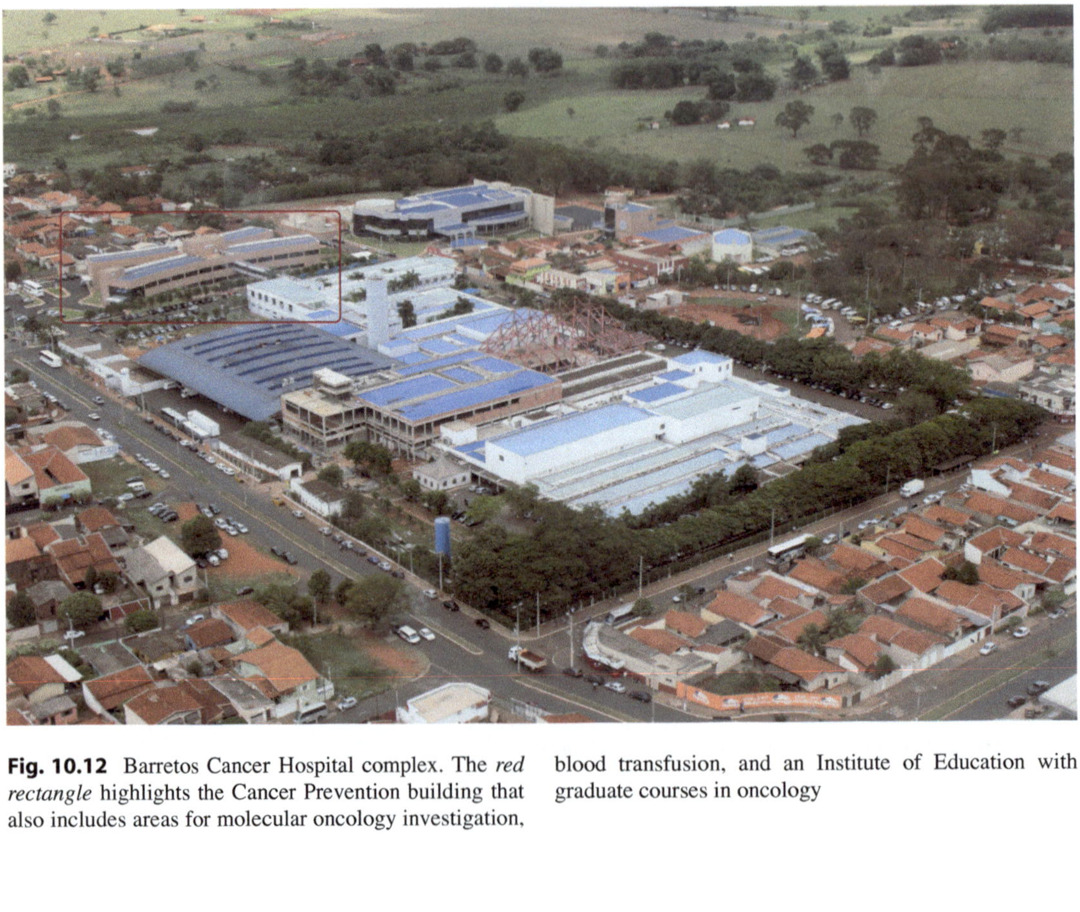

Fig. 10.12 Barretos Cancer Hospital complex. The *red rectangle* highlights the Cancer Prevention building that also includes areas for molecular oncology investigation, blood transfusion, and an Institute of Education with graduate courses in oncology

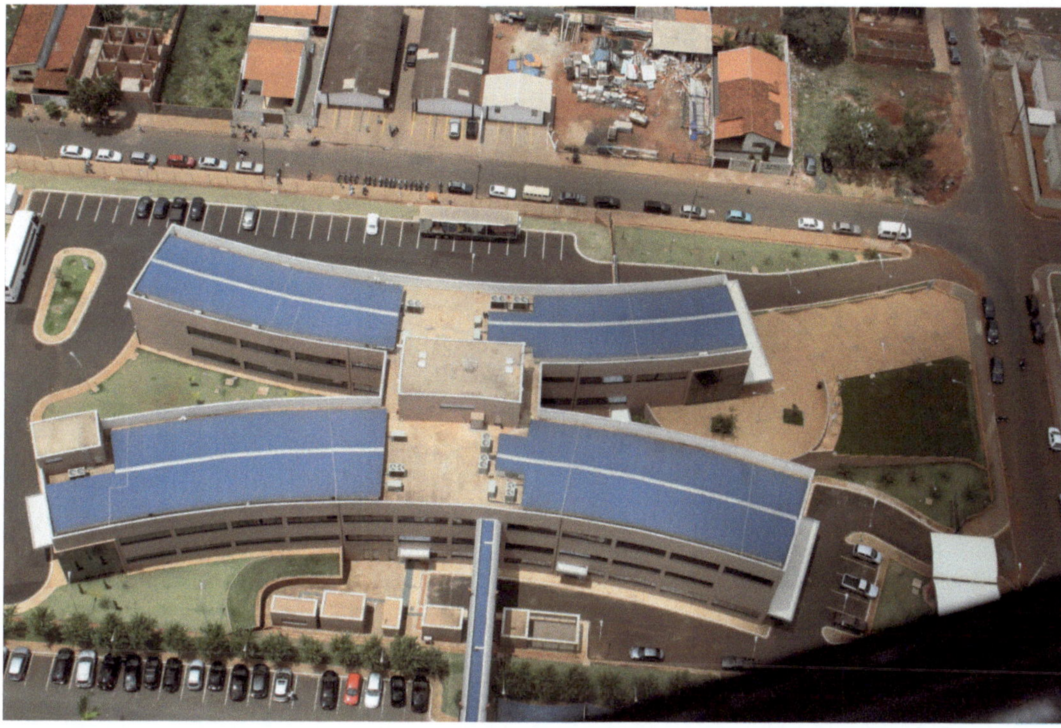

Fig. 10.13 Aerial view of the Cancer Prevention building

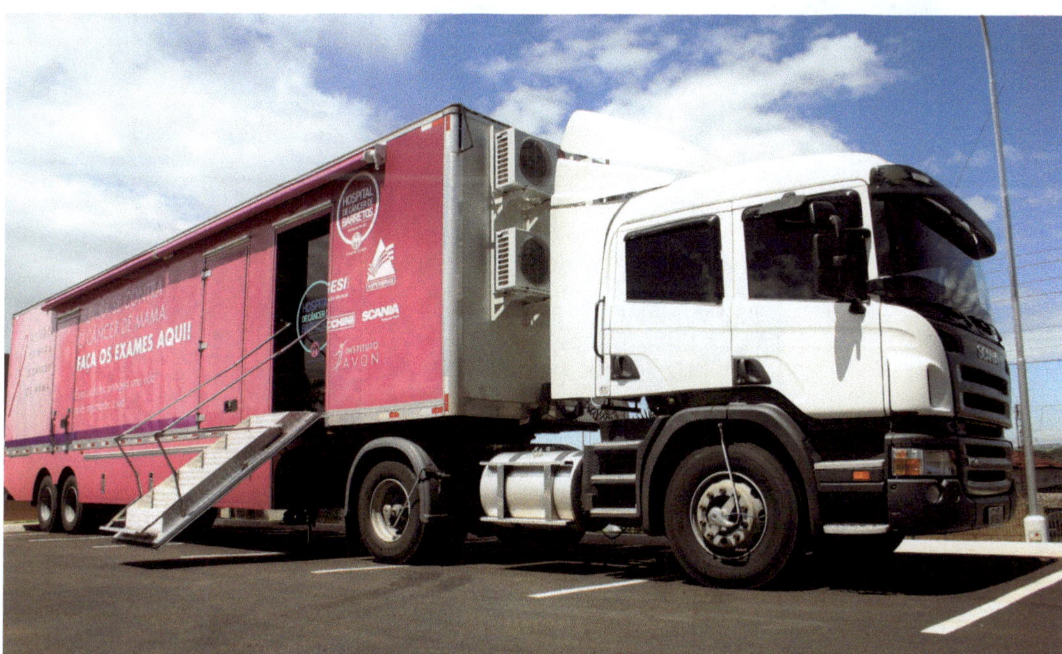

Fig. 10.14 The modern Mobile Unit 6 is a very robust vehicle with the capacity to cross remote rural areas with great autonomy

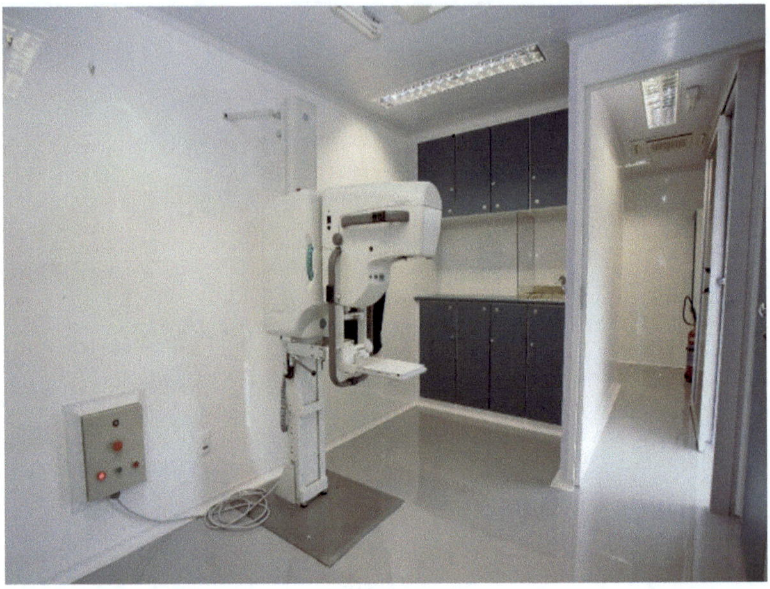

Fig. 10.15 Analog mammography equipment currently available to the poor population in mobile/fixed units in Barretos and Jales

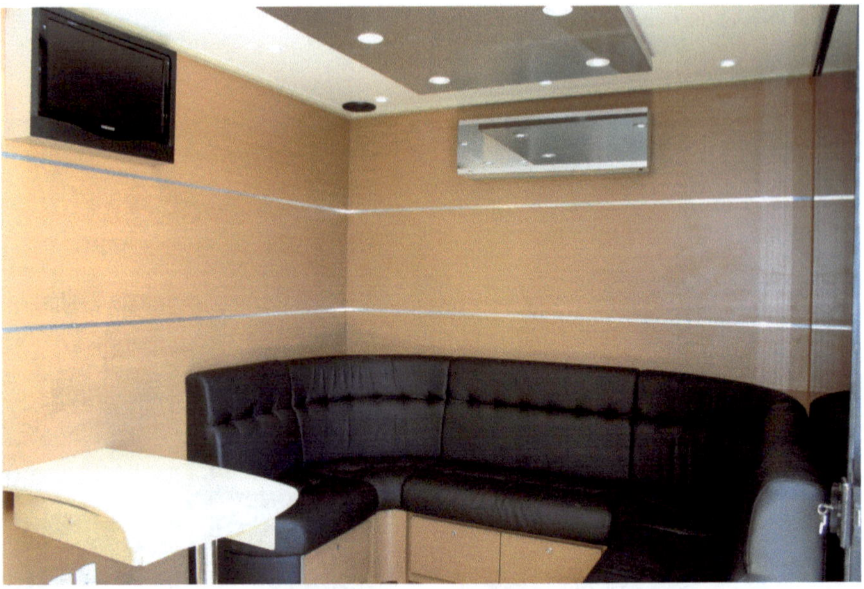

Fig. 10.16 Waiting room inside the Mobile Unit 6

Closing Remarks

Currently, besides the enormous physical and technological changes, the construction of new buildings for cancer prevention, and the modernization of equipment and long distance communication technology, we are experiencing an substantial increase in the quality of our partnership with the LRCB institute, which is responsible for the quality control of mammographic screening in Barretos Cancer Hospital. Due to this, the Department of Cancer Prevention has an external audit of international quality. This approach was critical in order to minimize errors in our enormous quantity of exams and maintain a high level of diagnostic quality. Similarly, the quality of cervical cancer screening has also improved with the introduction of Surepath™ (BD, Franklin Lakes, NJ), a liquid-based cytology technology, and Focalpoint™ (BD, Franklin Lakes, NJ), an automated imaging system primarily developed to assist in the screening of BD SurePath™ liquid-based cytology, but also a useful tool for the analysis of conventional preparations.

At present, the Department of Cancer Prevention has more than 120 employees, including physicians, nurses, technicians, radiology technicians, physicists, computer programmers, information technology personnel, researchers, and administrative staff. By the end of 2015, five new centers for cancer prevention in northern, southwestern, and midwestern Brazilian regions will have been built, demonstrating that there are no limits to this cancer prevention program. These new centers will carry out organized screening for breast and uterine/cervical cancer, in addition to prostate cancer screening and early treatment of skin cancer. Each of these five fixed prevention units will have a mobile unit to support mobile cancer prevention and facilitate medical assistance [4, 5].

The educational paradigm experienced a shift as well. In the near future, the first mobile cancer education mobile unit will be launched. Its purpose will be to disseminate continued education in cancer prevention in a context provisionally named Program of Knowledge and Culture Dissemination from Barretos Cancer Hospital. It will aim to educate children and adults about the options for cancer prevention (including behavioral options) and in the knowledge of different types of cancer, including cervical and breast cancer.

The Department of Cancer Prevention continues to grow in providing and amplifying medical assistance in rural and remote areas of Brazil. We started our journey using a bicycle, and now we are using six mobile units, trucks, buses, and new cancer prevention centers. The emerging high-technology for early cancer detection encourages us to hope for new developments such as HPV testing for cervical cancer prevention and, in the foreseeable future, our own company that will undertake the construction and launching of more mobile units.

Acknowledgements The authors are indebted to: Dr. Edmundo Mauad, head of the Department of Cancer Prevention of Barretos Cancer Hospital, for the constant encouragement and enthusiasm for cancer prevention activities; to Dr Cristovam Scapulatempo, director of the Pathology Department, and his colleagues who provide us with the best support for cytopathological examination; and to all the professional staff of the Department of Cancer Prevention and the professionals that travel in the mobile units for their unflagging commitment to cancer prevention.

References

1. Mauad EC, Gomes UA, Nogueira JL, Melani AG, Lemos DL, Hidalgo GS. Prevention of cervical cancer in a poor population in Brazil. Fam Pract. 2002; 19(2):189–92.
2. Shetty MK, Longatto-Filho A. Early detection of breast, cervical, ovarian and endometrial cancers in low resource countries: an integrated approach. Indian J Surg Oncol. 2011;2(3):165–71.
3. Mauad EC, Silva TB, Haikel Jr RL, Bauab S, Longatto-Filho A. Is community intervention in breast cancer screening in Brazil feasible? J Med Screen. 2011;18(1):51.
4. Mauad EC, Nicolau SM, Gome UA, Da Costa Vieira RA, de Castro Mattos JS, Longatto-Filho A, Baracat EC. Can mobile units improve the strategies for cervical cancer prevention? Diagn Cytopathol. 2010; 38(10):727–30.
5. Mauad EC, Nicolau SM, Moreira LF, Haikel Jr RL, Longatto-Filho A, Baracat EC. Adherence to cervical and breast cancer programs is crucial to improving screening performance. Rural Remote Health. 2009; 9(3):1241.

Cost-Effectiveness of Screening for and Early Diagnosis of Breast and Gynecological Cancers in Low-Income Countries

11

Sujha Subramanian

Abstract

Screening and diagnosis provided for breast and gynecological cancers in the low-resource setting should be based not only on cost-effectiveness but also on affordability to ensure that large-scale implementation is possible. Over the past two decades, with the growing importance of economic evaluations in informing health care planning, a large number of cost-effectiveness assessments have been published for high-income countries, but these studies unfortunately have limited generalizability to low- or even middle-income countries. Only a few studies have been published on cost-effectiveness of screening in the resource-limited setting for breast and cervical cancer. In general, these studies support the use of clinical breast exams for breast cancer screening and the use of visual inspection with acetic acid or human papillomavirus (HPV) DNA testing for cervical cancer screening. HPV vaccination of adolescent girls can also be cost-effective, but the cost of both HPV vaccination and HPV DNA testing has to be quite low to make them affordable in the low-resource setting. No study to date has directly addressed the cost-effectiveness of providing integrated cancer screening, that is, combining breast and cervical cancer screening along with diagnostic evaluation for other gynecological cancers into a single visit. Integrating cancer screening services for women can potentially result in lower costs due to efficiencies for both the provider and the patient. On the provider side, synergies can reduce health care costs as a person is seen once for several screening tests and not multiple times. For the patient, a single trip is efficient and can reduce transportation and child care costs. Targeted screening trials and cost-effectiveness modeling are urgently needed to fully understand the impact of packaging screening for multiple cancers on the overall cost and effectiveness in the low-income setting.

S. Subramanian (✉)
RTI International, Waltham, MA 02451, USA
e-mail: ssubramanian@rti.org

M.K. Shetty (ed.), *Breast and Gynecological Cancers: An Integrated Approach for Screening and Early Diagnosis in Developing Countries*, DOI 10.1007/978-1-4614-1876-4_11,

Introduction

In the low-resource setting, it is essential that screening and diagnosis provided for breast and gynecological cancers are affordable and can be implemented on a large scale. Therefore, it is critical to identify not only the most cost-effective screening tests but also the most efficient screening delivery procedures to make cancer screening viable with very limited funding. Inexpensive but effective screening tests that do not require complicated screening delivery procedures are ideal. Combined screening for multiple cancers has been advocated in the low-resource setting in an attempt to reduce the overall screening delivery cost [1, 2].

In this chapter, we provide an overview of the cost-effectiveness of screening for breast and gynecological cancers and offer recommendations to address the gaps in knowledge in order to move the field forward. We begin with a discussion of the key attributes of economic evaluation with the focus on cost-effectiveness methodology. After that, we provide a review of cost-effectiveness modeling studies that have been performed to evaluate interventions that should be adopted in low-resource countries to screen for breast and cervical cancers. Then we discuss the evidence required to assess the benefits of combining or packaging multiple cancer screening, and, finally, we conclude with a discussion of the role of cost-effectiveness analysis in formulating cancer screening policies in the low-resource setting.

Overview of Cost-Effectiveness Methodology

The impact of cancer screening needs to be measured along the continuum of cancer care to ensure a comprehensive assessment of the benefits and costs. Although much of the costs of cancer screening are experienced in the short term, the benefits, when measured in terms of mortality and health-related quality of life (HRQL), are observed over the entire life span. A framework for assessing the economic costs and effectiveness of cancer-related interventions is provided in Fig. 11.1.

With the initiation of cancer screening, the following benefits and costs can be anticipated:

- Earlier disease stage at diagnosis and better treatment response
- Higher screening/diagnosis cost but lower treatment cost
- Increase in HRQL
- Decrease in morbidity (less burden on family members and community)
- Decrease in mortality

Therefore, although assessment of intermediate costs and outcomes can provide valuable information on the impact of cancer screening, comprehensive and complete assessment of the cost-effectiveness of the interventions requires modeling the impacts over the entire life span.

Cost-effectiveness analysis can be performed using a number of different perspectives. The broadest and most comprehensive is the societal perspective, since it includes all costs and outcomes shown in Fig. 11.1. Analyses performed from the program perspective or the provider perspective consider a narrower range of costs and effectiveness measures. The findings from the economic assessment can differ based on the perspective selected and therefore is a critical methodological decision. All key guidelines on cost-effectiveness assessment have advocated for the use of the societal perspective, and, in instances when other perspectives are required, they should be reported in addition to the societal perspective [3–6]. The major obstacle to reporting the costs and outcomes using a societal perspective is the availability of valid information to populate all the data parameters required for the analysis.

Objectives of Economics Evaluations of Cancer Screening Interventions

The resources available for delivering health care services are finite, and, furthermore, in the case of low-resource countries, the funding available is very limited. Economic assessments play a key

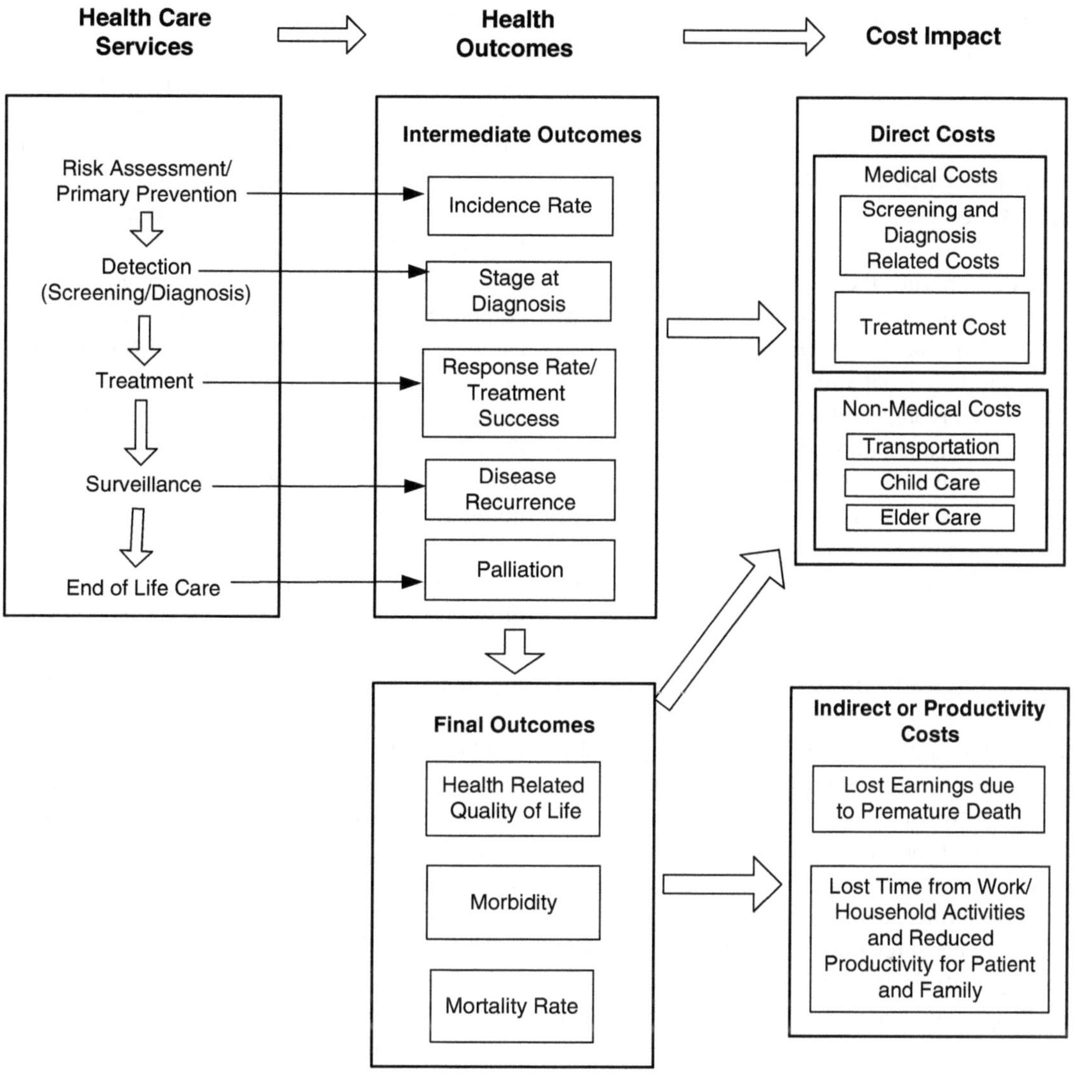

Fig. 11.1 Framework for assessing economic costs of cancer along the continuum of care

role in the selection of interventions and policies to improve cancer care and reduce the burden of cancer. Specifically, the objectives of economic studies are the following:

1. *To allocate resources efficiently*: Cost-effectiveness analysis allows the comparison of interventions in order to identify the ones that are the most cost-effective—that is, the interventions that provide the highest level of benefits for the resources expended
2. *To assess resource requirements*: Budget impact analysis provides information to estimate the costs required in various budget periods—critical for the successful implementation of selected screening tests and interventions
3. *To formulate cancer screening policy*: The information on cost-effectiveness and resource requirements assists policy makers to advocate for and allocate funding for cancer screening programs

In addition to informing the planning process, economic evaluations can be used to monitor the cost-effectiveness of screening programs using data from real-world implementation, and the findings can help to further improve the screening delivery process and make it more efficient whenever possible.

Weighing the Cost Versus Effectiveness

When comparing the cost and effectiveness of interventions, there are several possible scenarios. For instance, if an intervention has lower costs and better outcomes compared to another, then it is favored and should be selected; this principle is called dominance. If an intervention is more costly but yields better outcomes than the other, then additional assessment is required. The intervention is only cost-effective if the additional effectiveness justifies its additional cost. There are three methods to simultaneously consider the cost and effectiveness of an intervention: cost-effectiveness analysis, cost–benefit analysis, and cost–utility analysis. In each of these three approaches, the results are provided as a cost per unit of effectiveness and derived from the ratio of the cost divided by the effectiveness unit. Table 11.1 presents the differences between the three approaches. Cost-effectiveness and cost–utility analysis are commonly used to assess cancer screening intervention, while cost–benefit analysis is seldom used because of the challenges associated with reporting outcomes in monetary units.

Costs reported in cost-effectiveness assessment are presented in the local currency, US dollars, or "international dollar." The international dollar is the most appropriate for comparison between countries as it is a theoretical currency based on the purchasing power parity (PPP) of each country. PPP is the money that would be required to purchase the same goods and services in each country so valid comparisons can be made across countries. The base case comparison for the international dollar is the US PPP which is set to 1. International $1 has the same purchasing power as $1 has in the United States, but PPP adjusted figures are not expressed in US dollars to avoid confusion with nominal figures.

Health metrics that combine mortality, morbidity, and HRQL into a single measure are increasingly used by researchers and policy makers to assess the overall effectiveness. Several summary measures including the following are available: quality-adjusted life years (QALYs), disability-adjusted life years (DALYs), healthy life years (HLY), and years lived with disability (YLDs). All these measures are derived from two components: (1) life-expectancy or mortality estimates and (2) morbidity and HRQL impacts of the disease. The two measures often used in cost-effectiveness models are the QALY and DALY. There is no consensus on which outcome measure is the most appropriate to use in economic evaluation [7, 8].

The incremental cost-effectiveness ratio is required to evaluate the cost and benefits of the proposed intervention against the gold standard or "no intervention." In the case of cancer screening in the low-resource setting, the comparator chosen is usually the scenario with no screening available. When comparing two scenarios, for instance A (screening) and B (no screening), where A is more effective but also more costly, the ratio is simply the change in cost divided by the change in effectiveness of A and B:

$$\frac{\text{Cost}_{\text{Scenario A}} - \text{Cost}_{\text{Scenario B}}}{\text{Effectiveness}_{\text{Scenario A}} - \text{Effectiveness}_{\text{Scenario B}}}.$$

The resulting value is the cost to obtain each unit of increased effectiveness associated with program A. This incremental cost-effectiveness ratio for scenario A needs to be compared with the threshold for cost-effectiveness ratios to recommend adoption.

Based on the recommendations of the World Health Organization (WHO) Commission on Macroeconomics and Health [4], threshold values adopted for cost-effectiveness are based on the gross domestic product (GDP) data as these data are accessible indicators reported by all countries. The commonly accepted threshold values are highly cost-effective if less than GDP per capita, cost-effective if between one and three times GDP per capita, and not cost-effective if more than three times GDP per capita (see http://

Table 11.1 Comparison of cost-effectiveness, cost–benefit, and cost–utility analysis

Method	Cost measure	Effectiveness measure	Ratio
Cost-effectiveness analysis (CEA)	International dollar (Int. $)	Natural units, for example, life years saved (LYS)	Cost per LYS
Cost–benefit analysis (CBA)	Int. $	Monetary value (Int. $)	Cost per Int. $1 of benefit
Cost–utility analysis (CUA)	Int. $	Years of life gained adjusted for quality of life Quality-adjusted life years (QALY) or disability-adjusted life years (DALY)	Cost per QALY or DALY

www.who.int/choice/costs/CER_thresholds/en/index.html). In general, when considering the low-income, high-mortality countries in Asia and Africa, cost less than International $2,000 per unit of effectiveness (such as life years gained) can be considered highly cost-effective and cost between International $2,000 and $6,000 can be considered cost-effective.

Summary of Current Cost-Effectiveness Research

Over the past two decades, with the growing importance of economic evaluations in informing health care planning, a large number of cost-effectiveness assessments have been published. The majority of these studies on cancer screening have been targeted at assessing screening interventions in high-income countries. These studies unfortunately have limited generalizability to low- or even middle-income countries. A few studies though have been published on the cost-effectiveness of screening in the low-resource setting. In this section, we review these studies to understand the types of analyses that have been performed, the findings from these assessments, and their implications for cancer screening policies. We focused our assessment on modeling studies that allow for the inclusion of costs and outcomes over the entire life span. A targeted literature search was performed using PubMed, and citations of the manuscripts initially identified were reviewed to select additional publications. We only included peer-reviewed manuscripts in our final list of studies that were systematically reviewed. When multiple studies were available using the same model or similar studies for the same country, we selected the most up-to-date assessment [9–12]. In addition, we focused on studies related to adolescent girls and women only and excluded any studies that assessed HPV vaccination for boys [13]. The majority of the studies selected performed assessments directly related to low-income countries, but we did include a few models from middle-income countries as these may provide valuable lessons for cancer screening in the low-resource setting. For each study, we present the country or region of relevance, the interventions or tests compared, the intervention identified as the most cost-effective, and the incremental cost-effectiveness ratio of this intervention (generally compared to no screening).

Breast Cancer Screening

We identified seven studies that met our selection criteria, and these studies were published starting in the year 1998 to the present (Table 11.2). Five of the articles reported results based on parameters relevant to a specific country (Taiwan, India, Brazil, and Ghana) [14–18], while two of the studies focused on regions (Asia and Africa) [19, 20]. The interventions assessed ranged from media campaign to increased awareness, screening using either CBE or mammography, and offering only treatment when cancer was diagnosed. The studies varied in the age range recommended for screening, the interval between screens, and the types of interventions compared. A study on

Table 11.2 Cost-effectiveness studies on breast cancer screening and other interventions to reduce disease burden

References	Country	Interventions/tests compared	Most cost-effective intervention: Screening schedule	Cost-effective ratio
[14]	Taiwan	2 Rounds of screening mammogram 1 year apart for high-risk and mass screening	High-risk women 2 rounds of mammography 1-year interval age 35 and older	US$4,851 per LYS
[19]	Africa Asia	Treating each stage, all stages, extensive program (treating all stages, awareness program, and mammography)	Extensive program (mammography 2-year interval age 50–70, awareness program, and treatment)	US$75 per DALY averted US$77 per DALY averted
[16]	India	CBE annually age 40–60, CBE every 5 years age 40–60, CBE at age 50, mammography at age 50, mammography at varied time intervals	CBE age 50	Int. $794 per LYS
[17]	Mexico	Varied starting age (40–50 years), covered population, and frequency of mammography	Mammography 2-year interval (age 48 with 25 % coverage; age 40 with 50 % coverage)	Int. $10,027 to $15,508 per LYS
[15]	India	CBE and mammography at various intervals and age ranges	CBE 5-year interval age 40–60	US$450 per LYS
[20]	Sub-Saharan Africa South East Asia	Treating each stage, treating all stages, and optimal program (treatment and screening mammography)	Optimal program (mammography every 2 years age 50–70)	Approx. Int. $2,500 per DALY averted Approx. Int. $4,500 per DALY averted
[18]	Ghana	CBE, mammography, and mass media awareness rising	CBE 2-year interval age 40–69	US$1,299 per DALY averted

CBE clinical breast exam; *DALY* disability-adjusted life years; *Int. $* international dollar; *LYS* life years saved

Taiwanese women [14] was the only model that compared screening high-risk women vs. average-risk women using mammography, and the conclusion reached was that mammography was not a cost-effective option for mass screening. The most cost-effective option was to screen high-risk women 35 years and older using two rounds of mammography with a 1-year interval.

Two models that assessed screening and treatment options for the Asia and Africa regions (note: not specific countries) found programs that included mammography screening to be more cost-effective than providing breast cancer treatment alone. Although these studies reached the same conclusion, incremental cost-effectiveness ratios reported were very different and can be due to the parameter values and model assumptions. The final study on mammography in Mexico concluded that, with incremental cost-effectiveness ratios ranging from Int. $10,027 to $15,508 per life years saved, mammography screening was cost-effective for the Mexican setting. These ratios would not be cost-effective for low-income countries. It is important to note that none of these studies included CBE as a comparator.

The three studies that compared CBE and mammography [15, 16, 18] concluded that CBE was the most cost-effective approach. The CBE screening options reported as cost-effective were once in a lifetime CBE at age 50, CBE at 5-year interval between the ages of 40 and 60 years, and CBE at 2-year intervals from age 40 to 69 years. All the reported incremental cost-effectiveness ratios are below Int. $2,000 and therefore can be considered highly cost-effective in low-income countries.

Since the models did not compare the same interventions, it is not possible to reach firm conclusions based on the seven studies reviewed. CBE appears to be the most cost-effective option, but the most efficient screening schedule using CBE (age range and screening interval) is not clear. Further modeling assessments are required to clarify the optimal CBE schedule, and this schedule may differ among the low-resource countries due to country-level differences, which can include differences in cancer epidemiology and cost.

Cervical Cancer Screening

We identified 14 studies that met our inclusion criteria: two studies included only cytology testing and assessed cost and effectiveness of different schedules [21, 22], four other studies assessed HPV vaccination only [23–26], and the remaining eight studies compared multiple modalities which usually included VIA, cytology, and HPV DNA testing; two studies also included HPV vaccination (Table 11.3) [15, 20, 27–32]. Seven out of eight studies that compared multiple screening modalities concluded that either VIA or HPV DNA were the most cost-effective approach; one found that VIA, when followed by cytology between the ages of 50 and 60, was the most cost-effective [30]. Only one study found cytology to be the most effective option, but this study did not focus on a particular country and developed models for the South East Asian and Sub-Saharan African regions as a whole to represent high child and high adult mortality countries.

Among the studies advocating VIA and HPV DNA, multiple screening regiments were assessed, and there is no consensus on the one standard schedule that is the most cost-effective. The screening scenarios range from single lifetime VIA or HPV DNA testing to repeated testing every 5 years. There is also variation as to whether the screening and diagnosis should be performed in a single visit or multiple visits. All the incremental cost-effectiveness ratios reported are under Int. $2,000, and therefore these screening schedules are very cost-effective even in the low-resource setting. In some countries, cost as low as Int. $10 per life years saved is possible, making cervical cancer screening a highly efficient public health strategy. Multiple studies also found that even once-in-a-lifetime single visit VIA screening can be effective in reducing mortality and this is highly cost-effective and potentially affordable even in the very low-resource setting. Further research though is needed to understand to what extent compliance with screening recommendations will impact the cost-effectiveness of alternate strategies. A few studies did attempt to include patient compliance in the model estimation [21, 22], but this needs to be incorporated more consistently to provide valuable input to guide decisions related to cancer screening policies.

The six studies that modeled the use of HPV vaccination in general concluded that the vaccination would be cost-effective in low-resource countries if the price was favorable. The vaccine would be cost-effective in Asia if the cost of the three-dose HPV vaccination was Int. $10; that is about US$2 per dose. In the Central American and the Caribbean region, a higher vaccination cost of Int. $25 (about US$5 per dose) is cost-effective. The cost of even US$2 may not be affordable for low-income countries, and, therefore, even though the cost-effectiveness has been established, the funding may not be available to implement a program that is estimated to cost millions. The GAVI alliance countries may be eligible for obtaining the HPV vaccine at a subsidized price, and this may make it more affordable for countries to vaccinate adolescent girls.

Other Gynecological Cancers

We did not identify any literature relevant to diagnosing cancers such as ovarian and endometrial cancers in the low-resource setting. Research focused on the use of diagnostic technique to detect these cancers will be valuable in understanding the costs and benefits of encouraging better diagnosis of these gynecological cancers. Potentially, early-stage detection can result in better treatment response and improved outcomes for the patient.

Table 11.3 Cost-effectiveness studies on cervical cancer screening and other interventions to reduce disease burden

References	Country	Interventions/tests compared	Most cost-effective intervention: Screening schedule	Cost-effective ratio
Cytology only				
[22]	Vietnam	Cytology	Cytology 5-year interval age 30–55	US$725 per LYS
[21]	Taiwan	Cytology, annual and triennial screening with varying levels of compliance	70 % Compliance 100 % Compliance Cytology 3-year interval age 30–69	US$628 per LYS US$8,174 per LYS
Multiple testing modalities compared				
[27]	Thailand	VIA, HPV, and cytology	VIA 5-year interval age 35–55	US$517 per LYS
[28]	India Kenya Peru Thailand South Africa	Once, twice, or thrice per lifetime VIA, HPV DNA, or cytology	Single 1-visit VIA at age 35 Single 1-visit HPV DNA at age 35	Int. $10 per LYS Int. $134 per LYS Int. $124 per LYS Int. $109 per LYS Int. $467 per LYS
[31]	India	HPV vaccination or screening with HPV DNA, cytology, or VIA at various intervals and ages	HPV vaccination (I$10) followed by three 1-visit VIAs	Int. $290 per LYS
[32]	China	HPV DNA and cytology at various number of visits	Single 2-visit HPV DNA	US$50 per LYS
[30]	Thailand	VIA, cytology, and HPV vaccination; start age 30–40 years and 5–10 year interval	VIA (age 30–45) followed by cytology (age 50–60) at 5-year intervals	Cost saving

[15]	Brazil Madagascar Zimbabwe	1-Visit VIA with treatment, 2-visit HPV DNA, and 3-visit cytology	Single 1-visit VIA with treatment	Int. $113 per LYS Int. $167 per LYS Int. $140 per LYS
[29][a]	Kenya Mozambique Tanzania Uganda	VIA and HPV DNA testing at various intervals and ages (over age 30)	HPV DNA testing 3 times in lifetime for older women and adolescence	Int. $1,370 per LYS Int. $720 per LYS Int. $450 per LYS Int. $720 per LYS
[20]	Sub-Saharan Africa[b] South East Asia[b]	VIA, cytology, and HPV vaccination in various frequency and age ranges	Cytology at age 40 with lesion removal	Int. $307 per DALY Int. $142 per DALY
HPV vaccination only				
[25]	Multiple countries in the Asia Pacific region	HPV vaccination	Cost of Int. $10 per vaccinated girl (approx. US$2 per dose)	Int. $30 to Int. $540 per DALY
[26]	Multiple countries in Latin American and the Caribbean	HPV vaccination	Cost of Int. $25 per vaccinated girl (approx. US$5 per dose)	Int. $10 to Int. $390 per DALY
[24]	South Africa	HPV vaccination vs. current screening strategy	HPV vaccination added to current screening strategy	US$1,078 to $1,460 per LYS
[23]	Taiwan	HPV vaccination vs. current screening strategy (cytology)	HPV vaccination at age 12 (US$364 for vaccine administration)	US$13,674 per QALY

VIA visual inspective with acetic acid; *HPV* human papillomavirus; *DALY* disability-adjusted life years; *QALY* quality-adjusted life years; *Int. $* international dollar; *LYS* life years saved

[a]This study also evaluated HPV screening for girls under 12 years and reached similar conclusion as Goldie et al. [25]

[b]High adult and child mortality countries

Integrated Screening for Cancer

Combining cancer screening programs together should intuitively yield cost savings [33]. An example of this approach is the integrated cancer screening offered by Cancer Care Ontario which combines cervical, breast, and colorectal cancer screening in one visit. In Australia, the Victorian bowel, breast, and cervical cancer programs are considering the option of offering combined screening. In the low-resource setting, packaging of breast and cervical cancer screening along with diagnostic evaluation for other gynecological cancers during well women clinical visits has been advocated [2].

No study to date has directly addressed the cost-effectiveness of providing integrated cancer screening, but we did identify one study that evaluated the costs and effectiveness of packaging other services with cervical cancer screening [34]. The other services considered included screening for cardiovascular disease, breast cancer, depression, iron-induced anemia, and sexually transmitted diseases. The findings were that under conditions of constrained resources, lower cost interventions for screening depression and anemia should be packaged with cervical cancer screening.

As indicated on Table 11.4, integrating cancer screening services for women can potentially result in lower cost due to efficiencies for both the provider and the patient. On the provider side, synergies can reduce cost as a person is seen once for several screening tests and not multiple times. For the patient, a single trip is efficient and can reduce transportation and child care costs. Other cost savings can result from providing training to providers for all cancer screening and diagnostic testing in one combined section; funding can also be streamlined to reduce administrative costs, and data collection can also be combined. Furthermore, in addition to cost savings, increased patient compliance with screening recommendations can improve the overall effectiveness of the screening program. Patients may be more likely to obtain screening for multiple cancers and thereby increase overall compliance with cancer screening recommendations [35].

To fully understand the economic impact of implementing combining screening for multiple cancers, targeted studies in the low-income setting are essential. These studies need to be designed to ensure that costs and effectiveness are systematically assessed. An ideal approach would be to begin with a screening study that can be implemented as closely as possible to mimic the real-world setting, and detailed cost data should be collected along with the effectiveness measures. Cost estimation should include both direct and indirect costs in order to ensure a comprehensive assessment of the impacts. The finding from this study can serve as input parameters to a validated cost-effectiveness model that can assess long-term implications of the integrated screening approach. A key challenge would be to develop similar models for each cancer site screened and allocate costs (shared cost of service delivery with integrated screening) to each type of screening (for example, VIA and CBE performed during the same visit).

Cost-Effectiveness Analysis and Cancer Screening Policy

Cost-effectiveness analysis cannot inform cancer screening policy in a vacuum. Cost-effectiveness assessment can identify the most efficient screening approach (type of test, age groups, and testing interval) which needs to be considered in the context of the overall affordability and health care system factors. A screening test or vaccination may be very cost-effective, but the cost in that population may be prohibitive. Targeted interventions aimed at high-risk women may be a viable option that needs further research [36]. In addition, the design of the health care delivery infrastructure may result in barriers that make delivery of the screening test not feasible. There may also be instances when a test is generally low cost and effective but may not be ideal for the low-resource setting. For example, it has been argued that it is challenging to provide high-quality cytology testing in countries like India for mass screening programs [37]. Additionally, screening programs should not be launched without

Table 11.4 Direct and indirect costs related to health care delivery

Cost data elements	Potential impact of integrating cancer screening services
Core direct costs (health services related)	
• Screening (programmatic and clinical costs) • Hospitalization • Outpatient clinical care • Physician visits • Rehabilitation/home health care • Prescription and nonprescription drugs	• Screening costs related to planning and screening delivery could be reduced • Outpatient clinic costs may also be lower as the number of visits are reduced
Other direct costs (non-health services costs)	
• Transportation to health care providers • Child care related to obtaining health care services • Special diets • Lodging for remote treatment facilities	• Single visit instead of multiple trips can reduce costs associated with transportation and childcare
Core indirect costs (impact on patient)	
• Reduced productivity • Lost wages due to premature death	• Less time required to obtain screening translates to less time lost from work and homecare activities
Other related indirect costs (impact on family/friends)	
• Time lost from work and housekeeping by family members or friends	• Less time commitment needed from family members for child care coverage, etc.

adequate planning for providing follow-up diagnostic testing and treatment.

Even when funding and infrastructure are available to deliver cancer care and screening tests, the penetration rate of the screening program may be low due to barriers faced by women. Some of these barriers include cultural or religious beliefs, language barriers, and not having a regular source of health care [38]. Compliance with screening has been reported in the range of 75–85 % in screening trails, but these may not be reproducible in the real-world setting [39–41]. Compliance generally declines with each additional round of screening [39], and, therefore, this should be an important consideration in designing screening programs.

Sensitivity analysis and hypothetical scenarios are important features of cost-effectiveness modeling that can help inform health policy when true values are not available. Assumptions are often required in modeling, but it is important to follow up after implementation to collect appropriate data to ensure that the assumptions are valid; the model results should be compared with real-world findings to better inform future health care policies. Therefore, it is important that economic studies are not only included in the planning process but also in ongoing program evaluation to provide feedback to further improve the cancer screening delivery process and make the most efficient use of limited resources.

References

1. Xiang W, Zhao FH, Shi JF, Li ZX, Ma JF, Qiao YL, et al. Feasibility of packaging screening for cervical cancer, breast cancer, and reproductive tract infection in a rural area in China. Acta Acad Med Sin. 2009;31(5):616–9.
2. Shetty MK, Longatto-Filho A. Early detection of breast, cervical, ovarian and endometrial cancers in low resource countries: an integrated approach Indian. J Surg Oncol. 2011;2(3):165–71.
3. Commission on Macroeconomics and Health. Macroeconomics and health: investing in health for economic development. Geneva: WHO; 2011.
4. Edejer TT, Baltussen R, Adam T, Hutubessey R, Acharya A, Evand DB, et al. WHO guide to cost-effectiveness analysis. Geneva: WHO; 2003.
5. Gold MR, Siegel JE, Russell LB, Weinstein MC. Cost-effectiveness in health and medicine. New York: Oxford University Press; 1996.
6. Russell LB, Gold MR, Siegel JE, Daniels N, Weinstein MC. The role of cost-effectiveness analysis in health and medicine. Panel on cost-effectiveness in health and medicine. JAMA. 1996;276(14):1172–7.

7. Smith MD, Drummond M, Brixner D. Moving the QALY forward: rationale for change. Value Health. 2009;12 Suppl 1:S1–4.
8. Robberstad B. QALYs vs DALYs vs LYs gained: what are the differences, and what difference do they make for health care priority setting? Nor J Epidemiol. 2005;15(2):183–91.
9. Goldie SJ, Kim JJ, Kobus K, Goldhaber-Fiebert JD, Salomon J, O'Shea MK, et al. Cost-effectiveness of HPV 16, 18 vaccination in Brazil. Vaccine. 2007;25:6257–70.
10. Ginsberg GM, Edejer TT, Lauer JA, Sepulveda C. Screening, prevention and treatment of cervical cancer—a global and regional generalized cost-effectiveness analysis. Vaccine. 2009;27(43):6060–79.
11. Goldie SJ, Kuhn L, Denny L, Pollack A, Wright TC. Policy analysis of cervical cancer screening strategies in low-resource settings: clinical benefits and cost-effectiveness. JAMA. 2001;285(24):3107–15.
12. Dasbach EJ, Insinga RP, Yang YC, Pwu RF, Lac C, Elbasha EH. The cost-effectiveness of a quadrivalent human papillomavirus vaccine in Taiwan. Asian Pac J Cancer Prev. 2008;9(3):459–66.
13. Kim JJ, Andres-Beck B, Goldie SJ. The value of including boys in an HPV vaccination programme: a cost-effectiveness analysis in a low-resource setting. Br J Cancer. 2007;97(9):1322–8.
14. Lai MS, Yen MF, Kuo HS, Koong SL, Chen TH, Duffy SW. Efficacy of breast-cancer screening for female relatives of breast-cancer-index cases: Taiwan multicentre cancer screening (TAMCAS). Int J Cancer. 1998;78(1):21–6.
15. Brown ML, Goldie SJ, Draisma G, Harford J, Lipscomb J. Health service interventions for cancer control in developing countries. In: Jamison DT, Breman JG, Measham AR, Alleyne G, Claeson M, Evans DB, Jha P, Mills A, Musgrove P, eds. Disease control priorities in developing countries, chapter 29. 2nd ed. Washington, DC: World Bank; 2006.
16. Okonkwo QL, Draisma G, der Kinderen A, Brown ML, de Koning HJ. Breast cancer screening policies in developing countries: a cost-effectiveness analysis for India. J Natl Cancer Inst. 2008;100(18):1290–300.
17. Valencia-Mendoza A, Sánchez-González G, Bautista-Arredondo S, Torres-Mejía G, Bertozzi SM. Costo-efectividad de políticas para el tamizaje de cáncer de mama en México. Salud Publica Mex. 2009;51 Suppl 2:S296–304.
18. Zelle SG, Nyarko KM, Bosu WK, Aikins M, Niëns LM, Lauer JA, et al. Costs, effects and cost-effectiveness of breast cancer control in Ghana. Trop Med Int Health. 2012;17(8):1031–43.
19. Groot MT, Baltussen R, Uyl-de Groot CA, Anderson BO, Hortobágyi GN. Costs and health effects of breast cancer interventions in epidemiologically different regions of Africa, North America, and Asia. Breast J. 2006;12 Suppl 1:S81–90.
20. Ginsberg GM, Lauer JA, Zelle S, Baeten S, Baltussen R. Cost effectiveness of strategies to combat breast, cervical, and colorectal cancer in sub-Saharan Africa and South East Asia: mathematical modelling study. BMJ. 2012;344:e614.
21. Koong SL, Yen AM, Chen TH. Efficacy and cost-effectiveness of nationwide cervical cancer screening in Taiwan. J Med Screen. 2006;13 Suppl 1:S44–7.
22. Suba EJ, Nguyen CH, Nguyen BD, Raab SS. Viet/American cervical cancer prevention project. De novo establishment and cost-effectiveness of Papanicolaou cytology screening services in the Socialist Republic of Vietnam. Cancer. 2001;91(5):928–39.
23. Liu PH, Hu FC, Lee PI, Chow SN, Huang CW, Wang JD. Cost-effectiveness of human papillomavirus vaccination for prevention of cervical cancer in Taiwan. BMC Health Serv Res. 2010;10:11.
24. Sinanovic E, Moodley J, Barone MA, Mall S, Cleary S, Harries J. The potential cost-effectiveness of adding a human papillomavirus vaccine to the cervical cancer screening programme in South Africa. Vaccine. 2009;27:6196–202.
25. Goldie SJ, Diaz M, Kim SY, Levin CE, Van Minh H, Kim JJ. Mathematical models of cervical cancer prevention in the Asia Pacific region. Vaccine. 2008;26 Suppl 12:M17–29.
26. Goldie SJ, Diaz M, Constenla D, Alvis N, Andrus JK, Kim SY. Mathematical models of cervical cancer prevention in Latin America and the Caribbean. Vaccine. 2008;26 Suppl 11:L59–72.
27. Mandelblatt JS, Lawrence WF, Gaffikin L, Limpahayom KK, Lumbiganon P, Warakamin S, et al. Costs and benefits of different strategies to screen for cervical cancer in less-developed countries. J Natl Cancer Inst. 2002;94(19):1469–83.
28. Goldie SJ, Gaffikin L, Goldhaber-Fiebert JD, Gordillo-Tobar A, Levin C, Mahé C, et al. Alliance for cervical cancer prevention cost working group. Cost-effectiveness of cervical-cancer screening in five developing countries. N Engl J Med. 2005;353(20):2158–68.
29. Campos NG, Kim JJ, Castle PE, Ortendahl JD, O'Shea M, Diaz M, et al. Health and economic impact of HPV 16/18 vaccination and cervical cancer screening in Eastern Africa. Int J Cancer. 2012;130(11):2672–84.
30. Praditsitthikorn N, Teerawattananon Y, Tantivess S, Limwattananon S, Riewpaiboon A, Chichareon S, et al. Economic evaluation of policy options for prevention and control of cervical cancer in Thailand. Pharmacoeconomics. 2011;29(9):781–806.
31. Diaz M, Kim JJ, Albero G, de Sanjosé S, Clifford G, Bosch FX, et al. Health and economic impact of HPV 16 and 18 vaccination and cervical cancer screening in India. Br J Cancer. 2008;99(2):230–8.
32. Levin CE, Sellors J, Shi JF, Ma L, Qiao YL, Ortendahl J, et al. Cost-effectiveness analysis of cervical cancer prevention based on a rapid human papillomavirus screening test in a high-risk region of China. Int J Cancer. 2010;127(6):1404–11.
33. Bobadilla JL, Cowley P, Musgrove P, Saxenian H. Design, content and financing of an essential national package of health services. Bull World Health Organ. 1994;72(4):653–62.

34. Kim JJ, Salomon JA, Weinstein MC, Goldie SJ. Packaging health services when resources are limited: the example of a cervical cancer screening visit. PLoS Med. 2006;3(11):e434.
35. Cancer Care Ontario. Ontario cancer plan—progress report for 2009. http://www.csqi.on.ca/cms/One.aspx?portalId=40955&pageId=41076
36. Sankaranarayanan R, Budukh A, Rajkumar R. Effective screening programmes for cervical cancer in low- and middle-income developing countries. Bull World Health Organ. 2001;79:954–62.
37. Saxena U, Sauvaget C, Sankaranarayanan R. Evidence-based screening, early diagnosis and treatment strategy of cervical cancer for national policy in low-resource countries: example of India. Asian Pac J Cancer Prev. 2012;13(4):1699–703.
38. Winkler J, Bingham A, Coffey P, Handwerker WP. Women's participation in a cervical cancer screening program in northern Peru. Health Educ Res. 2008;23(1):10–24.
39. Dinshaw K, Mishra G, Shastri S, Badwe R, Kerkar R, Ramani S, et al. Determinants of compliance in a cluster randomised controlled trial on screening of breast and cervix cancer in Mumbai, India. 1. Compliance to screening. Oncology. 2007;73(3–4):145–53.
40. Nene B, Jayant K, Arrossi S, Shastri S, Budukh A, Hingmire S, et al. Determinants of women's participation in cervical cancer screening trial, Maharashtra, India. Bull World Health Organ. 2007;85(4):264–72.
41. Yip CH, Smith RA, Anderson BO, Miller AB, Thomas DB, Ang ES, et al. Breast health global initiative early detection panel. Guideline implementation for breast healthcare in low- and middle-income countries: early detection resource allocation. Cancer. 2008;113(8 Suppl):2244–56.

Challenges for Breast and Gynecological Cancer Control by Early Detection in Less-Developed Countries

12

R. Sankaranarayanan, K. Ramadas, K. Grosse Frie, and Y.L. Qiao

Abstract

Early detection and adequate treatment are important approaches in the control of breast, cervix, corpus uteri, and ovarian cancers as they significantly improve survival outcome and quality of life. Cancer early detection approaches include screening programs and early clinical diagnosis through improved awareness and health service infrastructure and accessibility. High level of public awareness and well-developed and accessible health services are vital for the success of both approaches. While there are screening programs for breast and cervical cancers in high-income and selected less-developed countries, screening programs for cancer of the corpus uteri and ovary have not yet evolved. Integrating cervix and breast cancer screening into the general healthcare services is challenging. Political will, funding, and well-developed health services are important requirements for screening programs, which are not readily met in many less-developed countries, with the result that such programs exist only in two low-income countries and in approximately 20 middle-income countries. A more widely applicable early detection approach relies on early clinical diagnosis among people with symptoms and signs. Development of health policy, appropriate advocacy, resource allocation, and investments in improving health services meet with several challenges. Most information about barriers for participation in early detection initiatives in less-developed countries has been derived from qualitative studies.

R. Sankaranarayanan (✉) • K. Grosse Frie
Early Detection and Prevention Section (EDP), Screening Group (SCR), International Agency for Research on Cancer (IARC), Lyon 69008, France
e-mail: sankarR@iarc.fr; grossefrieK@iarc.fr

K. Ramadas
Regional Cancer Centre, Trivandrum 695011, India
e-mail: ramdasrcc@gmail.com

Y.L. Qiao
Department of Cancer Epidemiology, Cancer Institute/Hospital, Chinese Academy of Medical Sciences, Peking Union Medical College, Beijing 100021, China
e-mail: qiaoy@cicams.ac.cn

M.K. Shetty (ed.), *Breast and Gynecological Cancers: An Integrated Approach for Screening and Early Diagnosis in Developing Countries*, DOI 10.1007/978-1-4614-1876-4_12,

Larger quantitative studies are essential to further address the challenges and opportunities for early detection of cancer in routine health services. Promotion of education, awareness, and empowerment of women to seek health care, development of infrastructure for early detection, diagnosis and treatment of cancer patients, and, when resources permit, organized screening programs are important to improve early detection and reduce the burden of breast and cervical cancer in less-developed countries.

Abbreviations

ASR	Age standardized rate
BSE	Breast self-examination
CBE	Clinical breast examination
CIN	Cervical intraepithelial neoplasia
HPV	Human papillomavirus
VIA	Visual screening with acetic acid
VILI	Visual inspection with Lugol's iodine

Introduction

Less-developed countries (synonyms: developing countries, third-world countries, low-resource countries) are characterized by low national income, less diverse and less robust economies, poorly developed infrastructures, a high rate of population growth and unemployment, a large gap between the rich and poor, and poorly developed public education and healthcare systems and services. Most nations in Asia, Africa, and Latin America belong to the category of less-developed countries.

Breast, uterine cervix, corpus uteri, and ovarian cancers constitute a major burden of cancer among women in less-developed countries [1] (Table 12.1). Together, they account for 40 % of all incident cancers and 31 % of all cancer deaths in women in less-developed countries. Early detection and adequate treatment are important approaches in the control of these cancers as they significantly improve survival outcome and quality of life. While invasive cervical cancer can be prevented by vaccination, early detection, and treating cervical cancer precursor lesions, preclinical invasive breast cancers can be diagnosed by early detection. All four of these cancers can be diagnosed in early clinical stages for which treatment is effective in improving survival. Despite these advances, these cancers are still diagnosed in advanced stages with poor survival outcomes [2, 3]. We discuss the major challenges facing early detection efforts for these cancers in less-developed countries in this chapter.

Early Detection Approaches

Cancer early detection approaches include screening programs and early clinical diagnosis through improved awareness and health service infrastructure and accessibility. A high level of public awareness and well-developed and accessible health services are vital for the success of both approaches.

The objective of cancer screening is to prevent death from invasive cancer and to improve quality of life by early detection and treatment of persons with early preclinical, asymptomatic cancers or precancerous lesions by the application of a relatively simple, inexpensive test to a large number of apparently healthy persons in order to classify them as likely or unlikely of having the disease of interest. The usefulness and applicability of screening as a control option for a given cancer will depend upon the suitability of the disease for early detection and treatment, the public health importance of the disease, the availability of suitable screening tests and effective treatment for early stages of disease, and well-developed health services with adequate infrastructure and healthcare providers. The critical components of successful screening programs are high coverage of the target

Table 12.1 Estimated incidence, mortality, and 5-year prevalence from four gynecological cancers in 2008 in less-developed countries

	Incidence		Mortality		5-year
Cancer	Cases	(ASR)	Cases	(ASR)	prevalence
All cancers (female)	3,453,635	(137.2)	2,122,704	(84.9)	7,782,387
Breast	691,521	(27.1)	269,048	(10.7)	2,380,310
Cervix uteri	453,531	(17.7)	242,077	(9.7)	1,288,686
Corpus uteri	144,869	(5.9)	41,165	(1.7)	542,313
Ovary	125,226	(4.9)	75,724	(3.1)	305,463

Data from Ferlay J, Shin HR, Bray F, Forman D, Mathers C, Parkin DM. GLOBOCAN 2008 v2.0. Cancer Incidence and Mortality Worldwide: IARC CancerBase No. 10 [Internet]. Lyon, France: International Agency for Research on Cancer; 2010. Available from: http://globocan.iarc.fr, accessed on 9 Sept 2012
ASR: Age standardized rate

population with accurate, quality-assured screening tests and, for screened-positive patients, availability of diagnostic investigations, treatment, and follow-up care and information systems embedded within the program to ensure monitoring and evaluation.

Screening programs may be either organized or opportunistic. Organized programs are characterized by centralized screening invitations to a well-defined target population, systematic call and recall for screening, delivery of test results, diagnostic investigations, treatment and follow-up care, centralized quality assurance, and a program database with linkages to other information systems such as population-based cancer and death registration systems for monitoring and evaluation of the program purposes. In opportunistic programs, screening tests are provided on request or coincidentally during routine health-care interactions with patients, and there is no predetermined eligible population or systematic invitation for participation.

Both cervix and breast cancers are suitable cancers for screening from this perspective. In developed countries, cervical cancer screening by cytology has been particularly effective in reducing mortality to the tune of 60–80 % within two to three decades from the initiation of programs [4, 5], whereas mammography screening trials have reported reduction in breast cancer deaths by 20–25 % [6]. However, ongoing cytology screening programs for several years since 1970s in many Latin American countries have had very little impact on cervical cancer incidence and mortality due to programmatic and screening test limitations [5]. There are effective alternatives to cytology such as human papillomavirus (HPV) testing and visual screening with acetic acid (VIA) for detecting and treating cervical intraepithelial neoplasia (CIN), and these have been shown to prevent the occurrence of and death from cervical neoplasia [7–10]. Early detection methods for breast cancer include mammography screening, clinical breast examination (CBE), breast self-examination (BSE), and breast awareness linked with early clinical diagnosis. Screening mammography is still the best approach available for the early detection of breast cancer, when adequate resources make its appropriate use possible, despite its less than perfect effectiveness, high costs, and complex technology. There is no evidence yet that systematic CBE or BSE leads to significant reduction in breast cancer mortality, and final results from ongoing CBE trials are awaited [11–13]. Unfortunately, the BSE trials were conducted in regions where considerable early diagnosis was already ongoing, and, thus, the educational interventions could not show further reduction in advanced stages or in breast cancer mortality. Many less-developed countries have very limited capacity to perform breast imaging, so the available imaging services should be used for diagnostic purposes. Organized breast cancer screening would thus have a lower priority in less-developed countries. Many would consider that the resources in those less-developed countries should be better spent on developing cancer education and awareness creation and diagnostic as well as treatment services to begin with, postponing the development of screening for cervical cancer as a program until when resources permit.

Screening as a public health approach to control cancer of the corpus uteri has yet to evolve, and screening programs or trials evaluating screening for this cancer do not exist. Screening for ovarian cancer with tests such as CA125 estimation and ultrasonography is associated with high false-positive rates, and there is no evidence yet that screening leads to reduced ovarian cancer mortality; this is currently being assessed in randomized trials in high-income countries. No population-based screening programs exist for ovarian cancer.

A more widely applicable early detection approach relies on early clinical diagnosis among people with symptoms and signs. This requires improved public awareness of the disease, its symptoms and signs, and health services available to support diagnosis and treatment in the region; it requires well-trained and empowered healthcare personnel in primary care who can promptly recognize and refer people with suspected signs and symptoms either for early diagnosis or to rule out disease in higher levels of health services. Symptoms and signs that may give an early warning of cancer, however, should also trigger an informed and empowered individual to seek medical care. Most cancers could be detected earlier if the index of suspicion of cancer on the part of primary healthcare workers was higher, particularly when providing care for persons known to be at high risk for cancer. Symptoms and signs such as a lump in the breast or bleeding after sexual intercourse are much more specific, and a high level of clinical suspicion can lead to physical examinations and laboratory tests necessary to exclude or confirm the diagnosis. Improved public awareness and early diagnosis and treatment significantly contributed to reduced mortality from cervical cancer even before the introduction of screening programs in developed countries [14, 15]. The frequency of advanced breast cancers fell considerably, and survival rates increased significantly in the United Kingdom before the introduction of the national breast cancer screening program; this also occurred in Connecticut, USA, before 1975 when widespread mammography screening was initiated mainly due to greater awareness [16, 17]. However, raising awareness is not a simple exercise, and there have been only limited attempts to raise awareness of cancer systematically with well-planned and implemented input measures and evaluation of outcomes in less-developed countries. Adequate knowledge of health beliefs in a given region is vital for successful implementation of public awareness programs.

Political Challenges

Political will, funding, and well-developed health services are important requirements for screening programs. Successful implementation and sustenance of cancer screening require political commitment, regular budget lines to support capital and recurring costs, adequately developed healthcare infrastructure for the identification and invitation of eligible women to screening facilities, provision of high-quality screening tests, the evaluation of those with positive screening tests, treatment of those with cancer, trained human resources, facilitation of the steps between different levels of the screening processes, and continuous monitoring and evaluation using health information systems, all of which involve considerable healthcare resources. Given the resource and healthcare infrastructure constraints, cancer screening programs are not feasible in many less-developed countries. Many less-developed countries do not have the equipment, trained personnel, or supplies to organize a national or even regional screening program. Thus, screening programs do not exist in any of the 36 low-income countries (per capita GNI less than US$1,026 in 2011); national cervical cancer screening programs exist in only 20 of the 108 middle-income countries (per capita GNI ranging between US$1,026 to US$12,745), and breast cancer screening programs

Table 12.2 Population-based national screening programs in less-developed countries

Country category	Cervical cancer screening programs	Breast cancer screening programs	Colorectal cancer/stomach screening programs
Low-income countries ($N=36$) (per capita GNI < 1,026 USD)	None	None	None
Low-middle income countries ($N=54$) (per capita GNI 1,026–4,035 USD)	Paraguay Bangladesh	None	None
Upper-middle income countries (per capita GNI 4,036–12,745 USD)	Argentina, Brazil, Chile, Colombia, Costa Rica, Cuba, Latvia, Lithuania, Mexico, Montenegro, Panama, Peru, Romania, Russian Federation, Serbia, Thailand, Uruguay, Venezuela	Brazil, Malaysia, Uruguay	Uruguay

are even fewer as shown in Table 12.2. Almost all screening programs in less-developed countries suffer from poor organization, inadequate coverage, suboptimal performance, and limited or no impact on the burden of cervical or breast cancers [10, 18–22], although recent reorganization of cervical screening programs in countries such as Chile has led to a reduction in cervical cancer mortality [18].

Mobilizing political will and ensuring sustainable financing mechanisms to support resource-intensive public health interventions, such as cancer screening, are major challenges. Unfortunately, however, political factors are more important than cost-effectiveness considerations in mobilizing such political will. The power of the actors, organizations, and individuals involved is a major factor in mobilizing political decision-making process. Quite often, the political decisions to initiate early detection programs are not supported by careful planning to allocate financial and human resources on a continuing basis. Healthcare financing considerations are often rudimentary in many less-developed countries. Focused efforts from a strong and forceful coalition of organizations involved in cancer control are critical to bringing about the policy changes that will drive early detection and control of these major cancers in women. Fortunately, today such a coalition is emerging.

Challenges Related to Health Service Organization and Infrastructure

Integrating cervix and breast cancer early detection efforts into the general healthcare services is challenging. Access to the public and private health services to avail of early detection breast and gynecological cancers is a major challenge for many women in low- and middle-income countries [23–26]. The ability to provide adequate and affordable access to screening services and physical examination by health workers is not a trivial obstacle in health services in many less-developed countries, given the consistent lack of adequate planning, investments, and resource allocation over several years. The ubiquitous neglect of any systematic investments in health services and improving trained human resources has made several health services totally nonresponsive to the needs of populations in less-developed countries. Indeed, in the vast majority of less-developed countries, the primary health centers currently do not have the capacity to provide VIA or visual screening with Lugol's iodine, let alone cytology and HPV testing, since no consumables are available, and they are not equipped with sufficient specula, light source, couches, or equipment to sterilize used and soiled instruments. Strengthening primary care services to enable early detection tests, such as a speculum examination, VIA and VILI for cervical cancer early detection, and CBE for breast cancer detection, and empowering primary healthcare personnel to deliver these competently and refer women for further management will go a long way in strengthening the capacity and reach of primary care services in providing early detection services.

It is obvious that directing cervical biopsies or providing cryotherapy is seldom possible as part of continuum of early detection services in most primary healthcare settings. The secondary healthcare facilities in many less-developed countries are also poorly equipped to provide screening, diagnosis, and treatment services for cervical cancer precursor lesions. By the same count, facilities to provide diagnostic mammography and ultrasonography imaging as part of diagnostic workup of women with suspicious breast lumps are extremely limited in secondary care services, despite the fact that they are expected to function as referral centers for investigating women with suspected breast lumps. Secondary and tertiary care facilities for treatment of invasive cancer and the means to subsidize or finance healthcare costs associated with diagnosis, staging workup, and treatment are inadequately conceived and developed in many less-developed countries, leading to a substantial proportion of cancer patients dropping out of treatment. Thus, a myriad of challenges to strengthening different levels of healthcare services remains to be addressed in less-developed countries. Unless careful planning and financial allocations from national resources and committed loans that will be repaid by national governments by cost recovery and sustainable resource generation (not from external aid which may be driven by an external agenda rather than national needs) driven by political will and motivation go hand in hand with increasing GNI, health services and educational sectors will not keep pace with economic progress, as has been the case with less-developed countries in sub-Saharan Africa.

Lack of healthcare providers and transportation facilities to reach health centers is a common problem, especially in rural areas or for women living in temporary dwellings and in slums. Difficulty in navigating through large and complex healthcare facilities can also be a problem. In countries where health service delivery is fragmented and highly underdeveloped, many patients first consult traditional healers. Traditional healing is a popular practice in several low- and middle-income countries and is also related to late-stage presentation. It is also commonly seen that cancer patients typically visit and seek care with multiple providers before they reach the referral hospital where adequate and good quality services can be obtained to rule out or confirm cancer and where appropriate treatment can be initiated [27, 28]. Such a long referral process can take time, and thus women present at a later stage or get lost in the system. Visiting traditional healers instead of or in addition to professional health services for treatment purposes can be motivated by different reasons, such as fear of surgery, influence of social networks and family, earlier bad experience in a hospital, trust in alternative therapies, financial problems, fear of health outcomes after treatment, not being aware of having cancer, and shyness about seeing a doctor [28].

Advocacy-Related Challenges

To improve healthcare systems effectively in order to reduce the burden of cervical and breast cancer in low- and middle-income countries, politicians and decision makers have to take over leadership in implementing national cervical and breast cancer screening programs and to ensure that these screening programs are of high quality and are available for all target women. Advocates play a major role in reminding decision makers of the importance of national cancer screening programs. Advocacy for cancer early detection involves concerted efforts by interested persons such as cancer patients, survivors, relatives of cancer patients, the general public, and activists to convince politicians and health service administrators to make policy decisions and to introduce and sustain cancer early detection programs in public health services. It provides opportunities for people to get involved in efforts to rally policymakers and the general public to fight against cancer.

Advocacy for cervical cancer is generally less intensive than that for breast cancer. Cervical cancer is a disease of poor women who have no voice in the political decision processes, while breast cancer is a disease of women with more socioeconomic and political clout. Furthermore, cervical cancer is associated with a sexually transmitted infection which is a taboo topic in the eyes of the general public. Thus, cervical cancer advocacy from among cervical cancer patients, survivors, and their relatives is much more limited than that from breast cancer patients and relatives. However, given the large number of advocates found for HIV/AIDS (which is a sexually transmitted infection and disease), the absence of such strong advocacy for cervical cancer is rather perplexing and strange. Another reason might be that cervical cancer is preventable through screening, and therefore getting diagnosed with cervical cancer can be seen as the patient's fault by advocates, forgetting that poor women do not often have the chance to get screened.

Another challenge is that advocates, if not fully educated and aware of the priorities in a given setting, may not advocate for the most appropriate action needed; instead, they may argue and advocate for an action that might be inappropriate and not cost-effective in that context. For instance, in a setting which deserves investments in cervical cancer screening as a priority rather than breast cancer screening, advocates prompted by technology and sophistication may argue introducing mammography screening. Similarly, when resources should be invested in creating breast awareness and early clinical diagnosis, advocates may prompt investments in mammography screening. Such advocacy could result in a waste of precious healthcare resources. In low-resource settings, advocates and policymakers would be well advised to invest in programs that target a high proportion of women, including the most vulnerable ones, focusing on the cancer contributing to the largest burden.

Challenges From the Perspective of the Target Population

In the following overview, further challenges for early detection in less-developed countries from the perspective of the targeted women are discussed. Major barriers are discussed in general without focusing on any particular country. The barriers predominantly apply to both breast and cervical cancers, but it is specified when they specifically refer to one cancer site. The major barriers are listed in Table 12.3. To improve or implement successful early detection programs, the local situation, the existing healthcare system, and the type of program that will be applied should be considered in order to address the challenges more specifically.

Cancer-Related Knowledge, Beliefs, and Awareness

A main barrier for early detection is the lack of or low level of knowledge and awareness of breast and cervical cancers, screening, and early diagnosis among women and their communities. In low- and middle-income countries, especially in rural areas, knowledge and awareness of breast and cervical cancers and screening are reported to be lacking or very low, which are major factors that keep women from attending cervical and breast cancer early detection initiatives [23, 29–36]. In several surveys from rural areas, women pointed out that they never had any information or education about symptoms and signs of breast or cervical cancer, methods of early detection of these cancers, or that screening is an important issue [23, 24, 30, 34]. Women named schools, churches, communities, primary health providers, or workplaces as possible sources from which they would expect information. Lack of awareness about what a symptom or sign could represent, in terms of health outcomes, may lead to undue anxiety, confusion, or denial [37].

Low knowledge about breast and cervical cancer among women and their communities is also related to several misconceptions regarding the causes and risk factors of these cancers, the screening, and the treatment. In general, these concepts are fatalistic and have in common that, from their point of view, cancer is neither preventable nor curable. Women reported that they avoid being screened for cancer because they believe it is not curable and, therefore, prefer not to know if they have cancer [23, 25, 32, 34]. Beliefs that screening or surgery can lead to total

Table 12.3 Main barriers for women in low- and middle-income countries to participating in cervical or breast cancer screening

Knowledge, beliefs, and awareness	Lack of knowledge about breast and cervical cancer, often due to missing information and education
	Misconceptions and beliefs about cancer etiology, screening, and treatment, which are generally fatalistic and deny the preventable and curable character of cancer
	No awareness of being at risk to develop breast or cervical cancer and of early signs of cancer
Psychosocial factors	Fear of screening tests, test results, and treatment
	Feelings of shyness and shame related to clinical examinations
	Cultural values about health and illness, including fear of stigma when diagnosed with cancer and lack of understanding for preventive use of health service in the community
Social status	Financial burden, including costs for screening, treatment, and drugs and lack of health insurance
	Indirect costs like time, traveling costs, loss of daily earnings, or loss of employment
	Lacking social support
	Low social empowerment and gender inequalities, including dependency on husband, failure to consider own health as a priority, and fear of not being able to fulfill the role of a wife as a result of cancer
Health services	Poor access to health services
	Bad navigation through the healthcare system, including women's own health-seeking behavior and a missing referral system
	Use of traditional healers
	Poor quality of provided health services, including inappropriate equipment, lack of hygiene, and low education and training of physicians and nurses
	Behavior of physicians and nurses, including lack of confidentiality about test results and rudeness
	Healthcare provider's sex or ethnicity

loss of breast or uterus, further spread of cancer which leads to death, or assumptions that total mastectomy is the only treatment option also keep some women from participating in screening or treatment [38]. In some cultures, cancer is related to witchcraft, and women remain of the conviction that only traditional healers can help them [39, 40]. Many women believe that there is no effective therapy for cancer, especially when all the people they have known with cancer have died [37].

Another barrier is that women are not aware of being at risk of developing cervical or breast cancer. Several studies reported that women do not necessarily distinguish between a screening and diagnostic test and do not attend screening because they do not think that they are at risk of developing cancer or that screening can prevent them from developing cancer [23, 29, 30, 32, 33, 35]. Even if family members have already had a cancer diagnosed, women's personal risk perception is sometimes not influenced by their relative's experience [29]. Especially in the case of breast cancer, for which no effective primary prevention exists, it is important that women be aware of early signs to be able to detect them and to seek prompt healthcare attention. But it was reported that, even if women notice lumps in their breasts, they are often unaware that the lump could be cancer or a benign disease, and they do not seek health care before symptoms eventually develop and the disease becomes locally advanced [27, 29].

Psychosocial Factors

A variety of psychosocial factors can influence a woman's perception and participation in early detection of breast and cervical cancers. Fear of the screening test itself, the consequences of the screening test outcomes, diagnostic procedures, and treatment may play a major role in prompting women to avoid going for breast or cervical cancer screening [23, 25, 30, 32]. Other factors that consistently emerged in several interview-based studies leading to nonparticipation were shyness and uneasiness concerning medical examination and feeling ashamed to expose private parts, especially when the early diagnosis/screening provider is a man [23, 24, 26, 32, 36]. It is likely that women who underwent screening also suffer from such feelings, but maybe to a lesser extent or they might have resources or strategies to overcome these feelings.

Psychosocial barriers can also be related to the culture of the community, including values about health and illness. Women reported that, even if they theoretically understood the possible health benefits of breast and cervical cancer screening and early diagnosis, it was simply not common in their community to visit a healthcare provider, especially when feeling healthy and when there was apparently nothing wrong with their health. They were worried that their partners or community might not believe them and start doubting their character/moral standards and social integrity if they went to seek preventive care for major illnesses or would assume that they are sick, leading to social isolation and stigmatization [24, 33, 35]. Women reported that they feel ashamed about being sick and were concerned about being stigmatized or excluded from the community if they presented for gynecological examinations or were diagnosed with cancer [29]. In areas where HIV is common, women were also afraid that others might think they had HIV if they were diagnosed with cancer [39, 40]. Cervical cancer and its relationship to sexual intercourse increase women's anxieties about being stigmatized as an immoral, promiscuous, prostitute, and as having had sex with multiple partners [39, 40]. Even when lacking specific knowledge about HPV and little awareness or details about cervical cancer, men seem to have a generic understanding of cervical cancer as a sexually transmitted disease and believe it occurs when the woman is immoral or that the disease has something to do with the woman's past behavior. When men who lacked knowledge about HPV and/or who had very vague knowledge about cervical cancer were asked about risk factors, they often reported "having multiple sex partners" as a common risk factor for cervical cancer [41] and women reported they were afraid that their partner would assume that they had been unfaithful and immoral if they were diagnosed with HPV or cervical cancer [42].

Social Status

Socioeconomic factors, social networks, and the status of women in their communities have a strong influence on women's screening behavior. Economic factors, especially when screening is not provided for free, have been reported in several interviews as a major barrier for screening and early diagnosis. Having no health insurance and having to bear the costs for screening or eventual treatment were mentioned several times as barriers. Even when screening is provided for free, women are not only worried about possible costs for treatment and drugs [23–25, 32, 43], but also indirect costs like traveling costs to visit healthcare providers, loss of daily earnings, or missing time for other life priorities; this keeps women from participating in screening [23, 30]. Women who were employed reported that they were not allowed to leave work without actually being ill and that they have no time to attend screening because of long working hours [28, 32].

Regarding health information and seeking health care a lot of women primarily rely on information and support from their family and friends and on close interpersonal communication networks, especially in societies where lives are more centered around family, village, country, and social group ties [28]. Lacking social support was mentioned as a barrier in studies because women do not want to visit screening services on their own, especially when they have to travel long distances to the place where the screening is provided [23, 30]. On the other hand, having a male partner who is supportive of cancer screening does help women to decide to take part in such screening [44].

In most low- and middle-income countries, women have very low social empowerment, and gender inequalities are one of the main barriers for taking part in screening. Women are often dependent on their husband's ability or goodwill to be able to take part in cancer screening, diagnosis, or treatment. Women reported that it was difficult for them to convince their partners to get financial or emotional support to visit healthcare providers for screening, especially if they are not visibly ill [23, 24, 29, 30, 32, 45]. In societies where women have not been used to fullfil their own needs, but the needs of their families, women's health tends to be regarded as trivial by the society and women reported that they themselves fail to consider their health as a priority, to adopt preventive behavior, or to pursue preventive health care [23, 25, 32].

When being treated with cryotherapy or cold coagulation after cervical cancer screening, women are routinely advised to avoid sexual intercourse for specified periods such as 3–4 weeks or to use condoms when sexual intercourse cannot be avoided. This advice quite often makes women uncomfortable and afraid because they think their husbands may not accept this, may start sleeping with other women or will simply leave. Women also reported that they are afraid that, as a result of cancer, they might be unable to bear children or to provide sexual pleasure to their husbands, which could lead to divorce or failure to get married at all [23, 24, 35].

Healthcare Providers

There are several aspects associated with healthcare providers and health centers that can influence women's participation in early detection and healthcare seeking behavior. Poor quality of health resources (e.g., low hygiene standards), mistrust in the healthcare provider's qualifications to perform early detection tests or to interpret the test results, and long waiting time were mentioned by some women as major barriers to seeking care [23, 25, 29]. Other reasons for not availing oneself of early detection services are providers' inability to maintain confidentiality of the test results, rude behavior of nurses and physicians, and concerns about privacy or confidentiality during screening [23, 25, 34]. In small communities, women are concerned about being screened by people they know or that others will find out about their test results later [39, 40]. If the screening provider is a man or from another ethnicity, it can also keep some women from taking part in screening [23, 30, 36].

Some women perceived that some healthcare providers do not provide early detection tests unless they have symptoms and signs and will refuse to provide screening if the women are apparently healthy [33]. Communicating information about diagnosis, treatment, and prognosis to patients with genital or breast cancer was also reported to be inadequate, which leads to undue anxiety and depression. The language used by physicians, lack of systematic consideration of a patient's autonomy, failure to respect the privacy of women and their feelings/sensitivities, and absence of mechanisms that can provide decision-making power to women were other major challenges impeding participation in early detection programs [40].

Implications

Knowledge about the causation, risk factors, prevention, symptoms, early detection, and treatment possibilities for cervical and breast cancer is essential for women in order to be able to decide about taking part in screening and to seek professional healthcare services if cancer symptoms occur. This is especially important when screening is not organized but opportunistic. Moreover, not only women but also their partners, communities, primary healthcare providers, and eventually traditional healers should be informed and educated about breast and cervical cancer screening in order to facilitate early detection when women seek services. Additionally, awareness of being at risk of developing cancer and of symptoms related to cancer must be generated among target women. The connotation with death exists in relation to cancer in most societies, and education should, therefore, emphasize that cancer is a preventable and treatable disease.

As knowledge and awareness about breast and cervical cancers are directly related to the general level of education and economic status, education programs and campaigns should be customized and targeted for women and communities of different social strata and should especially consider deprived and vulnerable groups.

Psychosocial barriers that keep women from participating in screening should also be considered when developing education and screening programs. However, these barriers might be the most difficult factors to generalize as they are related to the individual women and her community, and cultural beliefs might be only partly altered by education and information campaigns. Cancer is often stigmatized, which is in itself a barrier for many women to participate in screening or seek health services. Higher rates of cancer survivors and expanding access to quality cancer treatment will probably decrease the stigma related to cancer, but efforts to include networks of breast and cervical cancer survivors, their partners, and families in education programs and campaigns might speed up this process.

Economically disadvantaged women are at a higher risk of not participating in early detection and treatment. Offering screening and treatment free of cost for vulnerable socioeconomic segments of the population or increasing the coverage of health insurances that are providing breast and cervical cancer screening and care could help to increase the participation among economically deprived women. Improving access to screening and health services, shortening waiting time, and providing possibilities to bring family members or children to visits might also help to decrease indirect costs. Special possibilities for working women must be considered, e.g., offering health services at workplaces or allowing paid or unpaid leave to visit health services. Awareness that deprived women are at a higher risk for not attending screening or seeking health care for breast and cervical cancer should be created on different levels, and social workers, community leaders, healthcare workers, and primary healthcare providers can be integrated to socially support these groups to get adequate health care. Empowerment of women is another essential element that can decrease the burden of cervical and breast cancers since, in many low- and middle-income countries, women have a low social status and rely on men to make decisions for them. Increasing empowerment of women by focusing on women's ability to make decisions, access information, and use social and internal resources might, therefore, help to increase participation in early detection [46].

The extent and quality of health care provided are further essential aspects. Only adequate high-quality screening, follow-up, and treatment for cervical and breast cancer are able to reduce the burden of cervical and breast cancer in low- and middle-income countries. Training and support for healthcare providers to be able to communicate and practice breast and cervical cancer early detection and referral will help to encourage women to participate in early detection, to seek professional health care in case of symptoms, and to attend follow-up and treatment sessions without increasing distress and anxiety. Training for healthcare providers should also include psychosocial aspects of the interaction with patients and the importance of respecting privacy during and after visits. In several low- and middle-income countries, only very few cancer referral centers provide treatment, and it can be difficult for women to reach these centers because of problems in transportation and navigation through the health services. Enhancing local healthcare providers to provide at least adequate information about breast and cervical cancer, screening, and referral might improve access to cancer services for women.

Most information about barriers to participating in breast and cervical cancer screening and treatment in less-developed countries has been derived from interviews with women. The majority of studies have used qualitative or mixed methods approaches, which give a broad overview of women's perception about barriers. However, information most often derived from a few and selected groups of women and larger quantitative studies analyzing participation in screening, follow-up, and treatment from research and pilot projects might not reflect women's early detection and health-seeking behavior in the existing healthcare systems. Larger quantitative studies are essential to further address the challenges and opportunities for early detection of cancer in less-developed countries, and future research should investigate larger quantitative studies in routine health services. Such information will contribute to improving the healthcare system effectively and help policymakers facilitate this goal. Promotion of education, awareness and empowerment of women to seek health care, development of resource appropriate policies and infrastructure for early detection, diagnosis and treatment of cancer patients, and, when resources permit, organized screening programs are important to improve early detection and reduce the burden of breast and cervical cancer in less-developed countries.

References

1. Ferlay J, Shin HR, Bray F, Forman D, Mathers C, Parkin DM. Estimates of worldwide burden of cancer in 2008: GLOBOCAN 2008. Int J Cancer. 2010; 127(12):2893–917.
2. Sankaranarayanan R, Swaminathan R, Brenner H, Chen K, Chia KS, Chen JG, et al. Cancer survival in Africa, Asia, and Central America: a population-based study. Lancet Oncol. 2010;11(2):165–73.
3. Sankaranarayanan R, Swaminathan R. Cancer survival in Africa, Asia, the Caribbean and Central America. IARC Scientific Publications No. 162. Lyon: International Agency for Research on Cancer; 2011.
4. Gustafsson L, Ponten J, Zack M, Adami HO. International incidence rates of invasive cervical cancer after introduction of cytological screening. Cancer Causes Control. 1997;8(5):755–63.
5. International Agency for Research on Cancer. IARC handbooks of cancer prevention, Cervix cancer screening, vol. 10. Lyon: IARC; 2004.
6. International Agency for Research on Cancer. IARC handbooks of cancer prevention, Breast cancer screening, vol. 7. Lyon: IARC; 2002.
7. Sankaranarayanan R, Esmy PO, Rajkumar R, Muwonge R, Swaminathan R, Shanthakumari S, et al. Effect of visual screening on cervical cancer incidence and mortality in Tamil Nadu, India: a cluster-randomised trial. Lancet. 2007;370(9585):398–406.
8. Denny L, Kuhn L, Hu CC, Tsai WY, Wright Jr TC. Human papillomavirus-based cervical cancer prevention: long-term results of a randomized screening trial. J Natl Cancer Inst. 2010;102(20):1557–67.
9. Sankaranarayanan R, Nene BM, Shastri SS, Jayant K, Muwonge R, Budukh AM, et al. HPV screening for cervical cancer in rural India. N Engl J Med. 2009;360(14):1385–94.
10. Sankaranarayanan R, Boffetta P. Research on cancer prevention, detection and management in low- and medium-income countries. Ann Oncol. 2010;21(10):1935–43.
11. Thomas DB, Gao DL, Self SG, Allison CJ, Tao Y, Mahloch J, et al. Randomized trial of breast self-examination in Shanghai: methodology and preliminary results. J Natl Cancer Inst. 1997;89(5):355–65.
12. Mittra I, Mishra GA, Singh S, Aranke S, Notani P, Badwe R, et al. A cluster randomized, controlled trial of breast and cervix cancer screening in Mumbai, India: methodology and interim results after three rounds of screening. Int J Cancer. 2010;126(4):976–84.
13. Sankaranarayanan R, Ramadas K, Thara S, Muwonge R, Prabhakar J, Augustine P, et al. Clinical breast examination: preliminary results from a cluster randomized controlled trial in India. J Natl Cancer Inst. 2011;103(19):1476–80.
14. Ponten J, Adami HO, Bergstrom R, Dillner J, Friberg LG, Gustafsson L, et al. Strategies for global control of cervical cancer. Int J Cancer. 1995;60(1):1–26.
15. Gustafsson L, Ponten J, Bergstrom R, Adami HO. International incidence rates of invasive cervical cancer before cytological screening. Int J Cancer. 1997; 71(2):159–65.
16. Jatoi I, Anderson WF, Rao SR, Devesa SS. Breast cancer trends among black and white women in the United States. J Clin Oncol. 2005;23(31):7836–41.
17. Stockton D, Davies T, Day N, McCann J. Retrospective study of reasons for improved survival in patients with breast cancer in East Anglia: earlier diagnosis or better treatment. BMJ. 1997;314(7079):472–5.
18. Sepulveda C, Prado R. Effective cervical cytology screening programmes in middle-income countries: the Chilean experience. Cancer Detect Prev. 2005; 29(5):405–11.
19. Lazcano-Ponce E, Palacio-Mejia LS, len-Leigh B, Yunes-Diaz E, Alonso P, Schiavon R, et al. Decreasing cervical cancer mortality in Mexico: effect of Papanicolaou coverage, birthrate, and the importance of diagnostic validity of cytology. Cancer Epidemiol Biomarkers Prev. 2008;17(10):2808–17.
20. Murillo R, Almonte M, Pereira A, Ferrer E, Gamboa OA, Jeronimo J, et al. Cervical cancer screening programs in Latin America and the Caribbean. Vaccine. 2008;26 Suppl 11:L37–48.
21. Nessa A, Hussain MA, Rahman JN, Rashid MH, Muwonge R, Sankaranarayanan R. Screening for cervical neoplasia in Bangladesh using visual inspection with acetic acid. Int J Gynaecol Obstet. 2010;111(2):115–8.
22. Khuhaprema T, Attasara P, Srivatanakul P, Sangrajrang S, Muwonge R, Sauvaget C, et al. Organization and evolution of organized cervical cytology screening in Thailand. Int J Gynaecol Obstet. 2012;118(2):107–11.
23. Ngugi CW, Boga H, Muigai AW, Wanzala P, Mbithi JN. Factors affecting uptake of cervical cancer early detection measures among women in Thika, Kenya. Health Care Women Int. 2012;33(7):595–613.
24. Keshavarz Z, Simbar M, Ramezankhani A. Factors for performing breast and cervix cancer screening by Iranian female workers: a qualitative-model study. Asian Pac J Cancer Prev. 2011;12(6):1517–22.

25. Agurto I, Bishop A, Sanchez G, Betancourt Z, Robles S. Perceived barriers and benefits to cervical cancer screening in Latin America. Prev Med. 2004;39(1):91–8.
26. Watkins MM, Gabali C, Winkleby M, Gaona E, Lebaron S. Barriers to cervical cancer screening in rural Mexico. Int J Gynecol Cancer. 2002;12(5):475–9.
27. Dye TD, Bogale S, Hobden C, Tilahun Y, Hechter V, Deressa T, et al. Complex care systems in developing countries: breast cancer patient navigation in Ethiopia. Cancer. 2010;116(3):577–85.
28. Muhamad M, Merriam S, Suhami N. Why breast cancer patients seek traditional healers. Int J Breast Cancer. 2012;2012:689168.
29. Fort VK, Makin MS, Siegler AJ, Ault K, Rochat R. Barriers to cervical cancer screening in Mulanje, Malawi: a qualitative study. Patient Prefer Adherence. 2011;5:125–31.
30. Basu P, Sarkar S, Mukherjee S, Ghoshal M, Mittal S, Biswas S, et al. Women's perceptions and social barriers determine compliance to cervical screening: results from a population based study in India. Cancer Detect Prev. 2006;30(4):369–74.
31. Paolino M, Arrossi S. Women's knowledge about cervical cancer, Pap smear and human papillomavirus and its relation to screening in Argentina. Women Health. 2011;51(1):72–87.
32. Parsa P, Kandiah M, Abdul RH, Zulkefli NM. Barriers for breast cancer screening among Asian women: a mini literature review. Asian Pac J Cancer Prev. 2006;7(4):509–14.
33. Markovic M, Kesic V, Topic L, Matejic B. Barriers to cervical cancer screening: a qualitative study with women in Serbia. Soc Sci Med. 2005;61(12):2528–35.
34. McFarland DM. Cervical cancer and Pap smear screening in Botswana: knowledge and perceptions. Int Nurs Rev. 2003;50(3):167–75.
35. Duran ET. Examination with the health belief model of women's attitudes to cervical cancer and early diagnosis in Turkey: a qualitative study. Asian Pac J Cancer Prev. 2011;12(5):1179–84.
36. Ansink AC, Tolhurst R, Haque R, Saha S, Datta S, van den Broek NR. Cervical cancer in Bangladesh: community perceptions of cervical cancer and cervical cancer screening. Trans R Soc Trop Med Hyg. 2008;102(5):499–505.
37. Shulman LP. Gynecological management of premenstrual symptoms. Curr Pain Headache Rep. 2010;14(5):367–75.
38. Ma GX, Yin L, Gao W, Tan Y, Liu R, Fang C, et al. Workplace-based breast cancer screening intervention in china. Cancer Epidemiol Biomarkers Prev. 2012; 21(2):358–67.
39. Chirwa S, Mwanahamuntu M, Kapambwe S, Mkumba G, Stringer J, Sahasrabuddhe V, et al. Myths and misconceptions about cervical cancer among Zambian women: rapid assessment by peer educators. Glob Health Promot. 2010;17(2 Suppl):47–50.
40. Primo WQ, Garrafa V. Ethical issues of diagnosis disclosure and treatment in patients with genital or breast cancer. Rev Assoc Med Bras. 2010;56(4):397–402.
41. Maree JE, Wright SC, Makua TP. Men's lack of knowledge adds to the cervical cancer burden in South Africa. Eur J Cancer Care (Engl). 2011;20(5):662–8.
42. Fernandez ME, McCurdy SA, Arvey SR, Tyson SK, Morales-Campos D, Flores B, et al. HPV knowledge, attitudes, and cultural beliefs among Hispanic men and women living on the Texas-Mexico border. Ethn Health. 2009;14(6):607–24.
43. Smith RA, Caleffi M, Albert US, Chen TH, Duffy SW, Franceschi D, et al. Breast cancer in limited-resource countries: early detection and access to care. Breast J. 2006;12 Suppl 1:S16–26.
44. Winkler J, Bingham A, Coffey P, Handwerker WP. Women's participation in a cervical cancer screening program in northern Peru. Health Educ Res. 2008; 23(1):10–24.
45. Bingham A, Bishop A, Coffey P, Winkler J, Bradley J, Dzuba I, et al. Factors affecting utilization of cervical cancer prevention services in low-resource settings. Salud Publica Mex. 2003;45 Suppl 3:S408–16.
46. Luszczynska A, Durawa AB, Dudzinska M, Kwiatkowska M, Knysz B, Knoll N. The effects of mortality reminders on posttraumatic growth and finding benefits among patients with life-threatening illness and their caregivers. Psychol Health. 2012; 27(10):1227–43.

Funding for Global Healthcare Intervention: Initiatives Aimed at Controlling Cancer in Women in Low-Resource Countries

13

Kelli A. Cohen, Gustavo S. Azenha, Alessandra Durstine, Rola M.S.K. Shaheen, and Mahesh K. Shetty

Abstract

This chapter explores funding for the prevention and control of breast and cervical cancer in low and middle income countries (LMIC), including: existing patterns of financing for cancer within the context of global health financing trends; the challenges to resource mobilization for cancer control; and recommendations for diversifying and strengthening resource mobilization to ensure more robust, effective, and efficient cancer control efforts. Domestic financing for health in LMICs—government and out-of-pocket payments—is the primary source of global health financing. Multilateral and bilateral funding provides the second main source of global health financing. International and domestic private funding—both corporate and not-for-profit sources—accounts for a less significant proportion of global health financing, yet plays an important role in driving policy and systems changes. Cancer control has been severely underfunded in LMICs: cancer control financing is marked by severe inequities between countries, and cancer has received extremely limited support from development donors and major global philanthropic organizations.

K.A. Cohen (✉)
Diagnostic Radiologist, Locum Tenens, McGovern Center for Humanities and Ethics, University of Texas, Houston, TX 77030, USA
e-mail: kcohenfein@mfein.com

G.S. Azenha • A. Durstine
Department of Global Health, American Cancer Society, New York, NY 10001, USA
e-mail: Gustavo.azenha@cancer.org

R.M.S.K. Shaheen
Department of Radiology, Harrington Memorial Hospital—BIDMC, Harvard Medical School, Boston, MA 02115, USA
e-mail: rshaheen@bidmc.harvard.edu

M.K. Shetty
Woman's Center for Breast Care and MRI, Woman's Hospital of Texas, Houston, TX 77054, USA
e-mail: mshetty@womens-radiology.com

M.K. Shetty (ed.), *Breast and Gynecological Cancers: An Integrated Approach for Screening and Early Diagnosis in Developing Countries*, DOI 10.1007/978-1-4614-1876-4_13,

As a result, cancer prevention and control resources have been very limited and, where existent, more strongly beholden to domestic sources than other major global health challenges. In order to redress the grave disparities in cancer control financing and strengthen resource mobilization for cancer control, there is a need to fortify global and national cancer control policies, develop innovative domestic models for health financing cancer and other chronic diseases, more strongly leverage existing global and national health financing mechanisms to foster synergistic women's health and health systems strengthening initiatives, and cultivate greater engagement of corporate, nonprofit, and individual donors in global and domestic spheres. These multiple and complementary efforts will help ensure that resources are more equitable and adequate to the cancer burden, that resources are mobilized more effectively and efficiently, that resources are utilized in a manner better aligned with local stakeholder priorities, that resources limit redundancies and duplication of efforts, and that resources promote sustainability to ensure longer term progress on cancer control and global health.

A: Funding for Global Healthcare Intervention: Initiatives Aimed at Controlling Cancer in Women in Low-Resource Countries

Gustavo S. Azenha and Alessandra Durstine

Introduction

Funding for the prevention and control of breast and cervical cancers in developing countries has been insufficient to address the magnitude of the cancer burden and ensure equitable access to proven interventions. Resource mobilization remains one of the most critical challenges for strengthening health systems in LMICs to adequately and equitably address the global cancer burden. There is an urgent need to strengthen resource mobilization efforts of major actors—governments, multilateral organizations, international NGOs, local philanthropic NGOs, and the corporate sector—and develop novel models and strategies to raise and mobilize funding.

Technologies, infrastructure, and human resources for screening, diagnosis, treatment, and management of cervical and breast cancers can be quite costly, and cost barriers have been one of the principal challenges to strengthening cancer control in low and middle income countries (LMICs). While some interventions for breast and, especially, cervical cancer prevention and control can be fairly low cost, diagnostics and treatment can be expensive, especially when considered within overall health budgets and per capita health spending in LMICs. Where late presentation is common—the norm in LMICs—the costs of care can be particularly high, compounding the financial challenges of cancer control in developing countries. Although availability of resources is only one among many barriers to ameliorating breast and cervical cancer control, the limited availability of resources is a critical barrier that permeates the multitude of barriers at different levels and scales to increased availability, quality, and equity in cancer control services (e.g., including barriers such as public awareness, effective health promotion and communications strategies, health worker training, policy and guideline development, and access to screening and treatment technologies).

In this chapter, the authors provide a snapshot of funding and fundraising at various scales for the control of breast and cervical cancers in LMICs. The challenges to resource mobilization for cancer control are discussed, as well as major funding sources, strategies, models, and institutions. Particular emphasis is placed on local and international philanthropic organizations and their role in funding cancer control. The chapter closes with several recommendations to strengthen fundraising and increase efficiency in resource mobilization for breast and cervical cancers.

G.S. Azenha (✉) • A. Durstine
Department of Global Health, American Cancer Society, New York, NY 10001, USA
e-mail: Gustavo.azenha@cancer.org

The Challenge of Funding Cancer Control in Developing Countries

Cancer control resources in LMICs have come from a variety of sources including governments, out-of pocket payments, the private sector, and philanthropic NGOs. Unlike other major global health challenges, international development assistance from both multilateral and bilateral agencies for cancer control has been extremely limited thus far and played a fairly negligible role in cancer control financing in the developing world [1]. Development assistance for health in LMICs since 2000 has primarily targeted HIV/AIDS, tuberculosis, malaria, and maternal, newborn, and child health programs [1–3].

Funding for cancer control in LMICs has been relatively restricted and significantly out of line with the disease burden [1]. From 2004 to 2008, the estimated donor funding for cancer was only US$60 million [2, 4]. Although analyses of global cancer costs, funding, and spending have been absent and data are limited, the current picture is quite alarming. A recent report commissioned by the American Cancer Society and the Livestrong Foundation [5] and an article from the Harvard Global Task Force on Expanded Access to Cancer Care and Control in Developing Countries (GTF. CCC) [6] provide some of the first more comprehensive analyses of global cancer costs and spending. This incipient work points to stark inequities and a disconnect between the burden of cancer and resource mobilization patterns.

Global cancer medical spending has been "heavily skewed to high income countries" [1], with only 5% or less of global health spending on cancer control in LMICs, despite accounting for approximately 80% of the global cancer burden as measured in disability adjusted life years (DALYs) [5, 6]. Farmer and colleagues have pointed out that these inequities are even more glaring when we consider the most medically underserved regions. Global cancer medical spending is estimated at less than 1% in low income countries, less than 2% in lower middle income countries, and 2% in upper-middle income countries. The African region, for example, "accounts for only 0.2% of global cancer medical costs compared with just over 1% of global spending on health, 6.4% of new cancer cases, and 15% of the global population." Given the scarce availability of data for disease-specific spending in developing countries, information on per capita spending for cancer in developing countries is difficult to ascertain, but one analysis from Sri Lanka found that spending on malignant neoplasms was approximately US$2–3 per capita. In contrast, per capita spending in many high income countries is over US$150 [6].

The limited global resources applied to cancer control are, in part, a reflection of the lack of robust cancer control policies at global and national levels. The lack of stronger cancer control policies and comprehensive cancer control plans at global and national levels is indicative of a limited awareness and/or commitment to cancer control and serves as a strong impediment to resource mobilization efforts. Robust cancer policies and action plans are crucial to ensure relevance and support strategic and efficient resource mobilization at various scales. These limitations in resource mobilization and policies are themselves imbricated within a lack of awareness and persistent myths about cancer in the developing world, including the perceptions that the cancer burden is insignificant in LMICs and that cancer control is unattainable in LMICs because of the unaffordability of care and inadequate physical and human resources [7].

These resource mobilization and policy hindrances are not a cancer-specific phenomenon, but one which has characterized and impacted the prevention and control of non-communicable diseases (NCDs) more generally [1, 4]. In 2008, only approximately 0.5% of total development assistance in 2008 targeted NCDs [2]. According to a report by the Centre for Global Development, in real terms, financing for NCDs has risen (having more than doubled between 2004 and 2008), yet relative to other established global health priorities and to the NCD burden, global resource mobilization for NCDs has been negligible. In 2007, NCD funding in LMICS was only 2.3% of funding for communicable diseases. The development assistance targeting NCDs that did exist has come primarily from bilateral and multilateral agencies with the remaining coming from corporate funding and nonprofit donors [4].

The Role of Multilateral Organizations and Global Financing Initiatives

While in recent years innovative global financing initiatives (e.g., GAVI, the Global Fund, and the US President's Emergency Plan for AIDS Relief (PEPFAR)) have proven important for driving solutions to a variety of major global health challenges (including malaria, tuberculosis, HIV/AIDS, and vaccine preventable diseases in children), to date no innovative global financing mechanisms have been developed to specifically target cancer (and/or other NCDs). Innovative global financing mechanisms like GAVI and the Global Fund have not only helped in raising funds, but have also introduced innovations in resource use efficiency through pooling from different donor sources, strengthening accountabilities, promoting synergistic resource allocation, developing cost-saving procurement strategies, and fostering multi-stakeholder participation in resource allocation decisions [1].

It is important to note that donor governments have been the primary funders of innovative global financing mechanisms (GAVI and the Global Fund). For example, 95% of financing for the Global Fund have come from donor governments (with the bulk of the rest coming from the Bill and Melinda Gates Foundation). While GAVI is less dependent on development assistance, donor governments account for 39% of GAVI funding [1].

International development assistance for global health serves as a driver of policy change and local resource mobilization efforts of governments, the private sector, and civil society organizations, and, therefore, the lack of attention to cancer by international development donors has contributed to more limited local resource mobilization efforts. Leveraging existing global health and development financing initiatives or creating new ones is important to strengthen resource mobilization for adequately addressing the burden of breast and cervical cancers.

Although global health intergovernmental organizations, including the World Health Organization [8], its regional branches (e.g., PAHO), and International Agency for Research on Cancer (IARC) have been actively engaged in breast and cervical cancer control, budgets and human resources dedicated to cancer control efforts have been relatively limited and their role has been primarily restricted to research and technical guidance to member states and others for service delivery, cancer planning, and policy development. Nonetheless, they have played a critical leadership role in strengthening awareness of the cancer burden and strengthening cancer control efforts. In addition, they have been key partners in existing partnerships for the prevention and control of breast and cervical cancers with governments, local health institutions, global and local NGOs, and the private sector.

Despite the absence of innovative global financing mechanisms and strong financing for cancer control efforts, a variety of collaborative endeavors has brought notable impacts to the prevention of breast and cervical cancers in LMICs in recent years. Partnerships of various scales and stakeholder configurations have yielded improved surveillance and data, novel resource-level appropriate technologies and interventions, strengthened technical guidelines, and improvements in the quality and equity of services.

For example, HPV vaccinations projects have been launched by Mexico, Panama, Malaysia, Peru, Argentina, and other countries. Even with negotiated price drops with manufacturers, vaccine adoption by LMICs has been limited due to costs [9, 10]. Through its EPI Revolving Fund, the Pan American Health Organization's (PAHO) has been able to pool purchasing of HPV vaccine, thereby making HPV affordable ($14–15 per dose) for participating countries in the Latin America and the Caribbean (LAC) region [11]. While these costs are still considered prohibitive for many LMICs, the PAHO model of procurement provides a good example of innovative and concrete approaches to financing cancer control.

Given the funding scenario for cancer control in LMICs, there is an important need to identify new sources of funding beyond conventional official development assistance [1]. Importantly, innovative financing and resource mobilization efforts should encompass not only identifying additional funding and channeling new funds to countries, but also the more effective use of existing and new funds through pooling financial resources, developing new incentives for delivery and allocation at various scales, and implementation of programs through contracting, financing, and oversight [1, 12]. With the current challenges to cancer control financing—and global health financing more generally—improved efficiencies are crucial to improvements in cancer control in LMICs.

As recommended by the Harvard University *Global Task Force on Expanded Access to Cancer Care and Control in Developing Countries*, leveraging existing innovative global financing mechanisms (e.g., GAVI, the Global Fund, and the US President's Emergency Plan for AIDS Relief (PEPFAR)) and domestic health system funding are two of the main potential sources of new or enhanced revenue for cancer control [1].

The Role of Domestic Financing for Health in LMICs

Domestic governments play the primary role in cancer control financing in most LMICs; however, as indicated above, the resources invested in cancer control are largely insufficient to address the cancer burden. Limited resource mobilization by national and local (i.e., state and municipal) government is intimately connected to the absence or underdevelopment of cancer control policies. Governments play the primary role in provisioning healthcare in most countries and therefore play a leading role in mobilizing financial resources, human resources, infrastructure, and technologies for cancer control.

Establishment of cancer control as a health priority within legislative and executive policies plays an important initial step in catalyzing broader resource mobilization efforts. In addition, the creation of government cancer institutions plays an important role in strengthening resource mobilization and promoting more effective application of resources through coordinating efforts, strategic cancer planning, providing technical guidance, serving as educational institutions, and engaging in quality control. The creation and support of government cancer institutions are indicative of stronger commitment to cancer control and linked to more robust policies and resource allocation [13].

With the exception of the poorest countries (e.g., Malawi, Tanzania, and Mozambique), in most LMICs, total health expenditures are primarily from domestic financing. Approximately 99% of total health expenditures in middle income countries come from domestic sources, while about 74% of total health expenditures in low income countries come from domestic sources [1]. In most LMICs countries, government financing (e.g., through public health spending, social protection, or insurance schemes) and out-of-pocket spending account for the bulk of health expenditures. In many LMICs, out-of-pocket spending accounts for more than half of health expenditures [1, 14].

Many LMICs are "facing severe financial constraints, and their capacity to increase the availability and quality of health services over time will depend on their ability to increase funding from both domestic and external sources, and to use them efficiently and equitably." There is an "enormous variation in health expenditures between different countries," with the overall funding level for health in each country "determined partly by a country's wealth, the proportion of national income devoted to health, and inflows of funds for health from external partners" [15].

Average (weighted) per capita expenditure range in low-income countries is US$25 compared to US$4,692 in high income countries. Per capita expenditures range from US$48 in the WHO South-East Asia Region to US$3,187 in the WHO region of the Americas. Per capita spending for many LMICs (especially low income countries) falls below the suggested minimum cut off of US$44 to provide a set of essential health services (focusing primarily on HIV, tuberculosis, malaria, and maternal and child health, with some preventive activities targeting NCDs) proposed by the High Level Taskforce on Innovative International Financing for Health Systems [15].

To address the underfinancing of health in LMICs the WHO has recommended the following priorities to redress this issue: "raising more funds for health domestically," "reducing financial barriers to services by increasing forms of prepayment and the pooling of funds," and "improving efficiency and equity in the way resources are used" [15].

Domestic Financing and Cancer Control in LMICs

Cancer control financing replicates the broader patterns of health expenditure in LMICs.

Government funding is the primary source of cancer control resources in LMICs. This is especially the case in middle income countries where more robust public health systems exist and where the cancer burden is generally greater.

While data and analysis are limited, it is safe to assume that—as is the case for general health expenditures—overall and per-capita cancer expenditures vary widely between countries. Given the lack of information and the wide range of domestic health financing and domestic cancer control efforts, it is difficult to make generalizations, but a few common challenges emerge.

The socioeconomic burden, contribution to impoverishment, and often catastrophic consequences of out-of-pocket spending for health in low resource settings are general problems for health financing in LMICs [15], and these have especially problematic implications in the case of cancer. The often high costs of cancer and the chronic nature of cancer care place important limitations on the role of out-of-pocket expenditures for cancer control in LMICs, especially for underserved groups. Catastrophic hospitalization and chronic management costs due to cancer (and other chronic diseases) can be a major onus on individuals and families and important contributors to poverty where out-of-pocket costs are high [1, 16].

Levels of out-of-pocket spending on health as a percentage of total health expenditure by country vary widely. Only 47 countries fall below the 15% threshold considered to limit the incidence of financial catastrophe. Out-of-pocket payments account for more than 50% of total health spending in 36 countries. The WHO has recommended prepayment approaches (e.g., taxes and insurance) as a means to address the limitations of health financing models that are highly dependent on out-of-pocket payments. These prepayment approaches allow for pooling of resources and spreading risk [15]. The appropriate prepayment approach is contingent on the widely varying specific socioeconomic and health systems considerations within different countries.

To address the growing cancer burden, the increasing awareness of its health and socioeconomic impact, and the limitations of out-of-pocket payments for cancer control among low income populations, several middle income countries have devised innovative and effective reforms and innovations to improve resource mobilization for cancer control. There has been a trend in LMICs to reform health financing to "to offer population-wide financial protection to reduce the reliance on out of pocket spending." These types of reforms have been evident in many middle income countries as well as some low income countries. In several instances, these reforms have encompassed improved access to chronic disease care, including cancer screening and care [1].

Inclusion of a set of cancer prevention, early detection, treatment, and care as part of basic service packages of public health systems or insurance plans has increased access to cancer control in a variety of LMICs. Through prepayment and pooling, the negative implications of dependence on out-of-pocket payments are diminished. Financing for these packages have come from general public health financing pools or through creation of specific levies in some cases [1]. Improvements in resource mobilization in middle income countries have been driven by and imbricated within changes to cancer control policy changes that improve quality of care and address health equity concerns.

Several Latin American and Caribbean countries (e.g., Colombia, Chile, Mexico, Peru, and the Dominican Republic), for example, have reformed health financing through a variety of other health reforms (social insurance programs, separation of funds for public and catastrophic expenditures, the development of contributory and subsidized plans segmented to different socioeconomic groups, building and integrating social welfare programs) [1].

It is important to note that enhanced domestic government cancer control resource mobilization goes beyond increasing funds. Although amounts of investments are a key barrier, there are a variety of additional policy, planning, and operational barriers that inhibit resource mobilization and improved cancer prevention and care. For example, cytology-based cervical cancer prevention programs are inaccessible to most LMICs due to operational factors in addition to costs barriers [17].

An important challenge for governments in LMICs is the need to balance investments in different aspects of cancer prevention, screening, diagnosis (cytology and biopsies), treatment (surgical, radiotherapy, and chemotherapy), and palliation to ensure efficiency of resource mobilization, financial sustainability, and equity. For example, services and technologies need to be well defined in order to avoid overinvesting in costly treatments that do not significantly extend healthy life or impact outcomes at the expense of allocating funds to interventions that could save more lives (e.g., improving access to and quality of early detection) [1]. The challenges of rationalized planning that balances multiple cancer control needs are apparent when there is a lack of reliable epidemiological data and cost-benefit and other economic analyses of investments. There is also the broader challenge of weighing different disease priorities and interventions to maximize public health funds. Strengthening cancer planning and resource allocation decisions need to be undertaken within the context of overall health financing, health systems planning, and reforms to promote effectiveness and sustainability of cancer control efforts that support broader public health goals.

The Role of Health Institutions

With this broad overview of domestic financing and challenges in mind, it is important to understand the role of hospitals and healthcare institutes, which serve as the nexus of cancer services and cancer control efforts. While the financial resources, infrastructure, technologies, and specialized healthcare professionals are often insufficient to attend to the actual or potential demand for cancer control services in most countries, public healthcare facilities typically provide screening, diagnostic, and treatment services to the greatest numbers of people in developing countries.

University hospitals—which are typically publically funded and part of the public health system—often play an important role in provisioning screening and care as well as a critical role in training of healthcare professionals and cancer control research. Philanthropic hospitals and private hospitals can also play a very important role in cancer control in many countries. In many countries, philanthropic hospitals play a critical role in filling the lacunae created by limited or absent government facilities and services. Some philanthropic institutions may be affiliated with faith-based or culturally based organizations. Funding may come from hospital-driven fundraising activities or fundraising activities of organizations with which they are affiliated. Such hospitals may also be partially integrated into the public health systems and receive government resources (e.g., funding, staffing, infrastructure, and technologies) for their operation.

While private hospitals often serve a more restricted population and depend primarily on out-of-pocket expenses and insurance plan payments, in many cases they may also engage in philanthropic activities that provide access to screening and care to a wider population. The extent of the role of private hospitals in this regard is contingent on a variety of factors, including hospital leadership, the existence of laws and regulations that serve to stimulate or encourage attending patients from underserved populations, and the particular ways in which these private institutions are integrated with public healthcare networks. Private hospitals can also play an important role in driving local innovation in service delivery, promoting increased awareness and demand for cancer control services, and fomenting cancer research.

Government funding provides the bulk of financial resources for the operation of public hospitals and healthcare facilities in most countries. Depending on the country, these institutions may also receive some revenue from user fees. Government funding may also, to varying degrees, support cancer control activities of philanthropic hospitals and the philanthropic initiatives of private hospitals. While private hospitals may receive some government support and/or tax breaks, their primary support comes from user fees and private insurance plans from patients from more affluent socioeconomic backgrounds, which permit them to provide services at no cost or low cost to underserved groups.

While philanthropic hospitals may be integrated to some extent within public health systems and receive some government support, their cancer control facilities and services typically depend on additional fundraising activities targeting the private sector and the general public. Fundraising activities to support these philanthropic hospitals are contingent on support of local businesses and individual donors.

Additional sources of cancer control funding for public, university, philanthropic, and private health institutions are international health and research institutions. For example, institutions in LMICs sometime receive support from and/or have collaborative agreements with cancer hospitals (e.g., MD Anderson), academic institutions, professional associations, and public health institutions (US Centers for Disease Control and Prevention (CDC) and the National Cancer Institute (NCI) [18]) from high income countries. Such support has included resources and technical support for training, technologies, research, and service delivery. Intergovernmental agencies, including the WHO, the International Agency for Research on Cancer (IARC), and the International Atomic Energy Agency (IAEA), have also played a similar and important role.

The Role of Local Philanthropic NGOs

While government funding, insurance, and user fees play the most prominent role in funding cancer control in the majority of LMICs, philanthropic organizations occupy an important and growing niche. A variety of patient groups and other NGOs play an important function in resource mobilization for cancer control. Cancer leagues and other community-based, not-for-profit organizations often engage in fundraising activities to support philanthropic hospitals or philanthropic activities of private hospitals. Some cancer leagues and other NGOs often have strong affiliations with specific hospitals and are often created by hospitals administrators and staff as a means to strengthen fundraising efforts and engage volunteers.

A variety of NGOs that are independent of specific institutions have also come to play an important role in fundraising and resource mobilization for cancer control. They have also been critical to raising awareness, dispelling myths, and promoting policies and government accountability, all of which are closely intertwined with resource mobilization efforts. NGOs have become increasingly important as the cancer burden has grown, as organized civil society has grown, and as NGOs have increased their role in provisioning services, mobilizing resource for public health, and promoting policy change.

There is a wide spectrum of NGOs involved in cancer control efforts in LMICs, with a wide range of activities and a varying involvement in resource mobilization. Many cancer NGOs are volunteer-based organizations that focus on raising awareness, patient services, supplementing medical care through such services as emotional support, providing information about prevention, screening, and treatment, and/or organizing wig and prosthesis programs. Others may engage in community-based awareness and/or screening initiatives. While rarer—especially in low income countries—some NGOs actively focus on advocacy to strengthen policies and policy implementation to improve access to and quality of cancer screening and care. These organizations engaged in advocacy can play an important role in strengthening government resource commitments for cancer control at the national or local levels [19, 20].

The Expansion of NGO Engagement in Cancer Control in LMICs

For breast and cervical cancers, there have been three broad types of NGOs that have played a prominent role: general cancer NGOs, breast cancer NGOs, and women's and reproductive health NGOs [19]. Breast cancer civil society tends to have developed earlier in and be most prominent in high income settings, but breast cancer civil society organizations have become a notable presence in many low and, especially, middle income countries. While breast cancer civil society was not absent in other parts of the globe during the 1980s, during the 1990s and especially the 2000s, breast cancer civil society became more expressive internationally in middle and low income countries.

Over roughly the last 15 years, breast cancer advocacy movements "are emerging and gaining momentum in regions of the world with limited resources—Africa, Asia, Eastern Europe, and Latin America" [21]. For example, during the 1990s, breast cancer activists became the second largest group of patient advocates in Eastern Europe [22]. Breast Cancer NGOs exist in Argentina, Belarus, Brazil, Chile, China, Colombia, Ghana, Greece, India, Italy, Kenya, Japan, Malaysia, Mexico, Nigeria, South Africa, Venezuela, and many other countries throughout the world [21, 23].

Breast cancer groups have tended to be more focused on urban constituents in settings where incidence and mortality are higher and where screening, diagnostic, and treatment capacities are more robust, yet marked by inequities in access. Breast cancer groups in LMICs are primarily volunteer-based organizations and are often founded and staffed by breast cancer survivors [19].

Women's health and/or reproductive health and rights NGOs engaged in cancer control have been particularly active in cervical cancer control with a generally limited engagement in breast cancer control efforts. This pattern, in part, reflects the disease burden and health system engagements of their constituents; that is, their focus is typically on women in low resource settings (often, but not exclusively, rural) where access to and engagement with secondary and tertiary care facilities are limited. With their emphasis on primary care settings, health promotion, and preventative health, the relevance and synergies with cervical cancer prevention have been stronger than links with breast cancer control.

In general, there has been limited collaboration between breast cancer and women's health NGOs due to different constituencies and priorities. While the historical, socioeconomic, and health reasons behind this division are understandable, future efforts to control breast and cervical cancers will be more effective and utilize resources more efficiently with greater collaboration between these groups. Strengthened collaboration is important for more impactful and constituent-focused advocacy efforts for women's cancers as well as for developing more appropriate, efficient, and effective prevention, awareness, and service delivery efforts. More integrated breast and cervical efforts can help strengthen overall cancer policies, human resources for cancer control, and screening and treatment capacities. Such collaboration is also crucial to ensure that breast and cervical control efforts support broader health systems strengthening and women's health goals.

NGOs and Resource Mobilization in LMICs

Despite the expansion of cancer control civil society in LMICs and its critical role in raising awareness, advocating for strengthened policies, and provisioning important programs that attend to emotional and material needs of patients (transportation, food, childcare, etc.) and families, in general, NGOs have thus far not mobilized large amounts of local resources in LMICs.

Funding for NGOs engaged in cancer control in LMICs comes from a variety of sources. Government grants can be an important source of funds and in some national contexts may be the primary or exclusive source of funding. However, given the lack of attention to cancer control in many national contexts, government grant support may often be absent, inaccessible, or limited in other respects. Government grant opportunities specifically for cancer control are almost non-existent, and where government support is available, it typically comes from more general grant opportunities available for civil society groups or for public health efforts. The other main donors of local NGOs include private corporations, individual donors, and grants from international NGOs.

In the United States and Europe, NGOs have played a very important role in mobilizing resources for cancer, including resources for specific healthcare facilities, research, raising awareness about prevention and screening, supplementing medical care with other patient services (e.g., psychological care, emotional support, legal counsel, transportation, and childcare), and strengthening the provision of cancer prevention, screening, and treatment to underserved groups. This especially has been the case since around the 1980s with the growth and diversification of cancer NGOs and especially has been prominent in breast cancer control efforts [22–24].

Breast cancer organizations also developed more innovative, aggressive, and successful fundraising initiatives, with strategic fundraising campaigns targeting a variety of donors, ranging from individual to corporate donors. Fundraising efforts have used a variety of strategies and models, including cause-related marketing, event-based fundraising (e.g., walks, races, and galas), and direct solicitation. These models have been successful at garnering support from individual donors as well as private corporations (including pharmaceutical, medical equipment, insurance, food, clothing, cosmetics, and athletic equipment/sporting goods companies).

Fundraising through special events—which also play a role in building survivor communities and raising awareness—came to be adopted as a common strategy of many breast cancer organizations (e.g., Avon Walk, Komen Race for the Cure, ACS Making Strides Against Breast Cancer). Cause-related marketing also emerged as a widespread strategy among NGOs for fundraising and raising awareness. Another trend that accompanied the growth of NGOs and enhanced fundraising success was the growth of breast organizations that operated as foundations [22], raising funds not only for the organization's own programs but to support grants for research and community-based initiatives of other groups, with important implications for resource mobilization for cancer control.

Thus far in LMICs, the number and diversity of NGOs, the fundraising role of NGOs, and the scale of fundraising activities of these NGOs have been much more limited than in high income countries [20]. This reflects a variety of factors including the historical and contemporary cancer burden in these countries and the more limited role and size of the NGO sector. It also reflects a more challenging environment for philanthropy in LMICs.

NGOs in LMICs often have weak institutional capacity (e.g., staffing, management, evaluation and strategic planning). Organizations are often small, with limited community outreach, and have limited financial resources. Difficulties in fundraising stem from ad hoc funding strategies, donor portfolios with little diversity, and little experience with grant-writing at the national and international levels [20]. Additionally, from a corporate standpoint, given the size of the NGOs, they do not have enough national brand presence to warrant investment. Limited brand presence limits the perceived value of supporting cancer control efforts of NGOs to the public relations component of corporate social responsibility investments.

In addition to these organizational obstacles, the persistent stigma around cancer, limited cancer awareness, and the under-acknowledgement of the magnitude of the cancer burden in LMICs limit the identification and engagement of the public and corporate donors with the cancer cause, thereby contributing to challenges to cancer fundraising efforts. Furthermore, the culture of philanthropy varies greatly in different countries, with conceptions and models of philanthropy in many LMICs being distinct and not amenable to the same fundraising strategies that have been successful in high income countries. Lastly, the general economic conditions of countries and the tax laws for individual and corporate philanthropic donations shape local philanthropic practices in ways that present challenges for fundraising for social causes and NGO initiatives.

Where fundraising efforts of NGOs and philanthropic health facilities have been more successful, strong leadership has been a salient factor. Local political, economic, or cultural leaders who are survivors, have a personal connection to cancer, and/or have a professional link to cancer control have been important catalysts for more robust cancer fundraising efforts. Where political figures, doctors or other health professionals, local business leaders, religious leaders, actors, athletes, musicians, or other public opinion leaders have actively engaged in public support for cancer control, they have helped foster awareness, buy-in, and financial support for cancer control. Strong leadership has proven to be transformative for cancer control efforts at local levels, creating uncharacteristically strong cancer care in some municipalities and states that surpass the unfavorable national norms.

The Role of Private Sector Support for Local NGOs

As donor government funding for global health has leveled off in recent years, private sector financing has become relatively more important. The recent growth and globalization of the notion and practice of corporate social responsibility have brought increasing opportunities for support for NGOs from the private sectors. Often multinational companies have been drivers of trends in LMICs to develop explicit and organized corporate social responsibility programs, promoting and translating models of corporate social responsibility from global headquarters in high income countries to their regional and national offices in LMICs. However, local tax and fiscal policies similar to those in high income countries that serve to stimulate corporate philanthropy may be absent in many countries, thereby limiting the potential role of private sector donations for cancer initiatives of NGOs and philanthropic health facilities.

To date, the most active private donors for cancer control in LMICs have been pharmaceutical and medical technology corporations. Grants from pharmaceutical companies to NGOs have been important in LMICs. Not surprisingly, their role has been more prominent in middle income countries where there are stronger screening and treatment systems and larger potential markets. Pharmaceutical companies have supported cancer control efforts in LMICs through a variety of different partnership models and in a variety of ways, including grant support to NGOs, academic institutions, and health institutions for research, raising awareness, capacity building, screening and vaccination programs, and patient services. They have also contributed to breast and cervical control efforts through advocacy, donations of products (e.g., HPV vaccines), and negotiated price breaks for pilot programs. For example, HPV pilot projects have been developed with donated vaccines from manufacturers in a variety of countries. In the case of Rwanda and Bhutan, national scale pilot programs have been developed [9, 10].

While pharmaceutical donors have filled a critical void for cancer control and their funding has had positive impacts in many respects on cancer awareness, patient services, and cancer advocacy, it also presents some important dilemmas. For one, pharmaceutical funding poses some ethical challenges for NGOs and other grant recipients to ensure that patient and health system needs are not sidelined by marketing agendas of donors. This observation is not to be taken as a simplistic indictment of the pharmaceutical industry support as inherently problematic; rather, it is simply meant to point out that there are conflicts of interest to be considered.

The degree to which corporate social responsibility efforts of pharmaceutical companies are linked to marketing agendas varies quite widely and is contingent on the organizational culture of different corporations. These links also vary between different offices of multinational corporations and are also strongly shaped by government regulations established to ensure ethical industry standards and safeguard patient rights. Of course, conflicts of interest are not solely a concern for pharmaceutical company donors, but also relevant for other potential corporate donors (e.g., food and beverage industry).

In addition to presenting conflicts of interest, pharmaceutical and other corporate sources of financial support can also pose challenges from an organizational image standpoint. However ethical the terms of relationships between NGOs and donors, the existence of relationships can have negative repercussions for the legitimacy of NGOs and their programs among the public, the media, decision makers, and NGO constituents. Clearly defined government, corporate, and NGO conflict of interest policies are important to clarify relations and minimize potential issues and negative impacts on public perceptions.

Pharmaceutical funding also poses sustainability challenges for cancer NGOs and initiatives, as it can make these beholden to the overall industry economic health as well as the patent cycles of particular corporations. When more diverse sources of donations and funding are absent, it may be difficult to ensure longer term organizational sustainability that is necessary to develop stronger, more professionalized organizations with more impactful patient support, service delivery, and advocacy programs.

While pharmaceutical and medical technology companies have been the most prominent private donors thus far, there are other notable donors and there has been increasing support from other sectors of the corporate community with the expansion of corporate social responsibility programs. For example, Avon, through its Avon Foundation, is also a notable corporate donor in the cancer control field in LMICs, being especially active in supporting a variety of breast cancer activities (as well as other women's health issues). Other multinational corporations that have contributed funding to cancer control efforts include Carolina Herrera Perfumes, Dannon, Samsung, Nestle, and Caterpillar. It is worth noting that, outside of pharmaceutical company donations, corporate donations and cause-related marketing efforts for cancer control NGOs and initiatives in LMICs have primarily focused on breast cancer, with essentially no active programs in cervical cancer control.

The Role of International Cancer Foundations and NGOs

Other than pharmaceutical and medical technology support, the other major non-governmental source of funds for cancer control has come from international NGOs focused on cancer, women's health, reproductive health, or international health.

Examples of cancer NGOs that mobilize funds and support programs in LMICs include the American Cancer Society (ACS), the Susan G. Komen Foundation, the Lance Armstrong Foundation (LAF), and the Union for International Cancer Control (UICC).

There has been an increasing number of global health initiatives targeting breast cancer in LMICs [18]. Global initiatives for breast cancer control have included those of NGOs like the American Cancer Society, the Susan G. Komen Foundation, and oncology societies [18]. The growth and specific trajectories of breast cancer civil society have been in part due to the globalization of initiatives of established cancer organizations in the higher resource settings.

The Reach to Recovery Program, for example, was a pioneering initiative in this respect. In 1974, Francine Timothy and the American Cancer Society expanded Reach to Recovery to Europe. Reach to Recovery International became a program of the International Union Against Cancer (UICC) in 1994 and exists in over 100 countries around the world [25]. Reach to Recovery International has been an influential model internationally for peer support, emotional and psychological guidance, and education through survivors. The global influence of Reach to Recovery International has been facilitated by its volunteer-based, cost-effective model which has made the program successfully adaptable to a variety of resource settings [26].

During the 1990s and 2000s, civil society organizations based in the US and Europe have increasingly worked abroad, promoting awareness and supporting local NGOs through grants, trainings, technical assistance, information, and fundraising events. For example, European-based organizations (e.g., UICC, Cancer Research UK, and EUROPA DONNA) have engaged in a variety of international initiatives. During the last 15 years, numerous leading US organizations have expanded their activities oversees; The American Cancer Society, the Avon Foundation, the Lance Armstrong Foundation, Susan G. Komen Foundation, and the National Breast Cancer Coalition (NBCC) have all developed an international presence in the last 10–15 years. The geographic focus of activities has been different. The resource mobilization and programmatic strategies employed have also varied between organizations, but they have generally included one or several of the following approaches:

- Grants for research, capacity building, and/or community-based initiatives
- Trainings, meetings, and awareness events
- Education and awareness campaigns
- Advocacy activities directed at international institutions and/or national governments

These international NGOs have provided support for a variety of research, capacity building, service delivery, and advocacy efforts. In addition to providing grants, technical assistance, and trainings, these organizations have played an important role in connecting domestic NGOs with a variety of other local and international stakeholders, including donors (e.g., foundations and corporate donors).

International cancer organizations also play an important convening role for research, cancer planning, and advocacy. Examples include the UICC's World Cancer Congress and the Breast Health Global Initiative (BHGI). The American Cancer Society and UICC have also convened multi-stakeholder cancer planning forums that have helped strengthen cancer policies and cancer planning in several countries. Harvard University has also played a convening role through its *Global Task Force on Expanded Access to Cancer Care and Control in Developing Countries* (an initiative directed by the Harvard Global Equity Initiative, the Harvard Medical School, the Harvard School of Public Health, the Fred Hutchinson Cancer Research Center, the University of Washington, and the University of Washington School of Medicine). These convening efforts have proven important for raising awareness, strengthening policies, and fomenting resource mobilization.

International cancer NGOs have also helped promote awareness and strengthen media attention to cancer control in LMICs. The American Cancer Society, for example, has organized a variety of journalist summits on cancer control science and policy in Latin America, Africa, and Asia. The Lance Armstrong Foundation organized a Global Cancer Summit in 2010 bringing media, experts, and patient advocates together.

In global cervical cancer control, Cervical Cancer Action (CCA) has played a leading role. CCA is a coalition with the goal of preventing cervical cancer incidence and mortality globally. CCA is co-chaired by PATH and the American Cancer Society and includes the Pan American Health Organization (PAHO), the International Union Against Cancer (UICC), Cancer Research UK (CRUK), International Federation of Gynecology and Obstetrics (FIGO), the International AIDS Vaccine Initiative (IAVI), AIDS Vaccine Advocacy Coalition (AVAC), and the International Planned Parenthood Federation (IPPF) [27]. CCA has mobilized resource for advocacy, research, and service delivery.

The Alliance for Cervical Cancer Prevention (ACCP) has also had a significant impact. ACCP consists of eight partner organizations (EngenderHealth, IAEA/PACT (International Atomic Energy Agency's Programme of Action for Cancer Therapy), IARC (International Agency for Research on Cancer), Jhpiego, PAHO (Pan American Health Organization), Partners in Health, PATH, and UICC (Union for International Cancer Control) [28].

The Role of Other International Health Foundations and NGOs

A variety of international women's health and reproductive health organizations have increasingly engaged in cervical cancer control efforts. These international organizations have largely limited their engagements in cancer control to cervical cancer control and/or HPV vaccination. Increasing attention to cancer in the women's health and reproductive health arenas is part of an incipient shift towards a more holistic conception of women's health that focuses on both acute and chronic health needs throughout the lifecycle. These shifts are due to changing disease burdens in LMICs as well as increasing calls for more horizontal approaches to strengthening health systems to attend to diverse health needs of women.

Women's health and reproductive health organizations that support programs in LMICs include International Planned Parenthood Foundation and Jhpiego. There is increasing attention to cancer among these NGOs as well as a variety of other global leaders in women's health, including Women Deliver and Family Care International (FCI).

In Thailand, a collaborative pilot program focused on nurse training for screening and treatment methods for cervical cancer control (i.e., VIA and cryotherapy in single visit) was initiated in 2000 that included Jhpiego, the Ministry of Public Health, and the Royal Thai College of Obstetricians and Gynecologists, as well as support from the Alliance for Cervical Cancer Prevention (ACCP) and the Bill and Melinda Gates Foundation. Its success served as the foundation for a national program and the adoption of similar programs in other countries [9, 10, 27].

IPPF has helped develop and scale up HPV vaccination programs in Bolivia. In 2009, the Centro de Investigaci6n, Educaci6n y Servicios (CIES)—a member of International Planned Parenthood/Western Hemisphere Region (IPPF/WHR)—developed an HPV vaccine program in collaboration with the Ministry of Health and Sports and with technical support from IPPF/WHR. Vaccines for the initial pilot were secured through the Gardasil Access Program. The program has been successfully expanded to vaccinate over 80,000 girls throughout the country [9]. IPPF has recently added breast and cervical cancer screening to their charter.

In collaboration with UICC, IPPF/WHR is also leading a project on cervical cancer in countries in the LAC region (e.g., Guatemala, El Salvador, and Honduras) to support the systematic introduction of cervical cancer prevention into the agenda of civil society organizations that already work in women's health education, service provision, and/or advocacy. This initiative involves PAHO, local ministries, and domestic NGOs.

Other NGOs with a more general global health focus have also increasingly engaged in cancer control efforts in LMICs. Partners in Health (PIH) has, for example, been involved in ACCP and collaborated on cancer control programs in several countries (e.g., Rwanda).

PATH has long played a leading role in global cervical efforts. For instance, PATH has played an important role in HPV vaccine delivery models and in piloting other low cost interventions for LMICs (visual inspection, HPV test, improved precancer treatment via cryotherapy) [29]. PATH, with support from the Bill and Melinda Gates Foundation and in collaboration with local stakeholders (e.g., governments, research groups, and non-governmental organizations), began HPV vaccine pilot projects in India, Peru, Uganda, and Vietnam. This work has been an important foundation for subsequent vaccine program design and implementation [30]. PATH has also supported technical innovations for service delivery in LMICs; a collaboration between Qiagen and PATH has led to the development of a low cost, portable version of the HPV DNA test that requires minimal training [9].

While the resources mobilized for the prevention and control of breast and cervical cancers by international NGOs have been fairly limited relative to global health spending, efforts by US and European cancer and other health organizations have benefited NGOs and cancer control efforts in LMICS in numerous ways, including:

- Sharing of best practices (e.g., needs assessments, media engagement, advocacy campaign development, fundraising, relationship building, and volunteer engagement)
- Increased profile of cancer survivors and diminishment of stigma
- Enhanced dialog between medical professionals, policy makers, and patients
- Enhanced access to information and patient empowerment
- Promotion of policies for improved access to and quality of care

- Enhanced participation of civil society organizations in cancer and health policy formation and research
- Increased capacity and sustainability of NGOs
- Enhanced networking with organizations at national, regional, and international levels.
- Creation of pilot programs to test screening strategies and technologies in resource-limited settings

Current Scenario and Financing Priorities

In recent years, cancer has increasingly been acknowledged as an important global health issue within international development policies. There have been a variety of global resolutions calling for strengthened policies, resources, and technical assistance for cancer control: The Fifty-Eighth World Health Assembly Resolution on Cancer Prevention and Control (May 2005); UN Commission on Population and Development Forty-fourth Session Resolution (April 2011); and the Political Declaration of the UN High Level Meeting on the Prevention and Control of NCDs (September 2011). In addition, there are broader commitments to strengthen NCD prevention and control: the Johannesburg Declaration on Sustainable Development (September 2002); Political Declaration of the UN High Level Meeting on the Prevention and Control of NCDs (September 2011); the Rio Political Declaration on Social Determinants of Health (October 2011); and the Rio+20 Outcome Document (June 2011).

As global development policies, commitments, and metrics have historically had an important role in fostering resource mobilization efforts, international development assistance for cancer control may increase in the future and transform the current scenario in which international development assistance for cancer control efforts in LMICs is out of line with the magnitude of the health and socioeconomic burden of cancer; however, the current global financial crisis and dwindling donor funds have had important implications for global health funding, thereby limiting the short to medium term prospects of major increases in international development assistance directed at cancer control efforts [1].

Economic problems facing donor countries have led to a leveling of development assistance for health around 2010, and "increases in external financing for global health from traditional bilateral donors, the European Commission, and emerging economies is unlikely to materialize until 2015" [1]. The proportion of development assistance for health coming from individual donors, corporations, and foundations has increased in recent years (accounting for approximately 27% of total development assistance for health in 2007) [2].

With these trends in the traditional major sources of development assistance for health, the role of individual donors, corporations, and foundations is likely to remain an important factor in future global health funding, including for cancer control. While private sector contributions to cancer control "appear to be relatively small and uneven," they are important for "reducing country dependence on official contributions." Even small amounts of international financing "can play an important catalytic role in driving policy change and innovation in care delivery" [1].

Innovative Financing Frameworks and Strategies

Given the current global health financing scenario, innovative financing frameworks and strategies are necessary for strengthening domestic and global resource mobilization for cancer control. Innovative strategies aim not only to increase amounts of resources but to improve efficiency and impact of resource use.

Although the development of innovative financing mechanisms for cancer and/or NCD control would arguably provide the most impactful model to raise and channel resources for cancer control, there are several important barriers, including limited availability of donor funds, which make it difficult to establish new financing mechanisms.

Thus, for amplifying cancer control efforts in LMICs, one of the most important current strategies is to leverage existing financing mechanisms to address women's health, reproductive health, health systems strengthening, and other global health initiatives with potential synergies with breast and cervical cancers. For example, GAVI, the Global Fund, and the US President's Emergency Plan for AIDS Relief (PEPFAR) can be potential sources of new revenue for cancer control [1].

In addition to offering synergies that increase coordination and support health systems strengthening, leveraging existing partnerships and platforms is also beneficial since it reduces transaction costs and avoids to high initial startup cost for creating new innovative financing mechanisms [1]. Beyond potentially catalyzing increases in funding and creating incentives to promote funding, innovative financing mechanisms can lead to pooling of resources from different donors—donor governments, the private sector, philanthropic organizations, and other sources—and bring changes in resource allocation that create a variety of other benefits, including increased scale, enhanced country ownership, improved participation of diverse stakeholders in decision making, and the incorporation of performance-based funding principles [1].

There are three major examples of global health-related innovative mechanisms (GAVI, the Global Fund, and UNITAID) that go beyond raising funds for health and engage in resource mobilization, pooling, channeling, and allocation [1]. These can be leveraged for improvements in breast and cervical cancer control as well as serve as models for similar cancer or NCD-specific efforts. For example, the PAHO EPI Revolving Fund employs a model of procurement that employs elements of these global health financing platforms and serves as a good example of innovative approaches to financing cancer control.

The Harvard *Global Task Force on Expanded Access to Cancer Care and Control in Developing Countries* has suggested that the commitment-based model of the UN Secretary General's Every Woman Every Child Program could be adopted for increasing funding for the prevention and control of breast and cervical cancers [1]. The UN's Global Strategy for Women's and Children's Health has been able to garner considerable commitments from governments, private foundations, multilateral organizations, the UN, the private sector, and professional associations for reproductive, maternal, newborn, and child health [1, 31]. This platform can also be potentially leveraged for breast and cervical cancers. Linking interventions for cancer and other NCDs to those for reproductive, maternal, newborn, and child health can help promote a lifecycle approach to women's health and further efforts to move towards more horizontal approaches to global health that strengthen health systems [1].

Two main innovative financing mechanisms to address breast and cervical cancers have developed in recent years: the GAVI HPV vaccination initiative and the President's Emergency Plan for AIDS Relief's (PEPFAR) Pink Ribbon Red Ribbon (PRRR) initiative. Neither are novel platforms, but modifications of existing platforms to encompass cancer through integrated initiatives. While these efforts are rather incipient, they provide an important model for bolstering resource mobilization for women's cancers, establishing new partnerships and collaborations, and engaging cancer control efforts within efforts to promote broader global health goals.

GAVI HPV Vaccination Initiative

In November 2011, the GAVI Alliance announced its decision to include HPV vaccines among the vaccines it supports for developing countries in response to country demand. GAVI aims to support HPV vaccinations for two million girls in nine countries by 2015. GAVI has negotiated reduced prices with manufacturers, with prices being further subsidized by GAVI financing for qualifying GAVI countries [32].

The GAVI HPV initiative involves a variety of collaborating partners including: World Health Organization (WHO); United Nations Population Fund (UNFPA); International Agency for Research on Cancer (IARC); the Cervical Cancer Action (CCA) coalition;

Alliance for Cervical Cancer Prevention; PATH; vaccine manufacturers; and academic institutions. GAVI's HPV initiative explicitly supports the UN Secretary-General's Global Strategy on Women's and Children's Health and aims to foster synergies with other public health interventions (HIV prevention, reproductive health, family planning, and nutrition) [32].

In addition to meeting GAVI performance indicator criteria, vaccine support for national or demonstration projects is contingent on submission of an application that successfully demonstrates the ability of countries to effectively deliver the vaccines to girls, including a "costing analysis of the proposed delivery strategy or strategies and evidence of non-GAVI resources to support delivery." Selection criteria and applications aim to ensure that countries can adequately manage "vaccine procurement, supply chain, temperature monitoring, storage and transport capacities, and report regularly on progress against targets, stock levels, wastage rates, and use of funds" [32].

Cervical Cancer and HIV/AIDS

Public–private partnerships to enhance the availability of cervical cancer prevention services provide an important opportunity to expand cervical cancer screening in LMICs (e.g., the PRRR) [17]. The PRRR program—led by the George W. Bush Institute, PEPFAR, Susan G. Komen for the Cure, and UNAIDS—links cancer to HIV/AIDS platforms in sub-Saharan Africa and Latin America and provides one example of an innovative model for addressing women's cancers [1]. Integrating cervical cancer control programs with existing initiatives for HIV/AIDS provides resource efficiencies in resource constrained environments, through sharing of resources and infrastructure. Successful pilots have previously been developed in Zambia with support from PEPFAR and private donations [33].

These efforts to integrate cancer services within HIV/AIDS have been scaled up and expanded with the launch of the PRRR initiative in 2011. PRRR leverages existing HIV/AIDS programs to strengthen cervical and breast cancer screening and awareness for at-risk women in sub-Saharan Africa and Latin America. This initiative is part of PEPFAR, administered through the Department of State's Office of the US Global AIDS Coordinator, and co-sponsored by the Bush Institute, the State Department, the Susan G. Komen Foundation, and the UN's HIV/AIDS program [34, 35]. While still in its initial phases, this program can potentially improve access to screening and care for breast and cervical cancer in sub-Saharan Africa, while supporting established local and global health priorities.

Conclusions and Recommendations

The GAVI and PEPFAR initiatives provide interesting models for future resource mobilization efforts for cervical and breast cancers; however, these are insufficient to address the magnitude of the breast and cancer burden in LMICs, and there is a need for increased engagement and support from public and private stakeholders. In order to address the task at hand, funding strategies need to be more robust and diverse.

Domestic sources (e.g., government, insurance payments, and out-of-pocket payments) will continue to remain the chief source of financing in most countries. Domestic governments play the most important role in most countries, and, therefore, focusing international efforts on advocacy and technical assistance for strengthened national policies that provide adequate financing schemes for cancer and other chronic conditions is critical to developing adequate cancer control funding.

Donor government support is the second most important source of global health financing and should be more strongly leveraged for breast and cervical cancers, despite the current omission of cancer control among the priorities of most of these donors and despite the contemporary economic challenges to development assistance more broadly. The GAVI and PEPFAR initiatives represent a positive step in this regard.

With limited existing development assistance and domestic government support for cancer control, private sources of financing—including corporate, NGO, and academic—will remain important in order to address the void created by the lack of other funding sources and to catalyze broader policy and resource mobilization for cancer control. The relative contribution of corporate and nonprofit NGOs to global heath has increased in recent years and will continue to be instrumental for all global health issues, including breast and cervical cancer.

However, given the magnitude of the cancer burden and the relatively small financial contributions of corporations and NGOs to global health efforts, these sources of funding should not be viewed as the primary solutions to the current lack of cancer control funding. These donors must be one component of a broader and more diversified resource mobilization strategy if we are to develop adequate solutions for the task at hand. It is also important that philanthropic efforts do no duplicate or interfere with government initiatives. The activities of private organizations and their role within public–private partnerships need to be mindful of national and local policies, accountabilities, and commitments so that private organizations are not taking on tasks that are governmental responsibilities or that undermine government initiatives.

Public–private partnerships and other collaborations are also keys to pooling of resources and efficiently mobilizing scarce resources to maximize impact and equity. Collaboration is needed at all levels between governments, the private sector, and civil society. Collaboration is also needed between actors involved in cancer and other health priorities (e.g., women's health, HIV/AIDS). Cancer prevention and control require multisectoral strategies, and collaboration is also needed between different agencies and ministries at global and local levels (e.g., health, education, and women's rights).

The appropriate constellations of interventions, partnerships, and donors will vary according to specific resources and social contexts. In general, domestic government, the corporate sector, and local NGOs will be more significant in middle income countries. In these countries, there are often government cancer institutes, more robust civil society engagement, and more opportunities for funding from the private sector. In lower resource settings where domestic resources are more limited, donor governments, multilateral institutions, and international NGOs have played and will continue to play a more prominent role in breast and cervical cancer initiatives.

The network of partnerships and donors, and the resource mobilization efforts will also differ with the type of cancer, in some respects. With relatively low cost interventions, existing and strengthening buy-in from women's health and reproductive health stakeholders, and existing or potential integration into existing innovative public–private partnerships and financing platforms, cervical cancer efforts have received and will continue to receive greater support from development assistance and domestic government financing than breast cancer control efforts. In contrast, strides in breast cancer control will continue to depend more on other sources of financing (corporate sector, individual donors, and support from international non-profits). Cervical cancer efforts will also depend and benefit from these sources of funding, but these sources will continue to be more important for breast cancer which remains to be more fully embraced as a priority in the global health and development arenas.

It is essential to increase funding to meet the challenge of breast and cervical cancers in developing countries. While there are many barriers and no simple solutions to adequately mobilize resources to address the cancer burden, the following recommendations can help promote impact and efficiency in resource mobilization:

1. Promote leadership at global, national, and local levels. Strong leadership plays a catalytic role in raising awareness, resource mobilization, and policy change. Identifying leaders with diverse leadership roles and encouraging their active and vocal involvement in cancer control efforts can drive positive changes.
2. Strengthen multisectoral engagement at global, national, and local levels. Engage other government agencies or sectors as appropriate (e.g., education and women's rights).

3. Foster improved national and local cancer control policies and ensure availability of adequate resources to implement these policies. As government funds are the key source funding for cancer control, especially for underserved groups, advocating for national and local investments in cancer and health financing reforms appropriate for cancer care is critical to strengthening the capacities of health systems to address the cancer burden.
4. Advocate for increased cancer control funding among development donors. While the current funding climate is challenging, there is much room for improvement, and even modest increases among leading development donors can help drive other resource mobilization efforts and strengthened policies and governance. Advocacy for increased cancer control resources should target existing health and development priorities with potential synergies and co-benefits, being mindful not to destabilize support for established global health and development priorities. It is essential that efforts to leverage existing platforms and promote synergies not undermine that ability to serve multiple health needs and that these efforts are informed by the overall challenges of public health financing in developing nations. As Mwanahamuntu and colleagues have pointed out: "For cancer prevention initiatives to succeed in the developing world, programs must avoid placing additional burdens on health systems already stretched thin due to competing priorities" [33].
5. Develop new global public–private partnerships and/or expand the scope of existing public–private partnerships: Innovative public–private partnerships have played a central role in transforming and strengthening resource mobilization for global health in recent decades. While the economic climate has been relatively unfavorable, public–private partnerships continue to be important drivers of policy change, diverse resource mobilization efforts, and the strengthening of health systems and their governance. Even modest efforts to address cancer control through new or existing public–private partnerships can yield important benefits for cancer control in LMICs.
6. Cancer NGOs and institutions in high income countries should increase support for local efforts. Cancer NGOs and other institutions (e.g., philanthropic hospitals and public health institutions) need to continue and expand their efforts to support local cancer NGOs and initiatives. Funding is especially valuable when accompanied by other appropriate capacity building, training, and technical assistance efforts (e.g., cancer control science, health promotions, health communications, patient services, patient navigation, health worker training, advocacy, and fundraising). The combination of grant support and sharing of accumulated expertise by established NGOs in developed countries has been and should continue to be an important driver of the development of more strongly professionalized and sustainable organizations in LMICs and of the development of more strongly evidence-based awareness, education, patient services, and advocacy initiatives. It is important that such donors also ensure that funding priorities are in line with local priorities and needs and that decision making regarding granting priorities involves consultation and participation of local stakeholders and experts. Given the primary role of government funding in cancer control, donor support to enhance local advocacy capacity is important for strengthening cancer control efforts in LMICs. It is very challenging to fundraise for advocacy programs from corporate and individual donors, and international NGOs are one of the few potential sources for strengthening advocacy capacity.
7. Promote increased collaboration between cancer groups as well as between cancer NGOs and other health NGOs at global, national, and local scales (e.g., NCDs, women's health, and reproductive health). Identifying shared interests and synergies between groups and implementing collaborative initiatives can strengthen programs, service delivery, and advocacy efforts. Collaboration can promote efficiencies in financial and human resource use, help to avoid duplication of efforts, expand scale and impact of initiative, and aide in promoting overall health systems strengthening.

8. Promote the diversification of the donor base of NGOs in LMICs: While there are many challenges to increasing and diversifying the donor base, diversification is critical to ensuring organizational and health system resilience, stability, and sustainability. Cancer and other NGOs with an international reach can play an important role in sharing fundraising best practices and help NGOs in LMICS understand and adapt different fundraising models (e.g., corporate donations, cause-related marketing, individual donors, international foundation or NGO grants, and government grants) to local needs. All types of donor sources have their strengths and weaknesses, and there is no ideal portfolio of donors. The appropriate donor portfolio is contingent on the organization, its mission, cultural context, and health systems context. While the fundraising models employed by cancer and other NGOs with an international reach may not be entirely translatable, they can provide a framework by which to develop locally appropriate models. In addition, engaging local experts in fundraising can help promote the diversification and increase in donor sources. Inviting fundraising experts to serve on NGO boards and/or contracting or securing pro-bono fundraisers can provide important support for local fundraising efforts.
9. Where absent, regulations to minimize conflicts of interest between private donors and recipients should be promoted: Government policies that address conflicts of interest are important. The development of conflict of interest policies by individual NGOs, individual corporations, and industry associations should also be encouraged. These policies are important to help safeguard patient rights and interests and can support NGOs in effective mission delivery and in strengthening their legitimacy among constituents and other relevant stakeholders. These regulations can also provide benefits to donors by helping safeguard their public image and promoting greater transparency of corporate social responsibility efforts, thereby supporting public relations goals.

References

1. Atun R, Knaul FM, Akachi Y. Section 8: Innovative financing: local and global opportunities. In: Knaul FM, Frenk J, Shulman LN, editors. Closing the cancer divide: a blueprint to expand access in low and middle income countries. Boston: Global Task Force on Expanded Access to Cancer Care and Control in Developing Countries, Harvard Global Equity Initiative; November 2011. Available from: http://ghsm.hms.harvard.edu/uploads/pdf/ccd_report_111027.pdf.
2. Institute for Health Metrics and Evaluation. Financing global health 2010: development assistance and country spending in economic uncertainty. Seattle: Institute for Health Metrics and Evaluation; 2010. Available from: http://www.healthmetricsandevaluation.org/publications/policy-report/financing-global-health-2010-development-assistance-and-countryspending-economic-uncertaint.
3. Pitt C, Greco G, Powell-Jackson T, Mills A. Countdown to 2015: assessment of official development assistance to maternal, newborn, and child health, 2003–08. Lancet. 2010;376:1485–96.
4. Nugent RA, Feigl AB. Where have all the donors gone? Scarce donor funding for non-communicable diseases. Washington DC: Centre for Global Development. Working Paper 2008; 2010.
5. Beaulieu N, Bloom D, Bloom R, Stein R. Breakaway: the global burden of cancer—challenges and opportunities. A report from the Economist Intelligence Unit, 2009. Available from: http://www.cancer.org/acs/groups/content/@internationalaffairs/documents/document/acspc-026203.pdf.
6. Farmer P, Frenk J, Knaul FM, Shulman LN, Alleyne G, Armstrong L, et al. Expansion of cancer care and control in countries of low and middle income: a call to action. Lancet. 2010;376:1186–93.
7. Knaul FM, Frenk J, Shulman, LN, editors. Closing the cancer divide: a blueprint to expand access in low and middle income countries. Boston: Global Task Force on Expanded Access to Cancer Care and Control in Developing Countries, Harvard Global Equity Initiative; November 2011. Available from: http://ghsm.hms.harvard.edu/uploads/pdf/ccd_report_111027.pdf.
8. World Health Organization. WHO/ICO Information Centre on Human Papilloma Virus (HPV) and Cervical Cancer. Available from: www.who.int/hpvcentre.
9. Women Deliver. Delivering cervical cancer prevention in the developing world; 2011. Available from: http://www.womendeliver.org/assets/Cervical Cancer_final.pdf.
10. Cervical Cancer Action. Progress in cervical cancer prevention: the CCA report card; 2011. Available from: http://www.cervicalcanceraction.org/pubs/pubs.php.
11. Pan American Health Organization. Report on the Latin American subregional meeting on cervical

cancer prevention: new technologies for cervical cancer prevention: from scientific evidence to program planning; 2010 June. Available from: http://new.paho.org/hq/dmdocuments/2010/Panama_report_en.pdf.
12. Girishankar N. Innovating development finance: from financing sources to financial solutions. The World Bank. Policy Research Working Paper 5111; 2009. Available from: http://wwwwds.worldbank.org/servlet/WDSContentServer/WDSP/IB/2009/11/03/000158349_20091103112908/Rendered/PDF/WPS5111.pdf.
13. Nigenda G, González Robledo MC, González Robledo LM, Bejarano RM. Disparidades al descubierto: un estudio comparado sobre Políticas de Cáncer de Mama en América Latina. American Cancer Society and Instituto Nacional de Salud Pública, Mexico; 2011 May. Available from: http://ulaccam.org/wp-content/uploads/2012/03/reporte-Disaparidades-al-descubierto.pdf.
14. World Health Organization. The World Health Report 2010. Health systems financing: The path to universal coverage. Geneva: WHO; 2010.
15. World Health Organization. World health statistics 2012. Geneva: WHO Press; 2012. http://www.who.int/gho/publications/world_health_statistics/EN_WHS2012_Full.pdf.
16. Nikolic I, Stanciole A, Zaydman M. Chronic emergency: why NCDs matter. Health, Nutrition and Population Discussion Paper. Washington DC: World Bank; 2011. Available from: http://siteresources.worldbank.org/HEALTHNUTRITIONANDPOPULATION/Resources/281627-1095698140167/ChronicEmergencyWhyNCDsMatter.pdf.
17. Sahasrabuddhe VV, Parham GP, Mwanahamuntu MH, Vermund SH. Cervical cancer prevention in low- and middle-income countries: feasible, affordable. Cancer Prev Res (Phila). 2012;5:11.
18. Coughlina SS, Ekwuemeb DU. Breast cancer as a global health concern. Cancer Epidemiol. 2009;33(5):315–8.
19. Azenha G, Bass LP, Caleffi M, Smith R, Pretorius L, Durstine A, et al. The role of breast cancer civil society in different resource scenarios. Breast. 2011;20:S81–7.
20. Durstine A, Leitman E. Building a Latin American cancer patient advocacy movement: Latin American cancer NGO regional overview. Salud Publica Mex. 2009;51 Suppl 2:S316e322.
21. Errico KM, Rowden D. Experiences of breast cancer survivor advocates and advocates in countries with limited resources: a shared journey in breast cancer advocacy. Breast J. 2006;12 Suppl 1:S111.
22. Koon KP, Soldak T, Gralow JR. Breast cancer advocacy: changing perceptions. Salud Pública de Méx. 2009;51 Suppl 2:325.
23. Collyar D. Science and society: How have patient advocates in the United States benefited cancer research? Nat Rev Cancer. 2005;5:73.
24. Lerner BH. Breast cancer activism: past lessons, future directions. Nat Rev Cancer. 2002;2:225.
25. Reach to Recovery International. The history of reach to recovery. Available from: http://www.reachtorecoveryinternational.org.
26. Bishop A, Kovtun A, Okromeshko S, Karpilovskaya S, Suprun N. Lives renewed: the emergence of a breast cancer survivor movement in Ukraine. Reprod Health Matters. 2001;9(18):130.
27. Cervical Cancer Action. About us. Available from: www.cervicalcanceraction.org.
28. Alliance for Cervical Cancer Prevention. Available from: www.alliance-cxca.org/.
29. PATH. Equal protection from cervical cancer. Available from: http://www.path.org/our-work/cervical-cancer.php.
30. Cervical Cancer Prevention. Practical experience from PATH. Available from: http://www.rho.org/HPV-practical-experience.htm.
31. Partnership for Maternal, Newborn, and Child Health. The PMNCH 2011 report. World Health Organization; 2011. Available from: http://www.who.int/pmnch/en/.
32. GAVI Alliance. Human papillomavirus vaccine support. 2011. Available from: http://www.gavialliance.org/support/nvs/human-papillomavirus-vaccine-support/.
33. Mwanahamuntu MH, Sahasrabuddhe VV, Kapambwe S, Pfaendler KS, Chibwesha C, et al. Advancing cervical cancer prevention initiatives in resource-constrained settings: insights from the Cervical Cancer Prevention Program in Zambia. PLoS Med. 2011;8(5):e1001032.
34. Rosenthal ET. Why the U.S. has gone global in the fight. J Natl Cancer Inst. 2011;103(22):1648–50.
35. US Department of State. Pink Ribbon Red Ribbon. 2011. Available from: http://www.state.gov/r/pa/prs/ps/2011/09/172244.htm.

B: Role of Philanthropists

Kelli A. Cohen

Introduction

Cancer is a disease which continues to be plagued by stigma and discrimination within many communities across the globe and displays no discrimination in how it targets its victims. While it affects everyone either directly or indirectly, it is irrespective of age, gender, race, ethnicity, or religion; approximately two thirds of the annual cancer mortality worldwide occurs in low and middle income countries (LMICs). Clearly, the burden of disease is disproportionately faced by the poor who either have no access to cancer care at all or cannot afford the exorbitant costs associated with catastrophic illness [1]. Globally, funding for cancer is heavily skewed to high income countries. Though cancer in low and middle income countries accounts for 80% of the global cancer burden, only 5% or less of global spending on cancer is in LMICs [2]. The dearth of funding is staggering, given the increasing illness and rising number of deaths from non-communicable diseases (NCDs) including cancer in LMICs. Projections show that by 2030, NCDs will cause 74% of mortality and 64% of morbidity in LMICs [3]. Collaboration and international partnerships remain at the core of achieving any success against cancer.

K.A. Cohen (✉)
Diagnostic Radiologist, Locum Tenens, McGovern Center for Humanities and Ethics, University of Texas, Houston, TX 77030, USA
e-mail: kcohenfein@mfein.com

This section of the chapter will provide an in-depth look at a recent history of global funding for health in low-resource countries, and a definition of philanthropy including its role through governmental and non-governmental organizations (NGOs) as well as private philanthropic entities involved in the global women's healthcare effort. Various international foundation efforts and initiatives targeting early breast and cervical cancer diagnosis, increased awareness, empowerment of the indigenous female populations, advocate enrichment, and national and international collaboration are identified and delineated to better comprehend the global role of philanthropic synergy in the global health effort.

Sustainable development, social justice with multidimensional equity, and application of advancing science and technology for all-around human well-being are touted to become the hallmarks of civilization in the twenty-first century. Between 1990 and 2007, global assistance for health development rose from about $6 billion to nearly $22 billion. Some middle income countries are starting to become regional donors, and many governments in low income countries are increasing their budgetary commitments to health. Important technological progress in the areas of HIV, malaria, vaccinations, and diagnostics, as well as in mobile computing and communications technologies has occurred in recent years. The biggest challenge in global health is the growing gap between the effective and cost-effective action we know works and what we actually implement. These efforts will require additional investments in both personnel and public health institutions [4]. Adequate financial allocations for health remain a bottleneck, and, in the wake of dwindling resources and strained economies, there is a pressing need for increasing funding for health. In September 2000, 189 Global Leaders came together at the United Nations to adopt the United Nations Millennium Declaration, committing their nations to a set of Millennium Development Goals (MDGs) to reduce poverty and achieve a range of health and development targets by 2015. Through the work of Global Fund to Fight AIDS, Tuberculosis, and Malaria (GFATM) and the US President's Emergency Plan for AIDS Relief (PEPFAR), millions of poor people worldwide have had access to care that would have been unimaginable a few decades ago [5]. In 2011, the United Nations General Assembly (UNGA) held for the first time a High Level Meeting (HLM) on the Prevention and Control of Non-Communicable diseases [6]. The non-communicable diseases (NCDs), which include cardiovascular disease, chronic respiratory disease, diabetes, and cancers, are the dominant public health challenge of the twenty-first century [7]. Left unattended, NCDs compromise the Millennium Development Goals, thwart the eradication of poverty, and undercut economic growth. NCDs account for an estimated 63% of the global death toll [7]. By 2030, it is estimated that NCDs may account for 52 million deaths worldwide, nearly 5 times the projected number of deaths from communicable diseases [7]. Most (80%) NCD-related deaths, especially premature (<60 years of age) deaths, occur in low and middle income countries [7]. The key tangible deliverable of the HLM is the Political Declaration on the Prevention and Control of NCDs [8]. While this declaration designated the World Health Organization as the coordinator of the global response to the NCDs charged with developing a comprehensive global monitoring framework and designated the UN Secretary General responsible for considering relevant partnerships, monitoring the realization of HLM commitments and reporting on progress in the prevention and control of NCDs [9], expected funding pledges for this underfunded sector (<3% of global health aid) [10] did not materialize. The traditional donor-country partnership model has been replaced with one wherein traditional global health champions (e.g., national and multinational donors) assume a more limited role [9]. Nevertheless, the dozen years since the adoption for the Millennium Development Goals have been a period of great achievement and advances in public health in the poorest countries [11].

Public health data indicate that the global burden of breast cancer in women, measured by incidence, mortality, and economic costs, is substantial and on the increase. Worldwide, it is estimated that more than one million women are diagnosed with breast cancer every year, and more than 410,000 will die from the disease. In low and middle income countries (LMCs), the infrastructure and resources for screening mammography are often unavailable. In such lower resource settings, breast cancers are commonly diagnosed at late stages, and women may receive inadequate treatment, pain relief, or palliative care [12]. The Global Summit panels define countries with limited resources as those countries with low or medium level resources as described by WHO (2002) [13]. Breast cancer is commonly diagnosed in late stages in countries with limited resources. Efforts aimed at early detection can reduce the stage at diagnosis, potentially improving the odds of survival and cure, and enabling simpler, more cost-effective treatment. The questions of funding and resources continue to dominate the inevitable realities of bringing these efforts to fruition. The paradigm of global health assistance is shifting toward a world "beyond aid" [14]. NCDs are encountering the tipping point of a maturing aid reform movement willing to conceptualize a world "beyond aid" [15]. As we look to the future of healthcare, taking into consideration the uncertainty regarding health reform and the US economy, it is imperative to recognize that economic and financial issues have been dominating global policy making. Ultimately, health and inequalities in health should feature more strongly as economic and social developments have profound effects on health inequalities [16].

As many as 100 million people could die of cancer over the next 10 years, the majority of them in developing countries. In low income countries for example, cervical cancer kills more women than any other form of the NCD [17]. Yet, its initial stages and precancerous lesions can be detected through routine examinations, making it easy to cure. To prevent unnecessary deaths and to save lives, international organizations, civil society, and the donor community must work together to increase the resources dedicated to cancer prevention, early detection, treatment, or cure and palliative care in developing countries. The International Atomic Energy Agency (IAEA) took action to combat cancer in developing countries by launching a Programme of Action for Cancer Therapy (PACT) in 2004. PACT's mission is to improve cancer survival in developing countries by integrating radiotherapy investments into public health systems. PACT will meet its goals by building public–private partnerships, mobilizing resources from nontraditional sources, and ensuring the effective and sustainable transfer of radiation medicine. Radiation medicine includes both radiotherapy (and radiation oncology) and diagnostic imaging involving the safe use of ionizing radiation and nuclear medicine procedures. Acting on its mandate to "accelerate and enlarge the contribution of atomic energy to peace, health, and prosperity throughout the world," the IAEA has enabled many countries to establish safe and effective radiotherapy capabilities, and to provide higher quality treatment to cancer patients. The World Health Organization (WHO), in accordance with its mandate as the directing and coordinating authority on international health work, has developed the National Cancer Control Programme (NCCP) Strategy. WHO has been implementing this strategy for well over a decade to advise countries in the fight against cancer. Technical support to countries will be further strengthened with the recent endorsement by the 61st World Health Assembly of a global strategy for the prevention and control of NCDs [17]. A formidable public–private partnership will combat cervical and breast cancer for women in Sub-Saharan Africa and Latin America. In mid-September, the President's Emergency Plan for AIDS Relief (PEPFAR) joined the George W. Bush Institute, Susan G. Komen for the Cure, and the Joint United Nations Programme on HIV/AIDS as well as private sector partners to launch Pink Ribbon Red Ribbon [18]. The United States' contribution to the partnership will build on the PEPFAR program, which was established under President George W. Bush to fight AIDS globally. The Obama Administration has built on PEPFAR through the Global Health Initiative, increasing the number of people receiving prevention, treatment, and care for HIV. Through PEPFAR, the US will invest an additional $10 million through the partnership, on top of the $20 million already allocated over the next five years, to expand screening and treatment of HIV-positive women for cervical cancer in Sub-Saharan Africa [18]. In the developing world where there is a general lack of funding, education, and awareness, women's cancers are often neglected. To compound the problem, women's cancers may be culturally associated with a stigma that further discourages women from seeing a doctor. Globally, cervical cancer is the third most common cancer in women, with 530,000 new cases and 275,000 deaths each year. 85% of cervical cancers occur in developing countries, yet, according to the World Health Organization, fewer than 5% of these women have access to screening. Cervical cancer is four to five times more common among women who are HIV-positive, because HIV reduces the body's ability to fight infections that may lead to cancer. Thus, PEPFAR programs are ideally positioned to test women with HIV for cervical cancer, and to treat it if needed. As Secretary of State Hillary Rodham Clinton so aptly articulated in a recent related article, "If we want to make progress on some of the toughest challenges we face in global health (in terms of combating communicable and NCDs in low-resources countries), then investing in women must be at the top of the agenda" [18]. The Pink Ribbon Red Ribbon (PRRR) initiative is the first large-scale proposal launched by the Bush Institute and the first major post-presidential initiative of the institute's namesake. Building on the PEPFAR's success in reducing HIV/AIDS in Africa, PRRR is driven by the recognition that, "it's not enough to save a woman from AIDS, if she is then left to die of another very preventable disease" [19].

Philanthropy plays an important humanitarian and catalytic role in addressing global health challenges worldwide. The term "global health" focuses on the substantial and complex healthcare challenges faced by developing nations around the world. While corporate involvement in and government aid for health has been extensively analyzed and critiqued in the public health literature, less attention has been paid to the impact of private donors on public health [20]. Over the past decade, the bulk of new health aid designed to reach the Millennium Development Goals has come from individuals and corporations [21, 22]. The influence of this private philanthropy on global health is profound and transformative [23].

Philanthropic attention toward strategies to embrace the global burden of breast and gynecologic cancers presents new opportunities for an integrated approach in screening and early diagnosis of women's cancers in developing countries as philanthropic dollars continue to play a defining and guiding role in meeting humanity's needs. Philanthropy is derived from the Greek words *philein* ("to love") and *anthropos* ("human being"). Philanthropy is defined as a desire to help mankind, especially as shown by gifts to institutions [24]. Here in the United States, philanthropy is synonymous with American principles, history, and culture. The term "philanthropy" is also used to describe the granting of money to nonprofit organizations by foundations and corporations. This type of giving is often called organized philanthropy or grant-making. While philanthropy can be defined in many ways and remains an evolving and largely misunderstood entity, the idea of giving is derived from the ancient Greek meaning "love for humanity." Modern definitions include the concept of voluntary giving by an individual or group to promote the common good and improve the quality of life for fellow human beings who find themselves within vulnerable, impoverished, or marginalized communities. Philanthropy may be mandated or influenced by religion or faith. Some faiths believe in giving alms to the poor, while others believe service to mankind demonstrates love and thereby a connection to God, as God is perceived as love. The Hebrew term "tzedakah" roughly means charity, but more accurately it is translated into "righteousness or correctness," intimating that when one gives charity or philanthropy, personally or collectively, one is achieving a higher purpose in "doing the right thing." Philanthropy embodies social activism in this regard. To fully embrace a diverse interpretation of individual philanthropy, we inquired as to the germinal inspiration for philanthropic endeavors of several American transformational givers in the realm of local breast cancer screening, evaluation, diagnosis, intervention, and treatment of the indigent population here in Houston, Texas, and in the general well-being of an African community in Uganda.

Philanthropic Examples

The Lester and Sue Smith Foundation

As recently as April 2011, The Harris County Hospital District (HCHD) in Houston, Texas, announced the largest private donation in its history: a $15 million grant for cancer services at their new outpatient clinic [25]. The grant from Lester and Sue Smith of the Lester and Sue Smith Foundation, a rare instance of medical philanthropy targeted for the poor, will fund cancer diagnostic and treatment equipment at the ambulatory center under construction at the HCHD's administrative headquarters. "I've heard too many stories of people coming to Ben Taub General Hospital when it's too late, when the cancer's already spread," said Lester Smith, a Houston oil executive and two-time cancer survivor. "I want all of Houston to receive the level of care that Sue and I receive." Noting these are "hard economic times," Smith said he was motivated to give after learning of the hospital district's limited space and need to upgrade equipment. Hospital district officials had asked Smith to give $2 million. Smith said he responded, "Would you be disappointed if I didn't agree to $2 million?" and they said, "of course not." He said there was sobbing in the room when he said he wanted to give $15 million instead. Public hospital giving is so rare that organizations tracking philanthropy's biggest gifts don't keep a list of such donations. The largest is thought to be a $50 million pledge grant to Parkland Health & Hospital Systems in Dallas, Texas, in 2008. "Public hospital giving is unusual, but we could start seeing a shift in that direction," said Stacy Palmer, editor of *The Chronicle of Philanthropy*. "I think because of the economic downturn, a new generation of donors may look more favorably on safety-net institutions." The Smith gift is part of the district's effort to change the perception that fundraising isn't necessary at tax-supported institutions, said Stephen DonCarlos, chairman of the HCHD Board of Managers. The gift brings the district's 2-year-old campaign to $25 million; its overall goal is $35 million [25].

The clinic, scheduled to open in late 2012, is expected to host about 160,000 patient care visits per year. It will be named the Smith Clinic in recognition of the gift. HCHD officials said the Smith gift will do wonders for cancer patient access, cutting down on waiting times, making it unnecessary for the facility to send some patients to other institutions for radiation, and quadrupling the number of stations at which it gives chemotherapy by infusion. Smith said the clinic's cancer equipment will be the same as that used at the Baylor College of Medicine (BCM), whose doctors impressed upon him the hospital district's needs. Smith has given $40 million to BCM during the past decade, including $30 million for breast cancer research and $10 million to the urology department. BCM doctors treated him for bladder and prostate cancer at The Methodist Hospital [25]. When questioned specifically about the origins and evolution of their philanthropic ideals, Sue and Lester Smith responded:

Cohen: What is the germinal inspiration for your philanthropic endeavors?

Lester: I grew up in a small, tight-knit Jewish community in Wharton, Texas. I was inspired first by my parents and extended family who chose community service as a part of daily life.

Sue: We have been blessed with much, and we live our lives feeling a sense of responsibility to share our time, talent, and resources with others.

Cohen: What are your goals and what have you achieved philanthropically?

Lester: We have a unique approach to philanthropy, offering a "hand up" and not a "hand out" to organizations. We've worked hard to achieve what we have, and we recognize the importance of challenging organizations to do the same. Our model is based primarily on matching grants. Organizations willing to set goals and work hard are rewarded.

Cohen: Why did you choose these specific areas of medicine and cross-sections of population?

Sue: When Lester was diagnosed with bladder and aggressive prostate cancer, we were determined to help others impacted by those diseases. When I lost my sister to breast cancer, we turned our sadness into a strong commitment to fund critical breast cancer research. We've come to realize that everyone has been touched by cancer in some way, and we want to do our part to ease suffering, especially for those without access to timely and quality medical care.

Lester: When you are faced with your own mortality, your perspective changes. We want to cure cancer, and, to do that, we need to fund critical cancer research. We also need to help those who cannot help themselves. A diagnosis of cancer is devastating and a particular burden to those who cannot afford treatment. That's why we made transformational gifts to Texas Children's Cancer Center and Harris County Hospital District.

(continued)

Cohen: What is the most gratifying aspect of this work?

Lester: I have peer counseled hundreds of cancer patients and their families. As I often say, "it takes one to know one" and it is an honor and privilege to help others who face the unsure future of a cancer diagnosis. That I can offer a kind word, access to care, or just a listening ear is truly humbling. It's also incredible to meet the researchers who are at the bench day by day, working tirelessly to find the cures, and to see the doctors and nurses who take those discoveries and deliver them directly to patients at bedside.

Sue: Meeting other survivors who are facing the same challenge and knowing our funds directly impact their treatment and care is extremely gratifying. My work with the Susan G. Komen Foundation has introduced me to hundreds of survivors who are taking their own cancer experience and putting it to work helping others.

Cohen: What is the most challenging aspect of this work?

Lester: I am very impatient. I want to cure cancer today, not tomorrow or next year.

Sue: A diagnosis of cancer affects everyone, not just the patient. Our work at Texas Children's Cancer Center is particularly touching because it impacts children and their families.

Cohen: How do you hope to convey philanthropic mindfulness and participation to younger and future generations of your family and community?

Lester: We challenge other organizations and foundations to think outside the box by our philanthropic model. We work closely with organizations like the Baylor College of Medicine to mobilize a strong volunteer base, set high goals, and work alongside them to achieve them. It takes everyone working toward the same mission.

Sue: We believe our actions speak louder than words. We hope we've modeled that in our community in a way that inspires others to do the same [26].

Philanthropist Robin Young-Ellis

Philanthropist, humanitarian, and Texas business owner Robin Young-Ellis embodies philanthropic ideals as well:

Cohen: What is the germinal inspiration for your philanthropic endeavors?

Young-Ellis: My earliest philanthropic efforts began over a decade ago with scholarships for local Texas children. As I became blessed in my business and was fulfilled personally, professionally, and assured that I was establishing financial sustainability for myself and my family, I recognized that I could help make a difference by sharing my own blessings with others. My development started with my contributions at the Houston Livestock Show and Rodeo as a Grand Champion, Reserve Champion, and Champion buyer. These auction contributions afford Texas children the opportunity to attend Texas colleges and universities. I believe I have now sponsored more than thirty-four children in this decade.

In 2005, I was moved by my roots as a military child and then a military spouse. Recognizing that Houston was a recruiting city and that patriotism flew below the

(continued)

	radar, I founded Salute to Our Troops Houston which honors and shows appreciation to our active duty and reserve troops and their families. Those philanthropic endeavors reach down deep and tug at the heartstrings and began to spread arms that eventually reached into the international arena: Uganda. In 2010, out of curiosity about what I heard about Uganda, I traveled with Hope 4 Kids International. The trip was titled a mission trip but for me I found it to be an exploration and learning journey. What I found unnerved and unraveled me. While it was a place of unimaginable beauty, pride, and possibility, it suffered political upheaval, unfathomable despair, disease, and decay. The people of Uganda are among the most hospitable in Africa. The nation is a result of the unification of ancient kingdoms, as well as many independent chieftains. Their strong heritage lives on in the hearts of the people, and their traditional costumes, language, and practices are unmistakable in the life of Uganda today. I remember thinking and wondering if I would ever return and if that would be my one and only trip. But today, after three years, I find myself pulled to Uganda and its beautiful people. When I step off the plane, I feel like I have gone home to my second family and that I have a purpose to help and to make a difference in someone's life.
Cohen:	What are your goals and what have you achieved philanthropically? Why did you choose this specific country in Africa?
Young-Ellis:	Why did I choose Uganda? I believe Uganda chose me. I traveled to Uganda to learn more, to explore, and to see with my own eyes what I had read for years and had heard about through news and through Hope 4 Kids International. There are so many areas that need help. How you come to choose a place can often be due to fate and being at the right place at the right time. The timing was right for me: at a young age in my professional life I had achieve great success. This provided and afforded me the blessing to reach out and share the love. In my lifetime, as a military child, my father was stationed in many countries as well as in the US. This opportunity provided insight on many levels. With that, I found a comfort level in Uganda that was fresh and new to any other feeling I have ever experienced.
Cohen:	What have you achieved?
Young-Ellis:	Sponsored Bukirayi Village in 2010: drilled 2 boreholes (water wells), constructed a church and a small 2-room clinic. Blessed with Baby Esther Ruth Young Kahawa. In 2010, by chance (maybe fate) I met a baby that was 48 hours old and abandoned. Esther Ruth Young Amunot was born between 2:00 am and 4:00 am, July 18, 2010. Abandoned, naked, and left alone by her biological mother in a trash dump of a slum area filled with prostitution, opium drugs, and crime. How she survived is a God Send because the trash dump is located in a bad area where wild dogs and wild pigs rummage through trash for food. Within 24 hours of Esther's birth, my beautiful Ugandan sister, Pastor Ruth Kahawa rescued baby Esther. In the African culture, it is not uncommon for a child to have more than one mommy or papa, especially a child that has been abandoned and orphaned. Joe and I are blessed to share a special relationship with Esther

(continued)

	and her new African parents, Pastor Ruth and her husband, Basil, and their 9 children. We will share in the beauty of her life, see her as often as we can, and love her always. In 2011, I read about the effort and interest of the University of Texas in Austin (UT) School of Architecture and their desire to go global. They were designing a school for Tanzania. I called, just out of curiosity again (and to see if by chance if they would have an interest in working with me). That afternoon, after meeting with the graduate students and their professor, I left Austin on a personal high that is indescribable. By reaching out to UT, I gained a remarkable and beautiful new relationship with a professor of sustainable development and eight amazing and talented grad students. They were on board and excited at the opportunity to develop a school of sustainability, a life that would provide young Ugandan students with more than four walls and a dirt floor. We would take our design and reach out to Uganda by helping implement an education that incorporated academics, farming, a vocation, business, and self-sufficiency. In 2012, I led the UT grad team to Uganda on an exploration and site survey journey. We returned from our trip holding with us a business plan that now incorporates also a clinic (we determined heath is the primary and priority action that we need to take on first), a women's center (to help the single and widowed mothers of these children learn to be self-sufficient) as well as a vocational and academic school plan.
Cohen:	What are your goals?
Young-Ellis:	My goal is to reach out to as many medical organizations as I can so that I may find one (or multiples) that have an interest in reviewing the health needs of our children and mothers. Beyond that, we have a 10-year building development that will hopefully afford us the opportunity to bring together other humanitarian and philanthropic and resource organization, such as we have done with UT, that may want to share their expertise by joining us in an effort to bring health, education, and self-sufficiency to a country that has long been a dependent country.
Cohen:	What is the most gratifying aspect of your work?
Young-Ellis:	Knowing that you can make a difference in a life. That you can turn a child's life around who has faced disease, sadness, emptiness, and despair. That you can truly reach out and teach them how to survive. My position is not one of dependency but one of teaching and implementing self-sufficiency. When you help a person build confidence, pride, and honor, he or she will take that and make a better life for themselves and their families.
Cohen:	What is the most challenging aspect of your work?
Young-Ellis:	Time. Juggling my own workload and demands with that of local and international philanthropic and humanitarian desires and efforts. I have often considered retiring from my company if an organization could afford to pay me a reasonable amount to build these clinics and schools. I have fallen in love with the international work, but in reality I still must earn a living to sustain my future.
Cohen:	How do you hope to convey philanthropic mindfulness and participation to younger and future generations of your family and community?
Young-Ellis:	The best way to spread awareness is to be a living example. To be a living example, you live the life: walk the walk through whatever resources you can offer. To

(continued)

some that means funds, to others that may be your talent, expertise, and knowledge, and then to others it may be a full combination of all. Through my own life and my own journeys, I am confident that the message will speak softly to another one's heart. I may or may not ever know if I have touched someone else in this way, but I am pretty sure that by loving life and all that we embrace for the good and by being a true living example that the chances are high that someone else will follow. And in their own way, they will use their own talents and resources to help others [27].

These humanitarian leaders continue to light the way through life-affirming sharing. They are educating and teaching by the sheer example of their life missions. In sharing their perspectives, core values, and experiential knowledge, they are able to translate their purposeful actions into inspirational invitation and engagement to collaboration toward making a meaningful difference for mankind.

Their generous stewardship and leadership of humankind inspire me and our fellow communities near and far. Walt Whitman once said, "I do not give lectures or a little charity. When I give, I give of myself." The gift of sharing represents both a personal and global responsibility to help heal the world. In Judaism, this effort to repair the world is embodied in the concept of "Tikkun Olam," whereby each individual has a debt to repay to the world. We are not entitled to receive from the world but in fact we are obligated to help in some meaningful way repair a corner of the world.

Everyone involved in the process is implicitly enriched as we become more meaningfully connected with our fellow man. It is synergistic and powerful to be a part of all who give of themselves authentically, creatively, lovingly, and abundantly. The individuals, corporations, and collaborative efforts mentioned here are helping to embolden, redefine, and embrace humanity. It is incumbent upon us to enlist the help of all generations in every walk-of-life and every professional arena. May we continue to inspire one another, for, in the words of Robert Frost, "We have miles to go before we sleep."

Synergy Between Non-Govermental Organizations and Governments

Within the United States, philanthropy has invested millions of dollars to reduce disparities in healthcare and improve minority health. Grants to strengthen providers' cultural competence, diversify health professions, and collect data have improved understanding of and spurred action on disparities. The persistence of disparities in spite of these advances has shifted philanthropic attention toward strategies to change social, economic, and environmental conditions [28]. The persistence of disparities within the US in spite of these advances appears relatively minimal when compared with the vast disparities found in low-resource countries, particularly with respect to women's health issues. Breast cancer is commonly diagnosed at late stages in countries with limited resources. Efforts aimed at early detection can reduce the stage at diagnosis, potentially improving the odds of survival and cure, and enabling simpler and more cost-effective treatment. Early detection of breast cancer entails both early diagnosis in symptomatic women and screening in asymptomatic women. Key prerequisites for early detection are ensuring that women are supported in seeking care and that they have access to appropriate, affordable diagnostic tests and treatment. Public education and awareness can promote earlier diagnosis, and these goals can be achieved in simple and cost-effective ways [29]. According to the most recent numbers released by the Giving USA Foundation, philanthropic support of healthcare rose 3.8% between 2008 and 2009, representing 7% of the total giving to all philanthropic entities of $303.75 billion in 2009. This is good news, considering that overall giving was down 3.6%. While US hospitals are looking at charitable donations to fill in revenue gaps [30], the Task Force analysis of investment patterns for global health suggests that, to date, contributions from the private sector and innovative financing appear to be relatively small and uneven, yet play an important role in reducing country dependence on official contributions. Other promising innovative resource mobilization and service delivery initiatives are mobilizing HIV/Aids platforms and investments to expand cancer care and control (CCC), especially for women's cancers. This is achieved by linking and leveraging investments from new initiatives, such as the Pink Ribbon Red Ribbon (PRRR) initiative. What has worked in innovative financing in global health is the emergence of viable, innovative, integrated financing mechanisms, such as the Global Fund and Global Alliance for Vaccines and Immunizations (GAVI), which have effectively pooled, channeled, and managed investment of donor funds at global scale to achieve results based on performance [31]. In the interim, in order to better understand the global philanthropic infrastructure, it is also important to understand the synergy created with governmental and NGOs, many of which are currently engaged in this work.

Professor Akira Iriye defines an NGO as "a voluntary non state, nonprofit, nonreligious, and nonmilitary association" [32]. A NGO is a legally constituted organization created by natural or legal persons that operates independently from any form of government. The term originated from the United Nations (UN) and is normally used to refer to organizations that are not a part of the government and are not conventional for-profit businesses. The term is usually applied only to organizations that pursue wider social aims that have political aspects, but are not openly political organizations such as political parties. The term, "non-governmental organization" or NGO came into currency in 1945 because of the need for the UN to differentiate in its Charter between participation rights for intergovernmental specialized agencies and those for international private organizations. At the UN, virtually all types of private bodies can be recognized as NGOs. They only have to be independent from government control, not seek to challenge governments either as a political party or by a narrow focus on human rights, be nonprofit, and be non-criminal [33].

The structures of NGOs vary considerably. They can be global hierarchies, with either a relatively strong central authority, or a more loose federal arrangement. Alternatively, they may be based in a single country and operate trans-nationally. With the improvement in communications, more locally based groups, referred to as grassroots organizations or community-based organizations, have become active at the national or even the global level. Increasingly, this occurs through the formation of coalitions. There are international umbrella NGOs, providing an institutional structure for different NGOs that do not share a common identity. There are also looser issue-based networks and ad hoc caucuses, lobbying at UN conferences. At times, NGOs are contrasted with social movements. As much as proponents of social movements may wish to see movements as being more progressive and more dynamic than NGOs, this is a false dichotomy. NGOs are components of social movements. Similarly, civil society is the broader concept to cover all social activity by individuals, groups, and movements. It remains a matter of contention whether civil society also covers all economic activity. Usually, society is seen as being composed of three sectors: government, the private sector, and civil society, excluding businesses [29].

The number of nationally operating NGOs is estimated at 40,000 [34]. International numbers are even higher: Russia has 277,000 NGOs [35].

India is estimated to have around 3.3 million NGOs in year 2009, which is just over 1 NGO per 400 Indians, and many times the number of primary schools and primary health centers in India [36, 37]. Beginning in the mid-1980s, NGOs have been perceived by donors as being important actors in development, poverty alleviation, and as symbols of societal responsibility, democracy, and morality [38]. Evolution of synergy between NGOs and governments, national and inter-national is imperative to adequately address the growing burden of breast cancer.

Breast cancer is the most common cause of cancer-related death among women worldwide, with case fatality rates highest in low-resource countries. Despite significant scientific advances in its management, most of the world faces resource constraints that limit the capacity to improve early detection, diagnosis, and treatment of the disease [39]. Although incidence, mortality, and survival rates vary fourfold in the world's regions, in the world as a whole, the incidence of breast cancer is increasing, and in regions without early detection programs, mortality is also increasing. The growing burden of breast cancer in low-resource countries demands adaptive strategies that can improve on the too common pattern of disease presentation at a stage when prognosis is very poor [40]. One of the most insidious aspect of this vicious illness-impoverishment cycle is that, for many cancer patients, the out-of-pocket spending is wasted as it does nothing to improve health. First, the cancer is often detected late, and so the best and only useful investment is for pain control and palliation. Second, a substantial proportion of what is spent by patients is not effective because they receive low-quality, poor, or inappropriate care. Third, it is often coupled with prohibitive transportation costs and investments of time. These difficulties are more likely to occur with a disease like cancer, where primary-level physicians are ill-prepared for early detection and diagnosis, and care often requires travel and ongoing treatment [41].

There have been an increasing number of global health initiatives to address breast cancer including efforts by PRRR Bush Initiative, Susan G. Komen for the Cure, The Breast Health Global Initiative (BHGI), The US Centers for Disease Control and Prevention (CDC), the American Cancer Society, The National Cancer Institute (NCI), and the Harvard Initiative. The focus for the next section of the chapter will be primarily on the Bush Initiatives.

Bush Initiatives

PRRR (Pink Ribbon Red Ribbon initiative) is an innovative partnership formed by the George W. Bush Institute, the US Department of State President's Emergency Plan for AIDS relief (PEPFAR), Susan G. Komen for the Cure, and the Joint United Nations Programme on HIV/AIDS (UNAIDS) that leverages public and private investments and existing health infrastructure to combat cervical and breast cancer, the two leading causes of cancer deaths among women in Sub-Saharan Africa. Other members and partners include Merck, GlaxoSmithKline (GSK), B-D, QIQGEN, Caris Foundation, Bristol-Myers Squibb Foundation, IBM, Airborne Lifeline, and the National Breast Cancer Foundation. The George W. Bush Institute (GWBI) advances freedom by developing and supporting initiatives that expand opportunity for individuals around the world. The Institute places an emphasis on programs that support human freedom, education reform, global health, and economic growth. In all of its programming, the Institute empowers women and military service members. GWBI is the policy arm of the George W. Bush Presidential Center, which will include the Presidential Museum and Library, and is located on the campus of Southern Methodist University (SMU) in Dallas, Texas [42].

During a recent visit in July 2012 to the University Teaching Hospital in Lusaka, Zambia, President George W. Bush, Mrs. Laura Bush, First Lady of Zambia Dr. Christine Kaseba, Zambian Minister of Health Dr. J. Kasonde, and United States Ambassador to Zambia Mark Storella dedicated the African Center of Excellence for Women's Cancer Control. President Bush also announced the donation of a new electronic hub (e-Hub) at the Center of Excellence, on behalf of all PRRR members and partners [42].

In addition, President Bush announced assistance to PRRR from Airborne Lifeline, a nonprofit organization that will provide airfreight services for medical equipment and transport medical personnel and patients as well as the support of the National Breast Cancer Foundation, which has provided the funding for a Health Promotion Manager who will be hired and based in Africa to support PRRR activities. Liz Thompson, President of Susan G. Komen for the Cure, Colleen J. McGuffin, Vice President of Health Engagement and Customer Value at Merck Vaccines, and Dr. Allan Pamba, Director of Public Engagement and Access Initiatives at GlaxoSmithKline (GSK) were on hand to announce PRRR initiatives supporting the Republic of Zambia and the fight against women's cancers, demonstrating the deep commitment of PRRR members and partners in expanding the availability of vital cervical cancer prevention, screening, and treatment, and breast care education to those in need [42].

The vision of the African Center of Excellence for Women's Cancer Control is to reduce deaths of women's cancers in the African region by raising the standards of care through education, training, and research, with a focus on primary and secondary prevention and treatment of early stage disease. The e-Hub, also called the electronic matrix, is a unique platform that permits distance learning and point of care to support and narrow the health workforce gap that exists in Zambia and across many countries in Africa [42].

In 2007, then Zambian President Levy Mwanawasa opened a $10 million specialist cancer hospital which will enable patients to receive treatment at home for the very first time. Mwanawasa said the National Cancer Diseases Hospital (NCDH) was built following a growth in the number of cancer patients in Zambia who have previously had to be treated abroad at a cost to the state of an average of $10,000 dollars per person. He reflected on statistics culled from 1995 to 2004, indicating that of the 5,000 cancer cases that required radiotherapy abroad, only 350 received treatment and the rest died without any treatment as they could not gain access to any form of intervention. Treatment at the hospital was reported to be based upon a cost-sharing plan between the patient and the government. The ultra modern hospital was built with the financial support from several international donors, while the International Atomic Energy Agency and the oil producing and exporting countries will offer radiotherapy for cancer treatment. Health Minister Brian Chituwo said the hospital would also cater to patients from other African countries. Over 3,000 new cancer cases are being detected in every one million Zambians annually [43].

In Africa, George Bush is a hero: "No American President has done more for Africa," said Festus Mogae, who served as President of Botswana from 1998 to 2008. Several millions of lives were saved from the ravages of AIDS with the availability of retro-viral drugs that stopped the transmission of the virus from one generation to the next. Clinics were built, and doctors and nurses were trained. A wrenching cultural conversation about sexual practices broadened, fueled by American money promoting abstinence, fidelity, and the use of condoms [44]. Created by President George W. Bush in 2003, the President's Emergency Plan for AIDS Relief (PEPFAR) was "launched to combat HIV/AIDS" [45]. PEPFAR has been the largest financial commitment of any country to global health and to treatment of any specific disease worldwide. Building upon the success of PEPFAR, President Obama launched the Global Health Initiative (GHI), shifting the focus from emergency programs to sustainable programs and from measuring the success of global health aid based on inputs to substantive and meaningful health outcomes. Other programs, remote from the level of PEPFAR's financial investment, continue to make a positive impact upon global health as well [46].

Bush remains proactive in the fight for African health. In September 2011, he launched a new program known as the PRRR initiative designed to tackle cervical and breast cancer among African women. Delfi Nyankombe responded to a reporter when questioned about George Bush: "George Bush is a great man. He tried to help poor countries like Zambia when we were really hurting from AIDS. He empowered us, especially women, when the number of people dying was frightening. Now we are able to live" [44]. Many of the women who were once dying from AIDS have survived and are now at risk of dying from breast or cervical cancer.

Nyankombe, 38 years of age, is a mother of three girls. She admires President Bush because of his current campaign to corral cervical cancer. Few are screened for the disease which now kills more Zambian women than any other cancer. "By the time a woman knows (she has cancer), she may need radiation or chemotherapy that can have awful side effects, like fistula. This is a big problem in Zambia, and he (Bush) is still helping us" [44].

Bush continues to lead the fight against cervical cancer in his post-presidential years and has so far helped to raise more than $85 million dollars for the cause. He says: "I believe freedom is important for peace and I believe one aspect of freedom is for people to be free from disease. Laura and I are very much involved in this initiative." In July 2012, Bush worked alongside other volunteers in Kabwe, Zambia's second-largest city, to renovate a health clinic which specializes in the early detection and treatment of cervical cancer. "You're always the former president but I wanted to come here as a laborer … I do want to say that on this particular trip myself and friends have left behind a clinic and hope to inspire others to come and refurbish clinics as well," Bush said.

Bush believes that "quiet service is the best kind of service." In Zambia, George and Laura Bush also visited an orphanage where many of the children were born with HIV. The children are alive today because of President Bush's 2003 AIDS initiative in Africa that provided billions of dollars for retroviral drugs and treatment [47].

Speaking in Kabwe during the handover of Ngungu Health Centre, which was recently refurbished with help from his foundation, President Bush implored citizens to support women's healthcare and said leaders should be moved to act whenever they saw people suffering. Bush indicated that the newly refurbished clinic will give many people a new chance at life. The clinic will provide cervical and breast cancer screening to local communities, offering an important service in an area of healthcare which is severely underserved in Zambia. In an active show of compassion, Bush said, "We are putting up a cervical cancer crusade to save lives because every human life is precious" [48]. In his effort to build upon PEPFAR and the State Department's Malaria Initiate, Bush stated, "Our mission is to say that thousands of women who would have died of cervical cancer without our intervention now live." He described his personal involvement in refurbishing the clinic with volunteers from the United States America and local community as "a labor for love for humanity." The Co-Director of Cervical Cancer Protection in Zambia, Professor Pharmah Groesbeck, said Mr. Bush's personal involvement in the project under the Red Ribbon Pink Ribbon initiative is the most important thing that has ever happened on the continent with regard to the prevention of cervical cancer [49].

Former First Lady Laura Bush joined husband ex-president George Bush, along with daughters Barbara and Jenna on a whirlwind trip to three countries in Africa in December 2011 to raise awareness for cervical and breast cancer. Former president George Bush, Laura Bush, Jenna Bush Hager, and Barbara Bush visited Girls Leading Our World (GLOW) in Lusaka, Zambia.

USA TODAY spoke with Mrs. Bush about the couple's commitment to combating Africa's high cervical cancer rate with their $75 million PRRR initiative:

Kindness:	Tell us more about the Pink Ribbon Red Ribbon Initiative campaign and what inspired it.
Laura Bush:	It's such a different story from when George and I first visited Africa in 2003. What's happened now is that because women are now living longer [as a result of Global Fund and PEPFAR's work], they are much more likely to contract the HPV virus and develop cervical cancer. They are living with AIDS but are dying

(continued)

	from cervical cancer. You seldom hear about the connection between the two here in the US, because it is part of the normal pap smear screening and because the HPV virus vaccine is prevalent and available in the US. Cervical cancer is easy to test for in a basic healthcare set up, if discovered early. The initiative will greatly expand access to cervical screening and treatments, helping to reduce the death rates. It's a very exciting project, and everyone we met with [in Africa] was very receptive.
Kindness:	Tell us more about your goals for the initiative.
Bush:	Our very obvious goal is to save lives, to increase the numbers of people who are living because they received the treatment they needed. When we first started talking about the initiative and the statistics—how cervical cancer is the most predominant cancer in Africa —we didn't believe it could include a vaccine program, because it would be too expensive. And yet it took us one year to develop the program because the companies that produce the vaccines have decided joined us.
Kindness:	Why is this initiative of particular interest to you and the president?
Bush:	This initiative is so important to us both. When George first announced the commitment of his administration a decade ago in Congress, the program was primarily aimed at addressing AIDS across the most devastated regions in Africa. I hope the American taxpayer realizes how many millions of lives have been saved, as a result. They are grateful and aware of what we've done. George believes this is a moral issue. As blessed as we are as a country, why would we be willing to stand by and watch a continent die? We wouldn't. It's not in the moral interests or security interests of our country to do so.
Kindness:	If there was one thing every American could do to help, what would that be?
Bush:	Many Americans already support these efforts through their churches or synagogues. In fact, many of the projects we visited in Africa were founded by Americans. We hope that this work will continue, and that the US will continue to fund programs like PEPFAR.
In times of economic uncertainty, there is a tendency to draw inward than outward. That is a mis-	take. Yes, these countries are poor, but they are working hard to work against these diseases. It's important for us to do what we can to help the African countries pick up the slack. And hopefully one day, they'll no longer need this help.
Kindness:	Both of your daughters have made public commitments to giving back. (Barbara, 30, helps provide fellowships to college grads through the Global Health Corps organization, while twin sister Jenna reports on these topics for NBC's Today.) How does that make you feel as their mother?
Bush:	I'm very happy that they have found this path. The world seemed a lot smaller when I was their age, and I was not nearly as knowledgeable as they are about these issues. The girls were certainly inspired by their dad's commitment and by the opportunities they had to travel with us. I'm really amazed by them—them and their friends. So many young people I know want to move to Africa or work for an organization that is health- or environment-focused or for programs like Teach for America. It's very inspiring [49].

(continued)

The PRRR is a synergistic initiative to leverage public and private investments in global health to combat breast and cervical cancer. It is a partnership between a part of the PRRR alliance which includes the George W. Bush Institute, the United States government (the United States Department of State President's Emergency Plan for AIDS Relief (PEPFAR)), the Joint United Nations Program on HIV/AIDS UNAIDS, the Susan G. Komen for the Cure as well as several different private organizations, including different pharmaceutical companies [50]. Early detection of breast cancer entails both early diagnosis in symptomatic women and screening in asymptomatic women which can be augmented with education and routine breast exam, and cervical cancer is amenable to primary preventions through vaccination against HPV, which has been shown to substantially reduce the incidence of cervical cancer. With strengthening stewardship, leadership, and philanthropy to expand access to Cancer Care and Control (CCC), multilateral agencies as well as bilateral agencies need to be engaged along with increasing the engagement of private sector [51].

The capacity to suffer is, clearly, part of being human. What suffering needs to be taken care of first and with what resources? It is possible to speak of extreme human suffering, and an inordinate share of this sort of pain is currently endured by those living in poverty [52]. The World Health Organization acknowledges that poverty is the world's greatest killer. "Poverty wields its destructive influence at every stage of human life, from the moment of conception to the grave. It conspires with the most deadly and painful diseases to bring a wretched existence to all those who suffer from it" [53].

References

1. Knaul FM, Frenk J, Lawrence S for the Global Task Force on Expanded Access to Cancer Care and Control in Developing Countries. Closing the cancer divide: a blueprint to expand access in low and middle income countries. Boston: Harvard Global Equity Initiative; 2011, p. xviii.
2. Farmer P, Frenk J, Knaul FM, et al. Expansion of cancer care and control in countries of low and middle income: a call to action. Lancet. 2010;376:1186–93.
3. World Health Organization. The global burden of disease: 2004 update. Geneva: WHO; 2008. Available at: http://www.who.int/healthinfo/global_burden_disease/2004_report_update/en/index.html.
4. Frieden TR, Garfield RM. The cover. Dimensions of global health. JAMA. 2012;307(19):2006.
5. Bhutta ZA, Reddy KS. Achieving equity in global health: so near and yet so far. JAMA. 2012;307(19): 2035–6.
6. United Nations General Assembly (UNGA). High level meeting on prevention and control of non-communicable diseases. Sep 19–20; New York. United Nations website. Available at: http://www.un.org/en/ga/ncdmeeting2011/.
7. World Health Organization (WHO). Global status report on non-communicable diseases 2010. World Health Organization website; April 2011. Available at: http://www.who.int/nmh/publications/ncd_report2010/en/.
8. United Nations General Assembly (UNGA). Political declaration of the High-level Meeting of the UN General Assembly on the Prevention and Control of Non-communicable Diseases. United Nations website. Sept 16, 2011. Available at: http://www.un.org/ga/search/view_doc.asp?symbol=A/66/L.1.
9. Marrero BA, Bloom DE, Adashi EY. Noncommunicable diseases: a global health crisis in a new world order. JAMA. 2012;307(19):2037–8.
10. Nugent R, Feigl AB. Where have all the donors gone? Scarce donor funding for non-communicable diseases Working Paper 228. Center for Global Development website; 2010. Available at: http://www.cgdev.org.content/publications/detail/1424546.
11. Sachs JD. Primary health care in low-income countries: building on recent achievements. JAMA. 2012;307(19):2031–2.

12. Coughlin SS, Ekwueme DU. Breast cancer as a global health concern. Cancer Epidemiol. 2009;33(5):315–8.
13. World Health Organization. Executive summary. In: National cancer control programmes: policies and managerial guidelines. Geneva: WHO; 2001. p. i–xxiv.
14. Narayan KMV, Ali MK, Del Rio C, Koplan JP, Curran J. Global non-communicable diseases-lessons from the HIV-AIDS experience. N Engl J Med. 2011;365(10):876–8.
15. Beyond aid; Speech by World Bank Group President Robert B. Zoellick. World Bank website; September 2011. PK:34370~piPK:42770~the sitePK:4607,00.html. Available at: http://web.worldbank.org/WBSITE/EXTERNAL/NEWS/0,,contentMDK:23000133-page.
16. Marmot MG. Policy making with health equity at its heart. JAMA. 2012;307(19):2033–4.
17. PACT: Programme of Action for Cancer Therapy: 1–12. Available at: http://cancer.iaea.org/.
18. Fighting Women's Cancer: Public-private partnership will combat cervical and breast cancer for women in sub-Saharan Africa and Latin America. August 24, 2012. p. 1–3. Available at: http://origin.voapolicy.org/content/fighting-womens-cancer-131539868/1482765.html.
19. Pink Ribbon Red Ribbon®: A bold initiative to advance women's health in the developing world. Fisher, Matt. November 6, 2011. Available at: http://www.smartglobalhealth.org/blog/entry/pink-ribbon-red-ribbon-a-bold-initiative-to-advance-womens-health-in-the-de/.
20. Wikipedia. Conflict of interest. Wikipedia; 2011. Available at: http://en.wikipedia.org/wiki/conflict_of_interest.
21. Ravishankar N, Gubbins P, Cooley RJ, Leach-Kemon K, Michaud CM, Jamison DT, Murray CJ. Financing of global health: tracking development assistance for health from 1990–2007. Lancet. 2009;373:2113–24.
22. Ooms G, Stuckler D, Basu S, McKee M. Financing the millennium development goals for health and beyond: sustaining the 'big push.' Globalization and Health 2010; 6:17. Available at: http://www.globalizationandhealth.com/content/6/1/17.
23. McCoy D, Chand S, Sridhar D. Global health funding: how much, where it comes from and where it goes. Health Policy Plan. 2009;24:407–17.
24. Philanthropy: Webster's New World Dictionary and Thesaurus. 2nd ed. New York: Hungry Minds; 2002. p. 477.
25. Ackerman T. Houston oil exec gives hospital district biggest donation. Houston Chronicle. April 20, 2011. Available at: http://www.chron.com/news/health/article/Houston-oil-exec-gives-hospital-district-biggest-1688116.php.
26. Smith L and S. Personal communication. Sept 17, 2012.
27. Young-Ellis R. Personal communication. Sept 18, 2012.
28. Mitchell F, Sessions K. Philanthropy and disparities: progress, challenges and unfinished business. Health Aff (Millwood). 2011;30(10):2017–22.
29. Anderson BO, Braun S, Lim S, Smith RA, Taplin S, Thomas DB for the Global Summit Early Detection Panel. Early detection of breast cancer in countries with limited resources. Breast J. 2003;9(2):S51–9.
30. Alford J. Focus on philanthropy: more hospitals are looking at charitable donations to fill in revenue gaps; trustees can help (Msg 32–34). March 2011. Trustee—Health Forum.
31. Knaul, FM, Frenk, J, Lawrence S for the Global Task Force on expanded access to cancer care and control in developing countries. Closing the cancer divide: a blueprint to expand access in low and middle income countries. Boston: Harvard Global Equity Initiative; 2011. p. 183.
32. Iriya A. Global community: the role of international organizations in the making of the contemporary world. Berkeley: University of California Press; 2004.
33. Willetts P. What is a non-governmental organization? UNESCO Encyclopedia of Life Support Systems. City University London. Retrieved 18 August 2012. Available at: http://en.wikipedia.org/wiki/Non-governmental_organization.
34. Anheier H, et al. "Global Civil Society 2001." 2001. Available at: http://en.wikipedia.org/wiki/Non-governmental_organization.
35. Rodriguez A. Hobbled NGOs wary of Medvedev. Chicago Tribune; May 7, 2008. Available at: http://articles.chicagotribune.com/2008-05-07/news/0805060608_1_civil-society-russian-authorities-russian-president-vladimir-putin.
36. India: More NGOs, than schools and health centres; July 7, 2010. Available at: http://oneworld.net.
37. First official estimate: An NGO for every 400 people in India. The Indian Express; July 7, 2010. Available at: http://www.wilsoncenter.org/publication/making-international-ngo-partnerships-work-lessons-american-armenian-collaboration.
38. Anderson BO, Shyyan R, Eniu A, Smith RA, Yip CH, Bese NS, Chow LW, Masood S, Ramsey SD, Carlson RW. Breast cancer in limited-resource countries: an overview of the Breast Health Global Initiative 2005 Guidelines. Breast J. 2006;12 Suppl 1:S3–15. Available at: http://www.ncbi.nlm.nih.gov.ezproxyhost.library.tmc.edu/pubmed/16430397.
39. Smith RA, Caleffi M, Albert US, Chen TH, Duffy SW, Franceschi D, Nystrom L. Global summit early detection and access to care panel. Breast cancer in limited-resource countries: early detection and access to care. PMID 16430395. Available at: http://www.ncbi.nlm.nih.gov.ezproxyhost.library.tmc.edu/pubmed/16430395.
40. Knaul, FM, Frenk, J, Lawrence S for the Global Task Force on Expanded Access to cancer care and control in developing countries. Closing the cancer divide: a blueprint to expand access in low and middle income countries. Boston: Harvard Global Equity Initiative; 2011, p. 185.
41. United Business Media, PR Newswire. July 4, 2012. President George W. Bush and the First Lady of Zambia Dr. Christine Kaseba Designate the African Center of

Excellence for Women's Cancer Control [Press Release]. Retrieved from: http://www.marketwatch.com/story/president-george-w-bush-and-the-first-lady-of-zambia-dr-christine-kaseba-designate-the-african-center-of-excellence-for-womens-cancer-control-2012-07-04.
42. Zambia opens first cancer hospital. Lusaka Times. July 19, 2007. Available at: http://www.lusakatimes.com/2007/07/19/cancer-gains-on-zambians/.
43. Landers J. Bush is hero in Africa for AIDS fight. Dallas Morning News. June 8, 2012. Available at: http://www.bushcenter.com/blog/2012/06/11/icymi-bringing-africa-back-to-life-the-legacy-of-george-w-bush/.
44. Reauthorizing PEPFAR [press release]. US President's emergency plan for AIDS relief. Available at: http://www.pepfar.gov/press/107735.htm.
45. Emanuel E. PEPFAR and Maximizing the Effects of Global Health Assistance. JAMA. 2012;307(19):2097–100.
46. Padden B. George W. Bush Focuses On Quiet Service After Presidency. July 4, 2012. Available at: http://www.voanews.com/content/george-bush-africa-cervical-cancer/1363615.html.
47. Mwenya G. George W. Bush visits Zambia to Boost Women's Healthcare. Zambia Reports. July 4, 2012. Available at: http://zambiareports.com/2012/07/04/george-w-bush-visits-zambia-to-boost-womens-healthcare/.
48. Mwaanga D. George Bush in labour of love—without fear or favour. Zambia Daily Mail. July 4, 2012. Available at: http://www.xtremezambia.net/george-bush-in-labour-of-love.
49. Garton C. Kindness: charity, philanthropy and social responsibility. USA TODAY. Jan 11, 2012. Available at: http://yourlife.usatoday.com/mind-soul/doing-good/kindness/post/2012/01/exclusive-interview-with-laura-bush/600280/1.
50. Bright M. Bush arrives. The post newspapers Zambia; July 1, 2012. Available at: http://www.postzambia.com/post-read_article.php?articleId=28365.
51. Knaul, FM, Frenk, J, Lawrence S for the Global Task Force on Expanded Access to Cancer Care and Control in Developing Countries. Closing the cancer divide: a blueprint to expand access in low and middle income countries. Boston: Harvard Global Equity Initiative; 2011. p. 116–117, 217.
52. World Health Organization. Bridging the gaps. Geneva: WHO; 1995, p. 5. (Reprinted/quoted in Kleinman A, Das V. Social suffering. London: University of California Press; 1997. p. 280).

C: Role of International Foundations in Improving Breast Cancer Awareness in Middle East and North Africa

Rola M.S.K. Shaheen and Mahesh K. Shetty

Despite the significant, strong strides in the scientific achievements in multidisciplinary breast cancer care, breast cancer patients in low to middle income countries—including the Middle East and North Africa (MENA)—continue to have low survival rates of 10–50% compared to a more than 85% 5-year survival rate in high income countries [1–3]. While this bold fact is mainly due to constraints of resources in cancer care in general, there are some specific regional factors and barriers that may contribute to the greater fatality for breast cancer patients in low to middle income countries. Some of those interesting regional factors related to breast cancer are: the obvious rise in the incidence rates, the higher frequencies in the younger ages, the advanced stages at the time of presentation [4, 5], and the likely prevalence of more aggressive tumors resulting in greater fatality rates. One of the cultural barriers is the low popularity for the screening concept: "why look for trouble" is a common attitude, which makes screening for breast cancer a low priority for some women despite their knowledge that screening can save lives due to early detection [6]. Evidence-based research is needed to unveil some of the regional risk factors since the well-known risk factors (such as lack of breast feeding, starting parity at an older age, and alcohol consumption) are not applicable within most of the social sectors in the MENA. This warrants an international call for innovative strategies and interventions tailored to specific regional needs and cultural barriers.

There is no doubt that breast cancer in low to middle income countries has attracted the attention of health sectors and the media both at regional and international levels. Numerous rigorous collaborative efforts and international initiatives are moving forward to increase breast cancer awareness in the region. International initiatives have recognized the importance of empowering women and advocates in the Middle East to improve awareness. International collaboration and partnerships have contributed largely to the increased breast cancer awareness and improved breast cancer management.

In the following sections, we discuss examples of the efforts and initiatives of international foundations that target breast cancer awareness and improve its management in MENA. The authors have been directly involved in these.

R.M.S.K. Shaheen
Department of Radiology, Harrington Memorial Hospital—BIDMC, Harvard Medical School, Boston, MA 02115, USA
e-mail: rshaheen@bidmc.harvard.edu

M.K. Shetty
Woman's Center for Breast Care and MRI,
Woman's Hospital of Texas, Houston, TX 77054, USA
e-mail: mshetty@womens-radiology.com

Harvard Global Equity Initiative and Global Task Force on Expanded Access to Cancer Care and Control in Developing Countries

Harvard Global Equity Initiative (HGEI) had conducted a conference in November 2009 in Boston on breast cancer awareness in developing countries [7]. Among the multiple sessions and workshops during the meeting, a regional breakout session for the Middle East and North Africa region afforded experts a great platform for brainstorming. The session has resulted in consensus recommendations presented by the one of the authors (Shaheen) on the last day of the conference. The recommendations can serve as a road map to improve breast cancer care in the region. It was emphasized that, at the country level, the first step is to develop a country-specific cancer control plan utilizing the EMRO skeleton. Research recommendations had focused on [1] conducting a multi-central baseline needs assessment including statistics and barriers to early detection of breast cancer and treatment, and [2] developing a cancer registry. Educational recommendations included:

1. Developing a multidisciplinary healthcare team that provides local training and increases opportunity for international exchange
2. Reversing the brain drain
3. Utilizing available resources to build upon and move forward
4. Emphasizing the crucial role of having resources for treatment and palliative care services along with establishing a screening program
5. Utilizing media, the public power of survivors, and civil and religious leadership to increase awareness about breast cancer and target all policy makers, women, men, and their healthcare providers

The recommendations had also encouraged efforts among affiliations and partnerships to collaborate locally and internationally. A need to develop a quality assurance program that is tailored to the local needs and barriers, yet meets international guidelines, was emphasized. It was also suggested to adapt the Breast Health Global Initiative (BHGI) guidelines which provide a flexible framework that can address differences in resources in various countries.

Another project was presented during the conference by one of the authors (Shaheen). An early stage of a multifaceted project on improving early detection of breast cancer in the Gaza strip, which is an initiative conducted by a group of radiologists from the Harvard Medical School and partially funded by CARE International in West Bank and Gaza, was presented [8]. The project highlighted barriers to early detection of breast cancer for Gaza women. Subsequently, the advancing study was presented at a Global Summit on International Breast Health-BHGI Conference in Chicago 2010 and was published in February 2011 [6]. It was viewed as an innovative study with important global perspectives in which expatriates from a war-torn politically unstable region were compared to their in-country cohorts. It urges researchers and policy makers to consider the influence of place of residency and what role exposure to a new environment and access to an alternative healthcare system may play in shaping women's beliefs, attitudes, or healthcare seeking behavior [9]. Additionally, this study highlights the important role of international foundations, which may be the only hope for bridging the gaps and overcoming the geographic barriers encountered in politically unstable cities. It is important to mention that BHGI strives to develop an evidence-based approach, an economically feasible plan, and culturally appropriate recommendations reflected in the BHGI guidelines [10].

The United States-Middle East Partnership for Breast Cancer Awareness and Research

The United States-Middle East Partnership for Breast Cancer Awareness and Research was first launched by former First Lady Laura Bush in 2006 in United Arab Emirates, extended in 2007 to the Hashemite Kingdom of Jordan and the Kingdom of Saudi, further extended in 2008 to include Egypt, and in 2009 was launched in the Kingdom of Morocco and the Palestinian territories. It is a model of public–private effort that unites local champions in the United States, the Middle East, and North Africa who are leading the fight against breast cancer. It is the first collaborative effort to help countries in the Middle East and North Africa fight breast cancer through improved awareness, clinical resources, and care. The partnership supporters include: government representatives, breast cancer advocates, doctors, nurses, other medical professionals, educators, and business leaders [11].

It is an expanded and unified network of MENA women's cancer organizations, experts, and advocates that maintains collaborative linkages with regional and global partners to raise awareness and leverage resources resulting in the eradication of women's cancers, with a special emphasis on breast cancer. In other words, the mission is to serve as a unifying regional partnership that leverages resources and catalyzes international collaborations between breast cancer and other women's cancers organizations and individuals in their efforts to enhance advocacy, clinical research, capacity building, medical training, and public awareness, with an aim to improving women's health in the MENA region.

More than 4,000 regional advocates have directly benefited from the Partnership's advocacy and medical capacity-building and consultative activities, resulting in outreach to over 25,000 community beneficiaries. The Partnership's work has grown to engage more than 200 different organizations representing more than 7,500 people in 17 countries in the Middle East and North Africa. The Partnership's interactive online network has generated more than 440 members as of this writing and receives an average of 150 visitors per month. Among the multiple, fruitful, collaborative efforts of the partnership is a community-based breast health awareness and screening project that was conducted through the Breast Cancer Foundation of Egypt. The aim was to increase breast cancer awareness among women as a step to encourage them to participate in breast screening in underserved areas. The project had focused on capacity building in key organizations in underserved areas to develop a sustainable breast cancer project. In 2009, the first Egypt Race for the Cure was successfully conducted and attended by 10,000 participants. It took place at the pyramids, which were lit in pink on the eve of the event.

In June 2010, Susan G. Komen for the Cure Foundation agreed to support the partnership to help it meet its goals and objectives. This was an important milestone in the partnership sustainability.

East Mediterranean Regional Organization–World Health Organization

Cancer is the fourth ranked cause of death according to WHO mortality estimates within the Eastern Mediterranean Region (EMR), thus succeeding cardiovascular diseases, infectious/parasitic diseases, and injuries [12–14].

Apparently the largest increase in cancer incidence among the WHO regions in the next 15 years is likely to be in the EMR [15], where breast cancer is reported as the most common type of female malignancy in almost all national cancer registries [1].

Among their numerous projects supporting maternal health and breast cancer awareness in the East Mediterranean region, East Mediterranean Regional Organization–World Health Organization (EMRO–WHO) and Susan G. Komen for the Cure have recently co-sponsored, in collaboration with IARC (International Agency for Research on Cancer and IAEA/PACT (International Atomic Energy Agency/Program of Action for Cancer Therapy)), in January 2012 the First International Meeting of the Regional Comparative Breast Cancer Research Program that was conducted in Sharm El-Sheikh, Egypt. An impressive commitment of all involved parties was noted through the coordination process by the organizers. This had contributed to the success of the event despite all the regional political challenges during the Arab Spring, particularly in Egypt.

The objective of developing a regional comparative breast cancer research program is mainly to develop a national cancer registry. A national regional cancer registry for breast cancer will provide the essential breast cancer data, including stage, age-specific incidence rates, and survival rate. It also will allow for comparison of demographic characteristics, clinicopathological presentations, and management outcomes of breast cancer patients. There is no doubt that this will advance breast cancer research with evidence-based tools made available through accessibility to the regional data.

It is inspiring to have the different stakeholders meet and agree on a collaborative process of data collection through the different participating centers in a multidisciplinary care approach. This program illustrates the essential roles of international agencies in supporting, advancing, and sustaining such an important initiative that is very much needed in the region. For example, the leading role of WHO in the coordination of efforts and in bringing all stakeholders to the table gives much credibility to the program and facilitates access to comparative data. The participation of the international agencies such as IARC and IAEA/PACT, with their technical support and supervision of the training workshops, is valuable. Last but not the least, the valuable role of the Susan G. Komen for the Cure Foundation cannot be over-emphasized in promoting advocacy, empowering breast cancer research grassroots, and incorporating targeted community outreach and public awareness.

One day prior to the EMRO–WHO regional meeting in Sharm El Sheikh, a bundled one day workshop [16] on comparative baseline needs assessment for breast cancer awareness and management in the Middle East was sponsored by Susan G Komen for the Cure Foundation and lead by one of the authors (Shaheen). This was a collaborative effort among researchers and experts from nine Arab countries along with expert support from the IARC, and faculty members from Harvard Medical School, Yale University, and John Hopkins University. The workshop included individual regional presentations on the local status of breast cancer in each country. In addition to having an opening session on the global perspective on breast cancer screening and treatment, the workshop included sessions on research ethics, and on quantitative and qualitative research tools which were very well received by participants. The participating researchers, who had different enriching professional backgrounds yet all work with breast cancer, provided short presentations about the status of breast cancer in their specific geographic locations. These comparative presentations were eye openers to participating researchers as they directed their attention to the regional differences in local settings; some countries are well equipped with skilled manpower and labor force but lack the financial resources and other countries have the financial resources and tools but lack the gearing expertise. Common cultural barriers were identified, and success stories with effective interventions were shared. The variable needs across MENA countries in breast cancer management call for further collaboration at regional levels to consolidate bridging efforts that may increase access for breast screening, diagnosis, and treatment.

This is another great example of the crucial role of international foundations in providing a platform for stakeholders, researchers, and advocates to advance breast cancer research through these brainstorming sessions and training workshops.

Woman's Cancer Foundation (www.womanscancerfoundation.org)

The Woman's Cancer Foundation is a Houston-based nonprofit clinical health foundation established to implement an integrated cancer screening strategy as explained in detail in Chap. 17 [17]. The foundation provides project design and expertise in order to construct such proposed clinics in low-resource countries. Training for healthcare professionals staffing the clinic and telemedicine support is also offered. Telemedicine support will include consultations for breast, endometrial, and ovarian ultrasound as well as webinar-based training sessions for the staff at the well woman clinic. The foundation is currently seeking funding to set up a pilot project in Nova Andradina in Brazil in partnership with

Barretos Cancer Hospital. This site of the proposed well woman clinic is in a rural area about 40 miles outside the city of Nova Andradina in the State of Mata do Sul and 500 miles north of the city of Sao Paulo. The city has no organized screening program in place. There is no healthcare facility in the city to provide indigent care for a population of 80,000. The newly opened cancer hospital branch of the Barretos Cancer Hospital is at a distance of 200 miles and will act as a referral center for screen positive cases and for those who need additional testing. The foundation is accepting requests for provision of project design, oversight of implementation, and training of staff and telemedicine support from local stakeholders in low and mid resource countries who are seeking to implement integrated cancer screening and early diagnosis services for women.

In summary, the role of international foundations is extremely crucial in supporting awareness of breast cancer, breaking some barriers for screening to achieve early detection of the disease and thus improve survival, increasing access for diagnosis and treatment, providing training sessions, advancing research, and facilitating regional collaboration and cooperation on multiple levels among stakeholders including governments and health policy makers.

Without rigorous efforts to fight breast cancer through the support of international foundations, women in MENA will continue to die from a disease that has high survival rates in other parts of the world. Having the chance to live should not be an accident of geography [18]!

Acknowledgments Special thanks to the Susan G. Komen Global Health Team (Ms. Chelsea Kelley) for their contribution to this chapter.

References

1. GLOBOCAN. Lyon: International Agency for Research on Cancer; 2008.
2. Cancer control opportunities in low and middle-income countries. Washington, DC: Institute of Medicine of the National Academies; 2007. www.iom.edu/CMS/3722/23083.
3. Brower V. Developing nations face challenges as breast cancer rises. J Natl Cancer Inst. 2011;103(24):1812–4.
4. EMRO. Towards a strategy for cancer control in the eastern Mediterranean region. 1st ed. Cairo: Regional Office for the Eastern Mediterranean, World Health Organization; 2010.
5. El Saghir NS. Responding to the challenges of breast cancer in Egypt and other Arab countries. J Egypt Natl Canc Inst. 2008;20(4):309–12.
6. Shaheen R et al. Barriers and opportunities for early detection of breast cancer in Gaza women. Breast. 2011;20 Suppl 2:S30–4.
7. Breast cancer in the developing world: meeting the unforeseen challenge to women, health and equity. An International Meeting Organized by the Harvard Global Equity Initiative, the Dana Farber Cancer institute, the Harvard School of Public Health, the Harvard medical School, and the Brigham and Women's Hospital. Boston, 3–5 Nov 2009.
8. Shaheen R. http://www.hsph.harvard.edu/breastandhealth/files/dr_rola_shaheen.pdf. 2009.
9. Breast Health Global Initiative. BHGI Bulletin 2011;8:5.
10. Anderson BO et al. Breast cancer in limited-resource countries: an overview of the Breast Health Global Initiative 2005 guidelines. Breast J. 2006;12 Suppl 1:S3–15.
11. http://bcpartnership.ning.com.
12. WHO. National cancer control programmes, policies and managerial guidelines, 2nd ed. Geneva: World Health Organization; 2002. http://www.who.int/.
13. WHO. Revised global burden of disease (GBD), WHO 2002 estimates. Geneva: World Health Organization; 2003. http://www.who.int/healthinfo/bodgbd2002revised/en/index.html.
14. WHO. Cancer control in the Eastern Mediterranean Region. (EMRO Technical Publication Series 20.) Alexandria: WHO Regional Office for the Eastern Mediterranean; 1995.
15. Rastogi T, Hildesheim A, Sinha R. Opportunities for cancer epidemiology in developing countries. Nat Rev Cancer. 2004;4(11):909–17.
16. Shaheen R. http://menabcstudy.blogspot.com/p/workshop-participants.html. 2012.
17. Shetty MK, Longatto-Filho A. Early detection of breast, cervical, ovarian and endometrial cancers in low resource countries: an integrated approach. Indian J Surg Oncol. 2011;2(3):165–71.
18. Mired HD. HRH princess Dina Mired, in her opening ceremony speech at Breast cancer in the developing world: meeting the unforeseen challenge to women, health and equity. An International Meeting Organized by the Harvard Global Equity Initiative, the Dana Farber Cancer institute, the Harvard School of Public Health, the Harvard Medical School, and the Brigham and Women's Hospital, Boston, 3–5, Nov 2009.

14 Coordinated Training on Early Detection and Diagnosis of Breast Cancer Across Different Levels of Health Workers: An Example from Peru

Vivien D. Tsu, Jennifer L. Winkler, Benjamin O. Anderson, Gustavo Javier Sarria Bardales, and Jose Jeronimo

Abstract

As breast cancer rates increase worldwide, many low- and middle-income countries are seeking feasible strategies for providing screening and early detection programs, improving diagnostic imaging and pathology services, and ensuring basic treatment and palliative care. The limited availability of appropriately trained staff is a severe constraint on reaching rural and otherwise disadvantaged populations with essential breast health care. An innovative project in Peru, designed to bring breast cancer screening and early diagnostic services to women in a rural area of the country, illustrates many of the challenges and potential solutions for training various health workers, ensuring that they can acquire and maintain critical competencies and that the health system provides the infrastructure needed to support their performance. This chapter describes an iterative and collaborative process to develop curricula for four key functions: education about screening among women in the target age range, breast screening by clinical breast exam, a first diagnostic step using fine-needle aspiration biopsy, and supervision. Functions were matched with the type of health provider or community volunteer that was already in place in this rural context. Each curriculum defined learning goals and incorporated competency evaluation at the end, and special efforts were made to ensure that messages were consistent throughout the different curricula and followed national guidelines.

V.D. Tsu (✉)
Reproductive Health, PATH, Seattle, WA 98121, USA
e-mail: vtsu@path.org

J.L. Winkler • J. Jeronimo
PATH, Seattle, WA 98121, USA
e-mail: jwinkler@path.org; jjeronimo@path.org

B.O. Anderson
Fred Hutchinson Cancer Research Center,
Department of Surgery, University of Washington,
Seattle, WA 98109, USA
e-mail: Banderso@fhcrc.org

G.J. Sarria Bardales
Instituto Nacional de Enfermedades Neoplasicas—
INEN, Direccion de Control de Cancer, Lima, Peru
e-mail: gsarria97@gmail.com

M.K. Shetty (ed.), *Breast and Gynecological Cancers: An Integrated Approach for Screening and Early Diagnosis in Developing Countries*, DOI 10.1007/978-1-4614-1876-4_14,

Introduction

While breast cancer was not previously seen as a high priority health problem in low- and middle-income countries (LMICs), steadily rising incidence and mortality rates have moved it onto the agenda in recent years [1–3]. As countries begin to realize the implications of a projected increase in breast cancer deaths of more than 70 % between 2008 and 2030 [4], many are looking for feasible strategies to reduce the growing toll by providing screening and early detection programs, improving diagnostic imaging and pathology services, and ensuring basic treatment and palliative care. A clear limiting factor is the lack of availability of trained staff at all levels of care [5, 6] as well as the weak linkages between the levels to facilitate referral and ensure follow-up after initial diagnosis and treatment. Two of the most significant gaps identified are the lack of awareness in the community and the lack of culturally appropriate education about breast cancer and the benefits of early detection [7, 8].

Frontline health workers, whether based in primary care facilities or out in the communities, have critical roles to play, particularly in providing health education, conducting screening, and helping patients navigate the referral system [9]. In addition to screening, some types of tissue sampling and pathology analysis are needed before appropriate treatment can be determined. The interface between primary care workers and more specialized medical providers can be challenging to organize, especially in LMICs where pockets of specialists exist in urban areas offering sophisticated and technology-intensive care while rural areas are unable to draw upon such resources. In-service and preservice training must be carefully designed to reflect essential skills and the realities of the environment in which the trainees will function.

An innovative project in Peru, designed to bring breast cancer screening and early diagnostic services to women in a rural area of the country, illustrates many of the challenges and potential solutions for training various health workers, ensuring that they can acquire and maintain critical competencies and that the health system provides the infrastructure needed to support their performance.

Developing a Resource-Specific Strategy: The BHGI Approach

Healthcare providers and policymakers working in a limited-resource setting may be forced to make decisions contrary to their best medical knowledge. Despite knowing the optimal management for a given patient based on guidelines developed in wealthy countries, less-than-optimal solutions are offered to patients where diagnostic and/or treatment resources are lacking. The constraint of limited resources generates tension for the clinician who is unable to offer "gold standard" treatments to any or all of the patients. Does a clinician decide to treat ten patients with an older, less expensive chemotherapy regimen or to treat two patients with a newer, more efficacious but also more expensive regimen? Given these difficult resource allocation choices, it is important to ask questions about which resources commonly applied in resource-abundant countries are actually needed in limited resource settings, where patients commonly present with more advanced disease at diagnosis.

The guidelines development process for LMICs should offer practical solutions to the implausibility of applying breast cancer guidelines developed for high-resource countries to countries or regions within countries with more limited resources. Established in 2002, the Breast Health Global Initiative (BHGI) created an international health alliance to develop evidence-based guidelines for LMICs in order to improve breast health outcomes. BHGI held four Global Summits to address healthcare disparities (Seattle, Washington, 2002), evidence-based resource allocation (Bethesda, Maryland, 2005), guideline implementation (Budapest, Hungary, 2007), and optimizing outcome (Chicago, 2010) as related to breast cancer in LMICs. Modeled after the approach of the National Comprehensive Cancer Network (NCCN), BHGI developed and applied a consensus panel process, now formally endorsed by the US Institute of Medicine, to create resource-sensitive guidelines for breast cancer early detection [10] diagnosis [11], treatment [12], and healthcare systems [13], as related to breast healthcare delivery in LMICs.

The BHGI Early Detection Panel in 2007 concluded that public education and awareness are the key first steps in down-staging disease, because early detection cannot be successful when the public is unaware or has adverse misconceptions about the value of early detection [10]. The approach and scope of any screening program will determine the success of an early detection program, as measured by cancer stage at diagnosis, and will also drive the resource allocation needed for cancer treatment. The effectiveness and efficiency of screening modalities—including screening mammography, clinical breast examination (CBE), and breast self-examination—were reviewed in the context of resource availability and population-based need. The debates in high-income countries that commonly focus on the efficacy vs. the costs and morbidity of screening mammography have little relevance in LMICs where mammography is unavailable, unaffordable, and impractical and where the majority of women are not diagnosed until their disease is already advanced. Social and cultural barriers to breast cancer early detection must be considered in any context where early detection programs are being established. The selection of appropriate resource-sensitive guidelines is critical in shaping the content of training curricula and assigning tasks to the right cadres of health personnel.

The Model of Care Selected in La Libertad

We applied the resource-specific strategy described in the BHGI guidelines to the context of Peru and developed a model of care to improve access and quality of breast cancer screening, diagnosis, and treatment services at lower levels of the health system. An important goal of this model was to ensure that women complete as much diagnostic evaluation as possible before they invest time and resources for traveling to a cancer hospital. This is particularly important in breast cancer screening, as a significant proportion of palpable masses can be recognized as benign changes through a simple diagnostic test.

We worked in partnership with national and regional leaders to ensure that the model was in line with national breast cancer guidelines. This model has been implemented in the Pacasmayo health network within the region of La Libertad in northern Peru and is based on the use of CBE performed at the local health facility, followed by referral of women with suspected masses to the local hospital for evaluation using fine-needle aspiration (FNA) biopsy. Women with a confirmed diagnosis can be referred for appropriate treatment (surgery, radiotherapy, systemic therapy) to a city located 2 h away by car (Trujillo), where a new regional cancer center has been established for the northern part of the country (IREN-Norte).

An important first step in any curriculum development is to define clearly and explicitly the essential functions that each trainee must be able to perform. We identified four functions necessary for implementing this model: education about screening among women in the target age range, breast screening by CBE, a first diagnostic step (FNA), and supervision. We then considered what type of health provider or community volunteer was already in place in this rural context who might take on each function.

Throughout Peru, community health promoters work in collaboration with the healthcare system to share information and educate community members on health-related topics. This organized group of volunteers was identified as being well suited to take on the role of promoting breast screening among women in the target age group.

Much of women's health care in Peru, including family planning, prenatal care, and cervical cancer screening, is performed by professional midwives. General doctors also play an important role—particularly in larger healthcare facilities—in providing screening services to women. These two categories of professionals were selected to perform screening with clinical breast exam at the local health facility and were oriented to the diagnostic step of FNA, to which women identified with a mass would be referred.

The Peruvian regulatory framework requires that doctors perform certain types of diagnostic procedures, including FNA. Therefore, doctors at the local hospital were selected to perform the initial diagnostic step of FNA biopsy. At the regional cancer institute, a pathologist already had training and expertise in the reading of breast cytology. This existing capacity made it possible to implement FNA at the local hospital level, as the infrastructure for reading the results was already in place in a close-by city.

We had initially planned for clinical supervision of the midwives providing CBE to be the responsibility of breast cancer experts from the regional cancer institute, but it quickly became evident that the scope of their clinical responsibilities, and particularly their limited time and availability for travel, would make their direct supervision of CBE activities at the local level impossible. Instead, professional midwives located within the health network—with leadership abilities and interest in serving as supervisors—were selected to be trained in the use of the instruments and techniques for performing supportive supervision visits to midwives practicing CBE.

Curriculum Development and Implementation of the Training

An essential component of implementing this model has been the coordinated training for these four functions, both in process and content. Curriculum development was done collaboratively, and then training for each group was rolled out. We conducted the first round of trainings of health promoters, CBE providers, and FNA providers in June and July 2011 and the first training of supervisors in March 2012.

The development of each of the curricula shared a common process of defining learning objectives and technical competencies to be achieved, developing a preliminary draft of the training material, performing an initial validation of the drafted materials, compiling materials into a standardized format including a reference manual, a guide for participants, and a guide for trainers, and allowing for a broad review by experts contributing to the project. For each training curriculum, criteria for achieving competency were defined.

The training structure ensured that participants engaged actively with the material. This was accomplished through interactive dialogue with trainers, exercises where learners practiced their skills in a simulated environment, and participant demonstration of newly acquired clinical and supervisory skills in supervised settings.

The key messages were kept consistent throughout all four curricula, and references to the other curricula were included where they were relevant. For example, the messages for women and communities emphasized in the health promoters' curriculum were also described in the CBE training. This included an emphasis on women understanding what is normal for their own breasts, the specific signs and symptoms that signal the need for a clinical exam for women of any age, and the importance for women aged 40–59 to seek an annual clinical breast exam by a trained healthcare professional even if they do not have any symptoms or the self-examination is normal. The CBE training for midwives also incorporated an orientation about the FNA biopsy procedure that was consistent with the more detailed descriptions of the procedure used within the FNA training materials.

The courses were designed through an iterative process. For example, in the case of the clinical breast exam curriculum, the course was adapted from a curriculum previously developed for use in the Ukraine a decade earlier [14]. After it was translated into Spanish, it served as the starting point for the Peruvian course design. Peruvian breast experts at the national and regional level first came to an agreement on the basic learning objectives and competencies to be achieved in the training. Peruvian cancer experts then developed an initial set of slides based on the cancer epidemiology in Peru and their clinical experience. Following the first round of training, the training materials were compiled into a reference manual, a guide for participants, a guide for trainers, and a standardized set of slides. This package of materials was then reviewed by clinical breast cancer experts at both the national and regional cancer institutes and was validated in three subsequent CBE trainings for midwives and general doctors.

The *community promotion curriculum* was designed to orient health promoters to the use of the community materials (an outreach flipchart and accompanying manual) and strategies for successfully conducting community education sessions on early detection of breast cancer. The manual divided the educational session into its various components: receiving and welcoming participants, self-introduction of participants, introducing the topic, gathering existing ideas and experiences on the topic, sharing "new" information, evaluating whether information shared was clear and understandable, commitments to action, and closing. The "new" information covered in the session was focused on the following topics: (1) knowing our breasts: recognizing normal and suspicious changes; (2) breast cancer: identifying risk factors (particularly age); and (3) importance of early detection and of an annual clinical breast exam.

Two experts from the Department of Health Promotion, Prevention, and Cancer Control at the national cancer institute (INEN) provided training to 13 community health promoters at the local hospital in the area of our intervention. The interactive training took place over a 2-day period. The final curriculum built on the initial training and added a verification list and knowledge exam to evaluate competency.

The *clinical breast exam curriculum*, designed for midwives and general doctors, includes a reference manual and guides for participants and trainers. The topics covered included: breast cancer fundamentals, the breast cancer prevention and control program in Peru, normal breast anatomy and breast anomalies, the CBE, the algorithm for diagnosis and management of women with positive findings, information recording, FNA biopsy, breast cancer treatments, and counseling. The clinical competencies and learning objectives included:

1. Talking to women about breast cancer screening and diagnosis
2. Performing CBEs, including visual exam and history taking
3. Interpreting the results of the CBE process (asking, seeing, and feeling)
4. Appropriately referring patients for further diagnosis
5. Accurately recording CBE results and referral information on health information system (HIS) forms

To demonstrate competency, participants were required to obtain a score of at least 85% on a knowledge exam and demonstrate competent performance of the CBE by performing all of the actions described in a validation checklist.

The facilitators of the CBE course were two breast specialists from the regional cancer institute supported by specialists from the national cancer institute. Participants attended a 2-day training consisting of scientific theory, practical application, and patient counseling with respect to CBE. Participants had the opportunity to practice what they had learned by carrying out CBE on silicon models, conducting practice counseling sessions, and reviewing images of clinical breast anomalies (Fig. 14.1). At the end of the first day, participants took a knowledge exam to demonstrate their understanding of CBE. The second day of training was practical and included each participant completing the CBE procedure on patients under the supervision of an instructor who used a checklist to comment on their progress.

The *FNA curriculum*, for doctors at the local hospital, was also organized into a reference manual and guides for participants and trainers. In addition to clinical and counseling skills, the course covered the rationale for use of FNA, its history, and its diagnostic accuracy. The learning objectives for the course were that participants be able to:

1. Talk to women about breast cancer screening and diagnosis
2. Explain who should have a FNA biopsy
3. Perform FNA biopsy and understand potential side effects or risks
4. Smear and fix a sample

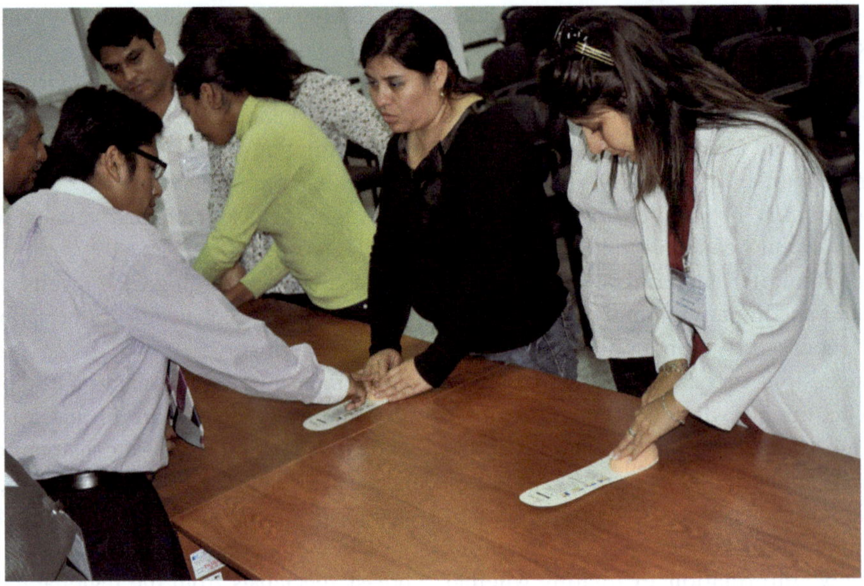

Fig. 14.1 Midwife trainees practicing clinical breast exam on silicon models

5. Evaluate the adequacy of a sample
6. Provide care and referral, as needed
7. Use recommended infection prevention practices to protect the woman, healthcare provider, and other healthcare workers
8. Accurately record FNA biopsy results on HIS forms

An external expert in FNA biopsy facilitated the 2-day FNA training, which took place in conjunction with the first CBE course. Sessions specific to FNA were offered to three physicians from the local hospital in the Pacasmayo network. These sessions included lectures on the theoretical context of FNA, when to use FNA and making appropriate referrals, FNA procedures, and how to judge the adequacy of the sample. It also included practice of the FNA technique using animal liver as a tissue stand-in. On the second day of the training, participants had an opportunity to practice under the supervision of the instructor.

The topics covered in the *supervision curriculum* and course material included definitions of traditional supervision vs. supportive supervision, criteria for accreditation and competency, planning a supervision visit, aspects of a supervision visit (programmatic and clinical), recording of information, techniques to understand the root causes of problems identified, and the closing meeting to report back to health facility leadership (the final step in a supervision visit). This 2-day training was intended to ensure that local and regional supervisors had the necessary skills and understanding to enable oversight and constructive support to improve clinical skills and competencies of providers, thereby improving the quality of services in health facilities providing clinical breast exams. The first day of the course was classroom-based, and the second included the performance of a supervision visit with support from the facilitators.

The learning objectives were that the participants would be able to:

1. Plan a supervisory visit
2. Know the criteria to be able to accredit the clinical skills of health providers that offer the CBE
3. Know and be able to use the data collection instruments used within the prevention and control of breast cancer program
4. Recognize the strengths in the provision of the breast clinical exam, to be able to replicate them in other health facilities

5. Identify and address the weaknesses of the facilities providing clinical breast exam, seeking solutions that would allow providers and the health facility to work effectively
6. Develop a work plan to ensure that CBE is provided adequately in a health facility
7. Know the appropriate indicators for monitoring the breast cancer prevention and control program
8. Assess and ensure the accuracy, completeness, and quality of program data
9. Demonstrate skills for effective supervision, including the ability to provide positive and specific feedback during and after a monitoring visit

The first supervision training was conducted by a breast cancer specialist with support from staff experienced in supervising other cancer prevention activities. The seven trainees had different backgrounds and experience, but all of them were involved in cancer prevention activities.

Challenges and Potential Solutions Identified

Common challenges across all the training activities were the limited availability of breast cancer experts to lead the training and difficulties in scheduling training sessions due to competing activities and obligations. It quickly became apparent that it would not be feasible to rely on breast cancer specialists for all levels of training. Appropriate local cadres who could serve as master trainers were identified for each type of training.

Health Promoter Training

There were several challenges for the training of health promoters, but the one that created significant delays was the limited time availability of the trainers and trainees. Because it was recognized that having high-level experts on breast cancer involved in the training of promoters would not be a sustainable option, the project decided to train a cadre of master trainers from the lower levels of the health system including community health promoters and health personnel with responsibilities in health promotion. Second, the trainees were people from the community with limited or no training related to breast cancer, and some of them had very limited education. Facilitators of the health promotion training noted a lack of scientific understanding of breast cancer among community health workers and suggested that an orientation to the topic be included in future trainings. Finally, the community materials (a flipchart and manual for promoters) had not yet been printed at the time of the first training, and we received feedback from the participants that these materials would be a valuable aid when making presentations to their communities (Fig. 14.2).

Clinical Training for CBE and FNA

The experience developed in northern Peru is one of the very few population-based screening programs for breast cancer screening using CBE. As in the case of developing trainers for promoters, we will need a core group of regional master trainers for CBE and FNA. A broader group of well-trained master trainers with CBE experience will be essential for bringing this model successfully to scale. An important challenge for the clinical training was to have sufficient women for the hands-on practice, both for CBE and for FNA. Since mobilizing women to come in for screening is best done by community promoters, it is necessary to coordinate the schedules so that health promoters are trained and mobilized first, a few weeks prior to the clinical training for health providers. They can then invite women to be screened as part of the clinical practice component of the training. To make best use of the time during the training session, one of the key recommendations was to ensure that written material is provided to participants ahead of time. It was also proposed that the CBE training and the FNA training for physicians be provided on different days so that the FNA session would not be required to go into the evening hours.

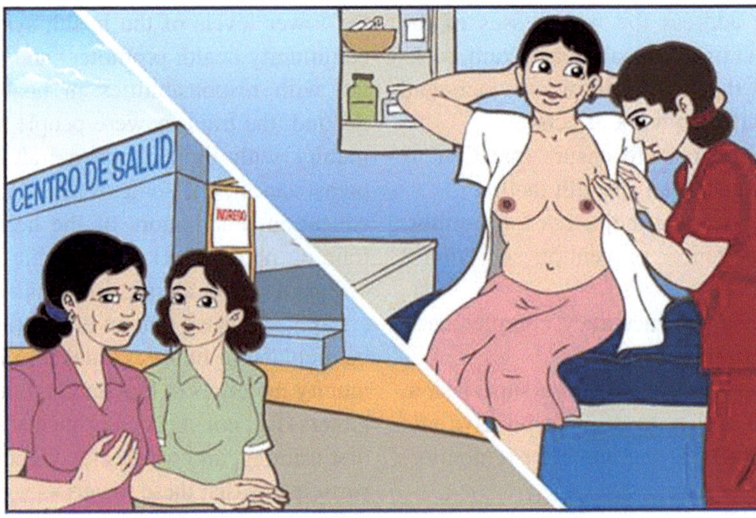

Fig. 14.2 Sample page from flipchart for community health promoters (Copyright 2011, Program for Appropriate Technology in Health (PATH). All rights reserved)

A challenge that has not yet been adequately addressed is the need for access to sufficient numbers of women with positive screening findings in a training environment to enable trainees to have hands-on practice and continuing education. While some breast abnormalities can be captured in pictures, important changes can only be identified through discussion with patients about their history, and others require the sensory experience of feeling the breast tissue. We are currently experimenting with the rotation of the trainees, each for 2 days, through the regional cancer institute to have direct experience with positive cases, but it is not clear whether this approach can be scalable to a national program. New strategies may need to be explored.

Supervision Training

Facilitators noted that participants demonstrated strong interest and dedication and performed well in the shared supervision visit. They also noted the commitment to and interest in the process on the part of the directors of the health facilities supervised. No challenges specific to the supervisory training were identified; some curriculum refinements are noted next.

Curriculum Refinements Made in Light of Experience

Experience from the first training sessions identified several ways in which future training can be improved. During the first trainings, it was possible to identify what parts of the materials were not clear enough for the trainees, where there was information irrelevant for work in the field, and what areas had insufficient information and needed to be expanded. As described previously, the training materials were refined and finalized after the completion of the first round of training sessions.

Health Promoter Training

Based on the recommendations that came out of the initial health promotion training, community materials were formalized. We also developed a training strategy to train a core group of master health promotion trainers within the health network. Materials for training master trainers were created to be able to standardize the process of training master trainers.

Clinical Training

In light of the initial training experiences, we consolidated and streamlined the material to put an emphasis on key messages. We shortened overview material considerably and reduced the number of slides that were used in presentations. The consolidated material included a stronger focus on the interactive components of the course. We developed and refined supporting materials for correctly recording breast cancer detection activities within the national information system. The training team noted that it would be helpful to have a complete materials list and standard set of slides for future trainings.

Supervision Training

Facilitators and participants agreed that, while the training was somewhat participatory, more time could be provided for group activities and interactive activities. Participants also identified suggestions for improving some of the forms used for recording the medical history and tracking of women referred for FNA. Facilitators also saw the need to further enhance the learning around how to conduct the closing meeting of a supervision visit. Participants expressed interest in further clinical information—particularly about FNA and common breast pathologies—and also requested a formal document recognizing their completed training as supervisors.

Incorporation into the Regional Health System

The initial plan considered the creation of special forms to capture detailed information from the patient breast health clinical history forms at the health facility level and then consolidate the information at the regional level. However, the regional ministry of health (GERESA) decided not to introduce any new specialized forms into the system. Previous experiences had shown them that a separate, parallel recording and reporting system creates additional burden on health workers and is not sustainable or efficient; often, health providers stop using the new forms or fill them insufficiently. Instead, they chose to use the existing HIS that records health worker daily activities to track breast health program indicators.

The HIS used by the Ministry of Health nationally in Peru records information for every provider encounter with a patient. Providers are usually very diligent in filling out the HIS forms because this information, which is entered into computers at the health center level, is used for tracking health worker productivity as well as targets for procedures set by the ministry at both national and regional levels. The coding of activities and findings from the CBE is done using the International Classification of Diseases. While this coding system is very extensive and complete, health workers are generally familiar with only a few commonly used codes. We saw that it was important to include an orientation to the codes that relate to breast health activities. We also encountered some challenges with the use of this system in that certain codes, such as FNA, had not been authorized within the HIS system and could not be tracked until they had been formally accepted and integrated into the national system. Once this approach was determined, the curriculum was reviewed again to be sure that terminology used in training was harmonized throughout with the terminology used in the HIS.

Discussion

Comparison with Training Elsewhere

This integrated approach to training health workers has not been described elsewhere to our knowledge, particularly in a limited-resource setting. In the Peru case, it has grown out of an integrated model of care that was designed to use different cadres of health workers to provide education and services related to breast cancer and its early detection. In those few LMICs that have recognized the difficulty of building a national screening program on mammography and have initiated services based on CBE, the efforts have generally been focused on CBE itself or community awareness-raising without a broad system approach. As a result, training has usually been directed at a single type of health worker with little or no coordination between physician, nursing, and community health worker sectors.

The few reports on training community-level workers to do CBE used an approach similar to the one employed in Peru, with a 1 or 2 day curriculum that includes lectures, photos, and hands-on practice with breast models and women. In Iran, rural community health workers called *behvarzes* had a day of didactic material and a day of practice supervised by a gynecologist [15]. *Behvarzes* work out of "health houses" and receive periodic visits from a doctor at a nearby health center. It is not clear what referral system was in place for women with a positive CBE. In Nepal, female community health volunteers (FCHVs) went through a 1-day training that included lectures, a video of CBE, a live demonstration, a manual on CBE, and practice on two women (observed by a surgeon) [16]. Out of 90 trainees, 14 scored well on the posttest and were selected for a research project that involved screening 1,340 women (with parallel screening by the surgeon), where there was good agreement on visual abnormalities and slightly lower agreement on identifying lumps. A pilot program in India trained rural auxiliary nurse-midwives to do community education around breast awareness and breast self-exam (BSE) [17]. The training consisted of two half-days with lectures and videos, practice on breast models, role play, and provision of an illustrated booklet. Again, there is no mention of any provisions for referral of women who identify an abnormality during BSE.

A program developed by the International Society of Nurses in Cancer Care has addressed the issue of training of master trainers in its Train The Trainer (TTT) breast health program [18]. This 2-day international workshop was directed at nurses who already had basic knowledge and experience working in cancer and who were expected to return to their countries and establish similar training programs. It covered a broad range of knowledge (epidemiology, risk factors, screening, diagnosis, treatment, and survivorship) and had skills workshops covering CBE, BSE, and support group facilitation. It has been replicated in Turkey by participants in the original TTT program [19]. One challenge with international programs is that they address only one part of the system and cannot change the environment to which the trainees return.

Implications for Scaling Up Within Peru

This pilot program is very consistent with Peru's national cancer control strategy and with its strong emphasis on prevention and early detection. In 2011, an initiative was launched focusing on reduction of five leading cancers (breast, cervix, lung, prostate, and gastric) and was started in ten regions. The government has invested significant resources in this effort and is looking for innovative approaches to overcome the current inequitable distribution of services and to ensure that rural and poor urban populations can benefit from appropriate and effective services.

The government of Peru and the National Cancer Control Program are planning to expand the experience from the Pacasmayo health network to multiple other provinces and regions. By 2013, all the health facilities in the region where the project is currently operating are expected to be included, and for 2014 they expect to have community promotion, CBE, and FNA available in 10 out of the country's 26 regions. The experience with the current project has identified some issues that need to be addressed in order to make the expansion of activities possible:

- Developing enough master trainers in each region for each part of the intervention before initiating the clinical activities.
- Improving the capacity for reading FNA samples; currently, the number of pathologists with training in breast cytology is limited, and there is a need for further training.
- Using the national identification number to track each individual from screening to diagnosis to treatment through the HIS recording system, thereby allowing the monitoring of

women screened and the completion of care for those with positive findings.

A special Training Excellence Center for breast cancer is being established within the national cancer institute which can lead the effort to scale up the coordinated package of four curricula developed so far. This center will ensure that the content is kept up to date with scientific and policy advances, and will work on the development of a cadre of certified master trainers in all the regions of the country. The Training Excellence Center will also coordinate and oversee quality control during implementation.

Implications for Other LMICs

The findings of the Peru CBE project are highly relevant to early detection in other middle-income countries where the economic feasibility of early detection strategies must be weighed against competing priorities and economic realities such as the costs of providing reproductive health care, treating infectious diseases, or managing other chronic non-communicable diseases like cardiovascular disease or diabetes [20]. Where referral systems for cancer care are still poorly developed, as is the case in most LMICs, building these linkages into the design of training programs is especially critical. While the selection of particular cadres of health worker will vary by country, the principle of defining essential roles and functions and then matching them to the most appropriate cadre available is also widely applicable. For example, female community health workers are ideally placed to raise awareness about breast health and screening among women in their communities, once they have appropriate training. In settings where nurses or midwives are authorized to insert intrauterine devices or do other complex procedures, they could also be trained to do FNA and assess specimen adequacy, as long as a microscope is available to them and a pathologist with cytology training and a specimen transport system are within reach. Where cancer specialists are limited but general physicians are more widely available, as in Peru, it may be more acceptable for doctors to take on the responsibility for FNA. Given the challenges all countries face in releasing health workers for extended training, the Peru experience suggests that short, competency-based training is feasible and well accepted. Only longer-term follow-up will determine whether such training leads to effective practice and good retention of skills.

Conclusion

As countries with limited resources turn their attention to the growing problem of breast cancer, it is critical that they not take a piecemeal approach. Before they launch into training for one cadre of health worker or another, a careful assessment is needed of the critical functions that will be required to ensure that women have the knowledge they need about breast health and screening services, that health workers have the skills they need for early detection and initial diagnosis, and that basic cancer treatment is available for those who need it. Bringing such services as close to the community level as possible will reduce the barriers for women, and using the lowest level cadre possible will increase the feasibility, affordability, and acceptability of such services. Coordinating the content of training for each level of health worker will help ensure that clear and consistent messages are conveyed and that women are smoothly referred from one level to the next. Developing curricula in a collaborative and iterative fashion promotes broader support for the content and capitalizes on learning from experience. Ultimately, for such training to be successful, it is critical that a national authority be recognized with responsibility for updating the curricula as scientific understanding or policy changes, guiding rollout of the program and overseeing implementation to ensure that standards are maintained.

References

1. Parkin DM, Fernández LM. Use of statistics to assess the global burden of breast cancer. Breast J. 2006;12 Suppl 1:S70–80.

2. Forouzanfar MH, Foreman KJ, Delossantos AM, Lozano R, Lopez AD, Murray CJL, et al. Breast and cervical cancer in 187 countries between 1980 and 2010: a systematic analysis. Lancet. 2011;378(9801):1461–84.
3. Akarolo-Anthony SN, Ogundiran TO, Adebamowo CA. Emerging breast cancer epidemic: evidence from Africa. Breast Cancer Res. 2012;12 Suppl 4:S8.
4. Ferlay J, Shin HR, Bray F, Forman D, Mathers C, Parkin DM. GLOBOCAN 2008 v1.2, Cancer incidence and mortality worldwide: IARC CancerBase No. 10 (Internet). Lyon: International Agency for Research on Cancer; 2010. http://globocan.iarc.fr. Accessed 12 July 2012.
5. Shetty P. India faces growing breast cancer epidemic. Lancet. 2012;379(9820):992–3.
6. Bello M. Awareness is the first step in battle against breast cancer. Bull World Health Organ. 2012;90:164–5.
7. Shulman LN, Willett W, Sievers A, Knaul FM. Breast cancer in developing countries: opportunities for improved survival. J Oncol. 2010;2010:595167.
8. Anderson BO, Cazap E, El Saghir NS, Yip CH, Khaled HM, Otero IV, et al. Optimization of breast cancer management in low-resource and middle-resource countries: executive summary of the Breast Health Global Initiative consensus. Lancet Oncol. 2011;12:387–98.
9. Wadler BM, Judge CM, Prout M, Allen JD, Geller AC. Improving breast cancer control via the use of community health workers in South Africa: a critical review. J Oncol. 2011;pii:150423.
10. Yip CH, Smith RA, Anderson BO, Miller AB, Thomas DB, Ang ES, et al. Guideline implementation for breast healthcare in low- and middle-income countries: early detection resource allocation. Cancer. 2008;113 Suppl 8:2244–56.
11. Shyyan R, Sener SF, Anderson BO, Garrote LM, Hortobagyi GN, Ibarra Jr JA, et al. Guideline implementation for breast healthcare in low- and middle-income countries: diagnosis resource allocation. Cancer. 2008;113 Suppl 8:2257–68.
12. Eniu A, Carlson RW, El Saghir NS, Bines J, Bese NS, Vorobiof D, et al. Guideline implementation for breast healthcare in low- and middle-income countries: treatment resource allocation. Cancer. 2008;113 Suppl 8:2269–81.
13. Harford J, Azavedo E, Fischietto M. Breast health guideline implementation in low- and middle-income countries (LMCs): breast healthcare program resource allocation. Cancer. 2008;113 Suppl 8:2282–96.
14. Zotov V, Shyyan R. Introduction of breast cancer screening in Chernihiv Oblast in the Ukraine: report of a PATH Breast Cancer Assistance Program experience. Breast J. 2003;9 Suppl 2:S75–80.
15. Naderi T, Bahrampoor A. Determination of sensitivity and specificity of breast tumor diagnosis by primary health care providers (Behvarz) using clinical examination by obstetrician as a gold standard. J Obstet Gynaecol. 2003;29(2):59–62.
16. Hyoju SK, Agrawal CS, Pokhrel PK, Agrawal S. Transfer of clinical breast examination skills to female community health volunteers in Nepal. Asian Pac J Cancer Prev. 2011;12:3353–6.
17. Rao RS, Nair S, Nair NS, Kamath VG. Acceptability and effectiveness of a breast health awareness programme for rural women in India. Indian J Med Sci. 2005;59:398–402.
18. Meneses KD, Yarbro CH. An evaluation of the train the trainer international breast health and breast cancer education: lessons learned. J Cancer Educ. 2008; 23:267–71.
19. Karayurt O, Gursoy AA, Tasci S, Gundogdu F. Evaluation of the breast cancer train the trainer program for nurses in Turkey. J Cancer Educ. 2010; 25:324–8.
20. Yip CH, Cazap E, Anderson BO, Bright KL, Caleffi M, Cardoso F, et al. Breast cancer management in middle-resource countries (MRCs): consensus statement from the Breast Health Global Initiative. Breast. 2011;20 Suppl 2:S12–9.

Telemedicine in Cancer Control Programs in Developing Countries

15

Karolyn A. Wanat, Kelly E. Quinley, and Carrie L. Kovarik

Abstract

The success of a cancer screening and early diagnosis program is critically dependent on the skill of the healthcare professionals involved. Initial training, continuing education, and consultation as needed are best achieved via telemedicine. The various components of such support for screening and diagnosis of breast and gynecological cancers are discussed.

Abbreviations

CCPPZ	Cervical Cancer Prevention Program in Zambia
CIDRZ	Center for Infectious Disease Research in Zambia
DAD	Data acquisition device
DART	Digital camera assessment of the reproductive tract
eC3	Electronic cervical cancer control
EDI	Enhanced digital imaging
HIV	Human immunodeficiency virus
HPV	Human papilloma virus
LEEP	Loop electrosurgical excision procedure
Pap	Papanicolaou
PIA	Photographic inspection with acetic acid
SMS	Short message service
VIA	of the cervix with acetic acid
VILI	Visualization of the cervix with Lugol's iodine, i.e., Schiller's test

Introduction

Developing screening programs for cancer in developing countries relies upon improving capacity of the local health systems for early detection and treatment of cancer as well as providing education to the population and preventative services [1]. There are multiple strategies to

K.A. Wanat • K.E. Quinley • C.L. Kovarik (✉)
Hospital of the University of Pennsylvania, Perelman School of Medicine at the University of Pennsylvania, Philadelphia, PA 19104-6056, USA
e-mail: Karolyn.Wanat@uphs.upenn.edu; kquinley@mail.med.upenn.edu; carrie.kovarik@uphs.upenn.edu

M.K. Shetty (ed.), *Breast and Gynecological Cancers: An Integrated Approach for Screening and Early Diagnosis in Developing Countries*, DOI 10.1007/978-1-4614-1876-4_15,

provide these services as part of cancer control programs, and one of the strategies is incorporating telemedicine for expanding access to care, providing educational services to providers and patients, diagnosing disease, and continuing management of these patients. This chapter highlights the use of telemedicine in developing countries for screening and diagnosis of breast, external genital cancer, and cervical cancer.

Breast Cancer

In developing low and middle income nations, there is a higher incidence of breast cancer, with an annual rise of at least 7.5 %, more than double that observed on a global level [2]. The challenges facing these countries and their women include access issues with prolonged wait times for diagnosis and treatment, and lack of education on the diseases and potential impact. The women in developing countries often present with more advanced disease associated with higher mortality, often due to lack of preventative and screening services and to the focus on infectious diseases of more acute onset [3]. In addition, misconceptions and stigma about the ability to treat, as well as the various treatment options available, exist and deter women in some populations from getting treatment. In other cases, women have awareness of breast cancer, but no programs exist for treatment [3]. For breast cancer prevention, screening with mammography and treatment of all stages have recently been demonstrated to be cost effective in sub-Saharan Africa and Southeast Asia [4]. Several methods have been explored to help expand access to these populations, including increasing awareness among the public and health authorities, increasing education about breast self-examination, improving access to rapid diagnosis, and improving education about the disease in order to remove any associated stigma [5]. Various telemedicine tools have been piloted and explored in this capacity.

The definition of telemedicine can be broad and applicable to various aspects of breast cancer education, screening, diagnosis, and management. The explosion of mobile phone availability has provided an inexpensive mode of communication, including to those individuals in remote areas. The improved access to this resource is one way to improve communication among physicians to each other and with patients. In addition, the increased access to internet availability also has provided increased means and modes of communication.

Diagnosis: Teleradiology

The ability to efficiently diagnose breast cancer requires access to imaging technology for evaluation of breast masses. In addition, breast cancer screening with mammograms is centered on medical imaging. According to the World Health Organization reports, the majority of the world population lacks access to health technologies, especially medical imaging technologies. In addition, even when medical imaging devices are available, they may be inadequate, nonfunctional, or personnel may lack expertise in management of the systems or interpretation of results. Broadly, teleradiology is a means of electronically transmitting radiographic images for interpretation at another site, and this can be an essential tool to increase access to interpretation of radiographic images in resource-poor settings. For example, in sub-Saharan in 2003, the majority of countries did not have a single radiologist.

The use of teleradiology has been utilized to increase access to services, but technology has been a limitation to its own incorporation. Recently, the feasibility of using mobile technology in order to create an integrated part of a medical imaging system for the interpretation of breast images has been demonstrated [6]. This technology consists of a simple data acquisition device (DAD) on the patient side, as well as an advanced image reconstruction unit at a central site. The mobile phone transmits unprocessed raw data from the patient site DAD to a central site where the end system would process the raw data; then the data would be interpreted by the end user and expert. This technology was tested on simulated breast cancer and shown to be feasible [6]. By dividing the imaging system into smaller components, the complexity and operation of the system at the remote patient site is decreased, and the data processing is centralized, thus increasing access to this state of the art imaging to patients who do not otherwise have access to advanced medical imaging. Earlier attempts at tele-mammography failed because of technical problems and the need for images to be processed at the site of the patient, but newer studies with more advanced technology have demonstrated that high-quality and multisite tele-mammography systems can exist within these technological constraints [7]. Increasing access to mammography in developing countries by centralizing data processing and interpretation would dramatically improve the ability to diagnose breast cancer in resource-limited settings.

Diagnosis: Telepathology

When a suspicious breast mass or nodule is identified, a tissue diagnosis is essential to confirm malignancy. Telepathology is the electronic transmission of digital images, either previously taken and stored ("store-and-forward") or live images, that can be used for education and diagnostic purposes. A successful store-and-forward system requires a microscope, digital camera or slide scanner, computer, internet connection, as well as the ability to process quality histology slides. The remote diagnosis of frozen sections, histology, and cytology from fine needle aspirations and surgical biopsies via telepathology is currently being practiced on a global level for multiple tissues, include breast lesions [8–11]. Although there are several roles for telepathology in the developing world, the use of telepathology as an alternative to an on-site pathologist for interpretation of fine needle aspiration or surgical biopsy specimens is attractive. Studies have demonstrated that the diagnostic accuracy of remote diagnosis of fine needle aspiration ranged from 80 to 95% with improvement to continued training and to use of the system [12, 13]. Reviewing specimens as part of a multidisciplinary team and having access to telepathology in general improve diagnosis and treatment of patients.

Although the ability to remotely interpret pathologic specimens may increase access to subspecialists, care must be taken in establishing this arrangement, as technical difficulties and time for transmission of the image can lead to frustrations with the system and impede timely diagnosis. The initial cost of a system set-up with a microscope and transmitting capacity is not minimal. Once established, having a local pathologist can help streamline diagnoses and interpretation of specimens, with more difficult samples sent for further interpretation. However, as systems become less expensive and more streamlined in transmission, telepathology will continue to be an important tool for diagnosing and establishing cancer centers in the developing world.

Management: Multidisciplinary Teams

In the developed world, multidisciplinary team management including a group of clinicians from different specialties or disciplines has been an important element in improving breast cancer outcomes [14]. These healthcare team members may not all be in the same location, and telemedicine provides a flexible platform to link professionals in different geographical locations, including more remote and further locations, and saves time and money associated with travel. In addition, it allows access to experts who are not in a geographic area in a more efficient manner. The feasibility of connecting multidisciplinary teams from cancer centers and remote cancer units with telemedicine was initially demonstrated for breast cancer, colon cancer, and lung cancer in Wales [15]. More recently, the TELEMAM trial consisting of a 473 patient discussion cluster randomized to telemedicine or in-person meetings to discuss breast cancer management demonstrated that there was similar clinical effectiveness between these two methods in Scotland [16]. The trial also studied the levels of satisfaction of the members of the multidisciplinary trial with the quality of the decision making, which were not statistically different between teleconferences and in-person meetings. Several other studies also have focused on health professional satisfaction with telemedicine and have found that to be generally supportive of tele-oncology [17–19]. One of the significant benefits highlighted was the reduced need for highly specialized clinicians to travel, which provided greater flexibility for meeting times. A challenge posed was technical support, which is an initial up-front cost [16]. In addition, telemedicine was shown to be clinically effective, in terms of the quality of decision making and adherence to best practices in the treatment of breast cancer.

Although this has not yet been studied in the developing world, similar principles of establishing multidisciplinary teams in a country with limited specialty physicians and staff would provide additional flexibility and increased access to these resources and services. Key components for success include technical performance of the equipment, quality decision making, communication between team members, and resource usage [20]. Establishing a multidisciplinary team or tumor board in a developing country to provide this specialized care for patients diagnosed with breast cancer is plausible. Remote physicians and subspecialists also could provide expert opinion and advice across countries and continents with this multidisciplinary approach and telemedicine.

Management: Compliance and Coordination of Care

After diagnosing and initiating treatment, the coordination of care and continued management of patients also are crucial in cancer control programs. Poor compliance and follow-up of patients after an initial visit to a physician are a problem in developing and low resource countries. Monitoring compliance and potential side effects of therapy is an essential component of oncologic care. In Nigeria, the mobile phone was used as a tool to improve communication and increase patient follow-up in African cancer patients, the majority having had breast cancer. High numbers (97.6%) of patients found the use of the phone worthwhile and preferred this mode of communication as it gave them a feeling that they had increased social support from their provider [21]. Because the majority of the patients in developing countries are poor, illiterate, and may travel long distances to be evaluated, access to a streamlined form of communication with their provider in between visits is helpful. Similar to compliance with antiretroviral and antituberculosis medications, adherence to treatment plans for breast cancer patients when using mobile technology has been shown to be effective. For women with breast cancer, this improved communication also is important from a cultural perspective, as in many developing countries women can travel to the doctor only when accompanied by or with permission from their husbands [21]. This mode of communication and social support relies upon the physician being able to speak patients' native language, which may be difficult in more resource-limited settings.

There is considerable ability to expand the use of mobile technology in resource-limited settings as a way to improve communication between providers and patients. This is essential in the care of breast cancer patients and coordination of cancer care, especially if therapy such as chemotherapy and radiation are employed. This extends from social support to counseling to coordination of care. Because cancer patients often have to manage a significant amount of information for coordination of their care, several mobile phone applications also exist to help manage care-related information, including applications that manage appointments, create reminders for taking medications, and communicate laboratory results [22]. Similarly, managing symptoms related to chemotherapy toxicity and potentially dangerous side effects can be difficult for both patients and physicians in any setting. A mobile phone-based advanced symptom management system was developed and demonstrated to be able to support the management of symptoms in patients with breast cancer who were receiving chemotherapy, increasing compliance and identifying patients who needed more emergent intervention [23]. Patients also reported significant benefit in using this system and felt more closely monitored and able to communicate with their physician [24]. This platform can extend from being a formal application to a simpler platform that can be incorporated on basic mobile technology.

External Genital Cancer

The incidence of external genital malignancies, including vulvar, penile, and anal cancer, has been increasing substantially in recent years in the both the developing and developed world. The association of the human papilloma virus (HPV) in these cancers is becoming stronger with current data suggesting HPV infection is potentially associated with 90–93% of anal cancers, 36–40% of penile cancers, and 40–51% of vulvar cancers. HPV is estimated to be involved in 5.2% of all cancers that occur worldwide [25, 26]. The human immunodeficiency virus (HIV) epidemic is also thought to play a role in the rising incidence of HPV infection and related malignancies, as these individuals are at increased risk for HPV-related cancers. This incidence is notable in the HIV-infected population, where rates can be 7–28 times higher than the general population and present as more advanced disease [27]. HIV-infected individuals have been reported to have a 35-fold increased risk of anal cancer among men, 15-fold increased risk of anal cancer among women, and a 5–6-fold increased risk of cancers of penis, vagina, and vulva [27, 28]. Because the rates of HIV are often higher in developing or underserved countries, these problems are becoming an increasing burden to these populations. Screening and diagnosis of external genital malignancies is lacking in developing countries, and specialists with expertise may not be available. Innovative strategies, such as telemedicine, may provide increased availability for screening and early diagnosis of these lesions in the high risk population. Because these malignancies are visually apparent, the use of telemedicine similar to that in dermatology is an attractive solution.

The use of telemedicine for patients with skin diseases and skin cancer screening in both developing and developed countries has been explored and shown to be an effective tool. Many projects and studies that initially incorporated teledermatology as a platform encountered barriers related to the information technology infrastructure and limitation of internet connectivity [29–31]. More recently, the use of mobile telephones or other handheld devices has been incorporated in various settings into dermatologic consultation, skin cancer screening, and the provision of on-going management for dermatologic diseases [29, 32–34]. In a resource limited setting within Egypt, a feasibility study of the use of a mobile telephone for teledermatologic consultation proved to be technically feasible and diagnostically reliable compared to in-person consultation for dermatologic diseases. Similarly, studies in resource-limited settings have demonstrated that the use of mobile phones to capture digital images for clinical diagnosis was feasible, provided good diagnostic accuracy, and served as comparable screening tools for diagnosing melanoma and non-melanoma skin cancers [35–37]. In these studies, high management decision making concordance between teledermatology and in-person consultation was observed, and this was of importance because of the direct impact it would have to patient care and outcomes [38].

Mobile teledermatology platforms could be applied for the screening, diagnosis, and even management of external genital cancers by incorporating the same principles used for screening melanoma or other skin cancers. Because these malignancies often present with visible abnormalities, digital imaging could capture the photos of lesions, which could then be submitted to a specialist for triage and management decisions. The portability and convenience of capturing high resolution clinical images with expanding technology and network coverage for expert opinion would be significant advantages in the screening and diagnosis of external genital cancers, similar to the more common skin cancers [38].

Patients have been extremely satisfied overall with care and accepted this platform as a means to care because of the increased access; some patients had reservations regarding photographs taken with identifying features, which would not be an issue for this type of screening system [39, 40].

Similar to melanoma and non-melanoma skin cancer screening, evaluating patients for external genital cancer requires a provider to evaluate these patients; however, one teleconsultant can reach multiple patients across multiple underserved areas. If screening is effective, then earlier detection of less advanced external genital cancers would allow for earlier and possibly simpler interventions and improved patient care.

Cervical Cancer

Background

Cervical cancer continues to play a major role in cancer-related mortality in the developing world, where it remains the number one cause of cancer-associated death among women [41]. In resource-poor areas, the degree to which the burden of this cancer falls upon women is due to insufficient laboratory, financial, and provider resources, which often lead to either inefficient screening programs or a complete lack of cervical cancer screening [42]. Pioneers in the field of telemedicine have identified the critical role that technology can play in filling current gaps existing in cervical cancer screening services, and they have begun to develop cervical cancer screening training, quality assurance, and provision of programs using telemedical approaches. These programs are helping to bring remote gynecological screening expertise to areas currently lacking sufficient numbers of women's health providers and experts.

Challenges of Conventional Cervical Cancer Screening in Resource-Poor Areas

Cancer screening programs utilizing conventional Papanicolaou (Pap) smear cytology, in conjunction with colposcopic cervical visualization, have proven highly effective and have markedly reduced mortality from cervical cancer in developed countries [43]. In Pap smear screening, cervical and endocervical cells are collected during a vaginal speculum exam, after which the collected cells are examined microscopically by a cytologist to determine whether cellular abnormalities suggest cervical precancerous or cancerous changes, usually caused by sexually transmitted HPV. In the case of the United States, Pap smear-based programs have reduced cervical cancer rates by 74% [43]. However, these cytology-based programs, which are standard of care for cervical cancer screening in the industrialized world, remain scarce in resource-poor countries where decreased awareness of cervical cancer, insufficient laboratory and testing facility infrastructure, substantial loss to follow-up owing to prolonged wait time for results, and the cost and need for trained gynecological experts and cytologists needed to interpret Pap smear results often render them not feasible [42, 44, 45]. HPV DNA testing frequently used in developed countries are also impractical in resource-poor areas, where its high cost makes routine implementation not feasible [46, 47]. Additionally, high rates of HIV-HPV coinfection contribute to the burden of cervical disease in many developing countries [45].

As upwards of 80% of cervical cancers may be prevented by routine screening [48] and simply screening women in resource-poor countries a single time, at age 35, has been shown to decrease the risk of cervical cancer by 25–36% [49], it is imperative for the health and longevity of individual women, as well as the cohesion of families, to continue to increase cervical cancer screening programs in these areas. Telemedicine specialists have stepped into this role and have pioneered programs specifically targeted to developing communities in order to increase the provision of cervical cancer screening services by bringing the providers' services to the patient, in a virtual fashion.

Current Cervical Cancer Screening Approaches in Developing Countries

In the developed world, colposcopy is used as an adjunct to Pap smears to visualize the cervix following abnormal Pap results; this enhances the sensitivity of cytology alone (which can be as low as 50%) [48]. To perform colposcopy, a medical provider uses a colposcope to illuminate and magnify the cervix between 10 and 40 times in order to visually evaluate the cervical tissue for precancerous or cancerous changes. In developing countries, however, many screening programs that lack the necessary resources for Pap smears are based solely on the "see-and-treat" method, where acetic acid and Lugol's iodine solution are used to grossly visualize the cervix without the use of cytology, and women with small lesions can be treated on site with cryotherapy. Those with larger lesions are referred to a tertiary referral center for a cervical biopsy or loop electrosurgical excision procedure (LEEP) [50].

To help visualize cervical dysplasia, acetic acid is applied to the cervix during a speculum exam. In this practice, called visualization of the cervix with acetic acid (VIA—also called Direct Visualization or Cervicoscopy), the acetic acid is applied to the cervix for 3–5 min; this serves to eliminate superficial cervical mucus to improve visualization and causes the whitening ("acetowhitening") of any superficial cervical cells that are abnormal or precancerous, as their higher than normal nuclear crowding causes cellular dehydration in the face of acetic acid (Fig. 15.1) [51].

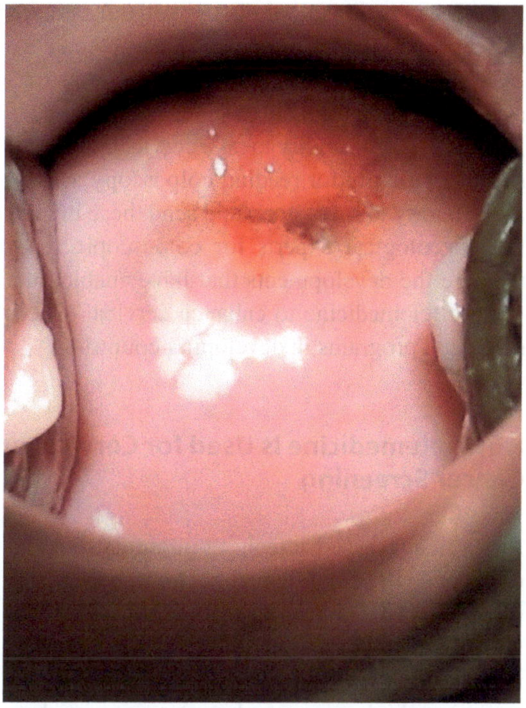

Fig. 15.1 Example of cervical acetowhitening following topical application of acetic acid

Lugol's iodine can also be placed on the cervix during speculum examination to enhance the identification of precancerous lesions. In visual inspection of the cervix with Lugol's iodine (VILI), also known as Schiller's test, glycophilic Lugol's iodine is applied to the cervical tissue and stains the normal, healthy squamous epithelium that has high amounts of glycogen brown, but renders precancerous and metaplastic regions of the cervix as well-defined saffron-colored yellow areas, as they contain abnormally low levels of glycogen and do not uptake the iodine [52].

Numerous studies from developing countries have illustrated largely divergent sensitivities and specificities for detecting early cervical cancer. However, trends show VIA to have superior sensitivity when compared to cytologic screening, with sensitivity of 50–90% vs. 44–85%, respectively; trends also show that VIA has inferior specificity, with VIA at 56–96% vs. cytology at 80–98% [49, 53–56]. Though VIA's low specificity can equate to high numbers of false-positives and raises concerns about overtreatment, resource scarcity often renders Pap smear cytologic screening not feasible. Thus, many programs in developing countries rely on VIA and VILI for screening, as these remain the most appropriate options in the face of resource scarcity.

VIA-focused programs and screening trials have been implemented in countries such as Ghana, India, Kenya, Peru, South Africa, Thailand, Zambia, and Zimbabwe [44, 49, 53, 57, 58]. There are also programs using VIA in conjunction with VILI in Botswana, China, Democratic Republic of the Congo, El Salvador, and India [50, 54, 55, 59, 60].

The high cost of colposcopes, which are needed to capture images of the cervix, as well as the need for trained specialists often preclude the use of a colposcope in developing countries [48, 61]. Programs in Botswana, El Salvador, and

Zambia have utilized store-bought digital cameras to approximate colposcopes and to capture images of the cervix, magnifying areas questionable for premalignant or malignant changes [44, 50, 60]. The ability to take cervical photos of sufficient quality for reading colposcopy as well as the ability to save, store, and send these images to gynecological experts for colposcopic readings are the developments that have enabled the field of telemedicine to enhance cervical cancer screening programs in developing countries.

How Telemedicine Is Used for Cervical Cancer Screening

As an image-based screening modality, colposcopy lends itself to telemedical approaches. The utilization of telemedicine for cervical cancer screening is founded on the basis of the capturing of digital cervical images (also called cervigrams), which are saved and transmitted to off-site gynecological experts where they can be viewed for distant real-time or delayed primary or secondary evaluation [44]. At the patient's bedside, these images can also be projected onto a television screen for patient viewing and for enlargement to more accurately characterize cervical lesions, often referred to as digital camera assessment of the reproductive tract (DART) [60].

Telemedicine is increasing women's access to cervical cancer screening services. Apart from laboratory and technology resources, one of the main resource scarcities for programs using VIA or VILI is the lack of available healthcare providers who have the knowledge and expertise to read cervical images. Therefore, one main advantage that telemedicine provides is the ability to transmit cervical images to off-site gynecological experts with the knowledge to diagnose precancerous or cancerous cervical changes. In this way, telemedical approaches help alleviate the shortage of women's health professionals who are needed to diagnose and triage cervical changes that may lead to cervical cancer.

Another advantage of telemedicine is its use in bolstering patient education on cervical anatomy and physiology as well as cancer etiology. This is of tantamount importance in areas with common misconceptions about the etiology of cervical cancer. In Botswana, for example, one study illustrated that a common belief is that intravaginal medicines and intrauterine contraceptive devices can cause cervical cancer [62]. The use of digital cervical images in DART to project a patient's cervix onto a television screen in the clinical setting can help educate the patient on the location and appearance of the cervix, as well as catalyze conversations on the reduction of cervical cancer risk factors by practicing protected sexual intercourse and taking part in smoking cessation programs.

Digital cervical images also contribute to more comprehensive medical records. They can be saved in patient charts, which in turn become part of medical databases containing more complete patient information that can be used to track progression of cervical changes as well as recurrence events and location of cervical biopsy sites.

Telemedical approaches to cervical cancer screening can greatly contribute to provider training as well as quality-control programs. Training nurses, midwives, and physician's assistants to be able to read and assess VIA or VILI enhanced cervical images can help alleviate the shortage of trained colposcopic providers in developing countries. Such approaches have been used in Zambia and Botswana [44, 50].

Telemedicine's use in cervical cancer screening can increase access to a colposcopic-like examination by providing an alternative to the use of expensive and often cost-prohibitive colposcopes. The use of store-bought digital cameras to capture cervical images and project them onto television or computer screens in DART and enhanced digital imaging (EDI) approaches, respectively, circumvents the need for colposcopes and provides a means of cervical visualization that is more affordable. Additionally, mobile health efforts in other areas of healthcare provision have extended medical services by using community health workers to address patient needs in the fields of HIV care, prenatal care, health education, and medication adherence, as seen with Dimagi, Inc., a global health

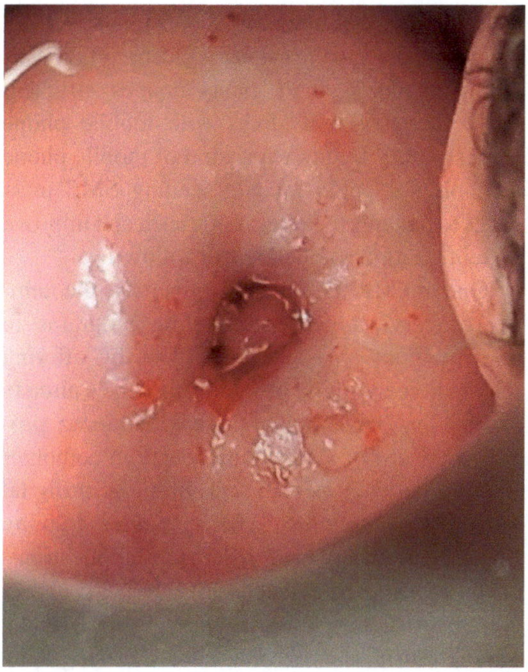

Fig. 15.2 High-quality cervical image taken by mobile phone camera

and technology company focused on mobile health [63]. A study in Botswana demonstrated that cervical images taken with mobile phone cameras were efficient for approximating colposcopy and provided images of high enough quality for remote diagnosis of premalignant cervical changes (Fig. 15.2) [45].

Overview of Telemedicine's Current Use in Cervical Cancer Screening

Though many community-based, hospital-based, and nongovernmental organizations are now utilizing telemedicine in such diverse fields as dermatology, ophthalmology, radiology, and critical care, current telemedicine programs focused on cervical cancer screening remain few in number. However, the Cervical Cancer Prevention Program in Zambia (CCPPZ) at the Center for Infectious Disease Research in Zambia (CIDRZ) provides the most successful model for a thriving see-and-treat approach to cervical cancer screening, which is based on telemedical remote consultations and trains providers from other areas in implementing similar telemedical cervical cancer screening programs worldwide.

Founded in 2006 in Lusaka, Zambia, the CCPPZ utilizes the see-and-treat approach to screening. This program was produced in collaboration with the University of Alabama at Birmingham, the University Teaching Hospital (UTH) in Lusaka, the research-focused CIDRZ, and the Zambian Ministry of Health, with the goal of creating a locally and nationally owned program with the support of foreign expertise and funding [46]. It is currently run by Dr. Groesbeck Parham, a gynecological oncologist from the University of Alabama at Birmingham. In 18 clinics, nurses utilize the electronic cervical cancer control (deemed "eC3") program to screen patients for cervical cancer and refer necessary cases to a tertiary hospital-based referral center [44]. The eC3 program is based on affordable mobile technology, where store-bought digital cameras are used to project real-time cervical images (following application of 5% acetic acid) onto large television screens for evaluation of cervical lesions; the images also serve as a background for patient education [44]. Digital cervigrams are taken with 6-megapixel resolution using store-bought digital cameras. Nurses bring these full size 6-megapixel images to weekly post-analysis quality-control training sessions for continuing education. The images can also be transmitted electronically to remote experts or to a secure website accessed by consultants for off-site evaluation (telecervicography, also known as photographic inspection with acetic acid—PIA [45]); the images can be resized to appear by default as a 1-megapixel image on the secure website, though they can be again enlarged to full size if desired. Images are also uploaded to the patient's electronic medical record [44]. Following the see-and-treat approach, patients eligible for cryotherapy are treated directly on site or referred to the UTH for cervical biopsy or LEEP. Since January 2006, the CIDRZ CCPPZ has provided over 100,000 screenings with the initiation of the see-and-treat prevention program.

The eC3 program is based on an image exchange using camera store-and-forward images, internet-based images, and mobile phone-based digital images. The program's remote consultation services currently rely on the program's secure consultation website, which was created by Dimagi, Inc., in 2008 using open-source Python software (Python Software Foundation, Hampton, NH) and is hosted on the internet server at the referral center in Lusaka. The goal of the website was to streamline the consultation process and increase the security of consult requests, which had previously relied on cervical images saved on laptop computers being uploaded and sent together with patient information in emails to consultants. Utilizing the store-and-forward approach, clinicians can now upload an image to the website directly from the digital camera and can add pertinent de-identified patient data, i.e., age, HIV-positivity, and qualitative assessment of cervical lesions. The website sends automated texts to on-call gynecological doctors notifying them to check the website for consultation cases. These consultants log on, make comments, and make final diagnoses; the on-site clinicians wait for these consultations. The website's physician interfaces allow for access to all patient records, whereas nurse interfaces are limited to their individual patient cohorts [44].

Mobile phones are helping accelerate the receipt of distant consultation, with the goal of obtaining expert opinions and treatment recommendations while patients are still in the clinic. Text messaging is utilized by the website, where a short message service (SMS) is automatically generated and sent to consultants on call, informing them of the images awaiting review; consultants can return a SMS to the nurse following review of the patient image and clinical history [44]. CCPPZ currently plans to expand the use of mobile phones to increase access to off-site consultation for remote clinics. Plans include identifying android phones with cameras or attachments capable of 50–70 mm angles of view and with minimal focal distances of 7–15 cm needed for viewing the cervix down the vaginal canal. The ultimate goal is for nurses to take cervical images with cellular phone cameras and then directly send the image to the remote consultant. A pilot study in Botswana previously illustrated the feasibility of taking high-quality images sufficient for accurate VIA readings with mobile phone cameras [45]. Future expansion of mobile phone technologies could include sending SMS messages to patients to increase outreach and improve patient treatment adherence or follow-up.

One of CCPPZ's goals is to increase the number of cervical cancer screening programs in resource-poor areas, which it does by offering telemedicine training programs to nurses already skilled in VIA and cryotherapy. Training programs consist of a weeklong course in computer training, as well as a 2-week training in digital photography training. The computer training focuses on the use of Microsoft applications, such as Word, Excel and use of Internet Explorer (Microsoft Corporation, Redmond, WA, USA), and the transmission of cervigrams. Cervicography training, which includes instruction on digital camera function, care, accessory use, and the taking of digital cervical photographs, focuses on mentoring participants to take high-quality cervical images with training on storing, resizing and tagging photos with patient identification numbers, as well as the creating of a standardized storage system [44].

Additionally, CIDRZ has published a guide listing the technological materials required for digital cervicography with the goal that future program clinicians will send consults to their website. Table 15.1 comprises their list of necessary hardware and materials, with associated cost, that clinicians would need to set up a similar eC3 program [44].

Limitations and Challenges of Telemedicine and Cervical Cancer Screening

Though telemedicine can extend screening services in resource-poor areas, there are limitations to telemedical approaches that utilize the see-and-treat screening method. Using a two dimensional digital cervigram instead of a live cervix for dysplasia evaluation makes it easier to

Table 15.1 Necessary equipment, with associated cost, needed to set up an electronic cervical cancer control program

	Average cost (US$)
Digital camera (e.g., Canon Powershot™ SX40 HS Digital Camera with built-in flash)	300
58 mm Canon Close-up Macroconverter Lens 500D	100
58 mm Canon SX40 HS Filter Adapter	9
Memory card(s) for cameras	50
Charger [e.g., Energizer® Rechargeable Compact Charger 2500 (NiMH/NiCd)]	20
Rechargeable AA batteries—8 or 12	2
Television or computer monitor (preferably at least 15 in.)	150
Cable for connecting camera to television or computer (usually included with camera)	5
PC Tuner card (if using camera with computer rather than television)	100
Extension cord/surge protectors	5
Laptop computers with external mouse	2,000
Software for integrating photographs into patient's electronic medical records (e.g., DBPix™; redistribution license)	350
Picture resizing software (e.g., Genius Picture Resize™; unlimited business license)	40
Internet source to share images and data electronically (optional)	Variable

Modified with permission from Parham GP, Mwanahamuntu MH, Pfaendler KS, Sahasrabuddhe VV, Myung D, Mkumba G et al. eC3—a modern telecommunications matrix for cervical cancer prevention in Zambia. J Low Genit Tract Dis 2010 Jul;14(3):167–173. Includes updates by Dr. Groesbeck Parham on May 12, 2012

miss three dimensional cervical changes such as ulcerations; this also makes the accuracy of a diagnosis heavily reliant on the quality of the cervical image [44]. Cervical cameras can become damaged or nonfunctional, and then they usually have to be sent abroad for repair [44]. Intermittent and unreliable internet connectivity can also compromise the speed with which remote consultation can be obtained.

The use of mobile phone cameras for taking cervical photographs presents its own set of challenges, as these phones often have automatic zoom functions. Clinicians using mobile phone cameras need extra training in the use of adequate and appropriate lighting, how to minimize glare from the metal speculum, and how to ensure the camera focus falls on the cervix and not the vaginal walls or hair; this will help them create a photo of sufficient quality to be used in PIA readings [45].

There are also inherent limitations of telemedicine owing to its use in conjunction with VIA. The test's low sensitivity compared to other screening measures increases the possibility of false-positive readings and overtreatment, and the subjective nature of diagnosis translates to a stricter need for well-developed quality assurance measures. However, the strength of VIA with cryotherapy is that it can be performed by many different levels of healthcare professionals, and it provides immediate results, allowing for the treatment of the patient during the same visit, and therefore limiting loss to follow-up of patients [61].

Summary and Conclusions

The adjunct of telemedicine in cervical cancer screening can greatly improve medical care for women in resource-poor areas by reducing barriers to the screening access [64]. The utilization of telemedicine is enabling the establishment of new quality-control programs, providing opportunities for continued development of diagnostic skills, and improving access to real-time gynecological expert advice [44]. The worldwide boom in mobile phone usage, both by patients as well as by clinicians aiming to use new technologies to improve medical care, promises to present new opportunities for increasing the extension of cervical cancer screening services in developing areas where they are most needed.

Tele-Education: Patients, Providers, and Communities

As part of cancer control programs, telemedicine can be an educational resource for patients, providers, and communities in general. This is especially important for some of the gynecologic malignancies that may be associated with a certain unfounded stigma.

For providers, telemedicine has been shown to be an effective and important educational tool in training younger and less experienced physicians to broaden their medical knowledge [31, 65, 66]. In addition, the use of virtual slide technology in providing an entire digital image of a biopsy from a glass slide not only will help with diagnosis but also will assist in pathologic education. This collection of digital images from telemedicine consultations can then create a resource for training local physicians in their home countries with the goal of self-sufficiency [67–69]. On a broader level, telemedicine platforms have been utilized to teach individuals in remote rural settings and to expand access to medical education, with the ultimate goal of improving patient care and survival [70–75].

With the increased access to cellular telephones and the internet, telemedicine also can be expanded to "tele-education" in order to educate individuals on the importance of healthy behaviors such as breast self-examination and basic information on malignancies, including HPV infection. Similar to programs that exist for patients with regards to heart failure, stroke symptoms, and chronic illnesses, tele-education can be applied successfully to teach individuals in developing countries about locally relevant diseases [76–78]. Limitations in developing countries or remote settings may include literacy and translation into multiple languages. However, using community health workers, messages and information can be shared in this innovative way. Similarly, text messaging or updates to general communities or community leaders also could be provided with regards to breast cancer screening importance or opportunities for vaccination against HPV that may help control extragenital and cervical cancer, if such programs are available.

The potential role of telemedicine in cancer control programs in developing countries is vast and adaptable to existing resources and specific demands of countries. Different aspects of the telemedicine program can be implemented and help strengthen the ability of developing countries to improve access and patient care in gynecologic cancers.

References

1. Sankaranarayanan R, Sauvaget C, Ramadas K, Ngoma T, Teguete I, Muwonge R, et al. Clinical trials of cancer screening in the developing world and their impact on cancer healthcare. Ann Oncol. 2011;22 Suppl 7: vii20–8.
2. Forouzanfar MH, Foreman KJ, Delossantos AM, Lozano R, Lopez AD, Murray CJ, et al. Breast and cervical cancer in 187 countries between 1980 and 2010: a systematic analysis. Lancet. 2011;378(9801):1461–84.
3. Igene H. Global health inequalities and breast cancer: an impending public health problem for developing countries. Breast J. 2008;14(5):428–34.
4. Ginsberg GM, Lauer JA, Zelle S, Baeten S, Baltussen R. Cost effectiveness of strategies to combat breast, cervical, and colorectal cancer in sub-Saharan Africa and South East Asia: mathematical modelling study. BMJ. 2012;344:e614.
5. Panieri E. Breast cancer screening in developing countries. Best Pract Res Clin Obstet Gynaecol. 2012; 26(2):283–90.
6. Granot Y, Ivorra A, Rubinsky B. A new concept for medical imaging centered on cellular phone technology. PLoS One. 2008;3(4):e2075.
7. Leader JK, Hakim CM, Ganott MA, Chough DM, Wallace LP, Clearfield RJ, et al. A multisite telemammography system for remote management of screening mammography: an assessment of technical, operational, and clinical issues. J Digit Imaging. 2006; 19(3):216–25.
8. Szymas J, Wolf G. Telepathology by the internet. Adv Clin Path. 1998;2(2):133–5.
9. Hitchcock CL. The future of telepathology for the developing world. Arch Pathol Lab Med. 2011; 135(2):211–4.
10. Hitchcock CL, Hitchcock LE. Three years of experience with routine use of telepathology in assessment of excisional and aspirate biopsies of breast lesions. Croat Med J. 2005;46(3):449–57.
11. Lopez AM, Graham AR, Barker GP, Richter LC, Krupinski EA, Lian F, et al. Virtual slide telepathology enables an innovative telehealth rapid breast care clinic. Semin Diagn Pathol. 2009;26(4):177–86.

12. Vazir H, Loane MA, Wootton R. A pilot study of low-cost dynamic telepathology using the public telephone network. Adv Clin Path. 1998;2(2):151.
13. Singh N, Akbar N, Sowter C, Lea KG, Wells CA. Telepathology in a routine clinical environment: implementation and accuracy of diagnosis by robotic microscopy in a one-stop breast clinic. J Pathol. 2002;196(3):351–5.
14. Sainsbury R, Haward B, Rider L, Johnston C, Round C. Influence of clinician workload and patterns of treatment on survival from breast cancer. Lancet. 1995;345(8960):1265–70.
15. Axford AT, Askill C, Jones AJ. Virtual multidisciplinary teams for cancer care. J Telemed Telecare. 2002;8 Suppl 2:3–4.
16. Kunkler IH, Prescott RJ, Lee RJ, Brebner JA, Cairns JA, Fielding RG, et al. TELEMAM: a cluster randomised trial to assess the use of telemedicine in multi-disciplinary breast cancer decision making. Eur J Cancer. 2007;43(17):2506–14.
17. Kunkler IH, Rafferty P, Hill D, Henry M, Foreman D. A pilot study of tele-oncology in Scotland. J Telemed Telecare. 1998;4(2):113–9.
18. Barry N, Campbell P, Reed N, Reid ME, Bower DJ, Norrie J, et al. Implementation of videoconferencing to support a managed clinical network in Scotland: lessons learned during the first 18 months. J Telemed Telecare. 2003;9 Suppl 2:S7–9.
19. Fielding RG, Macnab M, Swann S, Kunkler IH, Brebner J, Prescott RJ, et al. Attitudes of breast cancer professionals to conventional and telemedicine-delivered multidisciplinary breast meetings. J Telemed Telecare. 2005;11 Suppl 2:S29–34.
20. Kunkler IH, Fielding RG, Brebner J, Prescott R, Maclean JR, Cairns J, et al. A comprehensive approach for evaluating telemedicine-delivered multidisciplinary breast cancer meetings in southern Scotland. J Telemed Telecare. 2005;11 Suppl 1:71–3.
21. Odigie VI, Yusufu LM, Dawotola DA, Ejagwulu F, Abur P, Mai A, et al. The mobile phone as a tool in improving cancer care in Nigeria. Psychooncology. 2012;21(3):332–5.
22. Klasnja P, Hartzler A, Powell C, Phan G, Pratt W. Health weaver mobile: designing a mobile tool for managing personal health information during cancer care. AMIA Annu Symp Proc. 2010;2010:392–6.
23. Kearney N, McCann L, Norrie J, Taylor L, Gray P, McGee-Lennon M, et al. Evaluation of a mobile phone-based, advanced symptom management system (ASyMS) in the management of chemotherapy-related toxicity. Support Care Cancer. 2009;17(4):437–44.
24. McCann L, Maguire R, Miller M, Kearney N. Patients' perceptions and experiences of using a mobile phone-based advanced symptom management system (ASyMS) to monitor and manage chemotherapy related toxicity. Eur J Cancer Care (Engl). 2009; 18(2):156–64.
25. Parkin DM, Bray F. Chapter 2: the burden of HPV-related cancers. Vaccine. 2006;24 Suppl 3:S3/11–25.
26. Parkin DM. The global health burden of infection-associated cancers in the year 2002. Int J Cancer. 2006;118(12):3030–44.
27. Frisch M, Biggar RJ, Goedert JJ. Human papillomavirus-associated cancers in patients with human immunodeficiency virus infection and acquired immunodeficiency syndrome. J Natl Cancer Inst. 2000;92(18):1500–10.
28. Chaturvedi AK, Madeleine MM, Biggar RJ, Engels EA. Risk of human papillomavirus-associated cancers among persons with AIDS. J Natl Cancer Inst. 2009;101(16):1120–30.
29. Tran K, Ayad M, Weinberg J, Cherng A, Chowdhury M, Monir S, et al. Mobile teledermatology in the developing world: implications of a feasibility study on 30 Egyptian patients with common skin diseases. J Am Acad Dermatol. 2011;64(2):302–9.
30. Kaddu S, Soyer HP, Gabler G, Kovarik C. The Africa Teledermatology Project: preliminary experience with a sub-Saharan teledermatology and e-learning program. J Am Acad Dermatol. 2009;61(1):155–7.
31. Weinberg J, Kaddu S, Gabler G, Kovarik C. The African Teledermatology Project: providing access to dermatologic care and education in sub-Saharan Africa. Pan Afr Med J. 2009;3:16.
32. Massone C, Lozzi GP, Wurm E, Hofmann-Wellenhof R, Schoellnast R, Zalaudek I, et al. Cellular phones in clinical teledermatology. Arch Dermatol. 2005; 141(10):1319–20.
33. Schreier G, Hayn D, Kastner P, Koller S, Salmhofer W, Hofmann-Wellenhof R. A mobile-phone based teledermatology system to support self-management of patients suffering from psoriasis. Conf Proc IEEE Eng Med Biol Soc. 2008;2008:5338–41.
34. Shapiro M, James WD, Kessler R, Lazorik FC, Katz KA, Tam J, et al. Comparison of skin biopsy triage decisions in 49 patients with pigmented lesions and skin neoplasms: store-and-forward teledermatology vs face-to-face dermatology. Arch Dermatol. 2004;140(5):525–8.
35. Massone C, Hofmann-Wellenhof R, Ahlgrimm-Siess V, Gabler G, Ebner C, Soyer HP. Melanoma screening with cellular phones. PLoS One. 2007;2(5):e483.
36. Kroemer S, Fruhauf J, Campbell TM, Massone C, Schwantzer G, Soyer HP, et al. Mobile teledermatology for skin tumour screening: diagnostic accuracy of clinical and dermoscopic image tele-evaluation using cellular phones. Br J Dermatol. 2011;164(5):973–9.
37. Massone C, Brunasso AM, Campbell TM, Soyer HP. Mobile teledermoscopy—melanoma diagnosis by one click? Semin Cutan Med Surg. 2009;28:203–5.
38. Lamel SA, Haldeman KM, Ely H, Kovarik CL, Pak H, Armstrong AW. Application of mobile teledermatology for skin cancer screening. J Am Acad Dermatol. 2012;67(4):576–81.
39. Azfar RS, Weinberg JL, Cavric G, Lee-Keltner IA, Bilker WB, Gelfand JM, et al. HIV-positive patients in Botswana state that mobile teledermatology is an acceptable method for receiving dermatology care. J Telemed Telecare. 2011;17(6):338–40.

40. Scheinfeld N, Fisher M, Genis P, Long H. Evaluating patient acceptance of a teledermatology link of an urban urgent-care dermatology clinic run by residents with board certified dermatologists. Skinmed. 2003;2(3):159–62.
41. Parkin DM, Bray F, Ferlay J, Pisani P. Estimating the world cancer burden: Globocan 2000. Int J Cancer. 2001;94(2):153–6.
42. Roblyer D, Richards-Kortum R, Park SY, Adewole I, Follen M. Objective screening for cervical cancer in developing nations: lessons from Nigeria. Gynecol Oncol. 2007;107(1 Suppl 1):S94–7.
43. Saslow D, Runowicz CD, Solomon D, Moscicki AB, Smith RA, Eyre HJ, et al. American Cancer Society guideline for the early detection of cervical neoplasia and cancer. J Low Genit Tract Dis. 2003;7(2):67–86.
44. Parham GP, Mwanahamuntu MH, Pfaendler KS, Sahasrabuddhe VV, Myung D, Mkumba G, et al. eC3—a modern telecommunications matrix for cervical cancer prevention in Zambia. J Low Genit Tract Dis. 2010;14(3):167–73.
45. Quinley KE, Gormley RH, Ratcliffe SJ, Shih T, Szep Z, Steiner A, et al. Use of mobile telemedicine for cervical cancer screening. J Telemed Telecare. 2011; 17(4):203–9.
46. Mwanahamuntu MH, Sahasrabuddhe VV, Kapambwe S, Pfaendler KS, Chibwesha C, Mkumba G, et al. Advancing cervical cancer prevention initiatives in resource-constrained settings: insights from the Cervical Cancer Prevention Program in Zambia. PLoS Med. 2011;8(5):e1001032.
47. Sankaranarayanan R, Nene BM, Shastri SS, Jayant K, Muwonge R, Budukh AM, et al. HPV screening for cervical cancer in rural India. N Engl J Med. 2009;360(14):1385–94.
48. Chase DM, Kalouyan M, DiSaia PJ. Colposcopy to evaluate abnormal cervical cytology in 2008. Am J Obstet Gynecol. 2009;200(5):472–80.
49. Goldie SJ, Gaffikin L, Goldhaber-Fiebert JD, Gordillo-Tobar A, Levin C, Mahe C, et al. Cost-effectiveness of cervical-cancer screening in five developing countries. N Engl J Med. 2005;353(20):2158–68.
50. Ramogola-Masire D, de Klerk R, Monare B, Ratshaa B, Friedman HM, Zetola NM. Cervical cancer prevention in HIV-infected women using the "see and treat" approach in Botswana. J Acquir Immune Defic Syndr. 2012;59(3):308–13.
51. Van Le L, Broekhuizen FF, Janzer-Steele R, Behar M, Samter T. Acetic acid visualization of the cervix to detect cervical dysplasia. Obstet Gynecol. 1993;81(2):293–5.
52. Visual inspection with Lugol's iodine (VILI): Evidence to date. 2003. http://www.path.org/publications/files/RH_vili. Accessed 16 Apr 2012.
53. University of Zimbabwe/JHPIEGO Cervical Cancer Project. Visual inspection with acetic acid for cervical-cancer screening: test qualities in a primary-care setting. Lancet. 1999;353(9156):869–73.
54. Sangwa-Lugoma G, Mahmud S, Nasr SH, Liaras J, Kayembe PK, Tozin RR, et al. Visual inspection as a cervical cancer screening method in a primary health care setting in Africa. Int J Cancer. 2006; 119(6):1389–95.
55. Sankaranarayanan R, Wesley R, Thara S, Dhakad N, Chandralekha B, Sebastian P, et al. Test characteristics of visual inspection with 4% acetic acid (VIA) and Lugol's iodine (VILI) in cervical cancer screening in Kerala, India. Int J Cancer. 2003;106(3):404–8.
56. Sehgal A, Singh V, Bhambhani S, Luthra UK. Screening for cervical cancer by direct inspection. Lancet. 1991;338(8762):282.
57. Blumenthal PD, Gaffikin L, Deganus S, Lewis R, Emerson M, Adadevoh S, et al. Cervical cancer prevention: safety, acceptability, and feasibility of a single-visit approach in Accra, Ghana. Am J Obstet Gynecol. 2007;196(4):407.e1–8. discussion 407.e8-9.
58. Sankaranarayanan R, Wesley R, Somanathan T, Dhakad N, Shyamalakumary B, Amma NS, et al. Visual inspection of the uterine cervix after the application of acetic acid in the detection of cervical carcinoma and its precursors. Cancer. 1998;83(10):2150–6.
59. Shi JF, Canfell K, Lew JB, Zhao FH, Legood R, Ning Y, et al. Evaluation of primary HPV-DNA testing in relation to visual inspection methods for cervical cancer screening in rural China: an epidemiologic and cost-effectiveness modelling study. BMC Cancer. 2011;11:239.
60. Cremer M, Jamshidi RM, Muderspach L, Tsao-Wei D, Felix JC, Blumenthal PD. Digital camera assessment for detection of cervical intraepithelial neoplasia in rural El Salvador. Int J Gynaecol Obstet. 2005;91(1):42–6.
61. Sankaranarayanan R, Boffetta P. Research on cancer prevention, detection and management in low- and medium-income countries. Ann Oncol. 2010;21(10):1935–43.
62. McFarland DM. Beliefs about the causes of cervical cancer in Botswana: implications for nursing. Int Nurs Rev. 2009;56(4):426–32.
63. Dimagi: Mobile Health. http://www.dimagi.com/mobile-health/ (2012). Accessed 16 Apr 2012.
64. Ferris DG, Macfee MS, Miller JA, Litaker MS, Crawley D, Watson D. The efficacy of telecolposcopy compared with traditional colposcopy. Obstet Gynecol. 2002;99(2):248–54.
65. Williams CM, Kedar I, Smith L, Brandling-Bennett HA, Lugn N, Kvedar JC. Teledermatology education for internal medicine residents. J Am Acad Dermatol. 2005;52(6):1098–9.
66. Shaikh N, Lehmann CU, Kaleida PH, Cohen BA. Efficacy and feasibility of teledermatology for paediatric medical education. J Telemed Telecare. 2008; 14(4):204–7.
67. Dennis T, Start RD, Cross SS. The use of digital imaging, video conferencing, and telepathology in histopathology: a national survey. J Clin Pathol. 2005; 58(3):254–8.
68. Ayad E, Yagi Y. Virtual microscopy beyond the pyramids, applications of WSI in Cairo University for E-education & telepathology. Anal Cell Pathol (Amst). 2012;35(2):93–5.
69. Gongora Jara H, Barcelo HA. Telepathology and continuous education: important tools for pathologists of

developing countries. Diagn Pathol. 2008;3 Suppl 1:S24.

70. Latifi K, Lecaj I, Bekteshi F, Dasho E, Doarn CR, Merrell RC, et al. Cost-benefit analysis on the use of telemedicine program of Kosova for continuous medical education: a sustainable and efficient model to rebuild medical systems in developing countries. Telemed J E Health. 2011;17(10):757–62.
71. Condos SG, Stamkopoulos T, Selles JM, Merrell RC. Tele-affiliation in medical education: experience from the international program at Yale Office of Telemedicine. Methods Inf Med. 2002;41(5):382–6.
72. Mahapatra AK, Mishra SK, Kapoor L, Singh IP. Critical issues in medical education and the implications for telemedicine technology. Telemed J E Health. 2009;15(6):592–6.
73. Ricci MA, Caputo MP, Callas PW, Gagne M. The use of telemedicine for delivering continuing medical education in rural communities. Telemed J E Health. 2005;11(2):124–9.
74. Rafiq A, Merrell RC. Telemedicine for access to quality care on medical practice and continuing medical education in a global arena. J Contin Educ Health Prof. 2005;25(1):34–42.
75. Saiki Jr SM. The role of telemedicine in medical education. Hawaii Med J. 1999;58(12):326–7.
76. Schweickert PA, Rutledge CM, Cattell-Gordon DC, Solenski NJ, Jensen ME, Branson S, et al. Telehealth stroke education for rural elderly Virginians. Telemed J E Health. 2011;17(10):784–8.
77. Kobak KA, Stone WL, Wallace E, Warren Z, Swanson A, Robson K. A web-based tutorial for parents of young children with autism: results from a pilot study. Telemed J E Health. 2011;17(10):804–8.
78. Baker DW, Dewalt DA, Schillinger D, Hawk V, Ruo B, Bibbins-Domingo K, et al. The effect of progressive, reinforcing telephone education and counseling versus brief educational intervention on knowledge, self-care behaviors and heart failure symptoms. J Card Fail. 2011;17(10):789–96.

Breast Cancer Screening and Cervical Cancer Prevention in Developing Countries: Strategies for the Future

16

Kevin M. Kelly, Mahesh K. Shetty, and José Humberto Tavares Guerreiro Fregnani

K.M. Kelly
Pasadena Breast Ultrasound Center,
Pasadena, CA 91106, USA
e-mail: drkelly@ca.rr.com

M.K. Shetty (✉)
Woman's Center for Breast Care and MRI,
Woman's Hospital of Texas,
Houston, TX 77054, USA
e-mail: mshetty@womens-radiology.com

J.H.T.G. Fregnani
Center for Research Support, Teaching and Research
Institute, Barretos Cancer Hospital,
Barretos 14784-400, Brazil
e-mail: mdfregnani@terra.com.br

M.K. Shetty (ed.), *Breast and Gynecological Cancers: An Integrated Approach for Screening and Early Diagnosis in Developing Countries*, DOI 10.1007/978-1-4614-1876-4_16,

A. Future Strategies for Breast Cancer Screening in Developing Countries

Kevin M. Kelly and Mahesh K. Shetty

Abstract

Breast cancer is increasing 3.1 % annually. It is more deadly and more frequent in young women in developing countries compared to young women in the more developed countries. Important reasons for this increased incidence and lethality are poor nutrition (leading to decreased immunity to resist the advance of cancer), delayed access to health care, and poor quality of care when it is finally available. Early detection of breast cancer is the key to the control of its lethal effects. Increasing breast health awareness and clinical breast examination are key components of a screening program at the present time. Such a strategy is aimed at detecting Stage I and Stage II cancers and downstaging cancers from the now prevalent presentation at Stage III and Stage IV. For the future, however, a low cost methodology needs to be adopted in order to diagnose small node-negative cancers by screening the asymptomatic population. Organized screening mammography is not a feasible option for low and mid-resource countries, even in the future. A combination of low prevalence and the expensive infrastructure needed in terms of the equipment and trained health-care professionals makes this an unrealistic option and a potential drain and diversion of health-care funding resources in developing countries. The background of the situation that is currently in existence, problems thereof, and the potential for the use of whole breast ultrasound screening for breast cancer is discussed in this chapter.

K.M. Kelly
Pasadena Breast Ultrasound Center,
Pasadena, CA 91106, USA
e-mail: drkelly@ca.rr.com

M.K. Shetty (✉)
Woman's Center for Breast Care and MRI,
Woman's Hospital of Texas,
Houston, TX 77054, USA
e-mail: mshetty@womens-radiology.com

Status of Breast Cancer in Low Resource (LR) Countries

Breast cancer is a worldwide epidemic that is increasing 3.1 % per year, almost twice as fast as the increase in world population. Although only about half of the breast cancer cases occur in low resource countries, almost two thirds (63.5 %) of these cases occur in women under the age of 50, and almost three quarters (72.1 %) of the deaths from breast cancer found in this younger group occur in these developing countries [1].

Disproportionate Incidence in Young Women

The reasons for the increased incidence of breast cancer in younger women in LR countries and the disproportionate increased death rate among these women require complex explanations because of multiple causative factors. The overall incidence of breast cancer in the LR countries is not greater, and often is considerably less, than the incidence in the high resource (HR) countries. However, the incidence in women under 50 years of age in the developing countries is disproportionately high, probably for reasons discussed in the following sections.

Nutrition

The limited caloric intake of low resource women may have differing effects on cancer rates and the severity of cancer once established. Pre-cancer (in situ) and probably very early invasive cancer do not immediately establish an independent blood supply. Until they do, these proto-cancers must compete with the adjacent cells for nutrition. In the environment of low nutrients found in these women, cancer cells are at a disadvantage due to their higher metabolic rate, necessitated by the requirement to reproduce quickly. They may be unable to sustain themselves in this environment and fail to survive to establish a blood supply.

Compared to women from LR countries, women from HR countries with surfeits of nutrients form cancers which may more easily establish themselves, gain blood supplies, and go on to become clinically recognized cancers. Because of the increased sugar absorption in cancer cells, a Westernized diet may be particularly advantageous for cancer development [2]. This scenario may be true in China where the breast cancer rate has climbed greatly in the major cities over the past two or three decades due to the improved nutrition of these urban populations, with a diet including more free sugar than the traditional Chinese diet [3]. The cancer rate in the more nutritionally challenged countryside has not undergone the same marked increase. The countryside cancer incidence is less than half that of Shanghai, with the rate of increase accelerating faster in Shanghai for the past 30 years. The incidence of breast cancer in the urban areas is expected to be almost quadruple that of the countryside in 20 years [3].

The breast cancer rate will probably increase in women in all LR countries as their average caloric consumption increases, especially if this increase is accompanied by a disproportionate increase of simple sugars in the diet. At present, although the incidence of breast cancer is lower in LR countries, the mortality rate of these cancers is greater than those found in HR countries. The reasons are multiple.

Delayed Access to Health care

Obviously, where education is minimal and medical resources are scarce, cancers will be larger at discovery. These cancers would also be expected to be more aggressive and therefore more lethal as they enlarge [4].

Lower Quality Treatment

The lack of radiation and chemotherapy denies LR women any increased chance of survival once the cancer reaches the lymph nodes.

Decreased Immunity

Another important cause of the increased lethality of breast cancer in women of LR countries is that the body conserves energy when the diet is insufficient. The body is a multitasking organism, which, during times of extreme stress, including insufficient calories and other nutrients, will decrease its immunological defenses against infectious agents and cancer. Although it is more difficult for a breast cancer to recruit a blood supply in an undernourished woman, if it does succeed, it will likely grow faster and more aggressively than expected because of a reduced immunological resistance from the host [5] compared to women with better nutrition.

Hereditable Factors

The etiology of the majority of breast cancers is not well understood. Some breast cancer is clearly related to hereditary genetic defects such as BRCA1, BRCA2, and tp53, among many others. These genes are responsible for repair of strands of DNA damaged by ionizing radiation, free radicals, and other causes. If repair is impossible, some of these genes are responsible for the death of these damaged cells, thereby blocking unregulated reproduction of cells—in other words, formation of cancer [6]. However, at all ages, only about 5–10 % of breast cancer is explained by genetic abnormalities. The percentage of breast cancer related to genetic abnormalities is greater in the young, but it is insufficient to explain the preponderance of the young breast cancer cases in LR counties. Also, there is no reason to assume that the rate of hereditable factors would be greater in LR than in HR women.

Environmental Factors

Various environmental factors have been put forward to explain the increasing occurrence of breast cancer, such as exogenous estrogen, obesity, smoking, second hand smoke, alcohol consumption, and exposure to pesticides, but these factors do not explain the marked disparity between breast cancer frequency in women under age 40 in the HR and some LR countries.

Contagion

In 1936, Bittner [7] described transmission of breast cancer to normal mice through nursing from a strain of mice with a strong propensity for developing breast cancers. Once the originally normal mice developed breast cancer from this breastfeeding, their subsequent descendants did also. Since viruses had not yet been described, the etiology of this phenomenon was uncertain until the discovery of Mouse Mammary Tumor Virus (MMTV) as the causative agent [8].

Although some controversy still exists, Human Papilloma Virus, especially types 16, 18, 31, and 33, almost certainly is the underlying cause of up to 30 % of breast cancer in some regions of the world [9]. HPV-induced breast cancer, in the experience of the authors and others, is more aggressive and occurs more often in younger women [10] than would be otherwise expected. In the United States as in other countries, HPV infection peaks at a young age, usually under 30 [11] (Fig. 16A.1).

In general, the nutritional state of women is poor in LR countries relative to women from HR countries. Access to daily bathing is also compromised. Since HPV may persist in the pelvic region for many years without cancer of the cervix, the viral load of infective virus in the pelvic area will be considerably greater in those women who are able to cleanse themselves only weekly, monthly, or less.

Since common skin warts and all other HPVs are transmitted by an inoculum of the virus on broken skin or a mucous membrane, once established, the spread of the warts is by self-inoculation [12]. The chance of further self-infection is likely to be closely related to the amount of inoculum delivered to the susceptible site. Unlike HPV-induced malignancy at other sites, including cervix, anus, mouth, and pharynx, where the HPV is delivered to the site by and from a sexual partner, HPV-induced breast cancer may result from auto-infection through the nipple. This may occur from transfer of the inoculum from a woman's own perineum to her hands or the hands of a sexual partner and then to her nipple during bathing or other touching. Such auto-infection would be

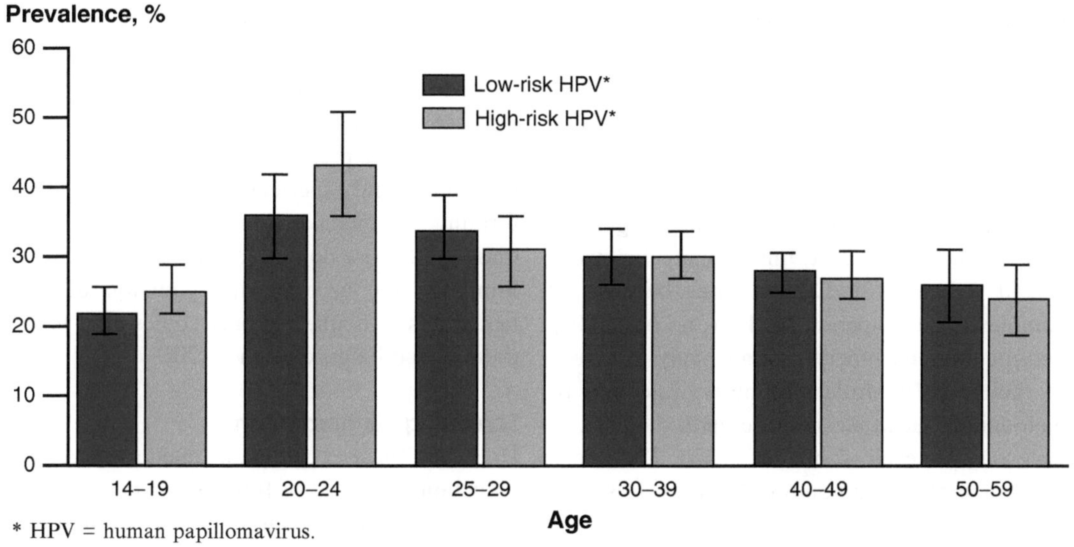

Fig. 16A.1 Human papillomavirus—prevalence of high-risk and low-risk types among females aged 14–59 years, National Health and Nutrition Examination Survey, 2003–2006. *HPV* Human Papillomavirus. Note: *Error bars* indicate 95 % confidence interval. Both high risk and low-risk types of HPV were detected in some females (reprinted with permission of Oxford University Press from Hariri S, Unger ER, Sternberg M, Dunne EF, Swan D, Patel S et al. Prevalence of genital HPV in the among females in the United States, the National Health and Nutrition Examination Survey, 2003–2006. J Infcct Dis 2011;204(4):566–73)

expected to be particularly increased in young women from LR countries who have a lowered resistance to infection and who, because of inability to maintain proper hygiene, would likely have more HPV available for transfer from their perinea. However, it is not certain if breast HPV infection may at times be secondary to blood-borne infection also. Pakistan has one of the highest rates in the world of both HPV infection and breast cancer in young women [13]. Further clinical research in this area is critically necessary in order to strengthen the logical argument that these findings are related.

Approaches to Decreasing Breast Cancer Morbidity and Mortality

There are three levels of attack to decrease morbidity and mortality: (1) prevention, (2) early discovery, and (3) improved treatment. Prevention and early discovery have the added benefit of being sufficiently economical to be feasible in large populations.

Prevention

As discussed previously, it appears that Human Papilloma Viruses are contributing to the problem of aggressive breast cancers in young women in LR countries. This virus may explain most, if not all, of the disproportional occurrence in young women from these countries, compared to similar women in HR countries. This is equivalent to the disproportionate morbidity and mortality of cervical cancer in LR countries. An intensive worldwide campaign of vaccination against HPV in all children ages 9–12, particularly girls, would significantly reduce the death rate from breast cancer in those women as they mature, in addition to increasing the lives saved from prevention of cervical cancer. The present HPV vaccine is effective against types 16 and 18, which are the HPVs most often found in association with breast cancer, as well as types 6 and 11, which cause genital and anal warts [14]. However, other types are common in Asia and may account for a significant number of young women's breast cancers in East and Southeast Asia [15].

Early Detection of Breast Cancer

Present Techniques for Detection of Breast Cancer

There are six possible methods for screening for breast cancer: physical examination and five imaging methods. Three of the imaging techniques can be dismissed immediately for widespread screening in LR countries because of complexity and expense. MRI has no portability and requires machinery costing many hundreds of thousands of dollars or more. Injection of gadolinium, an expensive rare-earth element, is necessary for each woman screened. The likelihood of performing contrast MRI for less than $200 in the near future is nil.

There are two nuclear imaging screening techniques, breast specific gamma imaging (BSGI) and positron emission tomography (PET), which use short-lived radioactive substances. The expense of the machinery and the unique rapid transportation requirements of the isotopes make these tests impossible in countries with poor technical infrastructures.

The three remaining breast screening methods need to be considered.

Physical Examination

The mean diameter of cancers discovered by non-imaging methods—including clinical breast examination (CBE), breast self-examination (BSE), and serendipity—is about 29 mm [16] in high resource countries. Recently, even in HR countries, BSE is considered not to decrease the average size of cancer discovered [17]. There is no study documenting the average size of breast cancers in asymptomatic LR women who are in a screening clinical examination program. Duffy and colleagues [18] predicted that screening for breast cancer with CBE alone in such a population would lead to a 13 % reduction in node-positive cases and a 12 % reduction in breast cancer deaths. The authors thought size reduction would probably occur only in cancers about 3 cm or larger because of the lack of well-trained examiners. As emphasized in Chap. 4 on screening for breast cancer, rigorous training in CBE is a key component of success. CBEs would miss most of the physically subtle, small cancers. Fine-needle aspiration (FNA) has been shown to be often over 90 % accurate in a meta-analysis [19], but many of the studies used image guidance, which would increase their accuracy over blind biopsy. Also, the FNAs were presumably more accurate due to the training and experience of the physicians performing the biopsies compared with the lower training of those doing biopsies in LR countries. Similarly, the accurate interpretation of FNA material is difficult, and only comes after proper training and long experience [20].

Screening Mammography

Dr. Lazlo Tabár [21] demonstrated about a 30 % reduction in mortality from breast cancer in the two-county Swedish study by discovering breast cancer two thirds smaller by volume at an average diameter of 1.8 cm compared with the 2.6 cm diameter average physical discovery without mammography. While this is a very significant decrease in mortality, it may be very difficult and expensive to replicate these results in LR countries. The two methods of recording mammographic images in wide use today are film-screen mammography (FSM) and digital mammography (DM), with both imaging technologies having significant base requirements. These two forms of mammography require a reliable source of high amperage and often high voltage electric current. FSM, the cheaper and easier form, also requires a source of clean water. DM requires a sophisticated computer installation, expensive viewing monitors, and many terabytes of data storage [22].

Mammography has some more pronounced disadvantages for women from low resource countries compared to women from higher resource backgrounds. LR women tend to be thinner and, therefore, more commonly have dense breasts with less fat to contrast with the fatless cancer (Fig. 16A.2). Up to 50 % of cancers in dense breasts will be visible by ultrasound before they are visible on annual screening mammography [23]. Since many of the cancers in LR women develop under the age of 40, not only is the percentage of women with dense breasts higher, but also routine screening mammography is not recommended in women younger than 40, partially because of the increased radiosensitivity of breast tissue below this age. For these reasons, the technical challenges of mammography

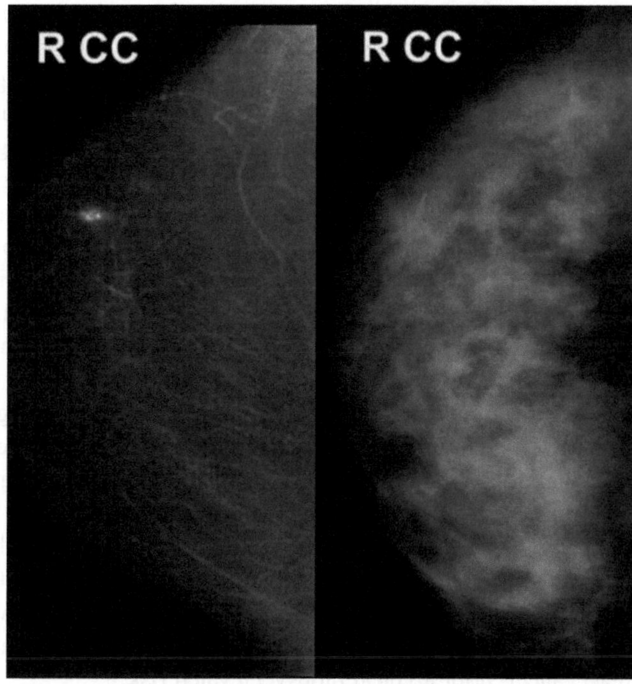

Fig. 16A.2 Left Image: Fatty breast appearing as dark tissue with an obvious white sub-cm cancer; Right Image: Mammographically occult 3 cm cancer obscured by the bright dense breast tissue

and its expected poorer performance in the LR setting compared with the HR model make it not the first choice for screening.

Breast Cancer Screening by Ultrasound

Breast cancer incidence is expected to rise in low and mid-resource countries in the coming decades. While mammography is likely to remain the backbone of screening for early detection of breast cancer in the developed countries, it is not a viable, cost-effective option for widespread implementation in developing countries. Screening for breast cancer using sonography may be a viable alternative to mammography. A case for potential use of sonography for population-based or opportunistic screening is discussed. Unlike mammography, a mortality rate reduction from breast cancer through the use of screening breast ultrasound will probably never be proven. Existing data on the value of screening breast ultrasound are based on studies conducted on women at higher risk for breast cancer and almost always as a complement to mammography.

Evidence for the use of ultrasound in breast cancer screening. It is neither possible nor practical to attempt to prove a mortality rate reduction from the use of whole breast ultrasound screening. Proof of mortality rate reduction will require a randomized controlled clinical trial involving a large number of women receiving screening with the new modality, who will then have to be followed for at least 15 years and be matched with a control group of women who receive the current standard care [24]. The new modality being tested would have to show mortality rate reduction over and above what has been achieved with screening mammography; this is unlikely to be the case anytime in the near future [24]. The use of breast ultrasound as a supplemental modality for breast cancer screening has been studied in women with dense breast tissue and in those with an elevated risk for breast cancer [25, 26]. A systematic search and review of studies involving mammography and ultrasound performed for screening of breast cancer found six cohort studies, of which only two had follow-up on patients with negative or benign findings. Screening ultrasound performed in women with American College of Radiology breast density types 2–4 identified primarily invasive cancers in 0.32 % of women. The mean tumor size was 9.9 mm, and 90 % of the cancers were node negative. Biopsy rate was high at 2.3–4.7 %, with positive predictive value of 8.4–13.7 % for those biopsied because of an abnormal finding on the ultrasound examination. The added benefit of using ultrasound to screen for breast cancers in women with a negative mammogram might be lower in women aged 50–69 years [25]. The most notable and the largest clinical trial of screening ultrasound to date is the American College of Radiology Imaging Network trial35 (ACRIN 6666). This study was a prospective multicenter trial randomized to one group receiving ultrasound and mammographic screening and one group receiving mammographic screening alone to compare the diagnostic yield of performance of breast ultrasound and mammography vs. mammography alone in women with elevated risk of cancer [26]. The criteria used in this study to determine an elevated risk for breast cancer included a personal history of breast cancer, prior atypical biopsy, elevated risk based on the Gail or Claus model, or both. A standard protocol and interpretive criteria were used. Mammography and ultrasound were performed and read independently, allowing for reducing potential biases in patient recruitment and interpretation. Data were analyzed from 2,637 patients who underwent imaging. Thirty-one cancers were detected in the study group, 11.8 per 1,000 women; the increase in the cancer detection rate because of addition of ultrasound was 4.2 per 1,000 women. The diagnostic accuracy for mammography was 0.78, for ultrasound was 0.80, and for combined mammography and ultrasound was 0.91 [26]. Ultrasound hence proved a useful supplemental modality, identifying additional small node-negative invasive cancers in this cohort of women at an elevated risk for breast cancer [26].

Breast sonography has never been studied or been advocated to be used as the only modality to screen for breast cancer. There is, however, some data from a study conducted in Japan that demonstrated the value of sonography when used as the only modality for screening of breast cancer in women <40 years of age [27]. This study was undertaken in the Ibaraki prefecture of Japan where the breast cancer screening recommendations include performing annual screening ultrasound and CBE in women of ages 30 through 56 and biannual mammography in women of ages 40 through 65. There were 12,359 women in the age group of 30–39 years who received annual screening breast ultrasound and did not undergo mammographic screening. Of these, 4,501 women also received annual CBE in addition to whole breast screening ultrasound. In young women, i.e., younger than the age of 40 years, as expected, the cancer yield was low, with a cancer detection rate of 0.04–0.07 %. In those women between the ages of 40–56 years in whom both mammography and ultrasound were used, the cancer detection rate ranged from 0.13 to 0.16 % for sonography and 0.1–0.22 % for mammography. Overall, 41,653 women underwent mammography, and 48,294 women underwent CBE and breast ultrasound. The rate of detection of stage I cancers was 72 % by ultrasound, 66 % by mammography, and 42 % by CBE [27].

Whole breast ultrasound screening: *pros and cons*. The benefits of ultrasound as a screening modality are that it does not use ionizing radiation, is well tolerated, and is optimally amenable for percutaneous biopsy guidance. Ultrasound is able to identify small non-palpable masses while undeterred by presence of dense breast tissue, which is an inherent limitation of mammography. Compared to mammography, the initial capital expense and resources needed to maintain equipment are significantly lower; there is also no need for stringent quality assurance and control required at multiple stages of screen film mammography, for example, training of mammography technologists and ensuring consistency and reproducibility in the quality of mammographic images (dependent on a host of factors including machine calibration, patient positioning, tolerance of breast compression, and the process of film developing). Mammographic viewing requirements, mammogram films filing, and storage are additional costs to be factored in. Overall, the cost to set up screen film mammography for breast cancer screening is expected to be several multiples of the costs required for breast ultrasound. However, unlike mammography, the vast majority of cancers that are seen on ultrasound are invasive cancers; DCIS is not usually identified by sonography [26]. It is debatable whether a screening examination that identifies small node-negative cancers is adequate or whether detection of DCIS is a more critical requirement of a screening test. There are limitations for the use of ultrasound in screening for breast cancer. Ultrasound has never been proved to reduce mortality from breast cancer. Limitation of ultrasound is the high rate of false-positive studies; the positive predictive value in those cases in which biopsy was performed was 8.8–8.9 %, compared with 23 % with mammography [26]. In this context, it is worthwhile keeping in mind that a false-positive ultrasound might not have the same consequence as that of a false-positive mammogram. As Kuhl points out in an editorial, a suspicious finding on a mammogram requires a much more expensive and time-consuming biopsy procedure than an ultrasound-guided core biopsy or a fine-needle aspiration biopsy that can be performed often immediately after the ultrasound examination [28].

The positive predictive value of screening ultrasound is low. Of 233 women for whom biopsy was recommended based on a suspicious ultrasound finding, only 20 (8.6 %) were diagnosed with breast cancer. However, in the same cohort, mammography, which is the accepted standard of care for screening, had a positive predictive value of only 14.7 % (20 of 136) [26, 28]. Ultrasound has the added advantage of being able to stage cancers by examination of bilateral axilla in women who are diagnosed to have cancer.

Optimizing use of whole breast ultrasound screening for breast cancer. As stated previously, a basic prerequisite for implementation of screening for any cancer should be a high prevalence of the cancer being targeted. Such organized screening programs must therefore be put in place once credible disease prevalence statistics have been established in the region that is targeted. The success of such a program is very dependent on the expertise of those performing and interpreting the sonograms. In developing countries, a cost-effective approach would involve training technologists to perform breast ultrasound, and, depending on available local resources, direct or remote supervision of breast ultrasound exams may be performed by a physician. Use of ultrasound has the added advantage of being amenable to telemedicine consultation via web-based link to remote centers of excellence. Training of nurses to perform ultrasound-guided percutaneous fine needle or core needle biopsy is a very feasible option with opportunity for real time supervision from remote sites. A successful 2 day training module has been established by the Educational Committee of the Japan. Participants are tested for ability to detect lesions using videos and ability to characterize lesions using static images [29]. A study compared 422 physicians and 415 technologists. Ultrasound technologists performed as well as physicians in recognizing and interpreting cancers on these tests.

Using criteria described in the Chap. 4 on screening for breast cancer, it is possible to minimize the false-positive rate for biopsy of ultrasound screen detected non-palpable solid masses. Since ultrasound screening has never been studied extensively as a modality by itself to screen for breast cancer, it may very well be a learn-as-you-go approach. A high false-positive biopsy rate is to be expected when ultrasound is used for routine screening. There may be ways of mitigating this limitation. One way would be not to biopsy non-palpable masses smaller than 1 cm that exhibit no malignant features and instead follow them on a yearly basis for 2 years. Another way to minimize false positives would be to offer annual screening ultrasound to women 50–69 years of age and biannual screening for women 40–49 years of age, since incidental benign abnormalities are more commonly encountered in younger women. The proposed methodology of using whole breast ultrasound is a novel one and its efficacy can only be validated by conducting large-scale observational studies. The aim of screening breast ultrasound would be mainly to identify stage I breast cancers, i.e., an invasive breast cancer that is less than or equal to 2 cm (T1), with no regional (axillary) lymph node metastasis (N0) and no distant metastasis (M0).

Screening sonography (ultrasound): handheld ultrasound screening. Handheld ultrasound examinations are used in most of the world—including Asia, Australia, South America, and parts of Europe—as a tool for screening for breast cancer. Handheld ultrasound has the advantages of being portable and not requiring elaborate base requirements as with mammography. All that is needed is a 110 V or higher electrical supply. However, there are significant problems in this manner of screening. Because there is no permanent record of the entire procedure, the study must be done by a skilled reader, usually a physician, who interprets the study as she is doing it. A less educated technician cannot be used, since she would have to interpret the results with her insufficient knowledge of the appearance of cancer. Ultrasound machines were designed for diagnosis rather than detection. This design prevents optimum imaging during breast screening, which is a pure detection task.

The ultrasound-machine monitors display very enlarged images suitable for review one-at-a-time for diagnostic inspection. Since the goal of breast screening is, or at least should be, the discovery of 5 mm or larger cancers anywhere in either breast, the entire image on the monitor must fit in the eye of the reader-operator during the motion of the transducer, since a 5 mm cancer may be anywhere in the image. While unique images are being displayed continuously, if the images are too magnified, eye movement will be necessary because of the eyes' inability to subtend the entire image. Inevitably, this will result in information being missed by the reader. Similarly, children who sit in the front row at the cinema think they will see better than everyone else, but in reality they cannot see the entirety of the images on the screen and are therefore sitting in the worst seats in the house.

Hand scanning is usually performed too rapidly to allow sufficient persistence of a 5 mm cancer for recognition on the monitor. The magnification of the lesion also decreases its contrast with the surrounding normal tissue. Typically, the contrast control on the ultrasound machine does not allow specifically for additional contrast in the grays between fat and cancer. If absolutely necessary in low resource countries, with insufficiently trained physicians or locations so remote that a fixed site with automated ultrasound for screening is not possible, then an alternative would be to simulate automated screening as much as possible by using a modified handheld technique. This possibility will be discussed in the recommendations that follow.

Automated whole breast ultrasound (AWBU). AWBU [24] is designed to find small cancers and to overcome the drawbacks of handheld screening. Although AWBU requires a fixed location for doing the examination, the advantages, described next, far outweigh this limitation.

The examination can be done by a minimally trained operator, since all the images are recorded for later review by a skilled reader, usually a physician who has been trained in breast ultrasound evaluation. The automated computer guidance is done by a machine (Fig. 16A.3) attached to the transducer of the ultrasound machine, which is detachable from the AWBU system, so that the ultrasound unit and the room can be used for diagnostic ultrasound of possible abnormalities found by AWBU and other tasks when breast screening is not being done.

The AWBU [30] system performs two of the four functions usually done by the operator of the ultrasound machine. The computer-driven arms (Fig. 16A.3) regulate the *position* and *speed* of the transducer as it passes over the breast. The *angle of incidence* of the transducer, and therefore the ultrasound beam, is controlled by the operator by means of a gimbal attached to the probe arm. The free-floating probe arm also allows the operator to apply the correct *pressure* on the breast to get optimum images.

Since the aim of AWBU is to record sufficient images for recognition of 5 mm invasive cancers anywhere in either breast, computer control of the gathering of the images is necessary to assure complete coverage of the both breasts. The speed of the transducer is synchronized to the generation of unique images, so that about 5 or 6 images will be recorded through a 5 mm cancer anywhere in the breasts. At the proper playback speed, the visual dwell time for a cancer this size will be about half a second, more than enough time for recognition of the abnormality (Fig. 16A.4). The images are gathered in linear rows with about 7 mm overlap of contiguous

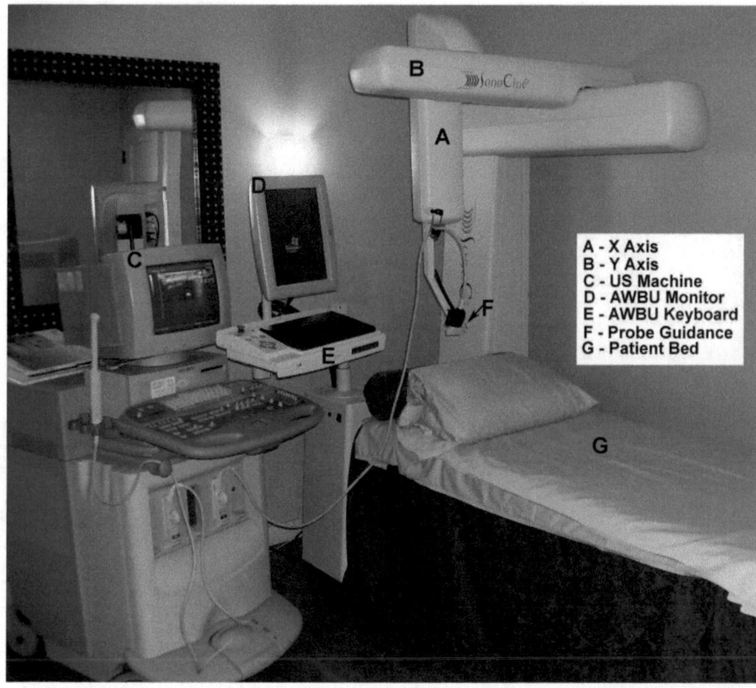

Fig. 16A.3 Automated whole breast ultrasound (AWBU) system with US unit attached (reprinted with permission of Elsevier from Kelly KM, Richwald GA. Automated whole breast ultrasound: advancing the performance of breast cancer screening. Semin Ultrasound CT MRI 2011;32:273–80)

rows (Fig. 16A.5). Because this pattern results in the least redundancy in scanning compared with a radial or anti-radial pattern, it is the quickest method to obtain complete breast coverage.

Because the location of all points in a breast can be calculated precisely relative to the nipple, the position of any abnormality identified by AWBU can be easily found on a later handheld ultrasound for follow-up or biopsy. Since the complete AWBU is stored permanently, comparison of a newly recognized finding with any previous examination is possible.

3D automated breast ultrasound (ABU). This type of automated ultrasound is performed with a single craniocaudad sweep from the subclavicular region to the inframammary fold with a 15 cm automated transducer. The patient examination is quicker to perform. 3D-ABU was not specifically designed to find 5 mm cancers. It is not a whole breast examination in that the axillary tail and lower axilla are not visualized completely. To obtain complete coverage, it depends on mammography to clear those areas [31].

The piezoelectric sensors (ultrasound recording elements) in a 3D-ABU 15 cm wide probe are further apart than in a typical 5 cm high frequency transducer. The 2D-ABU images, which are used for the 3D reconstructions, are almost three times further apart than AWBU images, 2.3 mm v 0.8 mm. Both of these factors reduce the sharpness and conspicuousness of small masses in the image stream or ciné. The ABU requires a sophisticated work station for 3D reconstructions. The file size of about 1 GB requires more expensive computer hardware to display and store these files. AWBU files are usually between 1/10 and 1/6 the size of the 3D-ABU files. At this time, there are no published, peer-reviewed, and multi-institutional studies of 3D-ABU. Consequently, the clinical results with this method are uncertain and are not comparable to AWBU.

Results of handheld and AWBU screening. There have been two large multi-institutional, published, peer-reviewed breast ultrasound screening studies performed, one handheld (ACRIN 6666) [26] and the other automated [23] (Table 16A.1). The handheld examinations were performed and read by academic radiologists specializing in breast imaging. The subjects in this study were all at high risk for breast cancer. Over half of these women had breast cancer previously. Of the cancers found,

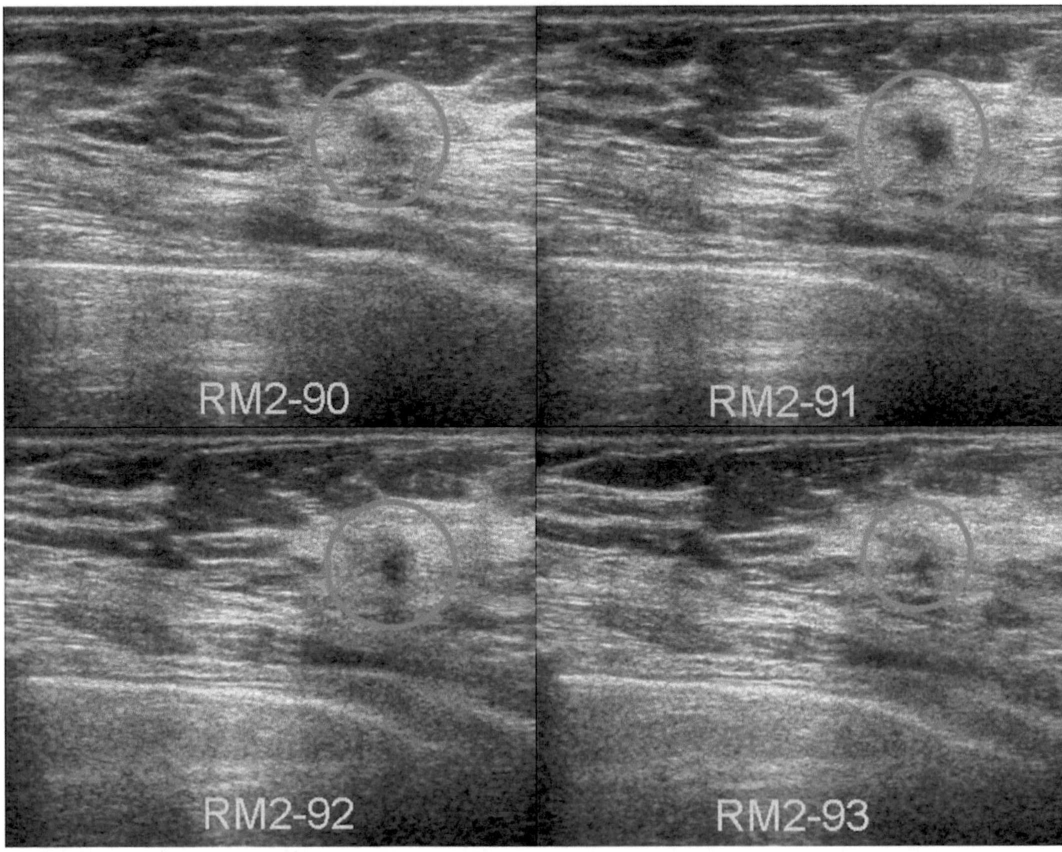

Fig. 16A.4 Sequential images through a 4 mm invasive lobular carcinoma

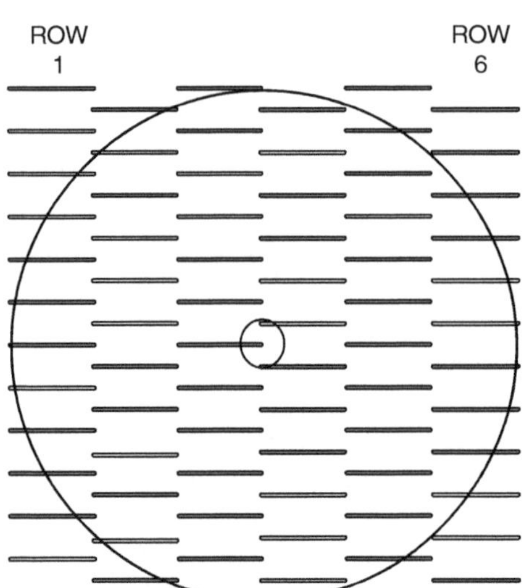

Fig. 16A.5 Contiguous craniocaudad rows with 800 μm image spacing and 7 mm overlap (reprinted with permission of Elsevier from Kelly KM, Richwald GA. Automated whole breast ultrasound: advancing the performance of breast cancer screening. Semin Ultrasound CT MRI 2011;32:273–80)

the authors did not state how many of the cancer recurrences were at or near the original surgery site. The cancers in the area of the previous cancer, although counted as screening discoveries, are, in another sense, not truly screening discoveries, since the locations of the scars are known and these areas will be explored more thoroughly as an area of great interest, as opposed to the rest of the breast tissue. The radiologists did well. They found 55 % more invasive breast cancers than mammography alone. The average diameter of the cancers was 1.2 mm. The average time to complete the scan was 19 min. Obviously, the radiologist must be available when the patient is present. A person of less training cannot do the scan because the detection of cancer occurs during scanning. If a technologist or a technician does not detect the cancer, it will not be in the images given to the radiologist. Also, the viewing at the bedside of a highly magnified image is not ideal for recognition of

Table 16A.1 Comparison of ACRIN6666 Handheld Screening US Study [25] and AWBU Study [24]

	Handheld			Automated		
Feature/finding	Total BC	DCIS	IBC	Total BC	DCIS	IBC
Sites	21			8		
Women	2,809			4,419		
Mammogram—US pair	2,809			6,425		
Dates	4/04–2/06			1/03–7/07		
Digital—film screen (%)	35	65		36	64	
Radiologist time	19 min average			5–7 min		
Not high risk (%)	0			29		
Previous cancer (%)	53			10		
Other high risk (%)	47			61		
Fat/mixed—dense/ED (%)	13	87		32	68	
Total BC–DCIS–IBC	40, 100 %	6, 15 %	34, 85 %	57, 100 %	7, 12 %	50, 88 %
Mammo visible	19, 48 %	5, 83 %	14, 41 %	23, 40 %	6, 86 %	17, 34 %
US visible	20, 50 %	1, 17 %	19, 56 %	38, 67 %	3, 43 %	35, 70 %
Both visible	31, 78 %	0, 0 %	11, 32 %	18, 32 %	2, 29 %	13, 26 %
Neither visible	9, 23 %	0, 0 %	9, 26 %	11,19 %	0, 0 %	11, 22 %
IBC ≤1 cm only on US %	6	18 %		14		28 %
All biopsy PPV	31/306	10 %		46/134		34 %
Mammo+biopsy PPV	20/136	15 %		23/59		39 %
US+biopsy PPV	20/233	9 %		38/99		38 %
Both+biopsy PPV	Not reported	–		15/24		63 %

Data from Elmore JG, Armstrong K, Lehman CD et al. Screening for breast cancer. JAMA 2005;293:1245–56; Nothacker M, Duda V, Hahn M et al. Early detection of breast cancer: benefits and risks of supplemental breast ultrasound in asymptomatic women with mammographically dense breast tissue: A systematic review. BMC Cancer 2009;9:1–9

AWBU automated whole breast ultrasound; *BC* breast cancer; *DCIS* ductal carcinoma in situ; *ED* extremely dense; *IBC* invasive breast cancer; *Mammo* mammography; *PPV* positive predictive value; *US* ultrasound; + positive

abnormalities. Interaction with the patient and the ultrasound machine are distracting. The proper transducer speed for identification of a 5 mm abnormality is about ½cm per second. Handheld scanning is much faster and allows less than the ½s necessary to recognize this size cancer. Unfortunately, the biopsy PPV for cancer was only 9 %, considerably less than what is customary in most major breast centers in the United States. Although not stated in the ACRIN article, there are probably two reasons for this low PPV.

All the women in the study were either at high risk for developing or already had had breast cancer, and they were understandably worried about developing another one. These women knew that the radiologists scanning them were the decision makers. It is my supposition that, during the scans, the radiologists might have stopped to look at difficult areas of breast tissue to clear them, and the women would notice and immediately ask "Can you biopsy this?" before the radiologist was even certain there was a true abnormality present. Once the biopsy question arises, it is hard to dissuade the nervous patient. These radiologists were not used to being put in this position, since they were not screening patients in their daily practice.

However, with screening mammography and diagnostic ultrasound, the radiologist has time to evaluate the imaging studies and formulate a plan before speaking to the patient. Consequently, with experience, the PPV of biopsy for screening ultrasound findings should be similar to the departmental PPV for diagnostic evaluation of breast abnormalities found mammographically or physically.

The AWBU study published in *European Radiology* in 2010 [23] found that the number of

Table 16A.2 Comparison of cancer diameters, volumes, doublings, and estimated 20-year survival among physical, mammographic, handheld ultrasound, and AWBU

Mode of discovery	Diameter (cm)	Estimated volume (cc)	Relative volume	Estimated doublings v AWBU	Estimated 20-year survival (%)
LR presentation	4	33.3	64×	6	38
HR presentation	2.6	9.14	17.6×	4.1	72
Screening mammography	1.8	3.0	5.8×	2.5	81
Handheld screening US	1.2	0.90	1.7×	0.77	93
AWBU	1.0	0.52	1×	0	95

LR presentation assumes no radiation or chemical therapy available
AWBU automated whole breast ultrasound; *LR* low resource; *HR* high resource; *US* ultrasound

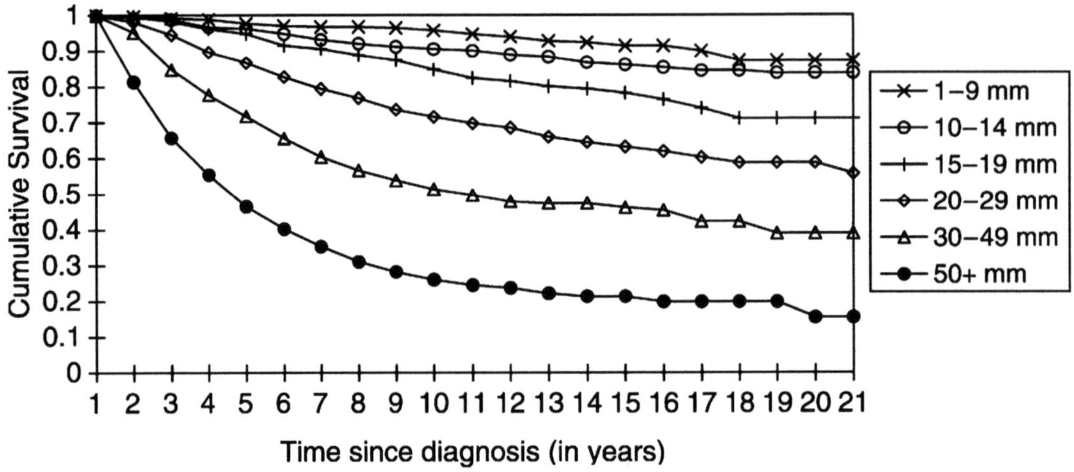

Fig. 16A.6 Survival of 2,294 invasive breast cancer cases by tumor size (reprinted with permission of Wiley from Duffy SW, Tabár L, Vitak B, Warwick J. Tumor Size and breast cancer detection: What might be the effect of a less sensitive screening tool than mammography? Breast J 2006;12 Suppl 1:S91–5)

cancers doubled and the number of 1 cm or less invasive cancers tripled from 7 to 21 when AWBU was added to mammography. The cancers found by AWBU average 1.0 cm compared with handheld ultrasound's average diameter of 1.2 cm, a three quarter larger volume (Table 16A.2). Duffy and colleagues [18] estimated that only about 10 % of women with breast cancers presenting up to 1.4 cm would die of their disease within 20 years (Fig. 16A.6). An advantage of AWBU is that the examinations, if done efficiently, can be conducted by lower trained personnel in about 15 min. Subsequent reading time by physicians trained in breast imaging is about 5–7 min [23].

Recommendations for Early Detection of Breast Cancer in LR Countries

Of the three possible methods of breast screening—clinical breast examination, screening mammography, and screening ultrasound—ultrasound will generally find cancers small enough that they may be cured by surgery alone, without radiation or chemotherapy, at a considerably less cost than screening mammography. This is an important consideration, since the LR countries have no practical way of obtaining significant amounts of these treatment modalities in the foreseeable future.

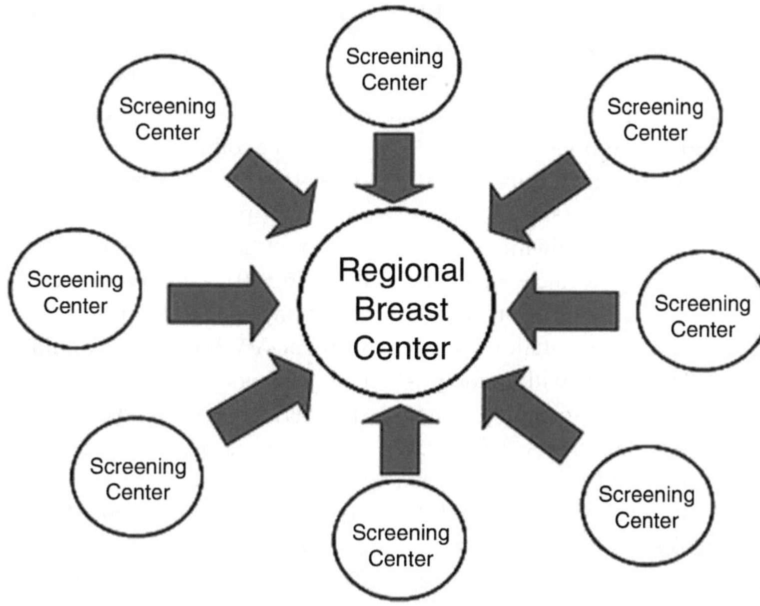

Fig. 16A.7 Schematic of a Central Regional Breast Center with a variable number of Satellite Breast Screening Centers using automated whole breast ultrasound

Mass Screening with Automated Whole Breast Ultrasound

In LR countries, maximum throughput will be important to minimize costs. AWBU will outperform handheld ultrasound, since the operator can be a lower skilled worker than the reader of the examination. The operator will be able to perform about four procedures an hour. A proficient reader can read about ten studies an hour, but will probably need to switch off about every 2 h to other less visually intensive tasks, such as diagnostic ultrasound or ultrasound-guided biopsies. If done efficiently, the AWBU procedure can be performed in about 15 min. Operating 6 days a week and 10 h a day, about 12,500 examinations could be performed annually per AWBU unit and ultrasound machine. If the prevalence of ultrasound-discoverable breast cancer were as high as the United States (6 per thousand) [23], as many as 60 cancers would be found the first year and probably 30 in the subsequent biannual rounds. In the United States, the annual incidence rate of breast cancer is about 0.3 % found at annual mammography. In China, the incidence rate appears to be about one-fourth that of the United States, but in the major cities the rate is rising and now may be nearly half the US rate. In that case, about 15 cancers would be found both in the first year and each succeeding biannual examination by each AWBU unit. The death rate from breast cancer over the next 20 years for women whose cancers were found at less than 1.5 cm would be about 10 %, compared to 40 % for cancers otherwise found. Although some uncertainty exists, probably beginning with the second round of screening 80 % of the cancers could be identified when they are less than 1.5 cm.

For a country with a high population density and a highly organized health-care system, the most efficient method for breast screening would be regional breast centers (Fig. 16A.7) distributed geographically throughout the country. Each regional center would be the diagnostic and treatment center for that geographic area. It would be staffed by radiologists reading the ABWUs done at multiple satellite screening centers throughout the geographic area as well as evaluating and needle-biopsing discovered abnormalities. The center's surgeons would perform lumpectomies or mastectomies on the women with cancer. The staff at the satellite screening centers would perform the AWBU examinations and transmit the data electronically or physically to the regional breast center for interpretation. The operators of AWBU equipment would need only minimal training. If each satellite breast center had four AWBU units, it would examine about 100,000 women each year. If the women had examinations every other year, 200,000 eligible women would be screened. Given that half the population is male and about half the female population is not between the ages of 35 and 75, with a compliance rate of 80 %, each satellite screening center could serve a general population of 1,000,000.

If each regional center had ten satellite centers, the center would read about 1,000,000 AWBUs annually and serve a base population of 10,000,000. As an example, for China to screen the entire country in this manner, it would have to create 130 regional centers to serve a population of 1.3 billion, of which 260 million would receive an AWBU biannually. In 2008, the annual number of new breast cancers in China was about 169,500 [32]. The increase of population plus the increase of the breast cancer rate are estimated at about 4.5 %, which, compounded over 4 years to 2012, would suggest that the number of cancers found in 2012 will be 203,400.

The estimate of 52,800 deaths for this year will underestimate the 20-year cumulative deaths for cancers discovered this year because 52,800 deaths are from cancers that were found anywhere from 1 to 20 years before, when the annual numbers of cancers were considerably smaller. Truer estimated 20-year mortality would be based on the average diameter of the cancer at discovery, probably about 3.0 cm for China. Using Dr. Tabár's 20-year longevity data (Fig. 16A.6), 40 % (81,360) of the 203,400 women learning they have breast cancer this year will die of this disease within 20 years if no effort at screening is made. Assuming 80 % biannual attendance of the eligible women at AWBU screening and that 80 % of the cancers are found at 1.4 cm diameter or less in these women, the death rate at 20 years would be reduced in those women from 40 to 10 %, since almost all these sonographically found cancers would be stage 1 with no lymph node involvement. Of the 130,176 women with cancers found at this size, 13,028 would be expected to die of breast cancer in 20 years. The other 20 % of attendees' cancers (32,544) would be found smaller than without AWBU, at probably 1.5–3 cm in diameter, with 20 % mortality expected at 20 years instead of 40 % (6,509). Obviously, the 20 %, who were non-attendees (40,680) and did not have their biannual AWBU screens would ultimately have a 20-year mortality rate of about 40 % (16,272). The overall result would be that instead of 81,360 women dying of their breast cancers within 20 years, only 36,809 would die and 55 % (44,551 women) would be saved. If 100 % attendance were achievable, theoretically the 20-year mortality would drop under 25,000.

Handheld Ultrasound Screening

In countries where there are not sufficient trained physicians for centralized reading of AWBUs or where transportation is not available to bring women to a screening facility or where there is inadequate governmental organization and/or funding to set up such facilities, handheld ultrasound screening remains a less efficient and less accurate option. To overcome the problems with handheld screening in the past, the technique had to be modified to mimic AWBU. The scanning must be done methodically and slowly so that sub-centimeter cancers can be seen. The rate of movement of the transducer must be approximately 1 cm per second. The operator should not interact with the woman during the scan so as not to be distracted. Any discussion should be done before or after the scan. The screening should be done in a fixed grid, radial, or anti-radial pattern (Fig. 16A.8) so that all the tissue is seen well *once*. Repetition only serves to increase the time of the scan and to put pressure on the operator to scan faster. With the least overlap, the grid pattern is the quickest and the easiest to learn. The retroareolar areas and the axillae should be examined separately. Any area in question should be marked

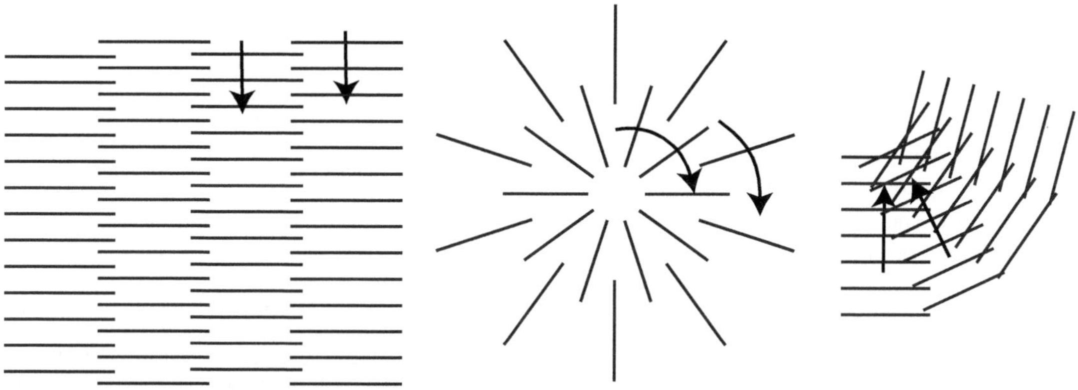

Fig. 16A.8 *Grid*; slightly overlapping craniocaudad rows from the infraclavicular line to the inframammary fold; *circular*: series of overlapping circles surrounding the nipple; *radial*: radial scans extending from the periphery of the breast to the nipple (modified with permission of Elsevier from Kelly KM, Richwald GA. Automated whole breast ultrasound: advancing the performance of breast cancer screening. Semin Ultrasound CT MRI 2011;32:273–80)

on the skin and examined as a diagnostic study at the end of the screening study so as to not interrupt the screening examination. Depending on breast size, the handheld screening examination will require between 10 and 20 min.

Clearly, the personnel performing the screening will need considerable training, which will take between 3 and 6 months. The personnel should be female, since the testing is being done away from a clinical setting. Because the operator is travelling to the women to be screened, any other testing necessary, such as Pap smears, should be done at the same time. These women also need to be able to recognize abnormal breast findings. This requires intensive instruction on how cancer appears sonographically. Fortunately, there are teaching cines that may be available from AWBU sites that simulate handheld scanning. Any country planning on implementation of such a program must be committed to the training and oversight that would be necessary.

Because of the difficulty of bringing women with any findings to a medical facility, the technician must be able to determine if the woman has cancer. Consequently, the technician will need to be able to do an ultrasound directed 14g needle biopsy or at least a FNA. In order to do either of these tests, the technicians need to learn basic sterile technique and limited local anatomy.

The advantage of a FNA is that it is safer and cheaper than a core needle biopsy, but it is more difficult to obtain a satisfactory specimen and to preserve the specimen correctly. The evaluation of the specimen requires an experienced cytologist, who may not be available in a very low resource setting. A 14 or a 16g biopsy delivers a better and more accurate specimen. It requires only immersion in formalin for preservation. It is more easily evaluated by a hospital pathologist, even in LR countries. However, the biopsy must be performed in a safe manner and is less forgiving of errors in technique. A disposable 14g needle is only a few dollars when used with a non-disposable spring-loaded gun.

Improved Therapy for Breast Cancer

Clearly, low resource countries are woefully lacking as regards the relatively recent advances in radiation and chemotherapy. Education of the medical providers and technical infrastructure is minimal in those countries. In the few places that they do exist to some degree, they are usually restricted to the influential and wealthy. What little capital is available is better spent on prevention and early detection.

Conclusion

Although in most developing countries there is minimal funding for programs to mitigate the effect of breast cancer, particularly in young women, early detection by sonographic discovery while the cancers are small enough that survival is highly probable even without radiation or chemotherapy is a feasible strategy for the future. Implementation of a HPV vaccination program would markedly lower the future incidence of cervical cancer in the young women who received their immunizations in their pre- and early teens. An unexpected bonus from a vaccination program may be a significant reduction of the disproportional incidence of breast cancers expected in these young women. Whole breast ultrasound may be a cost-effective alternative to organized screening mammography in view of lower prevalence of the target cancer and the massive investment in infrastructure and health-care personnel that would be required to implement a mammographic screening program. Unlike mammography, screening using sonography will aim to identify Stage I cancers; mortality rate reduction is unlikely to be ever proved with use of sonography. Use of sonography will need to be validated by undertaking observational studies in a large cohort of asymptomatic women. If the one drawback of the expected higher false positive rate with use of ultrasound can be overcome, sonography may very well prove to be a feasible low cost alternate to screening for breast cancer in developing countries.

References

1. Forouzanfar MH, Foreman KJ, Delossantos AM, Lozao R, Lopez AD, Murray CJ, et al. Breast and cervical cancer in 187 countries between 1980 and 2010: a systematic analysis. Lancet. 2011;378(9801):1461–84.
2. Pavelic L, Pavelic K, Vuk-Pavelic S. Human mammary and bronchial carcinomas in vivo and in vitro secretion of substances immunologically cross-reactive with insulin. Cancer. 1984;53:2467–71.
3. Ziegler RG, Anderson WF, Gail MH. Increasing breast cancer incidence in China: the numbers add up. JNCI. 2008;100:1339–41.
4. Polyak K. Breast cancer: origins and evolution. J Clin Invest. 2007;117:3155–63.
5. Satyaraj E. Emerging paradigms in immunonutrition. Top Companion Anim Med. 2011;26(1):25–32.
6. Farmer H, McCabe N, Lord C, Tutt AN, Johnson DA, Richardson TB, et al. Targeting the DNA repair defect in BRCA mutant cells as a therapeutic strategy. Nature. 2005;434:917–21.
7. Bittner JJ. Some possible effects of nursing on the mammary gland tumor incidence in mice. Science. 1936;84:162.
8. Ross SR. Mouse mammary tumor virus molecular biology and oncogenesis. Viruses. 2010;2:2000–12.
9. Akil N, Yasmeen A, Kassab A, Ghabreau L, Darnel AD, Moustafa A-E. High-risk human papillomavirus infections in breast cancer in Syrian women and their association with Id-1 expression: a tissue microarray study. Br J Cancer. 2008;99:404–7.
10. Kroupis C, Markou A, Vourlidis N, Dionyssiou-Asteriou A, Lianidou ES. Presence of high-risk human papillomavirus sequences in breast cancer tissues and association with histopathological characteristics. Clin Biochem. 2006;39:727–31.
11. Hariri S, Unger ER, Sternberg M, Dunne EF, Swan D, Patel S, et al. Prevalence of genital HPV in the among females in the United States, the National Health and Nutrition Examination Survey, 2003–2006. J Infect Dis. 2011;204(4):566–73.
12. Shenefelt PD. Nongenital warts. Medscape Reference Drugs Disease & Procedures. 2012. http://emedicine.medscape.com/article/1133317-overview
13. Khan S, Jaffer NN, Khan MN, Rai MA, Shafiq M, Ali A, et al. Human papillomavirus subtype 16 is common in Pakistani women with cervical carcinoma. Int J Infect Dis. 2007;11(4):313–7.
14. Center for Communicable Diseases. Epidemiology and prevention of vaccine-preventable diseases: human papillomavirus. The pink book: course textbook, Ch 10, 12th ed. Washington, DC: Public Health Foundation; 2012. p. 139–49.
15. Clifford GM, Smith JS, Aguado T, Franceschi S. Comparison of HPV type distribution in high-grade cervical lesions and cervical cancer: a meta-analysis. Br J Cancer. 2003;89:101–5.
16. Barth AJ Jr, Gibson GR, Mott LA, Becher RD, Poplack SP. Detection of breast cancer on screening mammography allows patients to be treated with less-toxic therapy. AJR. 2005;184:325–9.
17. Nelson HD, Tyne K, Naik A, Bougatsos C, Chan BK, Humphrey L. Screening for breast cancer: an update for the U.S. Preventive Services Task Force. Ann Intern Med. 2009;151:727–37.
18. Duffy SW, Tabár L, Vitak B, Warwick J. Tumor Size and breast cancer detection: what might be the effect of a less sensitive screening tool than mammography? Breast J. 2006; 12 Suppl 1:S91–5.
19. Yu Y-H, Wei W, Liu J-L. Diagnostic value of fine-needle aspiration biopsy for breast mass: a systematic review and meta-analysis. BMC Cancer. 2012;12:41.

20. Ljung BM, Drejet A, Chiampi N, Jeffrey J, Goodson WH 3rd, Chew K, et al. Diagnostic accuracy of fine-needle aspiration biopsy is determined by physician training in sampling technique. Cancer. 2011;93(4): 263–8.
21. Tabár L, Vitak B, Chen TH, Yen AM, Cohen A, Tot T, et al. Swedish two-county trial: impact of mammographic screening on breast cancer mortality during 3 decades. Radiology. 2011;260:658–63.
22. Keen C. SSPs take on larger role in digital mammography. Hefty data sets and multiple prior images threaten to put a strain on standard storage and network options. Diagnostic Imaging. 2005;27:S-23–31. http://www.diagnosticimaging.com/display/article/113619/1197582. Cited 17 Aug 2012.
23. Kelly KM, Dean J, Comulada WS, Lee S-J. Breast cancer detection using automated whole breast ultrasound and mammography in radiographically dense breasts. Eur Radiol. 2010;20:734–42.
24. Elmore JG, Armstrong K, Lehman CD, et al. Screening for breast cancer. JAMA. 2005;293:1245–56.
25. Nothacker M, Duda V, Hahn M, et al. Early detection of breast cancer: benefits and risks of supplemental breast ultrasound in asymptomatic women with mammographically dense breast tissue: a systematic review. BMC Cancer. 2009;9:1–9.
26. Berg WA, Blume JD, Cormack JB, et al. Combined screening with ultrasound and mammography vs. mammography alone in women with elevated risk of breast cancer. JAMA. 2008;299:2151–63.
27. Tohno E, Ueno E, Watanabe H. Ultrasound screening of breast cancer. Breast Cancer. 2009;16:18–22.
28. Kuhl CK. The "coming of age" of nonmammographic screening for breast cancer. JAMA. 2008;299:2203–5.
29. Tohno E, Takahashi H, Tamada T, Fujimoto Y, Yasuda H, Ohuchi N. Educational program and testing using images for the standardization of breast cancer screening by ultrasonography. Breast Cancer. 2012;19(2):138–46.
30. Kelly KM, Richwald GA. Automated whole-breast ultrasound: advancing the performance of breast cancer screening. Semin Ultrasound CT MRI. 2011;32:273–80.
31. Tabár L. Personal Communication. Santa Barbara, California. Summer 2011.
32. WHO International Agency for Research on Cancer. Breast cancer incidence and mortality worldwide in 2008 summary. 2008. http://globocan.iarc.fr/factsheets/cancers/breast.asp. Cited 17 Aug 2012.

B. Future Strategies for Cervical Cancer Prevention in Developing Countries: HPV Vaccine and Its Implementation Around the World

José Humberto Tavares Guerreiro Fregnani

Abstract

Cervical cancer prevention is a feasible option to control cervical cancer in low resource countries. In this chapter, the etio-pathogenesis of cervical cancer is presented. The types and role of HPV vaccine in cervical cancer prevention are discussed. The future strategy in preventing cervical cancer screening utilizing HPV cervical cancer vaccine is outlined.

Introduction

The human papillomavirus (HPV) infection is the most common sexually transmitted disease [1, 2]. According to the World Health Organization, there are approximately 440 million people affected by genital HPV infection around the world [3]. Among all diseases that HPV may cause, the one that has the greatest impact to public health is cervical cancer. Almost half a million cases globally are recorded annually, and 85 % of all the cases occur in developing countries. The highest incidences of the disease are recorded in Latin America, the Caribbean, Sub-Saharan and South Africa, and Southeast Asia [4, 5]. The World Health Organization estimates that cervical cancer cases will increase significantly in the coming years if no additional measures are taken, estimating that in the year 2030 around 775,000 new cases and 440,000 deaths will be recorded as a result of such tumors [6].

High-risk HPVs are not only linked to cervical cancer, but also to other types of cancer such as vulva, vagina, penis, anal canal, mouth, and oropharynx [7, 8]. However, even viruses considered to be "low risk" have some carcinogenic potential, although it is less common to see cancer caused by such viruses [9].

The Papanicolaou test, introduced in the 1950s as a cervical cancer screening method, is traditionally considered an example of a successful strategy for secondary prevention of cancer. Several countries reported dramatic reductions in the incidence and mortality coefficients due to cervical cancer after its implementation. But this phenomenon was observed especially in developed countries. In developing countries, cervical cancer screening programs did not present good results due to the low coverage offered by the Pap smear exam, poor quality of the cytological exam, and difficulty in getting access to health services [10]. These data justify the need for the incorporation of new strategies in the fight against cervical cancer.

One such strategy would be the use of an HPV vaccine in the primary prevention of cervical cancer. According to a manifesto by the

World Health Organization in 2009: "...routine HPV vaccination should be included in national immunization programs, provided that prevention of cervical cancer or other HPV-related diseases, or both, constitutes a public health priority; vaccine introduction is programmatically feasible; sustainable financing can be secured; and the cost effectiveness of vaccination strategies in the country or region is considered" [11].

However, critics argue that there is not enough evidence to conclude that the HPV vaccine will bring an effective reduction in the incidence of and mortality caused by cervical cancer. In order to achieve that, a period of 20–30 years would be necessary, since cervical cancer has a long natural history. Nevertheless, data from the Australian HPV vaccination program reinforce the idea that the HPV vaccine can be a tool for the primary prevention of cervical cancer. Brotherton and colleagues [12] showed a significant reduction in the incidence of high-grade cervical cytological abnormality in young Australian women. Since the natural history of cervical cancer is well known, one could infer that the reduction in the incidence of precursor lesions in cervical cancer will have a direct impact on the incidence of cervical cancer in the future. It is estimated that the HPV vaccine may reduce by 80 % the chance of cervical cancer developing during a woman's lifetime [11].

HPV Vaccines

Currently, there are two versions of the HPV vaccine, both of them developed with recombinant technology. They do not carry a live or attenuated virus or genetic material; therefore, they are not able to induce infection. Vaccines are comprised of VLP (virus-like particle), a particle similar to the virus capsid from the structural point of view [8, 13]. The quadrivalent vaccine (Gardasil® or Silgard®, Merck & Co, Whitehouse Station, NJ) protects against viruses 6, 11, 16, and 18, and the bivalent vaccine (Cervarix®, GlaxoSmithKline, London, UK) protects against viruses 16 and 18. One should remember that 70 % of cervical carcinomas are caused by types 16 and 18, and 90 % of genital warts by types 6 and 11. Both vaccines must be administered intramuscularly in three doses during a period of 6 months. The recommendation for the quadrivalent vaccine is that the second dose should be administered 2 months after the first dose and the third dose be administered sixth months after the initial vaccination. For the bivalent vaccine, the second dose is recommended 1 month after the initial dose. The current indication on the use of bivalent and quadrivalent vaccines approved by the Food and Drug Administration (FDA) is shown on Table 16B.1 [14].

There are no doubts regarding the safety of the bivalent and quadrivalent vaccines or their effectiveness in the prevention of precursor lesions of

Table 16B.1 Indication of the use of bivalent and quadrivalent vaccines according to US-FDA approval

Prevention of	Bivalent	Quadrivalent
Genital cancer caused by HPV types 16 and 18	Yes (cervical cancer)	Yes (cervical, vulvar, and vaginal cancer)
Cervical intraepithelial neoplasia (CIN) grade 2/3	Yes	Yes
Cervical adenocarcinoma in situ (AIS)	Yes	Yes
Cervical intraepithelial neoplasia (CIN) grade 1	Yes	Yes
Vulvar intraepithelial neoplasia (VIN) grade 2 and grade 3	No	Yes
Vaginal intraepithelial neoplasia (VaIN) grade 2 and grade 3	No	Yes
Genital warts (condyloma acuminata) caused by HPV types 6 and 11	No	Yes (girls and boys)
Target age	9–26 years of age	9–25 years of age

Data from FDA. Vaccines, Blood & Biologics. Vaccines. Approved products FDA; 2012 [cited 2012, Jul 20]. Available from: http://www.fda.gov/BiologicsBloodVaccines/Vaccines/ApprovedProducts/ucm172678.htm

cervical cancer [15–21]. The effectiveness of the vaccine is close to 100 % for the prevention of cervical intraepithelial lesions, and, in the case of quadrivalent vaccine, it also protects condyloma, vulvar, and vaginal intraepithelial lesions. The effectiveness of the quadrivalent vaccine decreases if women had a previous or have an infection by HPV at the time of vaccination [7]. Vaccines must be used only with a prophylactic intent, with no indication of treatment in cases of already established HPV-induced lesions [8]. Vaccines decrease the risk of precursor lesions, but they do not eliminate completely this risk since immunization does not cover all types of high-risk HPV. Thus, cervical cancer prevention by way of a Pap smear examination is still necessary even for those women that have been previously vaccinated for HPV [13].

Bivalent and quadrivalent vaccines have already been approved for use in more than 100 countries. However, not all countries included them in their public immunization program. Besides having questions about the best method of implementation, the cost of the vaccines itself is a relevant barrier for several countries, especially for low-income countries. Table 16B.2 highlights countries with national funding programs through mid-2012.

Table 16B.2 Countries with public funding programs for HPV vaccines[a]

North America	Canada
	United States
	Mexico
Caribbean & Central America	Panama
	Puerto Rico
South America	Argentina
	Guyana
Middle East & Africa	Kuwait
	Lesotho
	United Arab Emirates
Asia Pacific	Australia
	Japan
	Malaysia
	New Zealand
Europe	Austria
	Belgium
	Bulgaria
	Czech Republic
	Denmark
	France
	Germany
	Greece
	Iceland
	Ireland
	Italy
	Latvia
	Luxemburg
	Macedonia
	Netherland
	Norway
	Portugal
	Romania
	Slovenia
	Spain
	Sweden
	Switzerland
	United Kingdom[b]

[a]Last update: July 2012

[b]As of September 2012, bivalent vaccine was replaced by quadrivalent in the United Kingdom [14, 41]

Vaccination Strategy

One of the challenges to be overcome in HPV immunization programs is the age group that will receive the vaccine: teenagers. It is common knowledge that teenagers, especially the older ones, are less receptive and less adherent to vaccination programs. In the United States, for example, the overall coverage rate in 2009 among teenagers ranging from 13 to 17 was approximately 50 % for boys and 33 % for girls [22].

Currently, the discussion focuses on what would be the best strategy for the vaccination of teenagers: a school-based approach or one based on the health system. The European Centre for Disease Prevention and Control declared that school-based immunization: "…is likely to be the lowest cost option for the delivery of human papillomavirus (HPV) vaccines to preadolescent girls. However, local issues, such as whether school-based health services exist, funding arrangements for vaccine purchase and administration and obtaining parental consent may affect the feasibility of this approach" [23]. Regarding the immunization programs based on the health system, they considered that "a universally available additional or alternative option for HPV vaccine delivery. This may be more expensive than

Table 16B.3 Data from the Australian HPV vaccination program (school- and community-based)

	School-based (%)			Community-based (%)	
Age	12–13	14–15[a]	16–17[a]	18–19[a]	20–26[a]
Dose 1	83	84	81	64	52
Dose 2	80	79	75	53	42
Dose 3	73	72	66	38	30

Adapted with permission of the Australian Government from Immunise Australia Program. Human Papillomavirus (HPV). Information about the National Human Papillomavirus (HPV) Vaccination Program funded under the Immunise Australia Program: Australian Government. Department of Health and Aging. 2011 (updated Apr 04, 2011; cited 2012 Jun 30, 2012); Available from: http://www.immunise.health.gov.au/internet/immunise/publishing.nsf/Content/immunise-hpv#figure 2

[a]Catch-up vaccination programs were extended only up to December 2009

school-based immunization and monitoring of vaccine uptake may be more difficult here" [23].

It may be that no one single vaccination strategy is better than the other, but one strategy could be more adequate than the other according to each individual regional reality. The available literature provides examples of public HPV immunization programs that both succeeded and failed when each of the immunization strategies was applied.

Australia

The first country in the world to establish a national public HPV immunization program was Australia. In April 2007, they started the regular school-based vaccination program targeting girls aged 12–13. However, two other catch-up programs ran only up to December 2009, one of them being school-based and the other community-based. Women up to 17 years of age were vaccinated in schools, and older women or women who missed vaccination at school were vaccinated at community health agencies [24]. This particular program determined relatively high coverage rates for the school-based program [25]. The data presented by the Australian government may be seen on Table 16B.3. As of 2013, boys aged 12–13 will also be included in the school-based vaccination program.

Europe

Austria was one of the first countries in the world to have national immunization recommendation against HPV. Despite being the first country with regard to the recommendation, the country itself has never had a public policy for funding the vaccine. On the other hand, the majority of the European Community countries currently count on government funding for the HPV vaccine [26]. Different vaccination strategies were adopted in Europe, with considerable variation regarding targeted age groups, catch-up programs, and typc of vaccine. There is also a considerable variation in relation to the vaccine delivery, where the majority of programs are based on the health system (public or private). Few European countries adopted the school-based strategy for their vaccination programs. Table 16B.4 displays a summary of several European HPV vaccination programs.

In most European countries where the vaccine is given on demand, the general vaccine coverage rates are invariably lower than 90 %. In some countries, such as Belgium, the Netherlands, Germany, France, Norway, and Luxemburg, coverage rates are near or lower than 50 % [14, 26]. A few of the nonschool-based programs, such as the one in Denmark, reached higher coverage rates; the rate reached 80 % for the first dose of the vaccine for 12-year-old girls.

The Americas

Although the HPV vaccine has largely been approved for use in the United States and in the Caribbean, very few countries within this region have adopted public funding policies as of mid-2012, namely, United States, Canada, Mexico, Panama, Argentina, Puerto Rico, and the Guyana.

Table 16B.4 European countries with implemented HPV national immunization programs

	Regular vaccination program			Catch-up vaccination program				
Country	Start	Target age	3-Dose coverage % (year)	Start	Target age	3-Dose coverage	Type of program	Free of charge
Austria	2006	≥9					Private	No
Belgium	2007	12–18		2008	13–18		Private	Partially
Denmark	2009	12	58 (2010)	2008	15–17	73 (2010)	PHC	Yes
France	2007	14	24 (2008)	2007	15–23	30 (2008)	Private	Partially
Germany	2007	12–17					Private	Yes
Greece	2008	12–15					Private	Yes
Ireland	2010	12–13					SHC	Yes
Italy	2007/2008	11	56 (2009)	2007/2010	14–17/24		PHC	Yes
Latvia	2010	12					PHC+SHC	Yes
Liechtenstein	?	11–14		?	15–19		PHC	Partially
Luxemburg	2008	12	17 (2009)	2008	13–18	29 (2009)	Private	Yes
Netherland	2010	12		2009	13–16	45 (2009)	PHC	Yes
Norway	2009	12	30 (2010)				SHC	Yes
Portugal	2008	13	81 (2009)	2009	17	56 (2009)	PHC	Yes
Romania	2009	12		2010	12–24		PHC+SHC	Yes
Slovenia	2009	11–12					SHC	Yes
Spain	2008	11–14	70 (PHC)/84 (SCH)				PHC+SHC	Yes
Sweden	2010	10–12					SHC	Yes
Switzerland	2009	11–14		2009	15–19		PHC	Yes
United Kingdom	2008	12–13	80 (2009)	2008	14–17	32 (2009)	PHC+SHC	Yes

Data from Dorleans F, Giambi C, Dematte L, Cotter S, Stefanoff P, Mereckiene J et al. The current state of introduction of human papillomavirus vaccination into national immunisation schedules in Europe: first results of the VENICE2 2010 survey. Euro surveillance: bulletin europeen sur les maladies transmissibles = European communicable disease bulletin 2010;15(47); Limia A, Pachon I. Coverage of human papillomavirus vaccination during the first year of its introduction in Spain. Euro surveillance: bulletin europeen sur les maladies transmissibles = European communicable disease bulletin 2011;16(21)
PHC public health centers; *SHC* school health services

In the United States, bivalent and quadrivalent vaccines were approved for use in 2006 and 2009, respectively [14]. Currently, the country does not present a public funding program for the immunization of uninsured woman aged 21 or older. It is worth mentioning that, in the United States, 13 % of women between ages 9 and 18 and 27 % of those aged 19–26 are uninsured [27]. Uninsured girls up to the age of 18 benefit from the Vaccines for Children (VFC) Program [28]. This is a federal program that finances vaccines approved by the ACIP (Advisory Committee on Immunization Practices). Through this program, the CDC (Centers for Disease Control and Prevention) buys the vaccine directly from the manufacturer and distributes them to state health departments and public health agencies, which transfer the vaccines, at no cost, to public health clinics and to physicians' offices [29]. There are three additional public financing programs for women or girls who do not benefit from the VFC, namely, Immunization Grant Program, Medicaid, and State Children's Health Insurance Program [28]. In spite of these public immunization funding programs, the HPV vaccine coverage rate for one or more doses is only 45 % among North American girls [22]. It is worth mentioning that none of the described programs has a school-based approach.

In Canada, the quadrivalent vaccine was approved in July 2006 for women aged 9–26. The approval for the bivalent vaccine occurred in February 2010, for women aged 10–25. In an unprecedented way, in April 2011, Canada approved the quadrivalent vaccine for women up to 45 years of age, and in May 2011, the use of the quadrivalent vaccine for men aged 9–26 was approved [7]. In 2007, the Canadian government expended about 300 million dollars to provinces and territories as an incentive for an HPV national immunization program [30]. All provinces and territories have introduced HPV vaccine programs for adolescent girls into their immunization schedules since 2008. Noteworthy is the fact that each province/territory has its own HPV immunization program, but, in all those programs, vaccines are provided free of charge to girls through school-based clinics administered by local public health units [7]. Table 16B.5 shows the summary of HPV immunization programs in Canada. During the first year of the immunization program, coverage rates were variable: Newfoundland (85 %), Ontario (53 %), and Quebec (84 % for grade 4 and 87 % for grade 9). The coverage rate for the Atlantic provinces was approximately 80 % [31].

Table 16B.5 Characteristics of the HPV immunization programs in Canada

Province/territory	Year of implementation	Routine schedule	Catch-up program
British Columbia	2008	Grade 6	Grade 9
Alberta	2008	Grade 5	Grade 9
Saskatchewan	2008	Grade 6	Grade 7
Manitoba	2008	Grade 6	–
Ontario	2007	Grade 8	–
Quebec	2008	Grade 4[a]	9–17 years/grade 9
New Brunswick	2008	Grade 7	Grade 8
Nova Scotia	2007	Grade 7	Grade 8/grade 10
Prince Edward Island	2007	Grade 6	Grade 9
Newfoundland and Labrador	2007	Grade 6	Grade 9
Northwest Territories	2009	Grade 4	Grades 9–12
Yukon	2009	Grade 6	Grades 7–8
Nunavut	2010	Grade 6	–

Adapted with permission from Update on Human Papillomavirus (HPV) Vaccines. CCDR (Canada Communicable Disease Report) 2012;38:1–62

[a]Two doses in grade 4 and a third dose in Grade 9

In Latin America, information regarding HPV vaccination is still insufficient. As of mid-2012, only Mexico, Panama, and Argentina had implemented HPV public immunization programs. Of these countries, only Mexico showed data published about the HPV immunization program. The Mexican HPV vaccination program deserves mention because of the way it was implemented. In Mexico, the vaccine was approved for use in 2008. The HPV public immunization program did not cover the whole territory initially but only cities displaying the lowest human development index. This represented only 5 % of country's population. This program achieved a coverage rate of 85 % for the first dose in girls aged 9–12 (2009). In 2011, the Mexican government expanded the vaccination program to the entire country and included a school-based vaccination strategy for 9-year-old girls [32].

Until mid-2012, Brazil, the largest country in Latin America, had not implemented a public immunization program. Although quadrivalent and bivalent vaccines have been approved in Brazil in 2006 and 2008, respectively, at that time, both vaccines were available only in the private sphere. Nevertheless, a few municipalities by local political decision decided to offer the HPV vaccine for free. This was the case in São Francisco do Conde (BA), Campos de Goitacazes (RJ), Araraquara (SP), and Itu (SP). The first two municipal districts followed a school-based strategy, while the latter two opted for a local public health system strategy. None of these programs have data published regarding the coverage rates.

Barretos, a small Brazilian municipal district located in the state of São Paulo (southeast region of Brazil), recently participated in a school-based HPV vaccination demonstrative study. The study was designed and carried out by the Barretos Cancer Hospital, and it included girls attending sixth and seventh grades (average age: 12) enrolled in public and private schools in the city. From a total of 1,513 candidates for the immunization program, parents or legal guardians of 1,389 kids accepted participation for their girls in the program (91.8 % acceptance rate). The main reason reported by parents or guardians for refusing to participate was the fear of adverse events caused by the vaccine. The study confirmed high coverage rates for the three doses: 87.5 % (first dose), 86.3 % (second dose), and 85.0 % (third dose) (author's personal information). Peru also performed a demonstrative study involving a school-based vaccination strategy. This study involved approximately 8,000 girls attending the fifth grade and achieved a 88.9 % vaccination-coverage rate [33].

Funding for Vaccination Programs in Developing Countries

One of the main problems related to the HPV vaccine in developing countries is the cost of the vaccines. Mathematical models suggest that the HPV vaccine would be cost effective in low- and middle-income countries only if the three doses of the vaccine had a maximum cost of US$25 [11]. Considering that each dose of the vaccine has an average cost of U$120 [1], the magnitude of the problem can be appreciated. It is estimated that there are approximately 52 million 11-year-old girl candidates for HPV in developing countries and about seven million in developed countries [34]. Thus, low-income and many middle-income countries will have trouble implementing the HPV vaccine in the absence of a supporting funding program [29].

The main supporting funding programs currently available for the HPV vaccine are the ones described in the next sections.

GAVI Alliance (Global Alliance for Vaccines and Immunization)

Founded in 2000, this alliance is a public–private partnership with a global sphere of action whose main goal is to promote health through access to vaccines in countries that have low economic resources. Only countries with a gross national income lower than or equal to US$1,520 in 2009 (by the World Bank's classification) are currently candidates for GAVI's programs. According to such criteria, there are currently 57 GAVI-eligible countries (Table 16B.6). The alliance is comprised of members from the World Health Organization, UNICEF, the World Bank, pharmaceutical industries, research agencies, civil society, the Bill and Melinda Gates Foundation, the International Finance Facility for Immunization, in addition to developing country governments and donor governments. Today, the GAVI Alliance is the largest source of external funding for several immunization programs around the world [35]. In November 2011, complying with the demand of developing countries, the alliance included the HPV vaccine in their vaccine list. At this time, the quadrivalent vaccine manufacturer announced that they could supply the vaccine at a cost of US$5 per dose for the GAVI Alliance. In 2012, GAVI opened a round of applications for vaccine demonstration programs [36, 37].

Table 16B.6 Currently eligible countries for GAVI support

Afghanistan	Mali
Bangladesh	Mauritania
Benin	Mozambique
Burkina Faso	Myanmar
Burundi	Nepal
Cambodia	Nicaragua
Cameroon	Niger
Central African Republic	Nigeria
Chad	Pakistan
Comoros	Papua New Guinea
Congo	Rwanda
Côte d'Ivoire	São Tomé e Príncipe
Djibouti	Senegal
Eritrea	Sierra Leone
Ethiopia	Solomon Islands
Gambia	Somalia
Ghana	Republic of Sudan
Guinea	South Sudan
Guinea Bissau	Tajikistan
Haiti	Tanzania
India	Timor Leste
Kenya	Togo
Korea	Uganda
Kyrgyz Republic	Uzbekistan
Lao Lesotho	Viet Nam
Liberia	Yemen
Madagascar	Zambia
Malawi	Zimbabwe

Data from GAVI Alliance [cited 2012]. Available from: http://www.gavialliance.org/

Pan American Health Organization Revolving Fund

The Pan American Health Organization (PAHO) serves as the Regional Office of the World Health Organization in the Americas, and it provides a program for the acquisition of vaccines, syringes, and other immunization equipment for their 48 member countries. Countries pay for the vaccine, the cost of which is widely negotiated by PAHO with the manufacturers at a low price [36, 38]. In January 2010, the bivalent vaccine was offered to PAHO for a price of US$32. However, since then, there has been a significant reduction in vaccine prices. In 2012, the average prices for bivalent and quadrivalent vaccines offered to PAHO were US$13.48 and US$14.25, respectively [38]. The PAHO Revolving Fund is not truly a funding program, but it allows for a considerable price reduction for the cost of the vaccines for member countries.

Gardasil Access Program

The Axios Healthcare Development, a US nonprofit organization, manages the Gardasil Access Program (GAP). Through this program, Merck & CO has pledged to donate at least three million doses of the quadrivalent vaccine to organizations or institutions in developing countries. The guidances are provided by an independent advisory board comprised of public health experts. To date, more than a million doses of quadrivalent vaccine were donated to 22 participants in 20 countries (Bolivia, Kiribati, Honduras, Haiti, Guyana, Mali, Ghana, Cameroon, Lesotho, Tanzania, Kenya, Uganda, Georgia, Moldova, Uzbekistan, Nepal, Mongolia, Buthan, Cambodia, and Papua New Guinea). In this program, the doses of vaccines are donations, but, on the other hand, the costs related to the importation and to the whole cold chain are the responsibility of the participating organizations and institutions [39, 40].

Summary

The development of vaccines for HPV provides a new perspective on the primary prevention of diseases induced by the virus, especially cervical cancer. Although both versions of the vaccine currently available have been approved for use in more than 100 countries, the number of countries that implemented HPV public immunization programs is much lower. It is paradoxical to observe that the majority of countries that have an HPV immunization program already implemented are high-income countries with low cervical cancer incidence coefficients. Conversely, low- and middle-income countries, the ones with the greatest need for the vaccines, currently have limited access to the vaccines because of the high cost. Reduction of the vaccine cost is fundamental.

Programs that provide financial support, such as GAVI Alliance and PAHO Revolving Fund, are essential for the implementation of HPV immunization programs in countries that have few economic resources. Additionally, the development of a second generation of HPV vaccines, created using new production technologies at a lower cost, will make it easier to incorporate the vaccine in low- and middle-income countries.

References

1. Saslow D, Castle PE, Cox JT, Davey DD, Einstein MH, Ferris DG, et al. American Cancer Society Guideline for human papillomavirus (HPV) vaccine use to prevent cervical cancer and its precursors. CA Cancer J Clin. 2007;57(1):7–28.
2. Burchell AN, Winer RL, de Sanjose S, Franco EL. Chapter 6: Epidemiology and transmission dynamics of genital HPV infection. Vaccine. 2006;24 Suppl 3:S3/52–61.
3. WHO. Initiative for vaccine research (IVR)—viral cancer—HPV. World Health Organization. 2011. http://www.who.int/vaccine_research/diseases/viral_cancers/en/index3.html. Cited 30 Jun 2012.
4. Parkin DM. Global cancer statistics in the year 2000. Lancet Oncol. 2001;2(9):533–43.
5. Ferlay J, Shin HR, Bray F, Forman D, Mathers C, Parkin DM. Estimates of worldwide burden of cancer in 2008: GLOBOCAN 2008. Int J Cancer. 2010; 127(12):2893–917.
6. Ferlay J, Shin HR, Bray F, Forman D, Mathers C, Parkin DM. GLOBOCAN 2008 v1.2, Cancer Incidence and Mortality Worldwide: IARC CancerBase No. 10. Lyon: International Agency for Research on Cancer; 2011. http://globocan.iarc.fr. Cited 30 Jun 2012.
7. Update on Human Papillomavirus (HPV) Vaccines. CCDR (Canada communicable disease report) 2012;38:1–62.
8. WHO. Human papillomavirus and HPV vaccines: technical information for policy-makers and health professionals. Geneva: WHO Press; 2007. p. 43.
9. WHO/ICO. Human papillomavirus and related cancers in world. Summary report update. October 9, 2009. WHO/ICO Information Centre on HPV and Cervical Cancer. 2009.
10. Parkin DM, Bray F. Chapter 2: The burden of HPV-related cancers. Vaccine. 2006;24 Suppl 3:S3/11–25.
11. WHO. Human papillomavirus vaccines. WHO position paper. Weekly Epidemiological Record 2009;15: 118–31.
12. Brotherton JM, Fridman M, May CL, Chappell G, Saville AM, Gertig DM. Early effect of the HPV vaccination programme on cervical abnormalities in Victoria, Australia: an ecological study. Lancet. 2011;377(9783):2085–92.
13. Markowitz LE, Dunne EF, Saraiya M, Lawson HW, Chesson H, Unger ER. Quadrivalent human papillomavirus vaccine: recommendations of the Advisory Committee on Immunization Practices (ACIP). MMWR Recomm Rep. 2007;56(RR-2):1–24.
14. FDA. Vaccines, blood & biologics. Vaccines. Approved products FDA; 2012. http://www.fda.gov/BiologicsBloodVaccines/Vaccines/ApprovedProducts/ucm172678.htm. Cited 2012 Jul 20, 2012.
15. Garland SM, Hernandez-Avila M, Wheeler CM, Perez G, Harper DM, Leodolter S, et al. Quadrivalent vaccine against human papillomavirus to prevent anogenital diseases. N Engl J Med. 2007;356(19):1928–43.
16. Villa LL, Costa RL, Petta CA, Andrade RP, Paavonen J, Iversen OE, et al. High sustained efficacy of a prophylactic quadrivalent human papillomavirus types 6/11/16/18 L1 virus-like particle vaccine through 5 years of follow-up. Br J Cancer. 2006;95(11): 1459–66.
17. Quadrivalent vaccine against human papillomavirus to prevent high-grade cervical lesions. N Engl J Med. 2007;356(19):1915–27.
18. Paavonen J, Naud P, Salmeron J, Wheeler CM, Chow SN, Apter D, et al. Efficacy of human papillomavirus (HPV)-16/18 AS04-adjuvanted vaccine against cervical infection and precancer caused by oncogenic HPV types (PATRICIA): final analysis of a double-blind, randomised study in young women. Lancet. 2009; 374(9686):301–14.
19. Lehtinen M, Paavonen J, Wheeler CM, Jaisamrarn U, Garland SM, Castellsague X, et al. Overall efficacy of HPV-16/18 AS04-adjuvanted vaccine against grade 3 or greater cervical intraepithelial neoplasia: 4-year end-of-study analysis of the randomised, double-blind PATRICIA trial. Lancet Oncol. 2012;13(1):89–99.
20. Villa LL. HPV prophylactic vaccination: the first years and what to expect from now. Cancer Lett. 2011;305(2):106–12.
21. Villa LL, Costa RL, Petta CA, Andrade RP, Ault KA, Giuliano AR, et al. Prophylactic adrivalent human papillomavirus (types 6, 11, 16, and 18) L1 virus-like particle vaccine in young women: a randomised double-blind placebo-controlled multicentre phase II efficacy trial. Lancet Oncol. 2005;6(5):271–8.
22. Stokley S, Cohn A, Dorell C, Hariri S, Yankey D, Messonnier N, et al. Adolescent vaccination-coverage levels in the United States: 2006–2009. Pediatrics. 2011;128(6):1078–86.
23. Finn A. Strategy options for HPV vaccine delivery in EU countries. Guidance for the introduction of HPV vaccines in EU countries. Stockholm: European Centre for Disease Prevention and Control; 2008. p. 30–6.
24. Garland SM, Skinner SR, Brotherton JM. Adolescent and young adult HPV vaccination in Australia: achievements and challenges. Prev Med. 2011;53 Suppl 1:S29–35.
25. Immunise Australia Program. Human Papillomavirus (HPV). Information about the National Human Papillomavirus (HPV) Vaccination Program funded under the Immunise Australia Program.: Australian

Government. Depatment of Health and Aging; 2011 [updated Apr 04, 2011]; http://www.immunise.health.gov.au/internet/immunise/publishing.nsf/Content/immunise-hpv#figure 2. Cited 30 Jun 2012.
26. Dorleans F, Giambi C, Dematte L, Cotter S, Stefanoff P, Mereckiene J, et al. The current state of introduction of human papillomavirus vaccination into national immunisation schedules in Europe: first results of the VENICE2 2010 survey. Euro surveillance: bulletin europeen sur les maladies transmissibles = European communicable disease bulletin 2010;15(47).
27. HPV Vaccine: Implementation and Financing Policy. The Henry J. Kaiser Family Foundation. 2007. http://www.kff.org/womenshealth/upload/7602.pdf. Cited 2012.
28. The HPV Vaccine: Access and Use in the U.S.: The Henry J. Kaiser Family Foundation. 2011. http://www.kff.org/womenshealth/7602.cfm. Cited 2012.
29. IARC. Making cervical cancer vaccines widely available in developing countries: cost and financing issues. IARC. http://screening.iarc.fr/doc/IAVI_PATH_HPV_financing_brief.pdf. Cited 2012.
30. Smith LM, Brassard P, Kwong JC, Deeks SL, Ellis AK, Levesque LE. Factors associated with initiation and completion of the quadrivalent human papillomavirus vaccine series in an Ontario cohort of grade 8 girls. BMC Public Health. 2011;11:645.
31. Colucci R, Hryniuk W, Savage C. HPV vaccination programs in Canada: Are we hitting the mark? Report Card on Cancer in Canada [Internet]. 2010 Aug 11, 2012. Available from: http://www.canceradvocacy.ca/reportcard/2008/HPV %20Vaccination %20 Programs %20in %20Canada.pdf.
32. Progress toward implementation of human papillomavirus vaccination--the Americas, 2006–2010. MMWR Morbidity and mortality weekly report 2011;60(40):1382–4.
33. LaMontagne DS, Barge S, Le NT, Mugisha E, Penny ME, Gandhi S, et al. Human papillomavirus vaccine delivery strategies that achieved high coverage in low- and middle-income countries. Bull World Health Organ. 2011;89(11):821–30B.
34. Saxenian H. HPV Vaccine Adoption in Developing Countries: Cost and Financing Issues: International AIDS Vaccine Initiative/Program for Appropriate Technology in Health (PATH). http://www.iavi.org/HPVreport. Cited 2007.
35. Garland SM. Human papillomavirus vaccination: where to now? Sex Transm Infect. 2011;87 Suppl 2:ii23–4.
36. GAVI Alliance. http://www.gavialliance.org/. Cited 2012.
37. GAVI. Human papillomavirus vaccine support. GAVI Alliance. http://www.gavialliance.org/support/nvs/human-papillomavirus-vaccine-support/. Cited 2012.
38. PAHO. PAHO Revolving Fund. Pan American Health Organization; Available from: http://new.paho.org/hq/index.php?option=com_content&task=view&id=1864&Itemid=2234&lang=en.
39. Bonanni P, Levi M, Latham NB, Bechini A, Tiscione E, Lai P, et al. An overview on the implementation of HPV vaccination in Europe. Hum Vaccin. 2011;7(Suppl):128–35.
40. Ladner J, Besson MH, Hampshire R, Tapert L, Chirenje M, Saba J. Assessment of eight HPV vaccination programs implemented in lowest income countries. BMC Public Health. 2012;12:370.
41. GAP. Gardasil Access Program. 2012. http://www.gardasilaccessprogram.org/section/141. Cited 4 Nov 2012.

17 Well Woman Clinic Concept: An Integrated Approach for Screening and Early Diagnosis of Breast and Gynecological Cancers in Developing Countries

Mahesh K. Shetty and Jennifer C. Garza

Abstract

A vertical delivery of an integrated healthcare intervention to decrease mortality from breast and gynecological cancers is proposed for implementation through a Well Woman Clinic. The operations and logistics of such a clinic are discussed in this chapter. The pros and cons of horizontal and vertical delivery of healthcare services and the benefits of an integrated approach to screen for cancers in women are outlined. The methodology proposed is to screen for breast and cervical cancer and to diagnostically test symptomatic postmenopausal woman so as to detect endometrial and ovarian cancers at an early stage. The healthcare personnel required to carry out these tasks and the training and telemedicine support to ensure quality and consistency of services provided also are discussed. The need to have a robust and enforced referral system in place to provide a continuum of care for those women who are tested positive for malignancy and need definitive treatment and or surgery is emphasized. The methodology may need modifications for adaptation to individual countries and resources available; the core principle, however, of this proposal is integration of a well woman exam with screening and early diagnosis of multiple commonly occurring cancers affecting women. Some variation in the screening methodology, particularly for cervical cancer, is expected from one country to another and will be influenced by factors such as existing national or professional body guidelines or resource limitations.

M.K. Shetty (✉)
Woman's Center for Breast Care and MRI,
Woman's Hospital of Texas,
Houston, TX 77054, USA
e-mail: mshetty@womens-radiology.com

J.C. Garza, MS
Edinburg Regional Medical Center, Edinburg Children's Hospital, Edinburg, TX 78539, USA
e-mail: jc-garza@hotmail.com

Introduction

An integrated approach of providing a well woman examination in combination with screening for breast and cervical cancer as well as testing of symptomatic women for early diagnosis of ovarian and endometrial cancer is proposed.

M.K. Shetty (ed.), *Breast and Gynecological Cancers: An Integrated Approach for Screening and Early Diagnosis in Developing Countries*, DOI 10.1007/978-1-4614-1876-4_17,

While such a concept is applicable to a majority of women in low- and mid-resource countries with limited access to cancer screening and treatment residing in rural areas, the same may not apply to more affluent women residing in urban areas of mid-resource countries where a more robust cancer screening and early diagnosis approach may be available. These women then avail themselves of quality care based on personal resources.

A vertical program to deliver such an intervention is likely to be more effective than a horizontal delivery program through existing healthcare facilities that may not have the infrastructure needed for implementation of a cancer screening program in resource-poor settings. A well woman clinic can be set up as a free-standing clinic, as an addition to an existing primary healthcare center, or as a mobile clinic serving remote populations in low-resource countries who have only limited or no access to healthcare services.

Vertical Versus Horizontal Programs for Delivery of Healthcare Services [1, 2]

Horizontal programs are those that are implemented through existing health systems and receive funding through the government. These may include primary healthcare centers and/or regional hospitals and healthcare facilities. Incorporating a cancer screening service through a horizontal program has the theoretical advantage of using established facilities that are staffed to provide healthcare services to the population served. However, for such horizontal programs to succeed in implementing newly launched initiatives, the health system infrastructure has to be strong, well-funded, and well-staffed as is the case in developed countries. In resource-poor settings, healthcare facilities are often nonfunctioning and have poor infrastructure, making it nearly impossible to use them as a means to deliver new healthcare interventions. Vertical programs on the other hand are those that focus on a specific disease, and such programs are carried out in addition to primary care services. These programs are usually funded by an external donor for a finite period of time. There has been increased emphasis in recent years on vertical programs because they show quick results and are easier to operate than horizontal programs. Such programs have the best chance of being effective for cancer screening and early diagnosis interventions. Policy makers sometimes see vertical programs as draining and diverting limited personnel and financial resources in low-resource countries; they consider horizontal programs more sustainable and easier to manage. While this may hold true for providing basic services such as immunizations, cancer screening services are much more complex and would represent a challenge for successful implementation through an existing healthcare facility. Vertical programs on the other hand are more likely to be effective in low-resource countries. Sustainability of such vertical programs may be the greatest challenge due to funding requirements, and this needs to be addressed by policy makers and stakeholders.

Integrated Approach to Screening for Cancers in Women

A cost-effective strategy is a critical prerequisite of any new healthcare intervention in developing countries. Developing a strategy to diagnose multiple cancers afflicting women at a single site is a sensible approach to the integration of healthcare intervention services. This serves both the provider as well as the women in the target population well. The efficacy of integration of health services has been studied before. The Program for Appropriate Technology in Health (PATH) is a global health nonprofit that has advocated for and implemented integrated solutions for healthcare problems in developing countries [3]. The integration of HIV care services with maternal and child health in Kenya, HIV/AIDS with TB diagnosis in Tanzania, diarrheal disease and child nutrition in Vietnam, and the linking of agriculture and nutritional health in pregnant women in Kenya are some of the projects that have been very successfully implemented by PATH [1]. Such an approach is a departure from the usual traditional emphasis on specific health issues vs. attempting to provide a range of services to an individual. It makes practical sense to maximize the value of a woman's visit, particularly in rural settings, by addressing multiple healthcare concerns during a single visit. Such an approach makes sense both from a cost-effectiveness point of view as well as in terms of in maximizing compliance and participation in a cancer screening program. We propose an integrated approach for screening and early diagnosis of breast, cervical, endometrial, and ovarian cancer combined with a well woman examination that would involve providing a physical examination and routine blood/urine tests to assess the nutritional and general health status of women attending the cancer detection clinic. To date, such an approach has not been proposed or studied. There have been several reports on the benefit of combining breast and cervical cancer screening. Combined screening for breast and cervical cancer delivered through mobile clinics traveling to remote parts of Brazil has been reported with great success by the Barretos Cancer Hospital mobile cancer screening program, discussed in depth in Chap. 10 [4]. A study conducted in South Africa found that combining cervical and breast screenings led to an increase in cervical screening uptake [5].

Methodology and Rationale

Breast Cancer (Fig. 17.1)

The proposed strategy and rationale for screening for breast cancer are discussed in detail elsewhere in this book. A brief description is provided here. Annual screening commencing at 40 years of age and continuing until 69 years of age is suggested. As part of a well woman examination, screening for breast cancer is done by utilizing clinical breast examination that is performed by a nurse trained in CBE. There is considerable indirect evidence from studies that CBE can be recommended as an effective method for early detection of breast cancer. The examination is inexpensive, needs no special equipment, is easy to perform, is tolerated well by women, and healthcare professionals can be trained to perform it. CBE has been recommended as part of any global program for early detection of breast cancer [6].

CBE has never been studied in a randomized clinical trial such as has been done for mammography in order to prove mortality rate reduction. However, the effectiveness of CBE in breast cancer

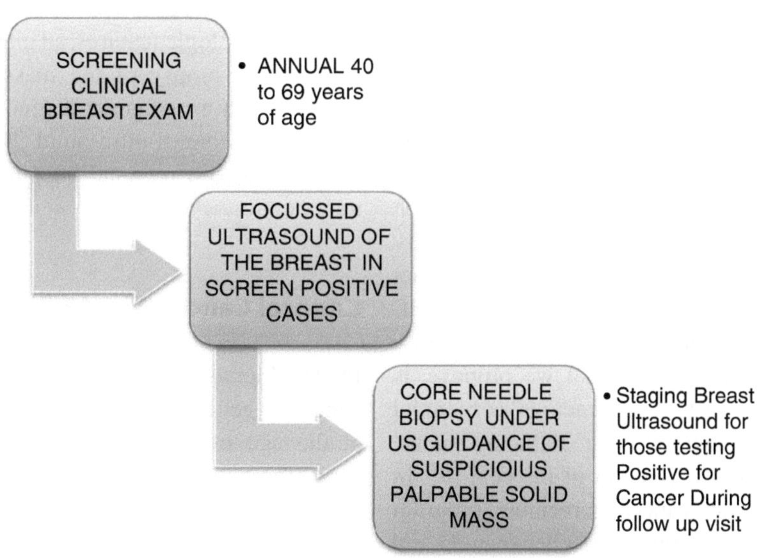

Fig. 17.1 Flowchart outlining methodology for breast cancer screening for breast cancer, single visit approach

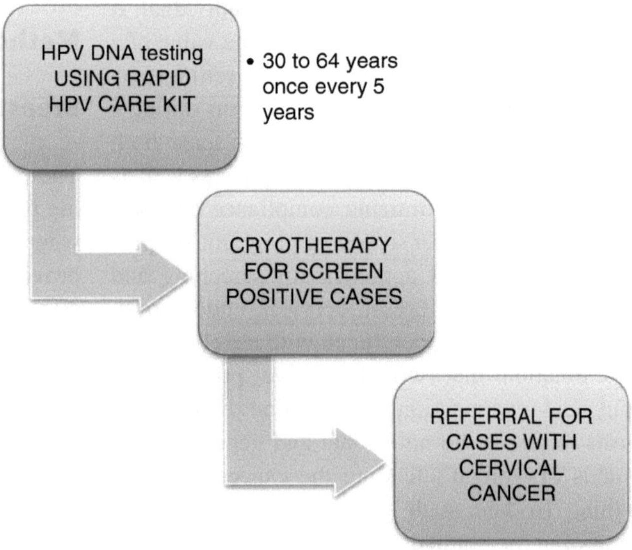

Fig. 17.2 Flowchart for cervical cancer screening, screen-and-treat approach, single clinic visit

screening and its role in reducing mortality from breast cancer have been reported in nonrandomized studies. A study conducted in Japan measured the effectiveness of breast cancer screening using CBE [7]. The change in the age-adjusted death rate from breast cancer for the period of 1986–1990 to 1991–1995 in the high coverage rate municipalities and comparable controls was studied. It was found that reduction of age-adjusted death rate was statistically significantly greater in those screened with clinical breast examination than those in the control group, suggesting that mass screening by physical examination contributed to the reduction of mortality from breast cancer [7]. The cost-effectiveness of CBE as a breast cancer screening modality has also been studied. It has been estimated that the mortality rate reduction was the greatest for programs that target women 40–60 years of age. Biannual CBE was expected to reduce breast cancer mortality by 16.3 %. Annual CBE, what we propose, is expected to be nearly as efficacious as biennial screening mammography for reducing breast cancer mortality at a fraction of the cost [8]. In the NHSS breast cancer screening program involving over a million women between 50 and 64 years of age screened with mammography, 60 % of the 5,000 cancers found were greater than 1 cm and therefore potentially detectable on CBE. In the US breast cancer detection demonstration project, 39 % of cancers under 1 cm in size were detected on CBE [9–11]. Following a CBE, all screen-positive women, i.e., women who have an abnormal finding on physical examination, are directed to the ultrasound examination room to undergo a focused sonographic examination of the palpable finding in the breast. In those with a solid mass demonstrating suspicious morphologic features, an ultrasound-guided core needle biopsy of the mass is performed. Patients with a malignant diagnosis are recalled for a staging breast ultrasound (BUS) and set up for referral to a regional hospital for definitive treatment.

Cervical Cancer (Fig. 17.2)

In developing countries, screening for cervical cancer is generally recommended to commence at the age of 30, as the maximum impact of screening has been shown to occur when women are screened in their thirties [12–14]. Screening of women in their 30s allows for identifying cancers in the preclinical phase, thereby maximizing the benefits of screening [13]. The optimal age group to be targeted for cervical cancer screening appears to be 30–59 years. Data published recently from a cluster randomized trial of 137,461 women studied in India demonstrated that even a single round of testing with HPV (Human Papilloma Virus) DNA resulted in significant reductions in the number of cases of advanced cancer and mortality from cervical cancer [12]. This study examined the efficacy of a single round of screening using visual inspection with acetic acid (VIA), cytology testing (PAP smear), and HPV DNA testing on the incidence of cervical cancer and associated death rates [13]. Women with a positive screening test were evaluated by means of colposcopy, and doctors reported the results as normal findings, inflammation, probable low-grade or high-grade precancerous lesions, or invasive cancer. Women with colposcopic findings of low-grade or high-grade lesions were offered immediate cryotherapy, if all the following criteria were met: the lesion could be covered by the cryoprobe and involved three quadrants or less of the cervix with no extension into the endocervix or vaginal walls; the squamocolumnar junction was fully visible; there was no suspicion of invasive cancer. Loop electrosurgical excisional procedure (LEEP) was offered to women with CIN lesions that were unsuitable for cryotherapy. Women with suspected invasive cancer were referred to the NDMCH or to the hospital of their choice for investigations and treatment with surgery, radiotherapy, or both [13]. Based on this large clinical trial and other previous studies, HPV DNA testing has been recommended for implementation as a method for cervical cancer screening in low-resource countries [14]. The cost-effectiveness of such a strategy has also been previously published. The most effective strategy—in terms of lives saved—was use of a single lifetime HPV test, followed by cryotherapy for women who tested positive. Such an approach demonstrated that the cost per year of life saved was $14, and the reduction of cervical cancer incidence was 32 % [15]. Although a single lifetime testing shows significant reduction in mortality, more frequent testing adds to the benefit of screening. Testing for HPV every 3 years has also been shown to be very cost-effective in saving lives [15]. HPV DNA testing can be undertaken in two-step processes, where during the initial clinic visit the test is administered and test-positive women are recalled for colposcopy. At colposcopy, women with abnormal findings undergo biopsy followed by treatment by means of cryotherapy or LEEP, depending on the size of the abnormality. Alternatively, use of single visit strategy may be adopted, which may be more beneficial in terms of cost savings, ensure better patient compliance, and minimize the risk of loss to follow-up. Single visit strategies are made possible by using HPV testing of self-collected samples or rapid processing of clinician-collected samples. A simple, affordable, and accurate HPV test (CareHPV™ test, Qiagen, Hilden, Germany) provides results within 3 h and was recently evaluated in China; in this study, the accuracy was found to be similar to that of the Hybrid capture 11 test, with a higher sensitivity than VIA. In the near future, this test kit should be available for use in low-resource countries. These two studies clearly demonstrate the appropriateness of using HPV testing as a primary screening method in low-resource countries [16]. The most cost-effective approach would involve use of HPV DNA testing and refer those women who test positive for cryotherapy. A randomized clinical trial of 6,555 nonpregnant women aged 35–65 recruited through community outreach and conducted between June 2000 and December 2002 at ambulatory women's health clinics in Khayelitsha, South Africa, clearly showed that such an approach was very effective [17]. Noncytology-based screening and treatment of positive cases, bypassing colposcopy, is a tremendous advantage in low-resource situations. When HPV rapid result kit is used, there is an opportunity for a screen-and-treat approach during a single clinic visit since results of the test are available in 2.5 h.

Endometrial and Ovarian Cancers (Figs. 17.3 and 17.4)

Unlike breast and cervical cancer screenings, the benefits of screening for ovarian and endometrial cancers have not been shown. These screenings are

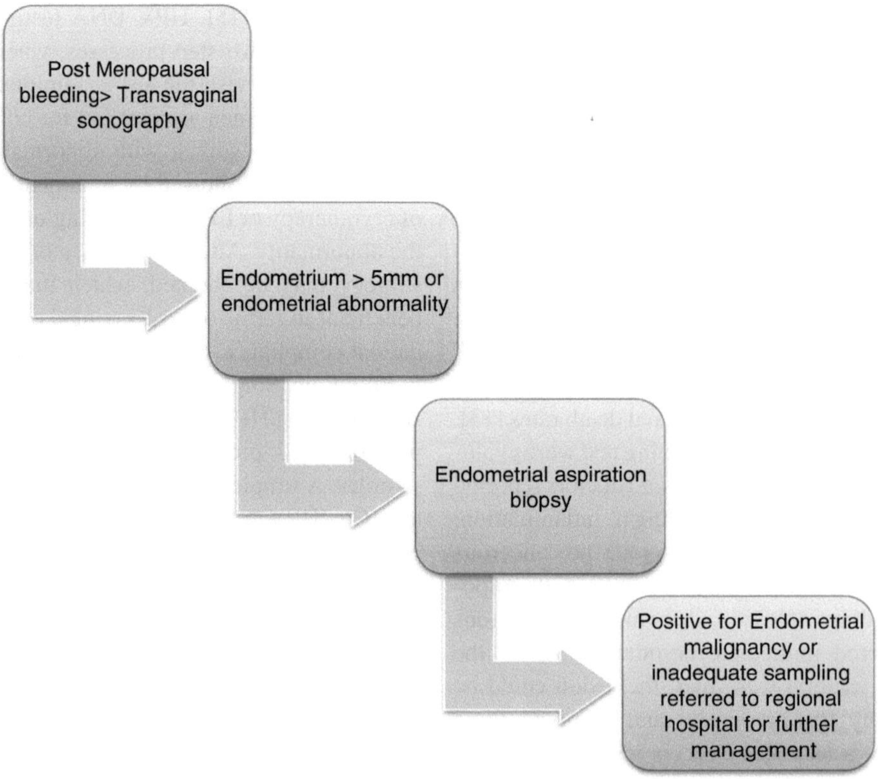

Fig. 17.3 Flowchart outlining methodology for early diagnosis of endometrial cancer

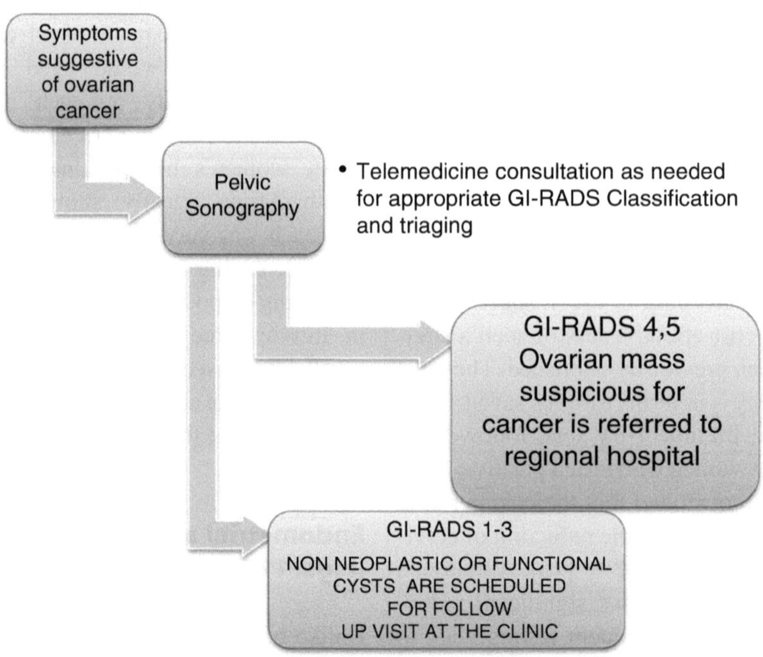

Fig. 17.4 Flowchart outlining methodology for early diagnosis of ovarian cancer

Table 17.1 Gynecologic imaging report and data system (GI-RADS) classification system for adnexal masses

GI-RADS grade	Diagnosis	Est. prob. malignancy (%)	Detail
1	Definitive benign	0	Normal ovaries identified and no adnexal mass seen
2	Very probably benign	<1	Adnexal lesions thought to be of functional origin, e.g., follicles, corpora lutea, hemorrhagic cysts
3	Probably benign	1–4	Neoplastic adnexal lesions thought to be benign, such as endometrioma, teratoma, simple cyst, hydrosalpinx, paraovarian cyst, peritoneal pseudocyst, pedunculated myoma, or findings suggestive of pelvic inflammatory disease
4	Probably malignant	5–20	Any adnexal lesion not included in GI-RADS 1–3 and with one or two findings suggestive of malignancy[a]
5	Very probably malignant	>20	Adnexal masses with three or more findings suggestive of malignancy[a]

[a]Thick papillary projections, thick septations, solid areas and/or ascites, defined according to IOTA criteria, and vascularization within solid areas, papillary projections, or central area of a solid tumor on color or power Doppler assessment. Est prob: estimated probability

Reprinted with permission of John Wiley & Sons Inc. from Amor F, Alcazar Al, Vaccaro H, Leon M, Iturra A. GI-RADS reporting system for ultrasound evaluation of adnexal masses in clinical practice: a prospective multicenter study. Ultrasound Obstet Gynecol 2011; 38: 450–455

not appropriate in countries with limited resources. However, there may be a potential to detect these cancers at an earlier stage by selectively examining postmenopausal women with symptoms suggestive of ovarian and/or endometrial cancers as part of a well woman examination. We recognize that the yield may still be low given the relatively low prevalence of these cancers; however, one has to keep in mind that performing these additional evaluations suggested next adds very little cost to the envisaged program and may have the potential to reduce the high mortality from being diagnosed at advanced stages of ovarian and endometrial cancers. It has been shown in several retrospective studies that the majority of women with ovarian cancer are symptomatic, even though some of these may be non-gynecologic in nature [18, 19]. Goff and coworkers have studied the value of using a symptom index to help in the early diagnosis of ovarian cancer. Women with ovarian cancer experienced symptoms more frequently, and these symptoms were of higher severity and of more recent onset than women with benign masses or those in the control population. A combination of bloating, increased abdominal size, and urinary symptoms was found in 43 % of those with cancer compared to 8 % of those without cancer presenting to primary care clinics. The authors of this study concluded that women with more frequent, more severe, and more recent onset of symptoms warranted further diagnostic investigation because they were more likely to be associated with both benign and malignant ovarian masses [18]. In another study, Goff and colleagues reported that symptoms associated with ovarian cancer were pelvic abdominal pain, urinary frequency/urgency, increased abdominal size and bloating, and difficulty eating/feeling full. These symptoms are particularly significant if present for less than year and present >12 days per month. A symptom index was considered positive if any of the following symptoms occurred >12 times per month and were present for <1 year: pelvic/abdominal pain, increased abdominal size/bloating, difficulty eating/feeling full. In the confirmatory sample, the index had a sensitivity of 56.7 % for early disease. The specificity was 90 % for women >50 years [19]. Based on these studies, we propose using the Goff symptom index to identify women who need additional diagnostic evaluation. Women in the age group of 50–69 with symptoms indicating increased risk for ovarian cancer may benefit from a pelvic examination followed by endovaginal sonography to assess the ovaries (Table 17.1).

Ultrasound evaluation of the endometrial thickness is the accepted method to assess endometrial abnormalities in postmenopausal women. About 10 % of postmenopausal women with abnormal bleeding are diagnosed with endometrial carcinoma. About 75–80 % of women with endometrial carcinoma will present with abnormal postmenopausal bleeding. In these patients, performance of transvaginal ultrasound for assessment of the endometrium identifies an abnormality in most women with endometrial cancer [20–24]. A large clinical study reported that 96 % of endometrial carcinomas will be detected in symptomatic postmenopausal women if additional procedures are performed only in those with an endometrial thickness of >4 mm [23, 24]. A thin and regular endometrial lining is very reliable for the exclusion of endometrial carcinoma in a postmenopausal patient with abnormal bleeding [24]. We recommend use of transvaginal sonography (TVS) in postmenopausal women with abnormal bleeding to identify those women who will need endometrial biopsy. An abnormal endometrium in a postmenopausal woman with bleeding detected on sonography is an indication for endometrial biopsy. As with screening methods for breast and cervical cancers, diagnostic assessment for early detection of endometrial and ovarian cancers can be accomplished during a single visit. Endometrial sampling is considered the gold standard as described in Chap. 8. Endometrial aspiration biopsy is easily performed as an outpatient procedure using a cannula. It is recognized that such a procedure may have limitations when abnormality as shown by ultrasound is focal; in such cases when endometrial aspiration biopsy fails, the patient can be referred for dilatation and curettage in a hospital setting.

Clinic Operation and Patient Flow

A typical floor plan of a well woman clinic is shown in Fig. 17.5a, b. The patient examination section of the clinic will require two rooms or cubicles: one for physical examination and obtaining samples from uterine cervix and a second room for procedures and biopsy as discussed next. The following sequence is suggested. Women would as a first step undergo a clinical evaluation including a well-performed CBE followed by a physical examination of the nutritional status and general well-being. Blood samples for CBC (Complete Blood Count) testing are then obtained. This is followed by cervical sampling for HPV DNA. Subsequently, those women with an abnormal finding on CBE then proceed to the procedure room for a focused BUS. Those who are triaged during clinical evaluation to receive TVS necessitated by symptoms indicative of either endometrial or ovarian cancer will undergo TVS in conjunction with the BUS. Endometrial biopsy is performed when an endometrial abnormality is identified. Those women in whom there is a solid suspicious breast mass on sonographic evaluation of a physical finding will undergo core needle biopsy under ultrasound guidance. Women who are tested positive for HPV DNA will undergo cryotherapy in the procedure room on the same day. Such a screen-and-treat approach has been studied and shown to be highly cost-effective; performing screening and treatment on the same day also serves to maximize compliance since a second visit is not required [11, 12]. Women undergoing breast biopsy will be advised to return for follow-up in 1 week. Those women with a malignant diagnosis will undergo a staging ultrasound; then they are set up to receive definitive treatment at a regional hospital with which the clinic has a preexisting affiliation in place for referral. Similar referrals to the regional hospital are to be arranged for women who may have a sonographic assessment that is suspicious for ovarian cancer or those who are diagnosed with endometrial cancer following an endometrial biopsy. The funding of the clinic should include provision for financial aid to enable the women to travel to the regional center and obtain treatment. Such arrangements should include transport, lodging, and meals for the patient and a member of her family, as the case may be. A preexisting agreement with a regional cancer hospital to treat patients diagnosed with cancer at the clinic should be in place when the well woman clinic commences its program. The downstream support is a critical component of this integrated strategy.

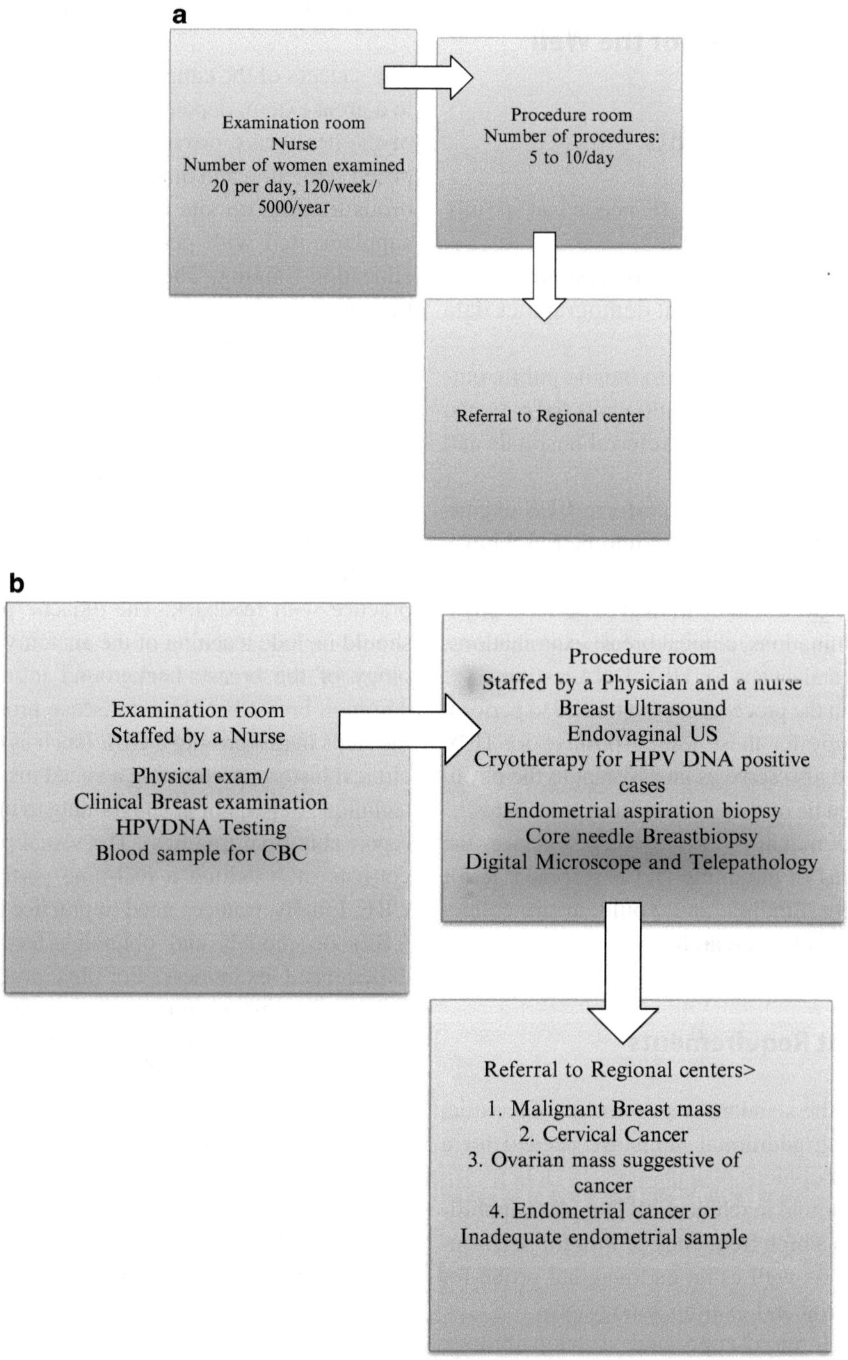

Fig. 17.5 (**a**, **b**) Flowchart outlining the operations of the well woman clinic

Resources Required for the Well Woman Clinic

Personnel Requirements

The following personnel are needed at a fully staffed well woman clinic:

- A receptionist who would be responsible for appointments and patient demographics data entry.
- A medical social worker to handle public outreach, coordinate follow-up visits for patients, and act as a liaison with referral hospitals and pathology labs.
- A physician who would perform BUS examinations, and breast and endometrial biopsy procedures.
- A nurse who would be trained to perform physical examinations, clinical breast examinations, and cervical swabs for HPV DNA testing.
- A nurse in the procedure room trained to perform cryotherapy for those testing positive for HPV DNA and also serve as an assistant to the physician when he or she is performing procedures.
- A clinic manager, who would oversee the operations of the clinic and is responsible for budgeting, funding, and would ensure collection of data for research.

Equipment Requirements

Apart from the standard requirements of a clinic, the following additional items are needed for a well woman clinic:

- An ultrasound machine with Doppler capabilities, with a high frequency probes for performing BUS as well as an endovaginal probe for endometrial and ovarian sonography.
- A digital microscope and a telepathology setup allowing for remote reads of histology specimens.
- Disposable core biopsy needles for percutaneous biopsy of breast masses.
- Endometrial aspiration biopsy cannula for endometrial biopsy.
- HPV DNA kits, including cervical samplers for obtaining cervical brush specimens.

Training of Clinic Healthcare Staff

The success of the cancer screening program will, to a great extent, depend on the skill and expertise of the healthcare providers carrying out the proposed screening and diagnostic studies. Initial rigorous training on site or off site will have to be supplemented with periodic continuing medical education training. The role of telemedicine and training in early detection of breast cancer is discussed at length in Chaps. 14 and 15.

As far as breast cancer screening is concerned, since the core of the proposed methodology is screening by clinical breast examination, training nurses and physicians at the clinic to perform consistently high quality CBEs is critical. There are three components of such a training program: a didactic presentation, a visual presentation, and practice with feedback. The didactic presentation should include teaching of the anatomy and physiology of the breast, background information on common breast health and disease processes, and the steps in performing a CBE (such as obtaining a clinical history, performing a visual inspection, the technique of palpation, and training to interpret and report abnormal findings). The visual presentation consists of watching a real-time performance of CBE. Finally, trainees need to practice performing CBEs on models and obtaining feedback from experienced examiners. For this portion of the training, live models provide the most realistic clinical experience. Measuring and demonstrating sensitivity and specificity of breast lump detection should also be a part of the training [25]. CBE training can improve sensitivity of breast lump detection and reduce false-positive rates. A program that studied effectiveness of a self-study manual and a 1.5 h skills-based curriculum reported an increase from 59 to 94 % in physicians detecting 60–100 % of lumps. The false-positive rate declined to 59 % of the pretest rate [26].

Quality assurance checks to monitor the screening methodology will determine the need and frequency of additional training. A telemedicine set up at the clinic is the best way not only to deliver periodic refresher course training but also to provide second opinion on test findings. Such a link is best established with regional referral hospitals or cancer centers and would need reliable Internet

Table 17.2 Measures of monitoring

Measure	Type of evaluation provided
Participation (compliance) rate	Indicates potential for effectiveness of screening program
Prevalence rate at initial screening test and rate of interval cancers	Provides estimates of sensitivity, lead time, sojourn time and predictive value
Stage and size distribution of screen-detected cancers	Indicates potential for reduction in absolute rate of advanced cancers
Rate of advanced cancers	Early surrogate of mortality
Breast cancer death rate	Final evaluation

Adapted with permission of Macmillan Publishers Ltd from Day NE, Williams DRR, Khaw KT. Breast cancer screening programmes: The development of a monitoring and evaluation system. Br J Cancer 1989;59:954–958

access as well as video conference capabilities. When local pathology lab support is not available, an additional investment in the purchase of a digital microscope is recommended with the capacity to remotely read the slides prepared by the nurse. Nurses are trained to process core biopsy or fine-needle aspirate samples and to mount the specimen slides on the digital microscope. A digital microscope and telepathology capability represent cost-effective solutions in the long run that help overcome the shortage of locally available pathologists or clinics in remote locations.

Referral System

A critical prerequisite of this program is an affiliation and/or an agreement with a regional hospital that has the capacity to perform additional testing of and treating of cancers diagnosed at the clinic. The medical social worker at the clinic and the clinic administrator should rigorously ensure that all women who are tested positive for breast, cervical, or endometrial cancers are treated at regional hospitals. Women should be provided with all and any assistance that is needed to ensure compliance and follow-up at facilities that provide definitive care. Women who are diagnosed with ovarian masses considered to be suspicious and those who have focal endometrial abnormalities with inadequate endometrial sampling and are in need of D & E will need to be referred to a specialist at the regional hospital. The overall success of this program depends on the existence of a robust and efficient system of referral for those who need treatment or additional testing. A clearly defined referral system for women with positive screen results and a system that ensures women receive appropriate treatment and follow-up should be in place and monitored. Any financial barrier to referral, treatment, and follow-up of women testing positive has to be overcome.

Monitoring Performance Metrics

A cancer screening program consists of a process that starts with identifying the target population, then invites women to participate, and ends with a negative examination or diagnosis and treatment of cancer, with outcomes documented. An attempt to follow up negatives and determine false-negative rate whenever feasible is also desirable. In the long term, observational studies will have to be conducted in a large patient population followed over many years in order to test the effectiveness of the program; however, in the short term, there are several indicators that can be monitored to determine effectiveness of the program. These are outlined in Tables 17.2, 17.3, and 17.4 [27]. During the first year of screening, performance benchmarks are expected to be lower than in subsequent years, due to existence of a greater proportion of advanced stage cancers in a previously unscreened population. For instance, the breast cancer detection rate is expected to be three times the incidence rates. A higher percentage of cancers will be diagnosed at a more advanced stage of the disease, and there will be fewer node-negative small cancers. As noted previously, a factor affecting performance metrics will be the skill level of the clinical staff, which is anticipated to improve over time. The success of the program is also critically dependent on the compliance and

Table 17.3 Indicators for assessing performance of a breast cancer screening program for women aged 40–69

Performance indicator	Acceptable (%)	Goal (%)
Participation rate	70	75
Pretreatment diagnosis of malignant lesions	70	90
Positive predictive value for biopsy		
Initial screen	50	50
Subsequent screen	75	75
Reinvitation rate within screening interval	95	100

Adapted with permission from the original table published in *European Guidelines for Quality Assurance in Mammography Screening,* 3rd Edition © European Communities 2001. Responsibility for the adaptation lies entirely with Mahesh K. Shetty

Table 17.4 Early surrogate indicators for monitoring effectiveness of screening for breast cancer 40–69 years

Surrogate indicator	Acceptable	Desirable
Interval cancers rate/background Incidence		
First year	30 %	
Second year	50 %	
Breast cancer detection rate		
Initial screening	3× incidence rate (3 per 1,000 women screened)	
Subsequent screen	1.5× incidence rate (1.5 PER 1,000 women screened)	
Stage >II/total cancers detected at screening		
Initial screening	25 %	<25 %
Subsequent screens	20 %	<20 %
Node-negative cancers/total cancers detected at screening		
Initial screening	70 %	>75 %
Subsequent screens	75 %	>75 %
Invasive cancers/total cancers detected at screening	100 %	100 %

Adapted with permission from the original table published in c 3rd Edition © European Communities 2001. Responsibility for the adaptation lies entirely with Mahesh K. Shetty

participation rate of the target population, and there are benchmarks to be monitored to ensure satisfactory compliance (Table 17.2).

Summary

Integrated screening of multiple cancers in women carried out in conjunction with a well woman examination and delivered through a vertical approach via free-standing clinics or through independently functioning additions to existing primary healthcare facilities may be a cost-effective solution to decreasing the mortality from breast and gynecological cancers in resource-poor countries. In reality, this may manifest itself as a mobile clinic in areas where access may be an issue due to remote locations.

Utilizing methods that are the least expensive and that are not resource intensive will help keep costs down. The challenges anticipated in implementation of this methodology will be funding for a vertical healthcare delivery system, sustainability, and availability of trained healthcare professionals to carry out the integrated clinical services outlined previously. Ensuring participation of the target population is yet another major challenge. A model clinic is being proposed to test the efficacy and practicality of such an approach; a Houston-based nonprofit organization, the Woman's Cancer Foundation (womanscancerfoundation.org), is leading this effort. Sustaining this challenge for the long term may necessitate that such projects be eventually integrated with existing healthcare facilities. The efficacy of such an approach requires validation through large-scale observational studies so as to demonstrate a case for widespread implementation of such an approach to reduce existing high mortality from breast and gynecological cancers in developing countries.

Appendix: Design, Layout, and Construction of a Well Woman Clinic in a Developed Country

Jennifer C. Garza

Introduction

The well woman clinic concept described previously may also be useful to help the underserved and/or indigent population in large cities of developing countries. The logistics of constructing a clinic in such a setting is described in this appendix. This description is in contrast to the bare bones approach outlined previously, keeping in mind that a clinic in a developed nation utilizing the same project design will have to meet certain minimum standards, and the funding available is significantly higher than in resource-poor settings (Fig. 17.6).

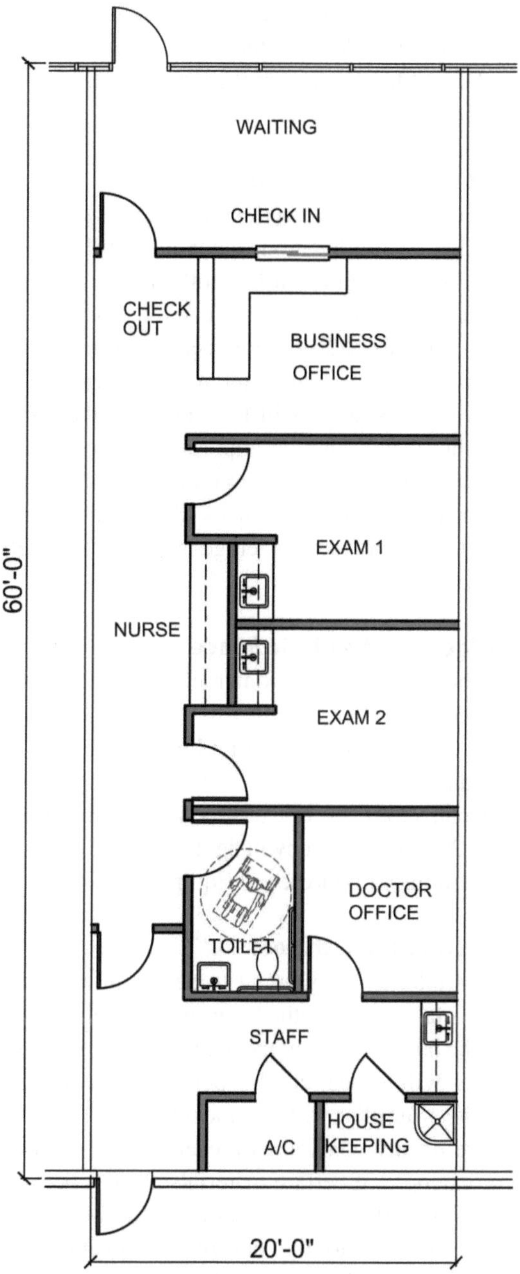

Fig. 17.6 Floor plan of a typical well woman clinic (Design by Robert Mason, Director, Architect, HCA/Gulf Coast Division, Houston, TX. Used with permission.)

Constructing a Well Woman Clinic

There are various factors to take into account when designing and building such a project. Building one from scratch, often called a "Greenfield" project, involves many steps. This appendix is designed to familiarize the reader with the various steps in the process. The process will vary depending on resources available at each specific clinic location.

Choosing a Location

It would be preferable to find a shelled out space in an existing building if one does exist. Also, an easily identifiable location will ensure the patient's ability to find the clinic and will ensure success. It is recommended to establish contact and work with local authorities to determine if land could be donated, if the determination is to build a free-standing clinic.

Cost to Build the Clinic

The cost for construction varies greatly and depends on the location, labor availability, and material availability. In US dollars, constructing medical office building space can range anywhere from $160 to $220/square feet in metropolitan areas. It will be important to determine what types of constraints will be present at the location, but it will also be important to speak with local architects and contractors to show you examples of completed work done along with cost to determine an average cost for the well woman clinic.

Budget for the Clinic Space

The budge for a well woman clinic space would include:

- Architect and Engineering Fees
- Land
- Contractor Fees for Construction and Build-out
- A 20 % contingency budget
- Furniture, Fixtures, and Equipment

Selecting an Architect

If possible, it is important to select an architect who is familiar with the location where the clinic will be built. Knowing the local building requirements will speed up the permit process. The architect familiar with the local area will also be aware of any constraints present in the market. For example, if certain materials are not permitted as part of the construction, the architect can make changes to the design specifications to allow for that. If certain utilities are not readily available, the architect can redesign the space to take into account these constraints. Architects also usually can recommend engineers for the project if necessary.

Architectural Design Process

There are several phases in the architectural design process. To cut down on costs, researching medical office floor plans and selecting one to base the clinic space upon will be beneficial. Many floor plans can be found on the Internet, and several should be provided to illustrate the medical office layout that should suffice for the well woman clinic. For purposes of the well woman clinic, most of the programming and schematic phases have been completed.

Programming

Programming is the activity of determining the set of needs the building or space needs to fulfill. In this part of the process, you define what exactly is needed; for example, the number of exam rooms, the lobby, the physician's office, etc.

Schematic Phase

Schematic phase is the first step in the design process for planning the clinic space. The architect will typically sketch out the space in this phase. This is a high-level design for the space and will generally specify the dimensions of the different components in the space. It will also show doorways and egress, and will allow you to look at the "flow" of the space.

Design and Development

During design and development, the scheme is refined into the final design. During this portion of the process, different sets of drawings for mechanical, electrical, and communication are designed and specified. For example, an issue that will be addressed will be the number of electrical outlets needed. Communication drawings show where data lines will be located or "dropped" in the various work spaces. Also, keep in mind the logistics of patients, family members, equipment, and personnel in the space when designing the different areas.

Construction Documents

The purpose of the various sets of drawings is to specifically spell out everything that is needed in order to construct the space. Construction documents typically are submitted to permit authorities. These authorities typically review the documents, and, in most cases, they will add comments and will prescribe required revisions to the design before the permit is granted. If the architect is familiar with the location, there will more than likely be a faster turnaround time to securing the permit.

Selecting a Contractor to Build the Well Woman Clinic

Before final construction documents are created, it is important to begin to identify a construction company or a contractor that will build-out the clinic. The contractor is in charge of procuring all the different trades needed for the project. For example, trades needed typically include flooring work, masonry, plumbing, electrical work, painting, cabinetry, etc. It is very important that a good working relationship exist with the contractor. It is suggested that one interviews several contractors. It is also important for them to demonstrate various completed projects. If possible, physically travel to locations where work was completed by these contractor candidates to determine the quality of their work.

Bidding Out the Project

If possible, the project should be bid out to at least three reputable contractors. The architect firm should be responsible for setting the "rules" for the bid. They should specify when the bid is due and the specific items that need to be addressed on the bid. For this part of the process, make sure contractors are as detailed as possible in the bid. Make sure all items have been addressed. If one contractor's price is significantly different from the others, it is more than likely that a component of the project was missed in the proposal. Other topics to take into consideration are the time it takes to order and receive supplies. It also is important to ask for an estimated time frame or schedule for construction completion. It is common to request a project timeline with key milestones identified. After questioning contractors and deciding on the price, it is customary to formally award the project to the contractor selected for the project in the form of written communication. In this communication, it is important to reference the project number if one was assigned and the total dollar amount that was agreed to. It is also customary to let the other contractors know by written communication that they were not selected for the project.

Change Orders

Change orders are changes requested after the original scope of the project has been agreed to. An example of a change order would be if it was decided to go with finished concrete for the flooring vs. ceramic tile flooring as bid originally. In this case, there very well may be a savings to the project because of the change in materials. If there is a savings, then a credit for the price specified in the original bid is due. Most projects have several change orders. Make sure both parties agree to a change order and sign off as well as date the change order. Adherence to this process will prevent any misunderstandings and arguments later. It is also important to decide how change orders will be paid and credited as the project progresses. This should be negotiated before the project commences.

Payment to Contractors

Usually, there is a payment at the beginning of the project in order for the contractor to procure supplies and labor. Generally, as the project goes through completion, there are different payment stages. It is important to negotiate the payment terms and schedule before the project is started. Again, proper documentation of these terms should be completed prior to the project commencing.

Contingency Budget

It is typical in a construction project that unanticipated issues previously not identified in the design process arise. For example, in an existing building, a wall may be demolished and then it is discovered that the plumbing will have to be rerouted or replaced due to its age. For this purpose, it is important to determine a contingency budget. It should be based on the overall project cost and can range from 10 to 20 % depending on the unknown conditions.

Well Woman Clinic General Layout

We provide schematics for typical clinic space with dimensions in the sections that follow. Sometimes, contractors can work with as little as this information to begin renovations or work. Again, it is important to know building code requirements in the local area. Generally speaking, the clinic should range from 1,000 to 2,200 square feet (Fig. 17.6).

Waiting Room Space

The waiting room space should be the first space that you walk into in the clinic. The size of the waiting room will be determined by the anticipated needs of the patients. If a large amount of family will accompany the patient, then it may be wise to develop a waiting porch area outside the clinic. "Gang" seating is also preferable. These types of chairs are connected to each other and make it difficult for visitors to rearrange the layout. A waiting room can be efficiently used and can be relatively small at 200 square feet. At 200 square feet, it could hold ten patients waiting at one time. At 400–500 square feet, the waiting room could hold well over 20 people at one time.

The patient would walk up to the check-in counter. The reception desk should consist of a walk-up counter. It could be enclosed or partitioned off with a transparent type of window, or it could be open to the public but partitioned off from the waiting room by the counter itself.

Exam Room [2]

Exam rooms should measure from 100 to 150 square feet. Exam rooms of this size should be large enough to fit a basic obstetrics exam table, an ultrasound machine, one or two seats, a counter with sink, and cabinets above the sink.

The clinic should have two exam rooms. One will be used for well woman examinations and various testing. The second exam room will be used for sonography and procedures.

Procedure Room [1]

The procedure room could be built larger than the exam rooms if necessary. For example, the waiting room could me made smaller so that one of the exam rooms could be made larger for use as a procedure room. This room would be used for cryotherapy and other clinical procedures.

Other Spaces

Other spaces to be included and planned are Office for Physician/Practitioner, Small Break Room/Lounge, and Closets.

Materials to Consider When Building the Clinic

Using durable materials is important for ensuring that the clinic hold up to patient use and possible harsh environmental factors. For the flooring, the sealed concrete floor should be sufficient. Ceramic tile throughout would also be a good choice. Walls should be built to local standards. Epoxy paint on cinder block will suffice for all areas. For a more decorative, yet cost-effective approach, ceramic tile could also be installed along the perimeter of the wall. This could serve as wall protection. For counters with sinks, it is highly recommended that a solid surface countertop be installed. Corian is a type of solid surface material that can be made for counters that will withstand water and is durable. Sometimes you will find laminate used in clinics, but laminate has a tendency to chip or warp with age. Another consideration is to pour out concrete countertops and seal them. This will be very durable and will be easy to clean in the long term.

Bibliography

1. Robert Mason, B.S. (Building Sciences), B.A., Architecture, Director, Facilities Services Group, HCA/Gulf Coast Division.
2. Ginger Baecker, Director of Satellite Clinics, Woman's Hospital Texas.

References

1. Msuya J. 2004 Horizontal and vertical delivery of health services: what are the trade offs? Making Services Work for Poor People' prepared for the World Development Report 2004/5. Available at http://www-wds.worldbank.org/external/default/WDSContentServer/WDSP/IB/2003/10/15/000160016_20031015125129/additional/310436360_200502761000211.pdf.
2. Atun RA, Bennett S, Duran A. 2005 Health systems and policy analysis: when do vertical (stand-alone) Programmes Have a Place in Health Systems? World Health Organization 2008 and World Health Organization, on behalf of the European Observatory on Health Systems and Policies 2008. Available at http://www.who.int/management/district/services/WhenDoVerticalProgrammesPlaceHealthSystems.pdf.
3. Directions in global health. 2011;8(2):8–12. Available at http://www.path.org/publications/files/ER_directions_8_2_winter11.pdf.

4. Nicolau SM, Moreira LF, Haikel Jr RF, Longatto-Filho A, Baracat EC. Adherence to cervical and breast cancer programs is crucial to improving screening performance. Rural Remote Health. 2009;9(3):1241–52.
5. Maree JE, Lu XM, Wright SC. Combining breast and cervical screening in an attempt to increase cervical screening uptake. An intervention study in a South African context. Eur J Cancer Care (Engl). 2012; 21(1):78–86.
6. Albert US, Schulz KD. Clinical breast examination: what can be recommended for its use to detect breast cancer in countries with limited resources? Breast J. 2003;9 Suppl 2:S90–3.
7. Kuroishi T, Hirose K, Suzuki T, Tominaga S. Effectiveness of mass screening for breast cancer in Japan. Breast Cancer. 2000;7(1):1–8.
8. Okonkwo QL, Draisma G, der Kinderen A, Brown ML, de Koning HJ. Breast cancer screening policies in developing countries: a cost-effectiveness analysis for India. J Natl Cancer Inst. 2008; 100(18):1290–300.
9. Mittra I, Baum M, Thornton H, Houghton J. Is clinical breast examination an effective alternative to mammographic screening? BMJ. 2000;321:1071–3.
10. Patnick J. 98 review NHS breast screening programme. Sheffield: NHS Breast Screening Programme; 1998.
11. Report of the Working Group to review the National Cancer Institute-American Cancer Society breast cancer detection demonstration projects. J Natl Cancer Inst. 1979;62:639709.
12. Sankaranaraynan R, Nene BM, Shastri SS, Jayant K, Muwonge R, Budukh AM, et al. HPV screening for cervical cancer in rural India. N Engl J Med. 2009;360(14):1385–94.
13. Wacholder M, Schiffman S. From India to the World—a better way to prevent cervical cancer. N Engl J Med. 2009;360(14):1453–5.
14. Goldie S, et al. Policy analysis of cervical cancer screening strategies in low-resource settings. J Am Med Assoc. 2001;285(24):3107–15.
15. Goldie SJ, Kuhn L, Denny L, Pollack A, Wright C. Policy analysis of cervical cancer screening strategies in low-resource settings clinical benefits and cost-effectiveness. JAMA. 2001;285(24):3107–15.
16. Qiao YL, Sellors JW, Eder PS, et al. A new HPV-DNA test for cervical-cancer Screening in developing regions: a cross-sectional study of clinical accuracy in rural China. Lancet Oncol. 2008;9:929–36.
17. Denny L, Kuhl L, et al. Screening-and-treat approaches for cervical cancer prevention in low-resource settings: a randomized controlled trial. JAMA. 2005;294(17):2173–81.
18. Goff B, Mandel LS, Melancon CH, Muntz HG. Frequency of symptoms of ovarian cancer in women presenting to primary care clinics. JAMA. 2004;291:2705–12.
19. Goff B, Mandel LS, Drescher CW, Urban N, et al. Development of an ovarian cancer symptoms index. Possibilities of early detection. Cancer. 2007;109:221–7.
20. Amor F, Al A, Vaccaro H, Leon M, Iturra A. GI-RADS reporting system for ultrasound evaluation of adnexal masses in clinical practice: a prospective multicenter study. Ultrasound Obstet Gynecol. 2011;38:450–5.
21. Van Den Bosch T, Van Schoubroeck D, Domali E, Vergote L, Moerman P, Amant F, et al. A thin and regular endometrium on ultrasound is very unlikely in patients with endometrial malignancy. Ultrasound Obstet Gynecol. 2007;29:674–9.
22. Smith-Bindman R, Kerlikowske K, Feldstein VA, Subak L, Scheidler J, Segal M, et al. Endovaginal ultrasound to exclude endometrial cancer and other endometrial abnormalities. JAMA. 1998;280:1510–7.
23. Tabor A, Watt HC, Wald NJ. Endometrial thickness as a test for endometrial cancer in women with postmenopausal bleeding. Obstet Gynecol. 2002;99:663–70.
24. Amant F, Moerman P, Neven P, Timmerman D, Van Limbergen E, Vergote I. Endometrial cancer. Lancet. 2005;366:491–505.
25. Saslow D, Hannan J, Osuch J, Alciati MH, et al. Clinical breast examination: practical recommendations for optimizing performance and reporting. CA Cancer J Clin. 2004;54(6):327–44.
26. Vetto JT, Petty JK, Dunn N, Prouser NC, Austin DF. Structured clinical breast examination (CBE) training results in objective improvement in CBE skills. J Cancer Educ. 2002;17(3):124–7.
27. IARC Handbooks on Cancer Prevention. WHO. Breast cancer Screening. 2008 Available at http://www.iarc.fr/en/publications/pdfs-online/prev/handbook7/Handbook7_Breast.pdf.

Index

M.K. Shetty (ed.), *Breast and Gynecological Cancers: An Integrated Approach for Screening and Early Diagnosis in Developing Countries*, DOI 10.1007/978-1-4614-1876-4,

MIX
Papier aus verantwortungsvollen Quellen
Paper from responsible sources
FSC® C105338

If you have any concerns about our products,
you can contact us on
ProductSafety@springernature.com

In case Publisher is established outside the EU,
the EU authorized representative is:
Springer Nature Customer Service Center GmbH
Europaplatz 3, 69115 Heidelberg, Germany

Printed by Libri Plureos GmbH
in Hamburg, Germany